# Developmental Dyslexia
# from Birth to Eight

*Developmental Dyslexia from Birth to Eight* takes a fresh approach to a condition which is often poorly understood and unjustly stigmatised. Illuminating the latest neurological advances in the field, this book will empower educational professionals to play a decisive role in supporting and encouraging children with dyslexia.

With an overarching focus on the ways in which practitioners can advance children's development and learning, *Developmental Dyslexia from Birth to Eight* recognises the varying guises in which this information-processing difference might present, and addresses the challenges that this creates for children and practitioners alike. Each chapter provides the reader with a thorough examination and explanation of dyslexia, along with reflective examples, case studies and relevant further reading. Areas of focus include:

- The origins and identification of dyslexia
- Intervention strategies and alternative therapies
- Observation and assessment
- Dyslexia and English as a foreign language
- Dyslexia-friendly settings
- National and global policy on provision for dyslexic children

An engaging and accessible guide, this book will be an invaluable resource for educational practitioners and childcare specialists seeking to enhance their knowledge and understanding of dyslexia, to better support the children in their care.

**Carol Hayes** has over 40 years' experience working as a teacher and tutor. She most recently held the post as Principal Lecturer in Early Years Education at Staffordshire University, UK.

# Developmental Dyslexia from Birth to Eight

## A Practitioner's Guide

Carol Hayes

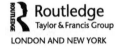
Routledge
Taylor & Francis Group

LONDON AND NEW YORK

First published 2018
by Routledge
2 Park Square, Milton Park, Abingdon, Oxon OX14 4RN

and by Routledge
711 Third Avenue, New York, NY 10017

*Routledge is an imprint of the Taylor & Francis Group, an informa business*

*British Library Cataloguing-in-Publication Data*
A catalogue record for this book is available from the British Library

*Library of Congress Cataloging-in-Publication Data*
Names: Hayes, Carol (Lecturer in early childhood studies), author.
Title: Developmental dyslexia from birth to eight : a practitioner's guide / Carol Hayes.
Description: Milton Park, Abingdon, Oxon ; New York, NY : Routledge, 2018. | Includes
    bibliographical references and index.
Identifiers: LCCN 2017051110 | ISBN 9780415786447 (hbk) | ISBN 9780415786492 (pbk) |
    ISBN 9781315211350 (ebk)
Subjects: LCSH: Dyslexia—Diagnosis. | Dyslexia—Treatment.
Classification: LCC RJ496.A5 H39 2018 | DDC 618.92/8553—dc23
LC record available at https://lccn.loc.gov/2017051110

ISBN: 978-0-415-78644-7 (hbk)
ISBN: 978-0-415-78649-2 (pbk)
ISBN: 978-1-315-21135-0 (ebk)

Typeset in Optima
by Apex CoVantage, LLC

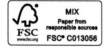

Printed and bound in Great Britain by
TJ International Ltd, Padstow, Cornwall

# Contents

# Acknowledgements

My thanks to Lewis Hayes the illustrator of this book, and for his willingness to share with you his experiences and feelings, openly and honestly.

I wish to thank Barry for his invaluable technical support, Sam for his support and encouragement, the staff and students at Staffordshire and Wolverhampton Universities, Francis and his clients at Farndon Dog Training School and Jenny and John (not their real names, but they will know who they are). Special thanks also to colleagues Ann and Debbie for their support, advice and encouragement.

Last but not least my husband who has been amazingly supportive on this journey.

# Foreword by Ruth Gill

Carol has worked in the early years sector as a teacher and tutor for over 40 years and my first encounter with her was via my setting staff who had just embarked on the final stage of their degree. Their knowledge and confidence grew enormously with tuition from Carol and their professional practice changed for the better. Some years later I was employed as a tutor in Carol's team and I could see why my setting staff flourished under Carol's tuition. I was, and still am, in awe of her dedication and passion to teach the next generation of educators everything they need to be an effective and responsive practitioner. Over the years I have come to fully appreciate Carol's expertise in the sector and her commitment to pushing the boundaries of knowledge and understanding in early years. Her PhD research into policy and prevalence of dyslexia in Wales in 2007 demonstrates her knowledge of the sector and the difficulties associated with getting the right support for children with dyslexia. Her more recent research presented in this book, along with other prominent research authors, suggests there is still some way to go to fully understanding dyslexia.

This book not only advances the knowledge and understanding of dyslexia for a range of educational professionals, but presents a 'fresh view' of what this means now for the sector and that childcare specialists need to support. Whether you work with very young children, adolescents or adults in education this book provides the answers we have patiently waited for. This long-awaited text is a passion of Carol's life and professional career, and we often discussed at length the need for such a text to highlight the struggles children and young people have in their education and future lives. Too many children have had their education and daily life affected by dyslexia and been made to feel that they are not capable, far from it! The mind of a person with dyslexia is creative and curious, with resilience that other children may not be able to display. Chapter 10 is a testament to these strengths.

Each chapter provides the reader with a thorough examination and explanation of dyslexia along with reflective examples, case studies and supporting additional reading to engage with. The golden thread running through all chapters is the influence of brain development and how advances in neuroscience are helping us to understand more about dyslexia. A more subtle thread noted is a greater appreciation for the nature of dyslexia and this takes hold as you progress through each chapter, each one with a fresh perspective of what we thought we knew but now know. You cannot help but be engulfed in the power of what Carol is communicating. I am reminded as I read each chapter of all the children I have educated; if only the knowledge I now have from reading this book was something I could have known 20 years ago. The indicators and manifestations presented by Carol in Chapter 5 are remarkable and will support a wide range of professionals in the sector in their daily interactions and assessments of children's needs. Carol uses the term information processing disorder to express the range of dyslexia related conditions that children display. Without this clarity how can we possibly give children the right support, at the right time?

This comprehensive and intellectually stimulating text is professionally relevant, not just for today but in years to come. The emphasis on how children with dyslexia feel about themselves and their belief in their own abilities is striking and makes me even more determined to ensure that the next generation of educators embrace the opportunity to make a difference.

Ruth Hudson-Gill
Senior Lecturer in Early Childhood

# The unidentified flying object of psychology

*'I wish you wouldn't keep appearing and vanishing so suddenly: you make one quite giddy.'*

*'All right,' said the Cat; and this time it vanished quite slowly, beginning with the end of the tail, and ending with the grin, which remained some time after the rest of it had gone.*

*'Well! I've often seen a cat without a grin,' thought Alice; 'but a grin without a cat! It's the most curious thing I ever saw in all my life!'*

Carroll, 2015: p. 84: original publication 1927

## Introduction

Defining dyslexia has always been, and remains to this day, controversial and divisive. Pumfrey and Reason (1991) remember the late Professor Meredith from the University of Leeds describing dyslexia as the 'unidentified flying object of psychology' (p. 6). This appears to describe exactly the nebulous and unformulated nature of the condition known as dyslexia. Like the cat, in the Alice in Wonderland story, which just keeps appearing and disappearing, just when you think you have an idea of what this condition really is, it just seems to fade away and remain unattainable. However, a lack of clear definition does not mean that it does not exist. It is possible to define some things which cannot exist, such as a disappearing cat; some things can be defined which could have existed, such as a UFO; and some things that exist for which we have no real definition, such as the universe. Dyslexia may well fall into the latter category.

There will always be limits to our understanding, but it is not logical to conclude that if we cannot define something then it cannot exist. It is only by pushing at these boundaries of understanding that we can develop a new and richer understanding of that which previously might have been unimaginable.

## Why should reading be a universal process?

Our first human ancestors probably emerged about 5–7 million years ago, but what we now recognise as modern man appears, from the fossil records, to be less than 200,000 years old. At this time there was very little language and certainly no one was reading. The human brain was developing and evolving but was not required to read.

The invention of written marks probably appeared around 3,400 BC, and was probably on clay tablets; it is likely that these were hieroglyphics and pictographic symbols, depicting what people saw at the time. An alphabetic script did not emerge until the second millennium BC and is thought to have been Phoenician (Tomasello, 2010). The advantage of this was that instead of hundreds and hundreds of pictures to learn and interpret, a phonetic system meant that a small number of symbols could represent all the sounds required to make up language. Those who could read at that time were highly valued as great masters, and reading was a very rare skill allowing civilisations to store and share knowledge.

It was not until the invention of the printing press by the German, Johannes Gutenberg, in the fifteenth century that reading was made more accessible. William Caxton is accredited with bringing the press to London in 1476, and he almost certainly mass printed the first book in English. Even so it was a very rare person who could read, and most were clerics and religious leaders. It was not until after the Reformation that a culture of books emerged and literacy became a popularist and necessary skill. In the eighteenth century, reading started to appear in the charity schools for the most impoverished children, but even then it was considered more important for boys to read than girls.

If you reconceptualise reading in terms of its historical evolution, then it is easier to understand that the human brain is not necessarily wired to deal with this extremely complex and multidimensional cognitive process, requiring interaction with the orthography of text and construction of meaning from it. It is unlikely that there is an area of the brain dedicated to reading in the same way that there seems to be for language, because we have not been reading for long in evolutionary terms, so the brain is born non-reading. Each person is unique, each brain individual, and the environmental and cultural context of each person is exclusive. If you start from this premise it is easier to see that each child will need to deal with the learning process in a different way. Essentially different brains will embark upon the process along distinctive routes and whilst there will be similarities in the way that children learn, there will also be wide variations. Reading is a cultural invention made relatively late in the history of humanity so the assumption that everyone *can* read is likely to be a false one.

# Dyslexia: the historical context

Acknowledging the very existence of dyslexia has in the past been an uphill struggle. Adolf Kussamaul, a German neurologist, has been accredited (Thomson, 1991) with being the first to notice the condition (1877) when one of his patients, who although intelligent and of good education, found it hard to learn to read. Kussamaul coined the term 'word blindness' which was later refined by the physician Rudolf Berlin to dyslexia ('dys', meaning difficult, and the Greek 'lexia', meaning speech and words).

By 1895 an ophthalmologist, James Hinshelwood, wrote in *The Lancet* about the case of a 58-year-old man who woke up one morning unable to read. Following on from this report William Pringle Morgan (1896), a physician, wrote in the *British Medical Journal* (BMJ) about a bright and intelligent 14-year-old who was still unable to read despite all his teachers' efforts. Moving on to 1925, Samuel Orton replaced the term 'word blindness' with strephosymbolia in an effort to explain the higher than average incidence of letter and word reversals and even mirror writing, seen in some children. Interestingly the first mention of 'word blindness'/dyslexia/strephosymbolia was by a neurologist (Kussamaul), but later reports were taken up by physicians (Orton and Morgan) and ophthalmologist (Hinshelwood), putting it apparently squarely into a medical context and in particular a visual difficulty. On the other hand, researchers and academics in the field of education have never been comfortable with a medical model for dyslexia, preferring to see this as an educational issue.

These early works were clearly instrumental in creating research interest in dyslexia, but it was not until the 1970s that this interest began to materialise into rigorous, validated research with the epidemiological study by Rutter et al. (1970). This study clearly showed that there was a category of children having a specific reading difficulty, as opposed to generalised poor readers, thereby validating a conceptual distinction between the two.

---

**CASE STUDY**

Having been unemployed since leaving school four years ago, John has finally secured a job with the local authority in the Parks and Gardens Department. They have explained to him that his wages will be paid directly into a bank account. John has never had a bank account, but he goes into a local branch and explains to the teller that he wants to open an account. Without looking up she hands him four closely typed forms and a pen. She asks him to complete these before processing his request.

John takes the forms, but all the new-found confidence that he had, which allowed him to go into the bank, was gone as he looked at the page of writing which meant very little to him.

The assumption of the teller was that everyone can read.

1. Consider how this experience made John feel.
2. Consider other similar scenarios that John may have experienced before.
3. What do you think happened next?
4. Potentially what impact could this everyday experience have upon John in the long term?

# Medical or educational?

Despite most authorities on dyslexia agreeing that dyslexia is inherent, congenital, and therefore present at birth, it is not now generally considered a medical issue, and forms no part of the medical training for doctors and nursing staff. It is certainly not a disease or an illness, therefore it receives no funding through the National Health Service (NHS). Its presence is usually confirmed by a Chartered Psychologist (educational or occupational psychologist), or a specifically trained dyslexia teacher with a postgraduate diploma in assessment of specific learning difficulties. However, you cannot escape the language used in connection with dyslexia; a quick look at the relevant literature will render words such as diagnosis, disability, symptoms, testing and treatment, all words associated with medical conditions. Certainly, the more that we understand about the neurological involvement (discussed further in Chapter 3), the gene studies and brain structures, the more a definition does move towards the medical camp, but as a difference and not an illness.

Traditionally the medical model holds that the problem is located within the individual. I would suggest that whilst the difference in information processing lies within the individual, it is the practitioners, teachers and wider society that create the problem. The interaction and epigenesis between the environment that the individual finds themself in, and the way in which they are able to process the information received. If you only see this as an educational issue surely that is belittling the experiences felt by the individual with dyslexia, implying that the problem lies with them not being able to learn in the 'correct' way. This brings to mind the very wise maxim, often attributed to Ignacio Estrada (director of grants administration at the Gordon and Betty Moore Foundation in America).

If a child can't learn the way we teach maybe we should teach the way they learn

Ott (1997) claims that 'dyslexia' is a medical term but 'specific learning difficulties' is educational, but considering the long list of words associated with dyslexia seen later in this chapter, it could be that this is just playing with words – a war of words. The British

Dyslexia Association describes 'specific learning difficulties (SpLD)' as an umbrella term to describe a number of different conditions such as dyslexia, dyscalculia, attention deficit disorder etc. On similar lines, Ott (1997) claims that the Orton Dyslexia Society (now known as the International Dyslexia Association) offered a helpful four-part analysis of this issue:

1. The differences between individuals are personal
2. The identification is clinical
3. The management is educational
4. The understanding is scientific

There is still much debate about whether it should be a medical or educational concern but I suggest that it is both, being medical in origin, but sensitive handling within an educational context could alleviate some of the difficulties that individuals with dyslexia experience; I have called this the interactionist model of difference.

> Many who work in the field no longer use the term 'diagnosis', nor do they talk about 'tests' and certainly not 'special tests'. They prefer to talk about assessment designed to expose where particular and persistent barriers to reading exist. In other words, terms which imply pass or fail result, when we are actually talking about degrees of difficulty in a range of areas are misplaced. Rather assessments should play an important role in planning and tailoring the best type of support that different individuals need.
>
> Rack and Rose (2014)

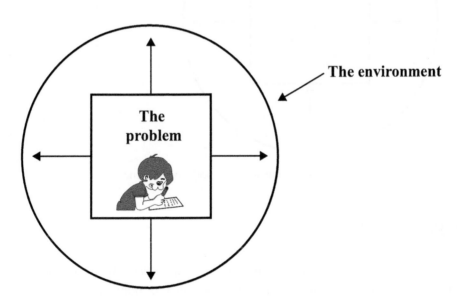

*Figure 1.1* Traditionally presented medical model

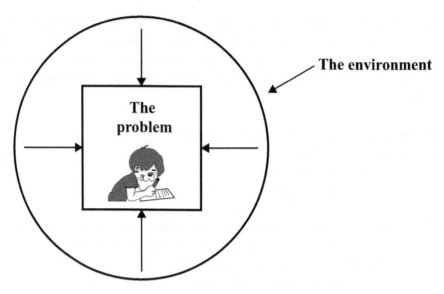

*Figure 1.2* Traditionally presented educational model

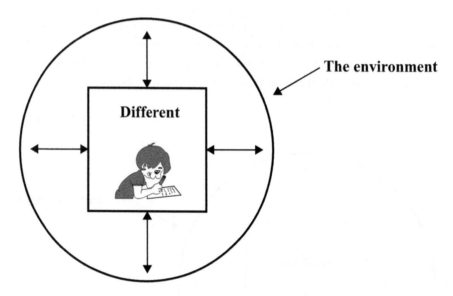

*Figure 1.3* Interactionist model of difference

## Defining dyslexia

The use of the word dyslexia implies that it is one easily definable condition, which is domain specific and therefore attributable to one area (or domain) of the brain. However, what the research into dyslexia has shown is that this is not the case, and instead it varies so much in its manifestations in different people that one definition is hard to achieve. Consequently, you will find an array of differing interpretations of dyslexia; however, the problem with a variety of definitions is that they often concentrate upon different aspects of dyslexia – some emphasise the neurological features, some the educational issues, and some the identification criteria. New research has also had the consequence that since Pringle Morgan (1896), the definition has changed and shaped from exclusionary definitions (concentrating upon what dyslexia is not), to discrepancy definitions (a discrepancy between expected reading levels and IQ), and finally to inclusive definitions (including all people regardless of IQ, poor school attendance etc.) and there are also variations to and overlap between these.

A piece of small-scale, independent research was undertaken for the writing of this book, which investigated the understanding of the definition of dyslexia by the general public. A random sample of general population adults (over 18 years) were asked, 'What does the word dyslexia mean?' The sample of 79 people overwhelmingly suggested that the condition was related to reading and literacy and the number of responses describing manifestations outside that remit, were very limited. The following figures show the results of this research.

However, the variation in definition can be seen in the following discussion of definitions currently in use by practitioners and educationalists.

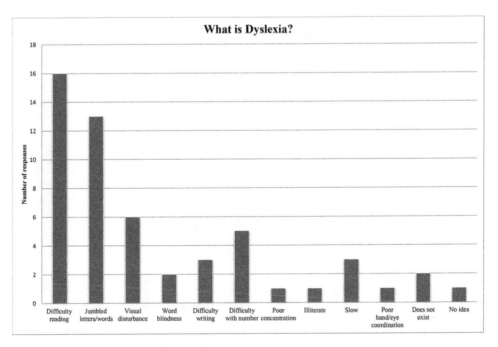

*Figure 1.4* Responses to the question 'What is dyslexia?'

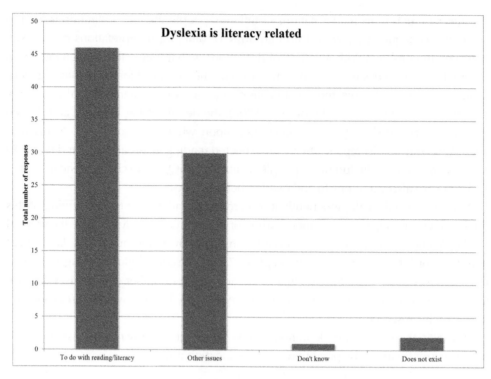

*Figure 1.5 Number of respondents that believed that dyslexia was literacy related*

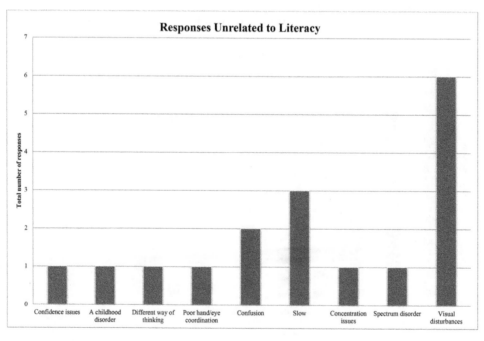

*Figure 1.6* Number of responses listing manifestations of dyslexia that were not literacy related

The British Psychological Society (BPS) offers the following definition:

> Dyslexia is evident when accurate and fluent word reading and/or spelling develops very incompletely or with great difficulty. The problem is severe despite appropriate learning opportunities . . . that is learning opportunities that are effective for the great majority of children.
>
> (British Psychological Society, 1999: online)

However, this definition leaves some unanswered questions, for example 'how severe is severe?' and what are appropriate learning opportunities? There is also no mention in this definition of any manifestations of dyslexia other than difficulties with reading and spelling.

The International Dyslexia Association (2002) offers another definition which is also adopted by the National Institute for Child Health and Human Development:

> Dyslexia is a specific learning disability that is neurological in origin. It is characterised by difficulties with accurate and/or fluent word recognition and by poor spelling and decoding abilities. These difficulties typically result from a deficit in the phonological component of language that is often unexpected in relation to other cognitive abilities and the provision of effective classroom instruction. Secondary consequences may include problems in reading comprehension and reduced reading experience that can impede the growth of vocabulary and background knowledge.
>
> (International Dyslexia Association, 2002: online)

This definition clearly identifies dyslexia as a neurological condition which implies that it is inherent; however, there are a number of issues with this designation which should perhaps be questioned, such as the very negative language prevalent in the definition, with words such as 'problems', 'difficulties' and the use of the word 'impede'. This is a deficit definition, relating firmly to the difference between expected abilities and achievement. This definition is again entirely focused upon literacy, reading and comprehension, with no mention of memory, co-ordination or concentration; if this condition is inherent and present at and even before birth, then such a definition could be seen as very unhelpful, until the child reaches an age at which society expects him/her to be able to read.

The definition still in use by the British Dyslexia Association (BDA) defines the condition as:

> Dyslexia is a specific learning difficulty which mainly affects the development of literacy and language related skills. It is likely to be present at birth and is lifelong in its effects. It is characterised by difficulties with phonological processing, rapid naming, working memory, processing speed and the automatic development of skills that may not match up to an individual's other cognitive abilities. It tends

to be resistant to conventional teaching methods, but its effects can be mitigated by appropriately specific intervention, including the application of information technology and supportive counselling.

(British Dyslexia Association, 2017: online)

Like the general public research (2016) conducted for this text (Figures 1.4, 1.5 and 1.6), the BPS and the International Dyslexia Association, the concentration of this definition is predominantly upon literacy and reading. Interestingly there is no mention in this definition of it being a neurological condition, although it does suggest that it is 'present at birth' but if this is the case and it is genetic, then it will be present even before birth, potentially from the moment of conception. In this early stage of human development no one would expect the baby/toddler to be literate, so how can the definition only relate to reading and literacy, in the way that the BDA definition and my small sample research suggest? The BDA definition could also be classed as a deficit model, suggesting that skills do not match cognitive abilities. However, it is believed that dyslexia can be found across all ages, genders and levels of intelligence (Reid 2016), although it may be said that it is easier to detect if there is a discrepancy between potential and actual ability. It is perfectly possible for individuals with low general ability to also have dyslexia, often resulting in a dual reason for their difficulties with reading and literacy.

A more inclusive definition is perhaps offered by Reid (2016):

Dyslexia is a processing difference, often characterised by difficulties in literacy acquisition affecting reading, writing and spelling. It can also have an impact on cognitive processes such as memory, speed of processing, time management, co-ordination and automaticity. There may be visual and/or phonological difficulties and there are usually some discrepancies in educational performance.

There will be individual differences and individual variation and it is therefore important to consider learning styles and the learning and work context when planning intervention and accommodations.

(Reid, 2016: p. 5)

Unlike the previous definitions Reid talks of differences rather than difficulties, acknowledging that individuals do think, react and process information differently, but he still refers to the discrepancies in educational performance, and the focus is still upon reading and writing and spelling. However, he does include manifestations such as memory, co-ordination, time management, automaticity and speed of processing.

Commissioned by the Labour government in 2009, the Rose Review sought to aid the identification and teaching of children and young people with dyslexia. Rose provided a detailed definition of dyslexia and one which is used primarily in schools in England and Wales today.

- Dyslexia is a learning difficulty that primarily affects the skills involved in accurate and fluent word reading and spelling.
- Characteristic features of dyslexia are difficulties in phonological awareness, verbal memory and verbal processing speed.
- Dyslexia occurs across the range of intellectual abilities.
- It is best thought of as a continuum not a distinct category, and there are no clear cut-off points.
- Co-occurring difficulties may be seen in aspects of language, motor co-ordination, mental calculation, concentration and personal organisation but these are not by themselves markers of dyslexia.
- A good indication of the severity and persistence of dyslexic difficulties can be gained by examining how the individual responds or has responded to, well founded interventions.

(Rose, 2009: p. 10)

I would suggest that Rose's definition, whilst trying to be inclusive in nature, is also attempting to be 'all things to all men', and in doing so has missed the point that some of those so called co-occurring difficulties could also be significant pointers for the identification and definition of dyslexia. The House of Commons Science and Technology Committee (2009) also criticised Rose for a definition that was too inclusive and failed to be useful as it was too 'blurred around the edges'. This definition concentrates almost entirely upon literacy and reading skills, which is possibly understandable when you remember that this was written for those working in schools and with children and young people whom you would expect to be reading and acquiring expertise in literacy. Notably there is no reference by Rose (2009) to a familial connection, inherent and genetic.

All these definitions exclude those who understandably cannot read because of age (babies and the very youngest children) and those who, through some compensated techniques, learn to read eventually, even if with great difficulty, but still have issues with personal organisation, co-ordination, visual memory etc. Reading difficulties clearly reflect only one dimension of dyslexia, rather than a categorical diagnosis. The problem with any definition is that we often want it to be measurable and identifiable, like a tick list, to enable us to compare one person with another, but is that a definition or simply a means of identification which could be very different. I believe, and the very premise of this book is, that dyslexia is not only about learning to read, it is so much more; that we should look back further to consider that dyslexia is in fact a variation of brain function, common to many people (6.3 million people according to Dyslexia Action, 2015). This implies that a part of the brain is working not in a deficit manner but in a different way to the majority of the population.

Looked at in another way, Eide and Eide (2011) suggest that the whole concept of dyslexia is a human invention to explain individuals who learn and process information differently from the majority of the population. I particularly like their analogy which suggests that it is like living alone on a desert island and finding a shiny cylindrical tube on the beach. When you examine it and look through it you begin to see an image of a miniature beach in front of you. You are amazed to think that you have discovered a device to make things look small. Eide and Eide (2011) use this analogy to show that, like the telescope, it can either expand and clarify our view of an issue, or used the wrong way can cause our view to contract. I am of the opinion that, like the telescope, we have defined dyslexia in too narrow a fashion, with the focus only upon literacy and reading difficulties, which is what has been seen in the past. Instead of narrowing the definition we need to turn the telescope around to use it in a different way, to expand the view to one that is more inclusive, better able to encompass more than just an individual who finds it hard to read, expanding the definition to the whole person across their entire life span, from conception to the grave.

There is certainly no shortage of eminent writers and researchers who claim to have defined dyslexia, and each definition and variation probably only contributes to the confusion about what it really is, leading to some 'doubting Thomas's' even today who, despite all the rigorous and scientific research, still question the validity of the whole concept. In 2009, writing on the entertainment and review website 'Manchester Confidential' the Labour MP Graham Stringer described it as a dyslexia 'myth' and a 'cruel fiction' blaming poor teaching alone for children's failure to read.

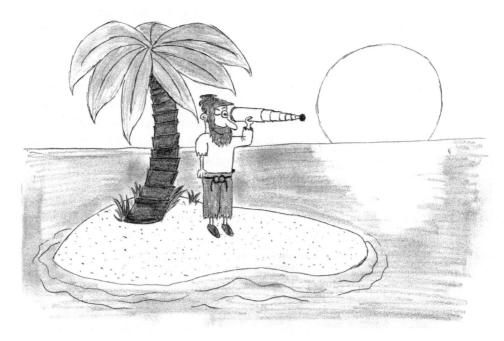

*Figure 1.7* The upside-down telescope

It is time that the dyslexia industry was killed off and we recognised that there are well known methods of teaching everybody to read and write.

(Stringer, 2009)

Despite Stringer's rather uninformed opinion, most authorities on dyslexia recognise that it is a clinical and neurobiological condition which is not caused by poor teaching, lazy children or inadequate enabling environments. For this reason, and to aid clarity when reading this book, I have adopted the following inclusive definition of dyslexia, which I hope will set the entire premise for the writing of this book for practitioners and families working with young children and babies.

> Dyslexia is a multifaceted neurobiological information processing difference, affecting the holistic development of the child from the moment of conception. It may require a more imaginative pedagogy to ensure that each individual reaches their inherent potential.

This definition refers to more than just literacy and reading but to much broader information processing, which could apply in many ways; it is inclusive and positive in its approach, recognising that each individual has ability and potential. There is no mention of failure, deficit or discrepancy. This can be classed as a working definition and not an operational one. It does not for example explain that symptoms are likely to be apparent according to age, for example it is quite normal for a two-year-old not to be able to read but quite unusual for them not to be reading by the age of eight. The manifestation of symptoms differs according to developmental stages and will depend upon quantification, quality and degree of environmental exposure. However, such an inclusive definition does provide a starting point for generating and testing a broad range of hypothesis as to causal explanations, allowing for a range of multi-variant explanations rather than a single causal factor.

---

**Reflect on this**

The definition of dyslexia that I have suggested above is clearly not quantifiable, not symptom based, it does not come with a checklist to compare one individual with another. It is an inclusive definition which some researchers and authorities may find difficult to work with.

- How important do you think a working definition of dyslexia is to the practitioner?
- With a colleague return to the definition from the Rose Review (2009). How does this definition differ from mine?

---

# Do we need a definition?

You may well ask why we need a definition, but without one which can be generally agreed and maintains some consensus, attempts to understand the condition and to implement the most appropriate forms of intervention will be hard to achieve. Only when we have an agreed definition will we be able to operationalise it and produce a working hypothesis, to enable practitioners, teachers, professionals and families to work together to optimise support for individuals with this condition.

One of the difficulties with a definition that concentrates upon reading and literacy as opposed to a more general view on information processing, is that there is a tendency to 'lump together' all those who have difficulties with reading, including those who have had poor teaching, those with poor motivation, those with poor environmental exposure, those with socioeconomic disadvantage and those with more general reading difficulties. This does children with dyslexia no favours, as it is like comparing apples with pears, confusing nature with nurture. Elliott and Grigorenko (2014) suggest that dyslexia should be seen as a subset of a larger pool of readers. Figure 1.8 shows how such a subgroup could sit within the sector of poor readers, but also demonstrates that capable readers are also included in the dyslexia subgroup.

A child who has no exposure to text is unlikely to achieve literacy, but the reason for this would not necessarily be due to dyslexia, which is why in 1997, Frith described dyslexia as a 'cultural phenomenon', and because at that time dyslexia was identified only with regard to literacy, he suggested that it would not be observable in non-literate cultures. This would also suggest that it would not be observable in the very youngest children, who by definition are not reading and often have limited exposure to text.

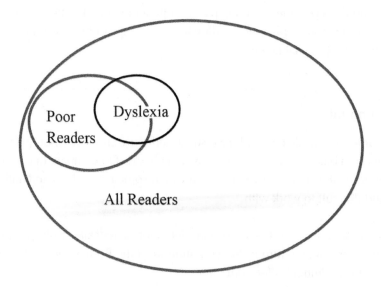

*Figure 1.8* Dyslexia as a subgroup of readers

The difficulty with Frith's (1997) assertion is that once again dyslexia is defined only in terms of reading and takes no account of the broader manifestations of the condition. If you examine a broader definition it accepts that a difference in information processing within the brain will have far a more wide-ranging impact upon the holistic development of the child, and is likely to either compromise or improve a broad array of abilities, including the process of learning to read.

---

**Reflect on this**

The following list of celebrities is often quoted as an example of individuals with dyslexia who have 'succeeded' in life despite the odds and is intended to be inspiring:

Whoopi Goldberg (winner of a Grammy, Academy Award and a Tony)

Steven Spielberg (film director)

Henry Winkler (actor, director and author)

Keira Knightley (actor)

Cher (singer, actor, winner of an Academy Award)

Jamie Oliver (celebrity chef and author)

Albert Einstein (scientist)

Agatha Christie (author)

Alexander Graham Bell (inventor)

Hans Christian Andersen (writer)

Leonardo Da Vinci (scientist, mathematician, engineer, inventor, artist, musician etc.)

How far do you believe that such a list provides a stereotype for learners who are dyslexic, which they would find hard to live up to?

Does this encourage us to believe that all people with dyslexia are really clever and creative, with high IQ and special talents?

---

# Acquired dyslexia

For many of you reflecting back on your experiences when learning to read it may have seemed naturally progressing and effortless, but make no mistake, it relies upon a highly complex series of interacting cognitive processes, probably set within distinct neural regions of the brain. When these areas of the brain are damaged or impaired in some way reading becomes much less effortless and appears as a mountain to climb.

In crude terms developmental dyslexia is considered to be genetic and inheritable, whereas acquired dyslexia occurs when previously literate individuals, who have sustained some form of brain trauma and damage, present with literacy and language disorders.

> Damage to general visual, phonological or semantic processing abilities are the root causes of acquired dyslexia.
>
> (Woollams, 2014: p. 1)

The article, written in *The Lancet* by Hinshelwood in 1895, first highlighted that dyslexia can be both acquired and developmental, and there have since been numerous reported and well documented case studies involving adults who were previously able to read appropriately, but lost that ability following severe head trauma or stroke. Whilst the main premise of this book is to focus upon developmental dyslexia, it is certain that those who study acquired dyslexia contribute enormously to our understanding of the elements and locations in the brain necessary for literacy and this is an area that will be returned to later in the book.

The use of the word 'dyslexia' implies that it is one definable condition which is domain specific, that it is attributable to one area (or domain) of the brain; what the work on acquired dyslexia appears to show is that reading is a highly interactive and dynamic process, hence damage to a particular area of the brain can cause variable differences in reading ability. Acquired dyslexia, as indicated by Woollams (2014), cannot be classified under one such umbrella, and she talks about moving away from a concept of a 'uniformity of the cognitive architecture across different individuals' (Woollams, 2014: p. 2). This results in identifiable differences in reading difficulty.

Woollams (2014) refers to three types of dyslexia brought about through acquired dyslexia:

- Phonological dyslexia: a difficulty in sub-word matching (letters and letter strings to sounds). Individuals with phonological dyslexia rely heavily on context and meaning to be able to read and find the production of non-words difficult. Such poor phonological awareness makes it hard to read out loud and individuals have difficulty with decoding, particularly with unfamiliar words.
- Pure alexia: sometimes called deep dyslexia, results in slow reading, where the number of letters in a word has a marked impact.
- Surface dyslexia: sometimes referred to as dyseidetic dyslexia or visual dyslexia, is a deficit in reading whole words particularly those with less visual spelling to sound mapping, for example the word 'enough'. Those with surface dyslexia need to be able to recognise words by sight.

What makes Woollams' work on acquired dyslexia even more complex is that she believes that individuals can have one or all of these difficulties in varying degrees, or indeed both developmental and acquired dyslexia.

One exciting result of Woollams' (2014) work is that she suggests that owing to the dynamic nature of reading deficits and the interactionist nature of the brain connectivity, the earliest identification of the condition could potentially produce alternative connective mappings in the brain allowing individuals with dyslexia to function in an outwardly normative fashion.

> Disruption to phonological representations before the onset of reading development will cause suboptimal mappings to develop between orthography and phonology. Once these mappings have been formed, remediation of the phonological representations alone will not directly affect them, hence why inclusion of a reading component in interventions is particularly important in older children. This work provides an elegant demonstration of the way in which connectionist modelling has the potential to influence the formulation of remediation strategies thereby helping to optimize treatment outcomes.
>
> (Woollams, 2014: pp. 8–9)

The study of acquired dyslexia clearly offers real opportunities for neurologists to study the nature of the cognitive and neural architecture of the brain and the processes involved when reading. Whilst procedures such as neuroimaging can reveal which broad areas of the brain are involved in the reading process, they cannot necessarily determine which areas are necessary for reading to occur.

> Through considering the striking reading deficits observed after different kinds of lesions, we can see what elements are necessary for fluent reading and where these processes are housed in the brain.
>
> (Woollams, 2014: p. 1)

This rather simplistic distinction between developmental and acquired dyslexia implies that they are two completely separate aspects of a similar condition, but this may be more complex than it first appears. If dyslexia is a neurological dysfunction, as researchers such as Frith (2002), Reid (2009) and Elliott and Grigorenko (2014) ask, where does the constitutional difference in the brain (the central nervous system) become different from tissue damage? It could be that such 'soft' neurological damage has been caused in utero and not as a result of genetic inheritance. In both cases it could be claimed that a child was born with dyslexia, but the causation could be very different, and very difficult with our present knowledge, to identify.

## It's all in a name

Not only can experts not agree on a universal definition of dyslexia, but even the name dyslexia is in dispute. In 2002, Doyle listed the terms shown in Table 1.1 used in books and articles about dyslexia; I have added a few more found in other sources.

With such a puzzling array of terms it is clear that the whole dyslexia industry has become a maze, needing demystification and elucidation to enable practitioners to see through the mist, and negotiate an appropriate pathway through the maze. However, the complexity of terms and definitions could, according to Pumfrey and Reason (1991), be more to do with the large number of differing professionals and professional organisations involved than the complexity of the issues themselves.

## Top down or bottom up?

The condition usually known as dyslexia can be viewed from a top-down or bottom-up approach. What this means is that you can look at the manifestations of the condition, for example difficulties with reading, difficulties with phonological awareness, messy handwriting, low self-concept, poor balance, poor organisation and time management etc., and attempt to cluster these together to produce one definition. This is a top-down

*Table 1.1*

| | | |
|---|---|---|
| Acquired dyslexia | Grapheme processor dyslexia | Specific learning difficulties |
| Acute Dyslexia | Hyperlexia | Specific reading difficulties |
| Alexia | Legasthenia | Specific learning differences |
| Attentional dyslexia | L-type dyslexia | Specific reading differences |
| Congenital dyslexia | Mind blindness | Specific learning disabilities |
| Congenital word blindness | Mixed dyslexia | Specific reading disabilities |
| Deep dyslexia | Morphemic dyslexia | Specific reading retardation |
| Developmental aphasia | Phonological dyslexia | Strephosymbolia |
| Developmental reading disorder | Phonological processor dyslexia | Surface dyslexia |
| Direct dyslexia | 'P'-type dyslexia | Traumatic dyslexia |
| Dyseidetic dyslexia | Primary reading disorder | Unexpected reading difficulty |
| Dyslectic | Semantic processor dyslexia | Visual dyslexia |
| Dyslexia | Specific developmental dyslexia | Visual processor dyslexia |
| Dysphonetic dyslexia | Specific dyslexia | Word blindness |

approach. The difficulty with that is that every individual is different and as you will see as you read further into this book, the way that dyslexia manifests itself can be different in different people. According to Frith (2002) it can even vary according to a range of characteristics such as:

- Age
- Gender
- Ability
- Motivation
- Personality
- Social support
- Physical resources
- Teaching systems and pedagogy employed
- The characteristics of the language and orthography being learned

This comes from a tick box mentality, the desire for a long list of indicators which when all are ticked means that you 'have dyslexia'. This would be so easy, and seems to make sense, but the so called 'experts' find that differing indicators cluster in slightly different ways, so they attempt to offer a word or new title for each differing cluster, hence the array of words to describe what they see. If you are not careful this wide variation of indicators can be classified into multifarious sub-groups of dyslexia, but it is debateable how useful this would be to understanding the condition, or how helpful to the practitioner or teacher when considering ways to manage the various sub-groups that might appear in their groups or classes. This top-down approach seems to hugely over-complicate the issues and produces questions from individuals such as: which cluster do I have? What label does this involve? Does this mean that I only have this label or can I have more than one?

Alternatively, you could consider dyslexia from the bottom up, in other words instead of looking at the identifiers of the condition, look instead at the cause, which I have already suggested is a difference in information processing. This seems to make more sense of the vast array of indicators of the condition, and as this different neurology of the brain interacts with the environment, so the way that the condition manifests itself will also vary. These environmental interactions could determine the ways in which the person with dyslexia exhibits this condition. An example of this might be a child with dyslexia who from birth has been exposed to a rich literate environment with lots of books, reading stories, rhymes, phonological games with highly supportive adults who understand and nurture his/her learning. It is likely that this child will learn to read and enjoy reading, albeit slowly and will achieve their goals, however this does not mean that s/he is not dyslexic and the manifestations of the condition may be different, such as poor short-term memory, sequencing issues, poor co-ordination etc. This is not a unique explanation, for example if you go to your medical doctor with a high temperature, sore throat and aching limbs, the doctor will not try to treat each symptom separately, but will attempt to identify the underlying cause. According to the NHS website (2015), there are potentially 86 different conditions associated with these symptoms from pharyngitis, Lyme disease, influenza, hepatitis to plague! Only when that underlying cause has been identified can the doctor recommend an appropriate course of action.

## Policy provision

Although there is no universally agreed definition or language to describe dyslexia, governments and legislators now recognise and accept that it does exist. There are 353 local authorities in England, 22 in Wales and 32 in Scotland each with responsibility to ensure provision for children with particular needs. Each has their own approaches and policies; Reid et al. (2005) undertook an audit of local authorities in Scotland and found that whilst all had some policy for dyslexia some policies were explicitly concerned with dyslexia, some were incorporated with other specific learning difficulties (SpLD) and some only mentioned dyslexia as part of a general teaching and learning policy. The inevitable conclusion of this is that it depends upon where you live as to the type and impact of the assistance that those with dyslexia are likely to receive and that brings with it the unpalatable concept of a postcode lottery.

In a snap shot review of 40 local authorities selected at random in England, conducted for this book in 2017, it was clear that the pattern in Scotland found by Reid et al. in 2005 was also evident in England today. Somewhat of concern was that all the policies reviewed concentrated upon literacy to the complete exclusion of all other manifestations of the condition, and mention of early years was only evident in two of the 40 authorities sampled. All accepted either the Rose Review or the British Psychological Society definitions. Interestingly one English authority had even changed the accepted Specific Learning Difficulties (SpLD) into Specific *Literacy* Difficulty.

Unpublished PhD research conducted in 2007 (Hayes) showed that within the principality of Wales there was a large disparity among the 22 local authorities and their approach to dyslexia policy, with very little joined-up practice. Each local authority was working independently, and opportunities were missed to establish a whole Wales policy for the identification and management of dyslexia. Even whole school policies were rare, it is possible that this was because teachers did not have dyslexia at the forefront of their minds. These findings were reiterated by Packer et al. (2016) in their research presentation to the British Dyslexia Association conference in Oxford 2016. Consequently, a postcode lottery of provision has grown up depending upon where the child is living.

Since the advent of the Coalition Government in 2010, schools in England have experienced increasing levels of autonomy with more school partnerships, and can exercise more powers over their policy and practice, free from the constraints of potential bureaucracy of a local authority. A research report for the department for education in 2014 by Sandals and Bryant admitted that:

> Approaches to supporting vulnerable children are evolving more gradually than school improvement and place planning. While there are innovative examples of schools-led approaches, there has not yet been a decisive shift to partnerships leading support for vulnerable children.
>
> (Sandals and Bryant, 2014: p. 7)

This same report suggested that school leaders were concerned about the capacity of local authorities to provide the right services for these vulnerable children.

Policies do not of necessity need to be written documents, especially in a small setting, but do need to be accepted corporate practice and often practice will come before a documented policy, rather than the other way around. Written policies are usually tested and trialled before they are set into concrete formats and implemented. As a consequence, documented policies need agreement and concordance and without that appropriate practice cannot be achieved. The reason for a written policy is to reconcile conflict where agreement needs to be in place, where there are incompatible and contradictory ideas and there is a need for common standards. There are many influences upon the process of policy making but cynically perhaps it could be argued that the economics of a policy are more influential upon whether a particular policy will come to fruition than the ideals behind it. This will depend upon how it influences staff numbers, premises, equipment and resources. The political acceptability of a policy will also influence whether a policy is accepted or not:

- how the public and professionals will view the policy
- how it fits with the cultural, religious and ethnic mix of the population
- previous political decisions and size of the Government majority and changes at election.

A policy statement for dyslexia needs to define good practice and be clearly set out to ensure that all practitioners are able to understand how to implement, maintain and evaluate the practice. It should offer unambiguous guidelines, which is likely to involve detailed and knowledgeable planning with 'joined-up' vertical arrangements between national government, local authorities, settings, staff and families. Horizontal integration of ideas from all agencies is also required and will involve parent partnerships and the concept of a holistic approach across the setting. With such devolved policy making between the local authorities, it could be that they are all attempting to 'reinvent the wheel', so opportunities are potentially being missed to establish an integrated policy for the identification and management of dyslexia.

## Chapter reflections

You have read in this chapter about the confusion that teachers, practitioners and families are going to have to negotiate if they believe that a child in their care has dyslexic tendencies. However, the fact that an agreed definition, or even agreed wording, has yet to be produced is, I believe, of little consequence to our understanding of the condition as it evolves. You have seen in this chapter that definitions abound, and most focus upon difficulties with literacy, nevertheless a broader view is beginning to take shape as the realisation of the impact on children's academic, physical, social and emotional development emerges. The term dyslexia is more than an issue to do with reading; this is one isolated indicator within a far more complex syndrome.

One aspect of a definition that I have not so far alluded to, but you will come back to in subsequent chapters of this book, is the issue of litigation. A vast industry has grown up around dyslexia and some teachers and practitioners are now fearful of the threat of litigation, should the children and their families feel that they have not had sufficient support to maximise their potential, and this is one reason why well researched and well-informed policy making is so important to safeguard all parties in the future.

Elliott and Grigorenko (2014) suggest that a definition of dyslexia is only necessary to meet the social, political and emotional needs of society, but I will argue in the next chapter, that whatever its weakness a definition serves a valuable purpose to ensure support, finance, legal protection and intervention for those directly affected by the condition.

> whatever exists, exists in a certain amount; and whatever exists in a certain amount can be measured. But many things that can be measured are not.
>
> (Turner, 1997: p. 13)

# Further reading

Elliott, J and Grigorenko, E (2014) *The Dyslexia Debate*. Cambridge: Cambridge University Press.

Julian Elliot really set the 'cat among the pigeons' in 2005 when interviewed for the Dispatches programme on Channel 4, by seeming to claim that dyslexia was a myth. This he says earned him hate mail! The Dyslexia Debate is a thought provoking book from two eminent psychologists, who examine and challenge many of the assumptions about dyslexia. The book reflects on the current research and attempts to redress the balance not by dismissing dyslexia out of hand, but by recognising the issues and attempting to open out the debate to understand that it is so much more than 'just' a reading difficulty.

# References

British Dyslexia Association (2017) *What are Specific Learning Difficulties?* Available online at: www.bdadyslexia.org.uk/educator/what-are-specific-learning-difficulties (accessed 17.07.17).

British Dyslexia Association (2017) Definitions. Available online at: www.bdadyslexia.org.uk/dyslexic/definitions (accessed 17.07.17).

British Psychological Society (1999) *Dyslexia, literacy and psychological assessment.* Report of a working party of the Division of Educational and Child Psychology. Leicester: BPS.

Carroll, L. (2015) *Alice's Adventures in Wonderland* (original publication 1921). London: Macmillan Children's Books.

Doyle, J. (2002) *Dyslexia an Introductory Guide* (2nd edn). London: Whurr Publishers Ltd.

Dyslexia Action (2015) *Facts and Figures about Dyslexia.* Available online at: www.dyslexiaaction.org.uk (accessed 19.06.16).

Eide, B. and Eide, F. (2011) *The Dyslexia Advantage: Unlocking the Hidden Potential of the Dyslexic Brain.* London: Hay House UK Ltd.

Elliott, J. and Grigorenko, E. (2014) *The Dyslexia Debate.* Cambridge: Cambridge University Press.

Frith, U. (2002) Resolving the Paradoxes of Dyslexia. In Reid, G. and Wearmouth, J. (eds) *Dyslexia and Literacy: Theory and Practice.* Chichester: Wiley and Sons Ltd.

Hayes, C (2007) *Policy and Prevalence of Dyslexia in Wales* (unpublished doctoral research).

Hinshelwood, J (1895) Word Blindness and Visual Memory. *The Lancet 2,* 21 December: 1564–1570. Available online at: https://archive.org/details/congenitalwordbl00hinsrich (accessed 21.07.17).

House of Commons Science and Technology Committee (2009) *Evidence Check 1: Early Literacy Interventions.* London: The Stationary Office.

International Dyslexia Association (2002) Definition of Dyslexia. Available online at: www.dyslexiaida.org/definition-of-dyslexia (accessed 04.07.17).

NHS (2015) *NHS Choices: Your Health Your Choices.* Available online at: www.nhs.uk/Conditions/Flu/Pages/Symptoms.aspx (accessed 21.09.17).

Orton, S.T. (1925) Word-blindness in School Children. *Archives of Neurology and Psychiatry* 14: 581–615.

Ott, P. (1997) *How to Detect and Manage Dyslexia: A Reference and Resource Manual.* Oxford: Heinemann.

Packer, R., Jones, C. and Williams, T. (2016) *Dwyieithrwdd a Dyslecsia/Bilingualism and Dyslexia: An Interactive Approach.* Presentation BDA: Oxford.

Pringle Morgan, W. (1896) A Case of Congenital Word Blindness. *BMJ* 7th November: 378.

Pumfrey, D. and Reason, R. (1991) *Specific Learning Difficulties.* London: Routledge.

Rack J. and Rose, J. (2014) *Dyslexia by any other Name . . .* Available online at: www.thedyslexia-spldtrust.org.uk/media/downloads/inline/dyslexia-by-any-other-name.1398777151.pdf (accessed 30.08.17).

Reid, G (2016) *Dyslexia: A Practitioner's Handbook* (5th edn). Chichester: Wiley and Blackwell.

Reid, G., Deponio, P. and Petch, L. D. (2005) Identifications, Assessment and Intervention: implications of an audit on dyslexia policy and practice in Scotland. *Dyslexia* 11 (3): 203–216.

Rose, J. (2009) *Identifying and Teaching Children and Young People with Dyslexia and Literacy Difficulties*. Nottingham: DCSF Publications.

Rutter, M., Tizzard, J. and Whitmore, K. (1970) *Education, Health and Behaviour*. London: Longman.

Sandals, L. and Bryant, B. (2014) *The Evolving Education System in England: A 'Temperature Check'*. London: Department for Education (DfE).

Stringer, G. (2009) *Manchester Confidential*. Available online at: www.manchesterconfidential.co.uk (accessed 08.08.17).

Thomson, M. (1991) *Developmental Dyslexia* (3rd edn). London: Whurr Publishers.

Tomasello, M. (2010) *Origins of Human Communication*. Cambridge, MA: MIT Press.

Turner, M. (1997) *Psychological Assessment of Dyslexia*. London: Whurr Publications Ltd.

Woollams, A.M. (2014) Connectionist Neuropsychology: Uncovering ultimate causes of acquired dyslexia. *Philosophical Transactions of the Royal Society* B 369. Available online at: http://rstb.royalsocietypublishing.org/content/369/1634/20120398 (accessed 17.07.17).

# 2 | Why does it matter?

*It is utterly meaningless. It is a pretentious word for 'thick'.*

Liddle, 2014

## Introduction

Continuing the discussion from the last chapter this section will question the need and desirability of a definition. It could be that a constrained definition, set in stone, is counterproductive for the individual, by not allowing for the many variations of the condition, thereby preventing individuals with difficulties, that fall just outside the definition, to be able to gain appropriate access to resources and support that they need. However, with no definition it makes it difficult to understand how prevalent the condition might be, and thereby the possible extent of the issues for society, as well as the individual.

This chapter will examine the impact of dyslexia on the holistic development of the child and dispel some myths about the gender imbalance and prevalence.

## Prevalence

The problem with a lack of clear definition (as you have seen in Chapter 1), is that without one it is almost impossible to assess its prevalence, in other words being able to understand how many people are impacted by this difference in information processing.

If you can't measure it you can't manage it.

(Ott, 1997: p. 12)

Estimates of prevalence rates vary wildly from 4–17% in the USA (Shaywitz, 2005), to the British Dyslexia Association (2016) which suggests that up to 10% of children in the UK have some degree of dyslexia, and in 4% of cases this is severe. A cautionary aspect is that in both these estimates the figures are only arrived at through examination of children in school that are already identified with dyslexia, and are based on a definition which almost exclusively relates to reading difficulties. However, even on these estimates, it means that in every nursery group of 25 children a practitioner is statistically likely to have at least two children with dyslexic tendencies, so in a primary school of 500 there are likely to be approximately 40, and in a medium sized comprehensive school of 1,500 children around 120 will be dyslexic. These numbers have to create an atmosphere of concern for all of you who work with young children, to ensure that you are taking account of the learning needs of all those within your care, as they clearly illustrate that this is not a rare condition, it is common and will affect the work of all schools, nurseries, home carers etc.

Another of the difficulties contributing to this seemingly impossible task is that not only is a definition difficult to arrive at, but so is severity. Most authorities do agree that the severity of the condition is on a continuum from mild to moderate to severe (Figure 2.1).

This is further compounded by the variety of sympathetic conditions which can indicate the presence of dyslexia, each of which can be indicated at different stages on the continuum. Ott (1997) therefore, described any prevalence figure as no more than a 'guesstimate', resulting in statistics which are fundamentally flawed. She called for a 'properly funded national enquiry to be taken of a large sample of the population' (p. 13). To date, 20 years on from Ott's request, no such research has been commissioned by the government, despite the issues over fiscal resourcing. I would suggest that however large the sample, without a clear and measurable definition it is an impossible task, as you do not know what you are measuring. Other difficulties, according to Miles (2004), are the practicalities of the time taken to undertake testing on such a mammoth scale, and the nature and accuracy of the tests used for assessment. This is compounded by the wide variety of diagnostic tests, methods and criteria currently used by professionals for an assessment, making it difficult to compare like with like. Once again, at the core of the current testing regime is assessing the child's ability to read, which eliminates children who, because of their young age, or lack of appropriate teaching, are understandably unable to read.

A further complication is that if, as is likely, dyslexia is normally distributed across the population of the UK in a similar way to height or weight (see Figure 2.2), and it falls on a continuum, it is difficult to make a decisive cut off point between those who have

Mild                                    Moderate                                    Severe

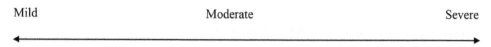

*Figure 2.1* Continuum of dyslexia

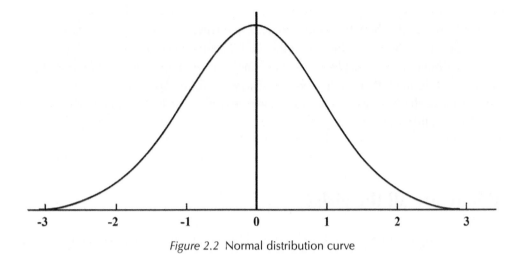

*Figure 2.2* Normal distribution curve

dyslexia and those who have not. A child with chickenpox is easily diagnosed as they either have it or have not. Dyslexia on the other hand relies on an arbitrary cut off point and it is almost impossible to say where that lies. Elliott and Grigorenko (2014) likened this to obesity (weight is normally distributed on a graph), however, at what point does a person on this chart become obese and who decides where that line falls? If this distribution also applies to dyslexia then the same dilemma occurs.

## CASE STUDY

Asher (aged 5 years) was bored . . . the teacher had been explaining a list of instructions to the class for them to do on a task for today. Asher listened so hard but had forgotten all but the first two tasks – 'get out your books' and 'turn to page 5'. He did not start the task like the others in his group because he did not know what to do, and whilst they were all working well, he was gazing around and flicking his pencil. The teacher noticed and came over, not as Asher had hoped, to show him what to do, but rather to reprimand him for flicking the pencil. As the teacher walked away Asher made a face at her and his friends saw and started to giggle. Asher was excited to have achieved such a reaction from his peers and smiled. It made him feel good, and there was precious little that he did in school that did make him feel good. He had already earned a reputation in his group for doing things that his peers did not dare feel able to, last week he swore at the teacher and his peers were in awe.

1.  How could Asher's behaviour escalate and why?
2.  What do you feel is the role of the adult in enhancing that escalation and of causing Asher to feel like a 'second class citizen', humiliated and frustrated?
3.  Do you think that the teacher's reaction could be classed as psychological abuse, by exposing Asher to anxiety and trauma? If so explain why you think that.

# Where are all the girls?

For decades dyslexia has been associated with boys and much of the research has been male orientated, even going so far as to exclude females from the research (Turner, 1997; Critchley, 1981; Naidoo, 1972). Estimates of the gender split in prevalence of dyslexia have for many years been between 4:1 and 6:1 in favour of males, creating an idea that girls rarely have dyslexia (Shaywitz, 2005). This male orientated approach has meant that thousands of girls have probably slipped through the net and gone through their education, even their whole lives, without understanding their differences. Research now indicates that there are probably as many females as males with dyslexia (Shaywitz, 2005). This suggests that girls can spend their whole formal education experience without their dyslexia being highlighted. Traditionally girls start to talk earlier than boys (Hayes, 2016) and are therefore able to talk about their thoughts and feelings, so there is possibly an underestimate of the impact that dyslexia has on them. Thankfully, research, such as Shaywitz (2005), has begun to catch up, and she suggests that there may not be such a differential between male and female prevalence rates. However, Shaywitz (2005) also suggests that girls with dyslexia often become socially isolated and feel powerless to change, even developing mental health problems associated with anxiety and depression. According to Alexander-Passe (2015), as many as 20% of children with dyslexia suffer from some form of depression, and another 20% a related anxiety disorder. The National Centre for Eating Disorders (2012) suggests anything in life that disturbs self-esteem, such as dyslexia, can lead to stress related difficulties, such as eating disorders and even suicide. However, the difference between the genders appears to be that girls, more often than boys, mimic good social behaviour and become withdrawn and quiet rather than noisy and rowdy; they are therefore often overlooked.

According to Reid (2009), although at school level many more males than females are identified as being dyslexic, at Higher Education level females outnumber males – how can this be? It is likely that there are more unidentified females in schools, 'hidden' by their greater social conformity. Boys are likely to be more disruptive in class when they become anxious and frustrated, and it is this anti-social behaviour that is causing them to be assessed more frequently than girls whose anxious behaviour tends to be manifested more by withdrawal and less confrontation. So rather than there actually being fewer girls than boys with dyslexia, what you are seeing is fewer girls being formally identified. Shaywitz (2005) also points out that most children are identified by teachers in schools and therefore the identification process is possibly skewed towards the boys who are more disruptive in class. As most subsequent research has been conducted on children with a formal identification, it has meant that in the past more research has been undertaken on males with dyslexia than females. Once again it must also be noted that confirmed identification of dyslexia has been done almost exclusively on a definition which assesses an individual's ability to read. All this would suggest that there are more males than females identified with dyslexia, however identified cases and the actual prevalence may be very different. The research undertaken by Shaywitz (2005) examined a representative sample of children rather than a school identified group. She showed that in the school identified group there were 3–4 times more incidence of dyslexia in the males than the females, but in the representative group there was, by contrast, very little difference in prevalence (Figure 2.3).

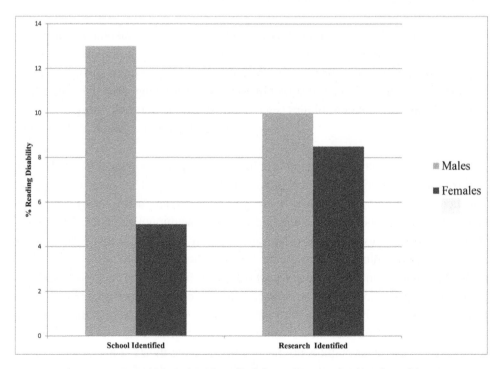

*Figure 2.3* Prevalence of reading disability in boys and girls (adapted from Shaywitz, 2005: p. 32)

Shaywitz (2005) suggests that the reason for this over-identification in boys is that teachers incorporate behaviour (even unconsciously) into their assessment and males tend to be more overtly poorly behaved than females, when bored, anxious or distressed. It is this poor behaviour that is causing increased referrals for evaluation. Girls who sit quietly in their seats are more easily overlooked, but are nevertheless failing to learn. However, she does make the point that set against this must be that in brain imaging scans (fMRI), brain activation patterns in males and females are different, perhaps demonstrating possible gender differences in brain organisation (this will be discussed further in Chapter 3).

# Labelling

Defining and knowing the prevalence of dyslexia is clearly important to educationalists, politicians, government officials and representatives who have to establish and allocate finance to those individuals and organisations working to assist with the condition. Under the Equality Act 2010 (Government Equalities Office, 2010), dyslexia is a 'protected characteristic' and classed as a disability, which means that those with dyslexia cannot be discriminated against. It is also recognised in the Children and Families Act 2014 (Gov.UK, 2014) as a special educational need.

> Disability has a broad meaning. It is defined as a physical or mental impairment that has a substantial and long term adverse effect on the ability to carry out normal day-to-day activities. . . . A mental impairment includes mental health conditions (such as bi-polar disorder or depression), learning difficulties (such as dyslexia) and learning disabilities (such as autism and Down's syndrome).
>
> (Government Equalities Office, 2010: p. 4)

According to Elliott and Grigorenko (2014) many psychologists still see the label 'dyslexic' as 'unscientific and conceptually problematic' (p. 182) despite recognising that there is something debilitating and severe that impacts many individuals. However, a definition is necessary to allow individuals, government and society in general, to understand that this condition is real and to allow them to formulate, provide and access appropriate intervention resources and strategies.

What is clear, when talking to adults who are identified with dyslexia, is the sense of relief that they feel. They often experience years of repression, years of believing that they are stupid, lazy and difficult; this falls away as they understand that there is a label for their condition, and that they share this condition with many other people. They are able to see that their plight is not necessarily down to their inadequacies or lack of effort, but is a discernible condition, which if it had been identified earlier in their lives could have avoided so much of the heartbreak and distress that many of them suffered throughout their lives.

Many who work in the field of education and in particular early years, resist the whole concept of labelling, they avoid going down the route of the 'self-fulfilling prophecy', whereby others' beliefs and predictions become your own and cause those expectations to be fulfilled. However, talking to adults with dyslexia, they believe that the label would have changed their lives for the better, and would far outweigh any potentially negative consequences.

> Early diagnosis should help to take away the burden of blame from the child, his parents, his teachers.
>
> (Ott, 1997: p. 25)

On the other hand Elliott and Grigorenko (2014) argue that a label for dyslexia should be abandoned as it is too imprecise, too poorly defined to make it useful. Early identification and labelling could also potentially lead to misdiagnosis, false positives and false negatives and possibly expectations that are too low for children who do not have dyslexia. Labels can certainly have both positive and negative effects with families, teachers and practitioners affecting their perception of a child and their expectations of success. For parents labelling their child can also be positive and negative, with parents liable to blame themselves for their child's difficulties (Elliott and Grigorenko, 2014).

A child who appears to read well can still be compatible with a label of dyslexia, but just because a child has reading difficulties does not necessarily label them as dyslexic, so to label a child dyslexic entirely on their ability to read would be wrong. Clearly to gain a label some form of assessment must be made, and this by its very nature will indicate both strengths and weaknesses across a whole range of issues. If dyslexia is only defined in terms of an ability to read, I can understand Elliott and Grigorenko's (2014) argument, but if you see dyslexia as a much wider and more complex information processing difference then conflating symptoms with definition makes no sense. A definition is not purely a list of presenting problems but an indication of the distinctive nature of something.

### Reflect on this

A child with a dyslexic label is often not expected to achieve academically although we know that many do, despite all the odds, and go on to university and other professional roles. In 2012/13 over 74,000 students declared a specific learning difficulty, representing 6% of the total higher education student population (Rodger et al., 2015).

1. Why do you think that some Higher Education students do not declare their dyslexia, despite the support (both financial and practical) that may be on offer?
2. How can you, as a practitioner, encourage aspiration in all the children in your care and in particular those that have been identified as being 'at risk' of dyslexia?

However, providing a label alone is not enough and is only useful if that label brings with it the resources and measures to put in place an appropriate course of action. Clearly the earlier that children can be identified as 'at risk' of dyslexia, the earlier such intervention can be started. Assigning a label to what the young child is experiencing can help to prevent the feeling of failure, which so many adults with dyslexia discuss; it is also likely to prevent that overwhelming feeling of helplessness, that many in my research talked about.

A label should ensure that a child receives reasonable adjustments to achieve their potential and should:

1. Help individuals make sense of their differences and understand that they are not 'just stupid'.
2. Allow adults, practitioners and teachers to relate to the label and ensure that appropriate intervention is in place.
3. Help the individual socially and emotionally to understand that they are not alone.
4. Attract additional resources to the individual.
5. Provide individuals with what Burden (2005) calls 'dyslexic identity', in other words self-identity – how you see yourself with that dyslexia label.

Burden (2005) believes that only when the label has been given can the individual begin to understand and negotiate it. This means knowing what it feels like to be dyslexic and this is vital to enable a child to deal with the challenges ahead. This is the first step to resilience, being able to rationalise their challenges and recognise their strengths and abilities over the weaknesses and deficits. This enables them to move away from what Burden (2005) calls 'learned helplessness' or the feeling that no matter what you do you cannot make it right, you cannot make a difference – 'If I am dyslexic I will never amount to much'.

If you get rid of the label dyslexia you could be opening the floodgates for those like Liddle (2014) who claim that these people are just lazy or 'thick'.

# Hidden effects of dyslexia

Hales (2001) talks about the emotional and social effects of dyslexia, with high levels of anxiety and frustration. He argues that dyslexia is so much more than a difficulty with reading, and that even if the practical problems of reading and spelling could be overcome there is a 'reciprocal relationship' between learning and living in the way that it affects a child's self-concept. Self-concept is perhaps one of the most important contributors to any learning, a self-belief that this 'thing' can be achieved. The effects of achievement on the body both physically and mentally can be seen every day as children learn and apply new things. Watching high class Olympic athletes shows this in stark contrast – the difference between the physical and mental effects of the athletes winning or losing. The impact of this in turn often relates to their willingness to continue, their determination to participate in their sport or to learn new things. A child who meets with constant failure eventually begins to believe that s/he cannot achieve, and this atmosphere of poor achievement can start in their very earliest years, almost without notice so that by the time that they start school they are already very familiar with a feeling of disappointment, let down and failure. This same attitude is likely to permeate into other areas of a child's life, outside of their academic

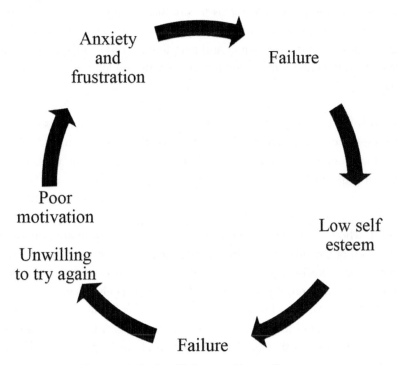

*Figure 2.4* Cycle of failure and low self-esteem

environment, as their expectation of success in any field diminishes. Pumfrey and Reason (1991) show that children with low self-concept often give up on tasks more easily and lack resilience and persistence when attempting a new task. If this starts in their early years then it could become habitual and they will become unwilling to risk embarking upon new things for fear of failure. This erosion of motivation in turn increases their chance of failure in the future, providing a vicious cycle of failure breeding failure (Figure 2.4).

It is likely that a child's perception of themselves is formed through their personal experiences as they interact with their environment and their close and significant others (parents, family, nursery workers, teachers, friends etc.). However, it is always difficult to judge whether poor self-concept is a cause or an effect of a lack of achievement, or an interaction between the two. Hales (2001) suggests that anxiety and the ability to manage the emotions are a factor consistent with the condition and not resultant from it. He believes that it is possible that individuals with dyslexia have an inherent vulnerability, which in time becomes learned behaviour. Pumfrey and Reason (1991) discuss the concept of 'learned helplessness', what Nicolson (2015) calls 'fear conditioning' or a sort of freeze response to threat (where the lack of success is attributed to external factors such as bad luck, poor teaching etc.), as a new experience becomes fear inducing. If you, like so many others in the population, are mystified by mathematics and number, bordering on phobic, you may also experience this. For some strange reason society seems to find it more acceptable for us to say that we are poor at mathematics, but not to say that we are poor at reading. For many, myself included, the whole concept of a mathematics test induces anxiety and fear, that in turn produces chemicals in the brain which lead to changes in subsequent behaviour and learning, leading to 'learned helplessness'.

> If these mental scratches [failure] are not allowed to heal by success or time, that is after a series of adverse, ongoing and inescapable failures, a 'mental abscess' is caused that is almost impossible to heal, and this eventually prevents any learning in that situation.
>
> (Nicolson, 2015: p. 68)

The child, who has to commit enormous effort and extraordinary perseverance just to keep up with others around him/her, often perceives no reward commensurate with the effort expended. If s/he is just achieving on the same level as their peers (quite a feat for some of these children) it is unlikely that they will receive any special recognition for their achievements. One level of that recognition is being able to explain to that child that there is a label for what they are experiencing, a label that can be applied to many of the frustrations they are experiencing and one that can be applied to many other people.

Ryan (2004) suggests that the majority of pre-school children in the UK are happy and well adjusted. The main problems only occur when their expected progress is not achieved and the frustration and anxiety experienced begin to increase as they realise that most of the other children around them appear to be able to achieve in an expected manner. This is then compounded when teachers, adults and parents also become anxious. Ryan (2004) considers that some will develop what he calls 'perfectionist expectations', that is believing that it is unacceptable to make mistakes, making the child with dyslexia feel inadequate and socially immature. When the feelings of failure become so entrenched within the child it is often difficult to reverse these feeling of disappointment and self-loathing. Clearly, we all make mistakes and silly errors, but being able to rationalise these and use them to progress our learning is a vital part of adult maturity and self-belief. If the child begins to anticipate failure, their willingness to take risks, that is to take on new challenges in new situations, begins to recede. We all tend to avoid situations that make us anxious or even frightened, and the child with dyslexia is no exception, but when this applies to so many everyday situations, new learning and new circumstances, then practitioners, teachers and families often misinterpret this as laziness and indolence.

Unfortunately, these anxiety-inducing situations can also provoke what appears to be anger, born out of frustration. As so often happens in human nature this sort of anger is often directed at those closest to us, parents and families. Children who contain their anger in school often allow it to erupt at home, where, ironically, they feel safest and most secure. This, understandably, can be very difficult for families to come to terms with. The social and emotional difficulties experienced by individuals with dyslexia are probably one result of the person being at odds with their environment (Ryan, 2004), so rather than part of the biological origins of dyslexia, they are possibly reacting to the consequences of the condition. Bruck (1986) described the social and emotional difficulties of dyslexia as:

> part or a manifestation of the same disorder as is responsible for academic failure.
>
> (Bruck, 1986: p. 362)

However, an artificial attempt to separate nature and nurture is very difficult, and Ryan (2004) also proposes that there is a possibility that children with dyslexia are inherently less mature and adept physically, emotionally and socially than their non-dyslexic peers. This, he claims, could in turn lead to poor social skills, with children unable to read the visual social cues of people's body language. This, combined with a problem with language, could result in children having difficulties relating to peers and adults, making friends and forming relationships. Clearly if this is correct it would be a very real argument for early intervention.

You could argue long and hard about whether the development of personality is nature or nurture, and probably not achieve a satisfactory answer. However, if you consider the new-born baby, most mothers will identify certain unique personality traits, the baby who is upset easily by stresses and tensions in their environment and cries constantly, or the placid, laid back baby that seems to cope with all that their new life throws at them calmly and easily. The great broadcaster and anthropologist Desmond Morris (2008) suggests that babies are hardwired with certain personality traits, variations that are inborn and not dependent on environmental differences. With these extremes at such a young age it would seem inevitable that some broad aspects of personality development are inherently based. Some children with dyslexia seem to have the resilience to cope better with the problems that society throws at them, whilst others become more anxious and frustrated. Frith (2002) goes so far as to suggest that these differences in personality and ability to cope could be the reason for the continuum from mild to severe in the children with dyslexia (Figure 2.1), as the manifestations are masked, or compensated for, by their ability to cope with the problems they perceive, thereby concealing the severity of the information processing difference.

The report *Dyslexia Still Matters*, produced by Dyslexia Action (2012), showed that a recent YouGov survey indicated that at school many children with dyslexia felt isolated, or even worse, felt bullied. More than 50% of the parents participating claimed that their children did not want to go to school, they felt different and school was a negative experience. Negativity from teachers was described by 37% of the parents surveyed, resulting in an impact on their child's self-esteem. Worryingly, 15% of parents in the survey reported that the teacher made public comments or made fun of their children when they made mistakes.

## CASE STUDY

Haf is seven years of age and struggles to manage effectively in school. She tries so hard to compete with her peers, but it seems that no matter what she does, she never quite manages to finish her work on time or make it as neat and tidy as the others in her class.

This morning she spent most of the time working on writing a sentence to accompany a picture that she had drawn about a trip to the zoo, that she had attended with her class. The other children had all finished but now it was break time. The teacher asked to see the work and after a few moments showed it to the rest of the class and asked them what they thought. She then tore up the paper and put it in the bin, telling Haf that she would need to redo the work after break when the others were doing other activities.

Working with a colleague, consider the following questions:

1. How do you think this made Haf feel?
2. How do you think that Haf will reflect upon this incident and how will she respond in the future?
3. Presumably the teacher felt that continuing with the same activity was going to benefit Haf and progress her learning. How else do you think that this situation could have been handled which could have been beneficial to Haf's learning experience?

Riddick (2009) examined levels of self-esteem in adults with dyslexia and found that their poor levels of self-esteem were not only confined to issues of reading and literacy, but were far more pervasive, infusing all aspects of their life. Like Hales (2001) she suggested that perhaps literacy is only one aspect of a much bigger picture.

# Dyslexia and stress

Mild anxiety can, if not addressed, lead far more seriously to stress. Stress can be both positive and negative; on the one hand it can be empowering, enabling you to confront situations that may be physically harmful (shall I run away from that tiger approaching me or take a chair and fight it off?) or psychological threat (shall I risk embarrassment and social rejection by reading aloud in class?). Stress is a physical and biological process with the production of stress hormones, such as adrenaline, enabling you to protect yourself and even keep you alive. However, when stress gets out of control, and when you feel unable to control your situation, that build up in the body of stress reactors can result in the brain going into 'freeze mode' where the brain shuts down and withdraws, as it is so confused it does not know how to proceed. For the child with dyslexia, who has been faced with failure on many occasions, this means that they are constantly faced with tasks that they believe are too hard for them to achieve. It is the perception of failure that is the problem, so if they believe that they are likely to fail again this will potentially induce this 'bad stress' response, no matter how much others tell them that they can achieve.

If this response becomes long-term then both physical and mental health can be impacted with an increased susceptibility to illness, heart disease, cancer, insomnia etc. Alexander-Passe (2015) suggests that it can also lead to unhealthy behaviour in later life such as smoking, excessive alcohol consumption, eating disorders, self-harm etc. High levels of stress can also prevent the child from engaging in normal childhood activities such as attending school and engaging with peers. Children whose dyslexia has not yet been identified are particularly at risk as they tend to blame themselves for their difficulties and regard themselves as stupid and unworthy. Alexander-Passe (2015) likens it to a child in a fight with 'one hand tied behind their back' (p. 119).

## Holistic development

If you consider the effects of dyslexia in a holistic sense, then you see that many children with dyslexia are also identified with coordination and physical function disorders. Some authorities, such as the British Dyslexia Association (2016), would attribute this to a completely separate and often co-occurring condition, frequently referred to as dyspraxia, or now more commonly referred to as developmental co-ordination disorder (DCD). However, its presence and common occurrence in individuals with dyslexia leads me to believe that this is possibly just another manifestation of the information processing disorder that we call dyslexia. The brain having difficulty linking information from the senses, muscles, joints, eyes etc., to activate and contract in the right order at the right time. This idea was also proposed by Nicolson et al. (2001), who argued that dyslexia cannot be defined solely in terms of reading and literacy, but is better described as a 'general impairment in the ability to perform skills automatically' (p. 508). These poor automatising skills are likely to impact the functions of balance, motor control, writing and even articulatory fluency. They may therefore be indicators of a cerebellar dysfunction.

> Poor motor skills may lead to difficulties with writing; poor articulatory fluency may have an impact via an impaired phonological loop on a reduced working memory and on phonological awareness and word reading, which may lead to difficulties with reading.
>
> (Haslum and Miles, 2007: p. 258)

The hypothesis of a cerebellar deficit is of course only one explanation for dyslexia, but it could also account for why motor skills and co-ordination appear to be affected in many individuals with the condition, as the cerebellum also scaffolds the skills such as speed and automaticity. What is not yet understood is whether there is damage to the cerebellum or a malfunction and whether it is possible to repair.

However, these findings are not universally agreed and have been disputed by Ramus et al. (2003), who gave only partial support to the presence of motor problems in children with dyslexia. However, following a very large sample study by Haslum and Miles (2007) of 12,950 children, they concluded that motor difficulty does occur in a significant number of children who also present with reading difficulties.

The number of children failing the motor tests increased with the severity of their underachievement [in reading].

(Haslum and Miles, 2007: p. 270)

Nonetheless, you must remember that motor skills problems do not cause dyslexia, but are likely to be associated with it in varying degrees, possibly because of the involvement of the cerebellum in some children with dyslexia, but it probably cannot be claimed in all children. In 2002, O'Hare and Khalid compared 136 typically developing children with 23 children with both co-ordination difficulties and reading and phonological awareness delays. Each child was asked to undertake three skills, catching a ball, jumping on a moving roundabout and handwriting. They concluded that all children with difficulties related to poor posture, balance and fast accurate control of movement should be also assessed for difficulties with phonological awareness. A follow up study by Pope and Whiteley (2010) suggested that whilst phonological processing difficulties are one indicator of dyslexia there may be others which manifest in deeper, underlying anatomical issues that originate in the cerebellar or vestibular areas of the brain, they do however caution that much more research is needed into this hypothesis.

To offer an example of the motor control difficulties that individuals with dyslexia might experience consider the task of lifting a pencil to begin drawing or writing. On the surface this appears to be a simple task, but, in reality, consider the true complexity of the task:

1. The eyes must co-ordinate to focus and search for the pencil on the table.
2. The brain must assess how far the pencil is from the body and its spatial position on the table. It must assess which direction to extend the arm and to grasp the pencil (hand-eye co-ordination).
3. The brain now informs the muscles of the arm to contract and extend the appropriate muscles to reach towards the pencil.
4. Once the arm reaches the pencil the brain informs the muscles of the fingers to open and close over the pencil. This fine motor movement is a precision movement and needs to be done accurately, opening the fingers to exactly the right amount and closing again to secure the pencil in the hand.
5. Once the pencil has been grasped the brain must instruct the fingers to adjust the grip on the pencil to achieve a secure pincer grip (Figure 2.5).
6. The strength of the grip is now important. Too loose and the pencil drops out of the grasp. Too tight and it becomes impossible to manipulate across the page to produce legible script.

With this level of complexity it is no wonder that many individuals have poor hand writing, messy paper and illegible print.

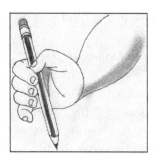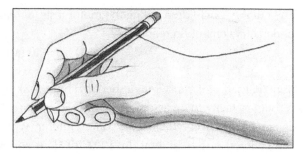

*Figure 2.5* Grasping a pencil (Hayes, 2016 *Language, Literacy and Communication in the Early Years*; pictures by permission of Critical Publishing)

# The tip of the iceberg

Unlike a physical disability, dyslexia cannot always be seen; it is not on show and therefore it has been in the past easy to deny its existence. It is surely difficult to manage something that you cannot measure. With such wide variations between the skills and challenges of the person with dyslexia, and even these being compounded with issues such as tiredness, stress or illness (Miles, 2004), it is almost impossible to allocate a cut-off point on that continuum or normal distribution curve, to distinguish the borderline dyslexic from the severe. Being able to measure something is a basic scientific premise, so if this is a condition which we are currently unable to measure, then no wonder that science finds its existence difficult to accept. The one clearly visible and measurable aspect of this condition is the child's ability to read, and as a society we have expectations of a child's facility to read. The English National Curriculum (2014) expects all children to undergo a series of tests at the age of seven years, to enable comparison of child with child, school with school and area with area. These form concrete statistics, scores which can be validated and are reputedly reliable and observable. As a consequence, the levels of delay in learning to read and spell have become the major focus for those wishing to study dyslexia. All other possible indicators of the condition have been pushed to one side in an effort to find a measurable sign.

Reid and Wearmouth (2002) suggest that there is a complex causal chain from biology to behaviour which, as yet, we do not fully understand.

The cause *may* be the neurodevelopmental syndrome of dyslexia.

(Reid and Wearmouth, 2002: p. 51)

However, if you consider a wider remit for the condition, as a neurodevelopmental disorder, then perhaps reading is just the tip of the iceberg – the visual context – just the bit you can see (Figure 2.6).

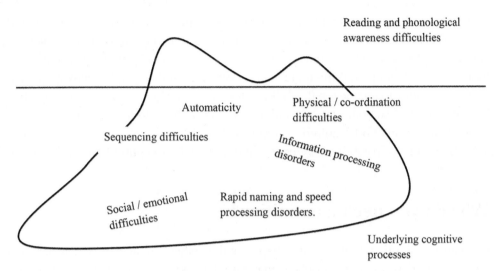

*Figure 2.6* The tip of the iceberg

Clearly if reading is to be the only defining feature of dyslexia the concept of early identification in babies and the pre-school child is unlikely, but to leave identification to the point where reading failure or a failure of academic performance occurs, is not only a failure of those around the child, and of society in general, it is immoral.

## Persistent primary reflexes

Primary reflexes emerge in utero and could be related to an evolutionary advantage in the newborn baby – sucking, rooting, breathing etc. McPhillips and Sheeny (2004) suggest that there could be over 70 such reflexes. In 1992, Blyth suggested that 85% of children identified with dyslexia have, what he refers to as, aberrant reflexes. That is reflexes which would be entirely normal in the newborn baby, but would not be expected to be present in the same child at 12 months or beyond. The transfer from reflex movements to learned behaviour is a significant landmark in a child's development. Blyth (1992) argued that their continued presence provokes neurodevelopmental delay and inhibits writing, reading, copying, attention and concentration by restricting the maturation of the brain. McPhillips and Sheeny (2004) undertook research into the asymmetrical tonic neck reflex (ATNR), which would not usually be seen in babies after three months of age; this is sometimes referred to as the fencing reflex (the newborn baby's face turns to one side and the arm and the leg on that side extend and the opposite side flexes). They suggested that primary reflexes that persist beyond twelve months of age could be linked to a range of learning difficulties. The results from the research by McPhillips and Sheeny (2004) appeared to indicate that

ATNR could play a part in early visuo-motor development, and its persistence could disrupt the development of physical skills such as rolling, crawling, riding a bicycle, catching and kicking a ball. They also suggest that when a child with persistent ATNR looks at their writing hand the reflex causes tension, and the child's reflex grasps the pencil too tightly to enable the flexibility of the muscles required to write or draw. This in turn produces excessive fatigue and muscle strain owing to the increased levels of concentration and effort required to complete a learning task. Such tiredness can also lead to emotional irritability, aggression and a greater susceptibility to physical and mental illness.

## Why do you need a definition?

To return to the original title of this chapter and whether it matters whether there is a definition for dyslexia or not, I believe that it is vital, and we must continue to strive for the answer for the following reasons.

An agreed definition will:

1. Ensure equality in the allocation of limited resources and support.
2. Make clear and dispel anxiety in all those with the condition and their families:

   - What is it?
   - What does it involve?
   - How can it be managed?

3. Demonstrate to families, practitioners and teachers how policy and practice may be developed to help them manage.
4. Allow society to understand the implications of this condition and what compromises may need to be made for a condition that they cannot always see.
5. Enable serious discrete research to be conducted that might aid early identification, management and understanding of the constitutional origins.
6. Bring together the vast range of interested organisations and services, such as educational psychologists, local authorities, schools, colleges, government departments, researchers and specialist organisations such as Dyslexia Action, British Dyslexia Association, International Dyslexia Association etc. to work together to ensure that all children can access their education equally.
7. Enable identification of possible fraudulent or misguided alternative therapies or interventions, whilst at the same time being open to new thinking and innovative management.
8. Encourage those who teach teachers and practitioners to include modules about dyslexia within their initial college and university programmes.

9. Persuade colleges and universities to engage with teachers, practitioners and settings to provide appropriate and realistically priced continuing professional development.

---

**Chapter reflections**

This chapter has attempted to put forward a hypothesis that considers dyslexia under a much broader banner than perhaps you have done until now. Dyslexia is frequently seen as a 'literacy problem', not only by lay people but also by teachers and practitioners (as has been shown in the primary research in Chapter 1). The argument made in this chapter is that this is not the full story. When people with dyslexia have difficulties with literacy skills this is because they are dyslexic and not the cause of it, and it is likely to be only one manifestation of a much more complex condition. Because this initial concern about literacy brought dyslexia to people's attention, somehow we have got 'stuck' in that mode, making it difficult to see that people with this condition are also likely to have difficulties with sequencing, order perception, map reading, maths, attention and concentration, time management, managing their possessions, difficulties with social interaction, confidence, anxiety, visuo-spatial skills, co-ordination and many other indicators. An over-concentration upon literacy skills could have masked the other, equally important manifestations of dyslexia.

The chapter has shown that dyslexia does not start and stop at defined points, but is an inherent part of a person's thinking process and remains on-going throughout life. If dyslexia is shown to be inherent and genetic, then the newborn baby is dyslexic and the toddler and the pre-schooler, long before they need to acquire the sort of literacy skills which are imposed upon them, according to our culture and place of birth. If we lived in a non-literate culture people would still be dyslexic, but we would probably see the condition in a completely different light, as positive, pioneering and original. Dyslexic babies eventually become dyslexic adults, having to adopt coping strategies to live within a literate society, but in a non-literate culture they would never have to cope or compensate for their differences and would probably be lauded for their differences. So what you see in dyslexia is not one thing but rather an amalgam of many. Elliott and Grigorenko (2014) call it a 'clearing-house' for the many manifestations of the condition with both strengths and weaknesses.

# Further reading

Reid, G. (2017) *Dyslexia in the Early Years: A Handbook for Practice*. London: Jessica Kingsley Publishers.

This book, written by one of the foremost authorities on dyslexia in this country, concentrates on the very practical identification and management of children at risk of dyslexia in the early years. The author's whole premise is based, not on a deficit model, but on the identification of need. Only when the practitioner understands these needs can the child be fully assessed for a dyslexic profile and management and resources adapted accordingly.

The practical nature of this text ensures that there are identified activities to help to meet the needs of the child, and he highlights websites where further activities and resources may be found. Reid emphasises that this is an ongoing process which is not about putting a label on a child, but rather to identify risk and support future learning. The text is written in an easy style and there is a useful explanatory glossary to help those who are less familiar with the technical terms.

# References

Alexander-Passe, N. (2015) *Dyslexia and Mental Health*. London: Jessica Kingsley Publications.

Blythe, P. (1992) *A Physical Approach to Resolving Specific Learning Difficulties*. Chester: Institute for Neuro-Physiological Psychology.

British Dyslexia Association (2016) *About the British Dyslexia Association*. Available online at: www.bdadyalexia.org.uk/about (accessed 30.07.17).

Bruck, M. (1986) Social and Emotional Adjustment of Learning Disabled Children: A Review of the Issues. In Ceci, S. (1986) (ed.) *Handbook of Cognitive, Social, and Neuropsychological Aspects of Learning Disabilities*. Hillsdale, NJ: Lawrence Erlbaum Associates.

Burden, R. (2005) *Dyslexia and Self Concept: Seeking a Dyslexic Identity*. London: Wiley.

Critchley, M. (1981) Dyslexia: An Overview. In Pavlidis, G. and Miles, T. (1981) (eds) *Dyslexia Research and its Applications to Education*. London: Wiley and Sons.

Department for Education (2014) *National Curriculum in England: Framework for Key Stage 1–4*. Available online at: www.gov.uk/government/publications/national-curriculum-in-england-framework-for-key-stages-1-to-4/the-national-curriculum-in-england-framework-for-key-stages-1-to-4 (accessed 20.07.17).

Dyslexia Action (2012) *Dyslexia Still Matters*. Surrey: Dyslexia Action.

Elliott, J. and Grigorenko, E. (2014) *The Dyslexia Debate*. New York: Cambridge University Press.

Frith, U. (2002) Resolving the Paradoxes of Dyslexia. In Reid, G. and Wearmouth, J. (2002) (eds) *Dyslexia and Literacy: Theory and practice*. Chichester: Wiley and Sons Ltd.

Government Equalities Office (2010) Equality Act 2010: *What do I need to know? Disability Quick Start Guide*. London: Crown.

Gov.UK (2014) *Children and Families Act 2014*. Available online at: www.legislation.gov.uk/ukpga/2014/6/contents/enacted (accessed 07.08.17).

Hales, G. (2001) Self-esteem and Counselling. In Peers, L. and Reid, G. (eds) *Dyslexia: Successful Inclusion in Secondary School*. London: David Fulton.

Haslum, M. and Miles, T. (2007) Motor Performance and Dyslexia in a National Cohort of 10-year-old Children. *Dyslexia* 13(4): 257–275.

Hayes, C. (2016) *Language, Literacy and Communication in the Early Years: A Critical Foundation*. Northwich: Critical Publishing.

Liddle, R. (2014) Dyslexia is meaningless. But don't worry – so is ADHD. *The Spectator* 15 March 2014. Available online at: www.spectator.co.uk/2014/03/dyslexia-isnt-real-but-dont-worry-neither-is-adhd/ (accessed 30.07.17).

McPhillips, M. and Sheeny, N. (2004) Prevalence of Persistent Primary Reflexes and Motor Problems in Children with Reading Difficulties. *Dyslexia* 10: 316–338.

Miles, E. (2004) Definitions of Dyslexia. In Johnson, M. and Peers, L. (eds) *The Dyslexia Handbook 2004*. London: BDA: 63–67.

Morris, D. (2008) *The Amazing Baby*. London: Firefly Books.

Naidoo, S. (1972) *Specific Dyslexia*. Bath: Pitman Publishing.

National Centre for Eating Disorders (2012) *Why People get Eating Disorders*. Available online at: www.eating-disorders.org.uk (accessed 30.07.17).

Nicolson, R. (2015) *Positive Dyslexia*. Sheffield: Rodin Books.

Nicolson, R., Fawcett, A. and Dean, P. (2001) Developmental Dyslexia: The cerebellar deficit hypothesis. *Trends in Neuroscience* 24(9): 508–511.

O'Hare, A. and Khalid, S. (2002) The Association of Abnormal Cerebellar Function in Children with Developmental Co-ordination Disorder and Reading Difficulties. *Dyslexia* 8: 234–248.

Ott, P. (1997) *How to Detect and Manage Dyslexia*. Oxford: Heinemann.

Pope, D. and Whiteley, H. (2005) The lost boys? A Case-history Study of Ten Very Able Children with Dyslexic Characteristics. *Educating Able Children* 8(1): 109–123.

Pumfrey, D. and Reason, R. (1991) *Specific Learning Difficulties*. London: Routledge.

Ramus, F., Pidgeon, E. and Frith, U. (2003) The Relationship between Motor Control and Phonology in Dyslexic Children. *Journal of Child Psychology and Psychiatry* 44(5): 712–722.

Reid, G. and Wearmouth, J. (2002) *Dyslexia and Literacy: Theory and Practice*. Chichester: Wiley and Son.

Riddick, B. (2009) The Implications of Student's Perceptions on Dyslexia for School Improvement. In Reid, G. (ed.) (2009) *The Routledge Companion to Dyslexia*. Abingdon: Routledge.

Rodger, J., Wilson, P., Roberts, H., Roulstone, A. and Campbell, T. (2015) *Support for Higher Education Students with Specific Learning Difficulties*. York: HEFCE.

Ryan, M. (2004) *Social and Emotional Problems Related to Dyslexia*. Michigan: International Dyslexia Association.

Shaywitz, S. (2005) *Overcoming Dyslexia*. New York: Vintage.

Turner, M. (1997) *Psychological Assessment of Dyslexia*. London: Whurr Publications Ltd.

# The neuro-biology of dyslexia . . . origins and research

*Everybody is a genius. But if you judge a fish by its ability to climb a tree, it will live its whole life believing that it is stupid.*

Argued to have been said by Albert Einstein . . . himself
thought to have been dyslexic

## Introduction

This chapter will look critically at a range of possible origins of dyslexia in the hope of 'busting a few myths' and comparing serious research threads. There might be one cause of dyslexia or even many contributing and overlapping causes, but it is likely that they will either be biological or experiential, or a combination of the two. If there is more than one cause they may take effect independently or in combination, as an interactionist model, and could interrelate dynamically or more slowly over a period of time, at different stages of development.

Since Hinshelwood (1895), research into the origins of dyslexia has escalated, from many different fields and disciplines such as medicine, psychology, sociology, pedagogy, genetics, neuroscience etc. The research has taken place not only in this country and the English-speaking world, but also across a global perspective as researchers in China, Arab and Middle Eastern countries, Scandinavia and Asia have come to recognise that there is an identifiable condition impacting people's ability to learn language. For this they all seek an explanation.

One of the greatest advances in this area of neurobiology in recent times has been the advent of brain imaging, meaning that no longer do we have to rely on dissecting post mortem brains to undertake research. Neuroscientists can now 'see' inside the active, living brain in a non-invasive manner, allowing a better understanding of brain structure, function, location and pharmacology.

A number of different systems can be deployed for differing types of research:

- fMRI (Functional Magnetic Resonance Imaging): This works by detecting changes in blood oxygenation and flow to the brain during neural activity. This method is less suitable for use with very young children, as the subject is required to remain very still.
- PET (Positron Emission Tomography): This uses small amounts of radioactive material to map functional processes in the brain as they become active. The major disadvantage of this method is that it is very expensive to operate.
- EEG (Electroencephalography): Electrodes are placed strategically across the outside of the head to measure levels of electrical activity. This is a non-invasive technique and is therefore well suited to use with very young children.
- MEG (Magnetoencephalography): This measures magnetic energy in the brain via sensitive devices called SQUIDs (superconducting quantum interference devices), determining various functions of different areas of the brain.
- NIRS (Near Infrared Spectroscopy): This is an optical technique used to measure blood oxygenation to the brain and provide an indirect measure of brain activity.
- CT Scan (Computerised Tomography): This projects X rays through the head and creates cross sectional images of the structure of the brain. However, it does not indicate brain function.

# Causal modelling

Before examining some of the research and theoretical input to explanations for dyslexia, it is useful to examine a framework into which all the explanations fall. Such a framework will enable you to better analyse and scrutinise the interrelationships between the competing theories. Frith (2002) talked of a biological origin to dyslexia leading to a cognitive deficit, resulting in a particular pattern of behaviour.

Frith (2002) talked about these as levels of explanation, with each level having their proponents and devotees (See Figure 3.1). To enable you to understand this complex condition you will need to consider these levels not as succinct and distinctive, but as domains that merge into each other and intermingle. Frith's levels can, of course sometimes operate independently, so for example the child who shows no difficulty with reading (behavioural level) may have their dyslexia masked by their excellent and progressive teaching, and their enabling environment. Equally there is the generally poor reader (behavioural level), who is not dyslexic, but has not had the appropriate environmental conditions to enable them to read.

Frith (2002) calls these levels – I have referred to them as domains, as levels tend to imply a hierarchy, one level taking precedence over the one below. It also implies that you can start with the behavioural signs and work backwards, for example poor reading

| Biological | Neurodevelopmental disorder with behavioural signs which extend beyond reading and written language. Genetics and neuroanatomical factors. | Cultural and Environmental Influences | Clinical manifestation of dyslexia | Remediation |
|---|---|---|---|---|
| **Cognitive** Including emotional factors, functional description of brain activity and phonology. | Information processing mechanisms. Visual and auditory. Perceptual processing. Motor and temporal processing. | | | |
| **Behavioural** | Observable. Characteristic features such as difficulties learning to read. | | | |

*Figure 3.1* Causal modelling diagram (adapted from Frith, 2002)

being accounted for by a range of different reasons, but perhaps a better scenario would be to work the other way up, from the biological to the behavioural.

## It's all in your DNA!

Every cell in your body probably contains 25–35,000 genes, carried on 23 pairs of chromosomes. In recent years more and more research has concentrated upon genetic factors having a causal link to dyslexia. Studies involving familial and inheritable evidence abound, and most writers in the field now acknowledge that genes play at least some part in determining whether a child will be dyslexic. Gilger et al. (1991) estimated that there was a 40–60% chance of a child being dyslexic if one parent also has the condition, and this percentage could be increased further if other family members are also dyslexic.

   Much of the research so far conducted has been based on a comparison between identical (monozygotic) and non-identical (dizygotic) twins, and appears to indicate that the monozygotic twins are more likely to have similar dyslexic inheritability issues than dizygotic twins. The focus upon twins has been an attempt to reduce the environmental influence, but clearly separating the genetic factors from the environmental factors (nature from nurture) is very difficult. This is so even for twins growing up alongside each other in a similar culture, eating similar foods and experiencing similar educational backgrounds etc. Although twin studies can potentially supply a great deal of very useful data, this type of research can also have many ethical challenges. Such challenges might be sampling problems, that may mean that it is not possible to generalise to the universal population and iatrogenesis (that it may lead to the self-fulfilling prophecy), where the research subject develops traits because they believe that they will manifest eventually. Another line of research has been with adoptees, where the risk of dyslexia has been linked to their biological but not their adoptive relatives (Wadsworth et al., 2001).

As you have already read, researchers in the twenty-first century are starting to ask whether dyslexia does have genetic origins. In the single gene model (autosomal dominant transmission), there would be one dominant gene for dyslexia, which only one of the parents would need to transmit to their offspring for it to be expressed. This would seem to be consistent with the prevalence rate, but would not explain why some individuals with dyslexia appear to have no affected relatives (Plomin et al., 2001). A single recessive gene would need to be passed on by both parents and would not be expressed in all their offspring, so some children would become carriers of the recessive gene, without manifesting any markers for dyslexia, but with the potential to pass it on to their children in the event of a union with another carrier. Therefore, Plomin et al. (2001) suggested that a multiple gene model was more justifiable, with the further possibility of hundreds of genes being involved. On the strength of current evidence available, it is debatable whether there is a single 'dyslexic gene' responsible for this condition, but there do appear to be several genes, carried on a small number of loci on the chromosomes, which could be causing an interesting reaction in the areas of the neuronal development necessary for reading.

It is very probable that genetics do play an important role in developmental dyslexia as they clearly play a vital role in the early development of the foetal brain, but this is a complex condition and probably not everything can be blamed upon the genes; it is more likely to be a complex and intricate interplay between genes and the environment.

Research into genetic linkage analysis (a way to pinpoint particular genes on a chromosome), and genetic mapping (Scerri et al., 2011), has identified broad genomic areas that could relate to the dyslexic condition, but these areas probably contain tens or even hundreds of potential candidate genes, making the intricacy of this research very difficult and time consuming. It is likely that this will also require multiple testing and screening to be able to identify a particular gene or gene area, and will require large samples with a heavy reliance upon statistical probability. Genetic linkage analysis conducted thus far does appear to have narrowed down certain areas of the genome that could be suitable for further research. From a large scale European study (the NeuroDys

Cohort) (Becker et al., 2014), four candidate genes in particular have sparked researchers' interest, although there are other culprits.

DYX1C1 on chromosome 15
ROBO1 on chromosome 3
KIAA0319 on chromosome 6
DCDC2 also on chromosome 6

This cross-linguistic research (Becker et al., 2014) looked at over 900 dyslexic participants in eight different European countries and 1,150 control candidates. The study showed quite weak links to the marker genes selected for the research, but the authors suggest that this could have been caused by the different ethnic origins of the sample. They also suggest that pre-school and nursery teaching methods, which differ widely across Europe, could have influenced the research. However, research by Taipale et al. (2003) appeared to show a number of susceptible genes for developmental dyslexia, which they claim could potentially disrupt protein function in the developing brain. Scerri et al. (2011) also showed strong associations between a number of genetic markers and reading skills, across the range of ability levels, but they concluded that

[t]he biological cause of RD [reading disability] and SLI [Specific Language Impairment] remains poorly understood, but it is clear that their manifestation is a result of multiple interacting factors, many of which have a genetic origin.

(Scerri et al., 2011: online)

One difficulty with all of these research projects is to ascertain definitively the identification of a dyslexia phenotype; otherwise they could be comparing apples with pears. It is notable that the inclusion of subjects for all of these research studies was taken entirely upon their word reading ability, and did not include manifestations of the whole spectrum of dyslexia related traits, which could have affected the results. It is of course possible, even likely, that in the future completely new loci will be identified, and with the tantalising idea of molecular genetic dissection (gene therapy), differing epistatic effects may become apparent. If heritability does play such a major role in determining children who are at risk of dyslexia, this is vitally important to the whole concept of early identification and early targeted intervention, before children reach the point of academic failure.

Our data suggest that the same genes contribute to reading impairment even in the background of different disorders. This would imply also that the same cognitive deficit is at the basis of reading problems regardless of other clinical diagnoses.

(Scerri et al., 2011: online)

Although dyslexia may be familial, family traits can also be transmitted culturally, so familiarity alone is possibly not a reliable indicator of genetic heritability. Elley (1994) suggested that the most reliable predictor of literacy achievement was the number of books in the home, school and library that the child was exposed to; this indicator is clearly environmental, but could also be influenced by parental genes. Most researchers in the field now agree that there is a genetic component to the origins of dyslexia, but it is also clear that we are still some way away from understanding the full molecular mechanisms responsible.

**CASE STUDY**

Marie is the manager of Puddleducks nursery, she has spent some time arranging a robust professional development session for the staff in the nursery, about dyslexia and identifying children at risk. She has organised an expert speaker for Friday evening after the children have left.

Jillian, a senior member of staff, does not want to stay and Marie overhears a conversation between Jillian and another, more junior, colleague.

Jillian: This is ridiculous; I have better things to do with my Friday nights! Anyway, why do we need to know about dyslexia . . . that is all about reading and I work in the baby room!

The pair go their separate ways, laughing.

What do you think that Marie should do?

What would you say to convince Jillian of the importance of attending the course?

If this is a signal that other staff are feeling the same, what do you think would change their minds?

# Neuro-biological factors: the magnocellular theory of dyslexia

Another possibility as a biological basis for dyslexia is some form of deficit to the sensory process, which could also explain why areas other than reading appear to be impacted in the person who is dyslexic.

As the newborn baby lies in their cot listening to adults talking, what s/he hears is a continuous stream of sound. Spoken language, unlike written language, has no spaces between the words, but the human brain appears to be hardwired to 'search' for language in the sounds that they hear; it is as though it is seeking meaning. Pinker (1994) calls this phonetic awareness a 'sixth sense'. The baby's brain starts to segment the sounds or phonemes, which when assembled in a particular order, make separate words with a particular meaning, giving the words distinctive boundaries.

To be able to read an alphabetic orthography a young child must be able to visually analyse (except in braille where the same analysis must be conducted from a tactile perspective) a series of characters in order to then translate these marks, or combination of marks, to sound. This requires an understanding that each character or letter has a consistent resonance but some combinations of letters carry a further sound such as:

| | |
|---|---|
| 'p' as in pig | 'c' as in cat |
| 'h' as in hat | 'h' as in hat |
| 'ph' as in tele*ph*one | 'ch' as in *church* |

To be able to read, the child has to identify the shape of the characters or letters and letter combinations that s/he sees in the text, and associate the shapes with the sounds that they hear – grapheme/phoneme mapping. Modern neurological scanning mechanisms have shown that this process relies upon the very small parvocellular neurons in the brain (often called P-Cells), which transmit nerve impulses between the brain and other parts of the body, in this case it is those that code for colour and detail including fine spatial aspects. These neurons, therefore, pass information from the eyes (primary visual cortex) to the visual word form area within the brain.

Not only is identification of phonemes important for reading but sequencing these quickly and accurately is essential for fluency (the fluency threshold for reading is thought to be 35 words per minute). This complex process is also dependent upon the magnocellular system (magnocells are over 500 times the size of the parvocells) and both conduct signals to the cerebral cortex (Stein et al., 2001).

> The M [magnocells] neurons form only 10% of the ganglion cells in the retina, but they are specialised for timing visual events by signaling movement rather than form or colour.
>
> (Stein, 2012: p. 32)

This stream of information is often referred to as the ventral stream, because it flows past the ventral part of the brain. This ventral stream is the pathway to the cerebral cortex associated with parvocells and is frequently referred to as the 'what' pathway, focusing as it does upon fine detail and colour. The magnocellular pathway, or dorsal pathway, is often referred to in the literature as the 'where' pathway, thought to focus on timing, sequencing, visual memory, contrast, eye movement, co-ordination of limb movements and motor function. It is therefore the magnocellular system that enables the eyes to guide visual attention and focus on the fixations necessary for reading. Thus if the magnocellular system is impaired in some way the young child is likely to have difficulty focusing their attention and controlling the convergence and binocular stability needed for eye fixation. According to this theory, it is likely to mean that the child will experience blurring of letters and movement of words on the page, with letters swirling or jumping about and other symptoms of visual stress.

Stein (2012) claims that the magnocells in the brains of people with dyslexia are up to 25% smaller than the magnocells in non-dyslexic brains. He suggests that these cells have migrated during foetal development into other layers of the brain. Snowling (2000) talks about a study by Lingston et al. (1991), which examined autopsy specimens from five dyslexic and five non-dyslexic brains. Whilst the parvocellular layers appeared similar, the magnocellular layers were smaller (reduced by up to 30%), and more disorganised. The magnocellular layers, which in the non-dyslexic brains were separate, in the dyslexic samples, were more merged. Clearly these autopsies were conducted on a very small sample, and it is unclear whether the brains were representative of dyslexic brains in general. It is also possible that the difference between the dyslexic and non-dyslexic brains examined could have been a consequence of dyslexia and not a cause. Whilst such post mortem findings suggest new and interesting areas for further research, they do not provide definitive proof. However, this sort of research could potentially provide anatomical and physiological evidence for the magnocellular theory.

It is vital that both the parvocells and magnocells cooperate to enable a reader to see a stationary image when their eyes move along the line of print. Information has to be combined from both the peripheral vision and the central vision. As you are reading this your eyes are not moving smoothly across the page as you may at first think, rather your eyes are moving in a series of stops and starts. When your eye settles on a word, this is called a fixation (which probably lasts for approximately 300 milliseconds), and when it moves across the next few words this is a saccade (Figure 3.2). Reid (2009) claims that these saccades take about 20–40 milliseconds and at that point vision is suppressed, enabling the content to be understood. Stein (2012) suggests that any reduced sensitivity

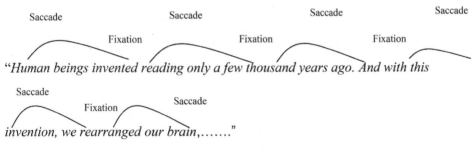

*Figure 3.2* Saccades and fixations (adapted from Wolf, 2008: p. 3)

in the magnocellular system could weaken that suppression, and as a consequence provide the reader with an excess of visual information, resulting in confusion and deterioration in visual acuity when reading. Pammer (2013) attributes this particularly to the speed of processing and therefore the fluency of reading.

During the saccade no detailed visual information is taken on board.

> Thus successful reading depends greatly upon achieving stable visual perception during each fixation on the word to be read and rapid shifts of visual attention to the next. The saccades between fixations and the drifts that occur during fixations cause letters to move around on the retina a great deal; yet, for good readers the print remains stationary on the page.
>
> (Stein et al., 2001: p. 67)

Later research conducted by Stein (2012) suggests that individuals with dyslexia also have difficulty with contrast thresholds; this issue will be returned to later in this chapter, but some researchers have suggested that this sensitivity can be ameliorated with the use of coloured overlays in up to 45% of the cases observed. Contrast sensitivity in reading is the ability to distinguish between the letters and their background. Contrast threshold is the minimum level of contrast required for someone to be able to discriminate the colour and brightness of an object. Consider trying to read in the dark where the contrast between the black of the print and the white of the paper is blurred – as the light fades it becomes increasingly difficult (see Figure 3.3).

However, there are critics of the magnocellular theory and Snowling (2000) points out that if there were direct relationships with visual impairment, then individuals with dyslexia would be likely to have more trouble reading continuous text than single words, but this does not generally appear to be the case. Snowling (2000) also suggests that replication of some of the findings from magnocellular theory research,

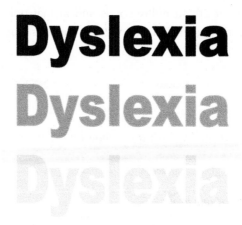

*Figure 3.3* Contrast thresholds (which is easiest to see?)

has been inconsistent. Fawcett (2001) believes that the theory does not explain why young children with dyslexia find it so hard to detect rhyme and time estimation, which do not require rapid processing. The greatest proponent of the magnocellular theory is Stein, but even he recognises that if magnocellular deficit does exist its effects are probably mild (Stein et al., 2001) and it occurs in only two-thirds of people with dyslexia. This implies that to see any statistical inference for this hypothesis, very large samples are required. Stein et al. (2001) also drew attention to what was called an auditory equivalent of the visual magnocellular system, which helps to detect frequency and amplitude of sound; this enables you to distinguish different sounds of letters or the phonology of reading. It is certainly true that individuals with dyslexia do appear to be less sensitive to modulation, variation of frequency and the development of phonological skills.

Fawcett (2001) took the magnocellular theory still further to suggest that sensorimotor skills are affected by the impairment of the cerebellum, which has a heavy input from the magnocells. Stein et al. (2001) proposed that the magnocellular system could also impact the immune system, with a higher than average incidence of conditions such as asthma, eczema, hay fever and glue ear being seen in dyslexic individuals.

Clearly this very complex theory requires far more research and investigation, but what we do not know is whether any of these brain structure differences are the cause or a consequence of dyslexia. However, it is likely that if there are neuronal changes in important regions of the brain, they could promote the formation of completely new reading and literacy circuits in the brain. Wolf (2008) suggests that the genetic circuitry of the brain could be compensating for the inefficiencies of the brain for reading.

> dyslexia will turn out to be a stunning example of the strategies used by the brain to compensate; when it can't perform a function one way, it rearranges itself to find another, literally.
>
> (Wolf, 2008: p. 197)

Wolf (2008) also talks of the experimentation on the brains of genetically selected mice.

> When the neuroscientist Glen Rosen at Beth Israel induced a small lesion in the auditory cortex of these mice, neuronal abnormalities formed in the thalamus, similar to those found earlier in the dyslexic brain. Most important, as a result of the lesions, the mice could no longer process rapidly presented auditory information.
>
> (Wolf, 2008: p. 204)

This research demonstrated how the migration, or perhaps a deficit of magnocells, could result in information processing difficulties. However, it must be emphasised that magnocellular theory is still highly controversial and researchers such as Elliott and Grigorenko (2014) and Singleton (2009) believe that it still does not have enough empirical evidence to describe this as any more than a complex but interesting finding, which currently offers a confusing picture. Certainly, there is insufficient evidence to offer a definitive causal link between magnocellular dysfunction and dyslexia.

## Visual stress

SSS – no, not a branch of the Special Forces, but a condition called scotopic sensitivity syndrome or visual stress or even Meares-Irlen syndrome. This is a theory that hypothesises that some people have low-level visual disturbances or unpleasant visual experiences when they are reading. According to Singleton and Henderson (2007), there are more reported incidents of visual stress sensitivity to text in individuals with dyslexia than in non-dyslexics, and those with dyslexia that experienced visual stress often found that it was significantly improved with the use of coloured overlays. These overlays are sheets of transparent coloured Perspex, usually A4 in size, which can be placed over the text to be read.

Singleton and Henderson (2007) believe that visual stress could also be attributed to magnocellular deficits, or cortical hyperexcitability, which is a condition that possibly affects up to 20% of all children and 65% of children identified with dyslexia. Cortical hyperexcitability is thought to be caused by pattern glare, and is not an unusual phenomenon in both those identified with dyslexia and those who are not. It can result in sore and tired eyes, headaches, photophobia (an over-sensitivity to light), visual distortions, perceptions of moving text and instability, but also can evoke seizures and migraine. Those that experience this condition often claim that words on a page swirl, jump up and down, have poor print resolution, have letters that overlap or have a halo effect or just become blurry and difficult to read. It must however be emphasised that this is not an optical problem but a perceptual one. Irlen (1991) claims that these symptoms can be alleviated with the use of the coloured filters, to remove the glare. Randomised double-masked placebo-controlled trials have supported the existence of visual stress and the effectiveness of the coloured filters for some individuals (Robinson and Foreman, 1999).

Wilkins (1995) speculates that the wavelength of light affects neuronal sensitivity and colour can reduce this glare and the cortical hyperexcitability, thereby reducing the unpleasant symptoms and perceptual distortions. Wilkins (1995) also emphasises that visual stress is not peculiar to dyslexia, and can often be identified in non-dyslexic readers, but the coloured filters and manipulation of letter size (larger print) and spacing, appears to offer a significant improvement in reading fluency and comprehension of the dyslexic readers.

Despite the term visual stress, not being a visual difficulty but a perceptual one, Irlen (1991) claims that there are five essential components of visual stress:

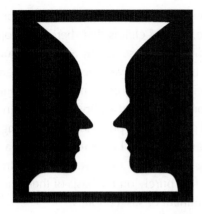

What can you see? A vase or two faces?

Where does the black become dominant to the white, or the other way around?

*Figure 3.4* Colour dominance and perception

1. Light sensitivity – glare, brightness and certain light conditions such as flicker. Very young children can be seen trying to get into a comfortable position with sufficient light to be able to identify the print.
2. Inadequate background contrasts – dealing with high contrasts such as black and white, where the white background can become dominant to the black letters (see Figure 3.4).
3. Poor print resolution – letters that dance and move. As the size of the print reduces from the books seen in the nursery/pre-school setting, to more advanced and smaller typefaces, this can become more apparent.
4. Restricted span of recognition – makes it difficult to move smoothly from line to line or to skim read – sometimes called 'tunnel reading'.
5. Needs frequent breaks – easily tired.

One major difficulty when identifying visual stress is that if a child has always experienced such visual distortions from a very young age, they come to accept it as 'normal' and do not report its existence. Often they only recognise that they have a problem when the symptoms are alleviated. Singleton (2009) and others point out that in the research to date, not all children with visual stress appear to benefit from the coloured filters, and some children who do not complain about visual stress do appear to benefit. He criticises some of the research for a lack of objectivity when it comes to identifying what constitutes reading improvement. For example, does reading improvement relate to the speed of reading, or the propensity for children to read more frequently due to a reduction in the stress, what is sometimes called the 'Matthew effect' (Stanovich, 1986)? The inclusion of undiagnosed dyslexics in the samples could also have artificially inflated the number of non-dyslexics diagnosed with visual stress.

A further complication with this theory is ascertaining the 'right' colour for a particular person, as it does appear that the colours that people find work best are often different. Irlen (1991) admits that some colours can make things better, but for other people it could make the visual stress worse, so she claims that there is an optimal colour for each person which needs to be individually assessed by an expert, qualified in the use of an 'intuitive colorimeter'. This highly sensitive piece of equipment will be able to assess an ophthalmic tint according to the person's sensitivity. The intuitive colorimeter enables colour and light saturation to be varied without a change in luminance. This will also allow for precisely tinted glasses to be prescribed, thus doing away with the need for cumbersome filter sheets, and allowing better reading from a white board and when writing. Unfortunately, probably due to expense, most children are not given a full colorimeter test and are identified purely on the basis of their choice of colour which clearly is not an objective determinant of susceptibility.

> a full understanding of visual stress is unlikely to be achieved without an account of its relationship with dyslexia. However the link between dyslexia and visual stress may not necessarily be causal.
>
> (Singleton and Henderson, 2007: pp. 130–151)

Once again there is controversy over this theory and great care must be exercised when attributing visual defects to dyslexia. Contrary to the general public's belief (see Chapter 1), children with dyslexia are probably no more likely to see letters and words backwards – 'bs' for 'ds' and 'was' for 'saw' (Shaywitz, 2003), than any other child, it is a normal process of development in the 4–5-year-old child, which I am sure that you have all seen with the children in your care.

# Glue ear

Glue ear, or more correctly Otitis Media, is an inflammation of the middle ear which is very common in early childhood, and normally clears up of its own accord as the child approaches puberty. Normally the middle ear is filled with air to enable sound waves to vibrate the ear drum (tympanic membrane), causing vibration of the fluid in the cochlea to ripple and an electrical signal to be carried to the brain – auditory perception. In children with Otitis Media the space in the middle ear is filled with a sticky, viscous fluid, which accumulates to the point that it pushes the ear drum taut, and can even result in a very painful perforated ear drum. At its most extreme it may be necessary for surgeons to put a small hole in the tympanic membrane and insert a tiny tube called a grommet, to allow the fluid to drain. However, according to Peer (2009) even when the grommets have been inserted, complex audio-processing deficits can persist for some time. Daly (1997) noted that in the UK, the incidence of Otitis Media was running at 20–30% of all children, which was significantly higher than many other countries, although no explanation has been offered for this.

Extensive research, undertaken by Peer (2002), showed an unusually high percentage of children identified with dyslexia (over 70%) had also suffered with glue ear at some point in their life. She concluded that it was possible that the symptoms of glue ear, with significant intermittent hearing loss, inconsistent acoustic information and possible stays in hospital, were mimicking dyslexia. If you consider that the average pre-school child will normally be learning approximately four to five new words a day, being able to hear accurately could potentially have a significant impact on their language learning, and in particular their phonemic awareness. The symptoms described by children with glue ear are:

- Pain and an inability to sleep.
- Loss of concentration and attentiveness resulting in tuning out of conversations.
- General language and communication difficulties. This is particularly likely when there is extensive background noise such as in an early years' room or school setting.
- Mishearing words, making it difficult to keep up with conversations.
- Confusing certain fine sounds and general auditory perception; in particular the soft vowel sounds of a, e, u.
- Reduced auditory processing speeds.
- Difficulties remembering and mapping sounds to words making it difficult to apply phonic rules or follow patterns.
- Poor spelling because they cannot hear the sounds.
- Difficulties for children in multi-lingual settings, such as Welsh medium and Welsh bilingual schools and nurseries – having to distinguish a wider range of sounds and phonemes.
- Tiredness, irritability and consequent behaviour issues owing to the constant struggle to hear accurately.
- Poor short-term memory (Gathercole and Pickering, 2000).
- Feelings of insecurity leading to poor social skills, withdrawal, social isolation and loneliness.
- Can become quiet and withdrawn.
- Problems with balance and ocular motor difficulties.

It must be remembered that not all children with glue ear will suffer from all or even most of these symptoms. Peer (2009) showed that when glue ear is apparent in babies under the age of one year, it is likely to persist for far longer than if it starts in the school-aged child. This finding was consistent with Wolf (2008), who showed that frequent ear infections and subsequent hearing loss in the first two years of life, could result in impaired development of both expressive and receptive language, ensuring a significant disadvantage to literacy development when starting school. Peer (2009) also suggested that there may be links to allergic reactions, particularly milk allergies, with subsequent possible weaknesses in the auto-immune system.

This intermittent hearing difficulty can be especially hard for a young child in a busy, noisy nursery, where there is a variety of background noise, such as chairs scrapping, children talking and shouting and a variety of activities all going on at the same time, making sound discrimination potentially very difficult. For the child with significant information processing difficulties, this additional slowness of auditory processing could place further stress on their ability to learn in the early years. So whilst glue ear is undoubtedly a medical problem, it brings with it educational, social and emotional difficulties.

> It may be that glue ear, occurring at a time when auditory and vestibular skills are developing rapidly, may of itself be sufficient to lead to symptoms of dyslexia.
>
> (Peer, 2009: p. 40)

# Ciliogenesis

This is a very new and exciting research area for dyslexia. Ciliogenesis is the process by which small hair-like structures called cilia, on cell walls, develop and move fluids from one place in the body to another by rapid and rhythmic beating, thereby contributing to neural migration. Neural migration is the process, seen in the developing foetus, by which neurons are moved from the place that they first develop to their final differentiated position in the brain, to enable them to interact appropriately. Virtually all the neurons are formed before birth and gradually migrate to their appropriate locations. However, according to Pinker (1994)

> head size, brain weight, and thickness of the cerebral cortex (gray matter) where the synapses (junctions) subserving mental computation are found, continue to increase rapidly in the year after birth. Long distance connections (white matter) are not complete until nine months, and they continue to grow their speed-inducing myelin insulation throughout childhood. Synapses continue to develop, peaking in number between nine months and two years (depending on the brain region), at which point the child has fifty percent more synapses than the adult!
>
> (Pinker, 1994: pp. 288–289)

The exact process by which dyslexia and ciliogenesis are linked is still very poorly understood, but mutations of some of the candidate genes (DYX1C1) for dyslexia also appear to have a contributory impact on cilia formation.

Primary Ciliary Dyskinesia (PCD) is a genetic disorder of the cilia. The motion of the cilia is thought to be responsible for organ placement in the developing foetus, and defective neuronal migration may result in aberrant connectivity between cells, which could be the key to understanding cognitive defects such as developmental dyslexia (Tarkar et al., 2013). Sensory neurons in the visual and auditory system have highly modified primary cilia, potentially causing levels of deafness, glue ear, sinus congestion, laterality defects and visual disturbances of the type seen in the child with dyslexia. The research into this area may well produce some exciting results in the next few years, but further peer reviewed research is required.

## Cerebellar deficit

The cerebellum is an area at the rear of the brain, long thought to be associated with dyslexia. When undertaking neuroimaging pictures, Fawcett and Nicholson (1992) showed that dyslexia was associated with cerebellar deficit in over 80% of the cases reviewed. According to Reid (2016), it is one of the first structures of the brain to differentiate in the embryo, and one of the last to mature, continuing to develop even after birth. This structure accounts for 10–15% of the total weight of the brain, 40% of the surface area, and contains 50% of the neurons; interestingly it is proportionately larger in humans than in any other primate.

The main role of the cerebellum is to coordinate muscle activity, in particular rapid skilled movement, and to maintain body posture by storing learned sequences of movements. In people with damage to the cerebellum there is frequently a change in their body posture, balance, limb rigidity (the inability to relax muscles normally), poor coordination and poor time estimation. However, the most important feature of the cerebellum is its plasticity, it has a remarkable capacity to regenerate itself very quickly, by changing its structure and function to adapt to new physical and environmental conditions.

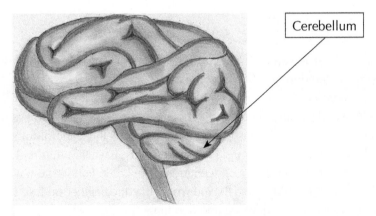

Cerebellum

*Figure 3.5* Location of the cerebellum in the brain

Fawcett and Nicolson (1992) argue that the cerebellum is responsible for automatisation, that is the ability to be able to do something routinely, without having to concentrate, such as walking, talking, maintaining body posture, thereby allowing you to undertake more than one activity at a time – the child running around the nursery, manipulating an airplane with their hands and making the brumming noise. The research conducted by Fawcett and Nicolson (1992) suggested that reading and writing were also subject to automatisation and noted that children with dyslexia have great difficulty with this process.

According to the theory of cerebellar impairment, a very young child with this condition will have motor delays, such as being slower to sit up, slower to walk, difficulty with fine motor control and difficulty with controlling the articulatory muscles, resulting in delayed babbling and deferred speech. Once the toddler starts to walk and talk this is likely to take up far more of their inner resources, causing tiredness and allowing less time and attention for other sensory feedback. Snowling and Hulme (1994) argue that processing phonemic information may therefore be less likely, leading to a loss of awareness of onset (the initial consonant or consonant blends of a single syllable word – cat), rime (the vowel and any final consonants – cat) and phonemes (the smallest unit of sound in speech). This ability to detect onset, rime and phonemes is, according to Goswami (1986), vital in the pre-school child, to enable him/her to eventually learn to read.

[D]ifficulties appear to be specific to reading and spelling because they involve a combination of phonological skills, fluency, automatization, and multi-tasking – a combination of all the skills that dyslexic children find difficult. Why does performance appear to be normal in other skills? Because literacy is of such critical educational importance it is examined minutely, whereas other skills are largely overlooked.

(Fawcett and Nicolson, 2001: p. 100).

## CASE STUDY

James is now married and in the army but describes here some of the difficulties he has encountered in his life with dyslexia:

When I was very young and at my first school I really struggled with reading and spelling and I really could not tell the time on a clock face, I was at the bottom of the class. The teachers used to tell me that I was thick and shouted at me a lot and I found that frustrating and I would get angry, have tantrums and cry a lot. The teachers said that I was not concentrating, but I didn't understand what I was being taught. . . . I couldn't understand words that the teacher said, so I suppose I mucked about a lot . . . drawing and doodling.

I was really unhappy at that time and did not want to go to school. One day the teacher screamed right in my face until he went bright red. . . . I really felt belittled and worthless. My perception of teachers was that they were always 'angry' and I was frightened. Being shouted at became so normal, I no longer wanted to try . . . why bother?

When I went to my new school I was eight years old and they quickly realised that I had problems. . . . They gave me work, but they asked if I understood. I had an assessment and when I was diagnosed with dyslexia it became easier . . . it gave me something so that if I didn't understand I didn't feel stupid, and it was easier to come forward and ask questions. I still got frustrated though when I would read an entire page with no understanding. I enjoyed biology but couldn't continue with it because of all the big words.

I still hate reading aloud as there is pressure if someone is waiting for me to read or write. When I left school, there were so many jobs that I knew that I did not have the confidence to do. . . . One of the good things about the army is that there are all sorts of people there and they do not take the mick or make it embarrassing. When they show me jokes on their phone I have to pretend to read, and laugh anyway. I have to adapt and do things differently because I am slower, and I avoid doing things in front of others.

Sometimes spoken words are hard to come out, I know what I want to say but cannot get it out. I have developed facilities to help. . . . The telephone is a good resource with the predictive text. I do enjoy reading if there are no other distractions. . . . I must be interested in it . . . a good story . . . but it is hard work and does not relax me so I tend to watch TV.

When I look back there are some respects in which I am better off, I would not have done things like photography and art without dyslexia and I find it hard to understand why other people struggle with these things.

# Cerebral asymmetry

The brain is divided into two distinct parts or hemispheres and in general the right hemisphere controls the left side of the body and the left hemisphere controls the right side.

It is also thought that the two sides process information in different ways (Eide and Eide, 2011). The two sides are usually asymmetrical, but interestingly in post mortem studies of brains from people with dyslexia, a higher level of symmetry was seen (Gerschwind and Galaburda, 1985), and there appeared to be an excess of cells in the right hemisphere. This is a very complex picture, but it should be noted that the post mortem studies only involved a very small number of brains. Further studies using MRI scanning

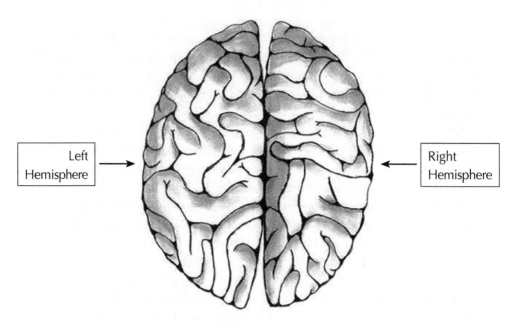

*Figure 3.6* Hemispherical nature of the brain

methods (in vivo studies) have not always demonstrated this consistently (Knight and Hynd, 2002). Although there are clearly differences of both structure and function there is no uniform pattern of asymmetry and in the general population there are about three in four people with left hemispheres greater than right, but one in 12 have no detectable asymmetry and about one in eight have right greater than left (Shapleske et al., 1999). Researchers are not able to confirm whether this is inherited or environmental, although there is always the possibility of an inherited susceptibility to environmental hazards before birth.

The brain is made up of approximately 80% grey matter which consists mostly of nerve cells or neurons (that is what we see when we examine a human brain), and white matter which is deeper into the brain and mostly consists of connective fibres to carry electrical impulses to facilitate communication between the nerves, transferring information around the brain (Pinker, 1994). Research by Booth and Burman (2001) indicates that there tends to be less grey matter in people identified with dyslexia than in the non-dyslexic brain. They claim that this could result in a greater difficulty when information processing, particularly sound and language. However, Pinker (1994) suggests that the brain is not only sculpted by increasing neurons, but also by losing some.

> Massive numbers of neurons die in utero, and the dying continues during the first two years before levelling off at age seven. Synapses wither from the age of two

through the rest of childhood and into adolescence, when the brain's metabolic rate falls back to adult levels.

(Pinker, 1994: p. 289)

Gerschwind and Galaburda (1985) showed that in the post mortem brains of people with dyslexia there were a number of misplaced cells (ectopias or brain warts), and these appear to have migrated to the outer layer of the cortex, which is normally cell free. The ectopias were found particularly in the left hemisphere of the brain, in areas normally associated with language activities. However, of necessity, post mortem studies have very small samples, which makes it difficult to know whether they are representative of the dyslexic brain in general or that the differences are specific and exclusive to dyslexia. On the other hand, the problem with in vitro studies using MRI scans is that they cannot detect the microscopic differences that can be examined in the post mortem studies.

Clearly this is an area of great complexity but there is a growing body of research (Shaywitz, 2003; Wolf, 2008) that suggests that people with dyslexia often use their hemispheres differently to non-dyslexics, with the right hemisphere being used more frequently for different processing tasks, including reading. Of course, it is not possible to know whether these differences are cause or effect. Rice and Brooks (2004) give the example of London taxi drivers who need to master 'The Knowledge' of the routes and locations. Both functional and structural differences in the area of the brain associated with spatial awareness have been observed in the brains of these taxi drivers. It is probably reasonable to assume that this is not something that they are born with, but has developed due to their exceptional experiences and brain plasticity.

---

**Reflect on this**

With a colleague consider the following questions and then compare your answers:

1. How important do you think it is for you, as a practitioner in early years, to understand more about the origins and aetiology of dyslexia?
2. How do you think it might help you to better identify and support a child at risk of dyslexia?
3. Consider two of the research approaches in this chapter and decide how they are different and how they are similar. Which do you find the most convincing and why?
4. List the skills that are most important to a child under the age of two years. How would each of these be impacted by the various theories put forward in this chapter?

**Chapter reflections**

This chapter has put forward a number of differing theoretical perspectives for the aetiology of dyslexia and current research strands. Whilst these may appear very different on the surface, what they most have in common is the idea that there are significant differences in the brains of people with this information processing disorder, either in structure or function or an interaction between the two. What is also clear is that nothing is clear, and once again I have to conclude that more research is needed to increase understanding. With that understanding comes the tantalising prospect of very early identification and thereby the ability to put in place appropriate targeted support, to ensure that case studies such as that of James are reduced to a minimum. Also with such research will come an indication of what that support needs to look like. Attempting to define dyslexia as a single entity is probably not achievable, and more likely Frith's (2002) domains of Biological, Cognitive and Behavioural need to be interwoven to offer various causal models, which contribute to a dyslexic syndrome within a cultural context.

One clear conclusion is the importance of children's early years, in some cases even before birth, to identification and remediation. However, it is positive to know that considerable progress has been made into dyslexia research, although probably creating more questions than illuminating answers.

# Further reading

Wolf, M. (2008) *Proust and the Squid: The Story and Science of the Reading Brain*. Cambridge: Icon Books.

Although published in 2008, this book is a classic of its time. The text looks at the history of early writing, through to the neuroscience of literacy. This is a book written for the general public, so whilst dealing with some highly complex ideas, the author manages to make it both readable and to guide the non-specialist through the complex twists and turns of the subject, explaining the scientific language and offering extensive notes to aid the reader. Maryanne Wolf is a teacher of child development and cognitive neuroscience, and it is this unique combination and merging of knowledge, that enable her to put reading into the context of a lifelong experience, from cradle to grave. In this book she encourages you to reconsider things that you may have long taken for granted, and to synthesise interdisciplinary research with a passion for the subject area.

# References

Brandler, W.M. and Paracchini S. (2014) The Genetic Relationship Between Handedness and Neurodevelopmental Disorders. *Trends Mol Med.* 2014 Feb; 20(2): 83–90. Available online at: www.ncbi.nlm.nih.gov/pmc/articles/PMC3969300/ (accessed 01.08.17).

Becker, J., Czamara, D., Scerri, T., Ramus, F., Csépe, V., Talcott, J., Stein, J., Morris, A., Ludwig, K., Hoffmann, P., Honbolygó, F., Tóth, D., Fauchereau, F., Bogliotti, C., Iannuzzi, S., Chaix, Y., Valdois, S., Billard, C., George, F., Soares-Boucaud, I., Gérard, C., Van der Mark, S., Schulz, E., Vaessen, A., Maurer, U., Lohvansuu, K., Lyytinen, H., Zucchelli, M., Brandeis, D., Blomert, L., Leppänen, P., Bruder, J., Monaco, A., Müller-Myhsok, B., Kere, J., Landerl, K., Nöthen, M., Schulte-Körne, G., Paracchini, S., Peyrard-Janvid, M. and Schumacher, J. (2014) *Genetic Analysis of Dyslexia Candidate Genes in the European Cross-linguistic NeuroDys Cohort.* University of St Andrews. Available online at: https://risweb.st-andrews.ac.uk/portal/en/researchoutput/genetic-analysis-of-dyslexia-candidate-genes-in-the-european-crosslinguistic-neurodys-cohort(9686c026-3c78-49b4-8f39-cb250e860cd0).html (accessed 01.08.17).

Booth, J.R. and Burman, D. (2001) Developmental Disorders of Neurocognitive Systems for Oral Language and Reading. *Learning Disability Quarterly* (24): 205–215.

Daly, K. (1997) Definition and Epidemiology of Otitis Media. In Roberts, J.E., Wallace, I.F. and Henderson, F.W. (1997) *Otis Media in Young Children: Medical, developmental and educational considerations.* Maryland: Paul Brook Publishing.

Eide, B.L. and Eide, F.F. (2011) *The Dyslexia Advantage: Unlocking the Hidden Potential of the Dyslexic Brain.* London: Hay House.

Elley, W. (1994) (ed.) *The IEA Study of Reading Literacy: Achievement and Instruction in Thirty-Two School Systems.* Oxford: Pergamon.

Elliott, J. and Grigorenko, E. (2014) *The Dyslexia Debate.* New York: Cambridge University Press.

Fawcett, A. (2001) (ed.) *Dyslexia: Theory and Good Practice.* London: Whurr.

Fawcett, A. and Nicolson, R. (1992) Automatisation Deficits in Balance for Dyslexic Children. *Perceptual and Motor Skills* 75: 507–529.

Frith, U. (2002) Resolving the Paradoxes of Dyslexia. In Reid, G. and Wearmouth, J. (2002) *Dyslexia and Literacy: Theory and Practice.* Chichester: John Wiley and Sons.

Gathercole, S. and Pickering, S. (2000) Working Memory Deficits in Language Disordered Children: Is there a causal connection? *Journal of Memory and Language* 29: 336–360.

Gerschwind, N. and Galaburda, A. (1985) Cerebral Lateralisation. Biological Mechanisms Associations and Pathology: A hypothesis and a programme for research. *Archives of Neurology* 42: 428–459.

Gilger, J.W., Pennington, B.F. and DeFries, J. (1991) Risk for Reading Disability as a Function of Parental History in Three Family Studies. *Reading and Writing* 3: 205–218.

Goswami, U. (1986). Children's use of Analogy in Learning to Read: A developmental study. *Journal of Experimental Child Psychology* 42, 73–83.

Hinshelwood, J. (1895) Word Blindness and Visual Memory. *The Lancet* 2, 21st Dec: 1564–70.

House of Commons Science and Technology Committee (2009) *Evidence Check 1: Early Literacy Interventions.* London: The Stationery Office.

Irlen, H. (1991) *Reading by Colours: Overcoming Dyslexia and Other Reading Disabilities through the Irlen Method.* New York: Perigee Books.

Knight, D. and Hynd, G. (2002) The Neurobiology of Dyslexia. In Reid, G. and Wearmouth, J. (2002) *Dyslexia and Literacy: Theory and Practice.* Chichester: John Wiley and Sons.

Lingston, M.S., Rosen, G.D., Dislane, F.W. and Galaburda, A.M. (1991) Physiological and Anatomical Evidence for Magnocellular Defect in Developmental Dyslexia. *PNAS* 88: 7943–7947.

Pammer, K. (2012) The Role of the Dorsal Pathway in Word Recognition. In Stein, J. and Kapoula, Z. (2012) (eds), *Visual Aspects of Dyslexia*. Oxford: Oxford University Press.

Pammer, K. (2013) Temporal Sampling in Vision and the Implications for Dyslexia. Available online at: www.ncbi.nlm.nih.gov/pmc/articles/rmc3925989 (accessed 25.11.17).

Peer, L. (2002) *Dyslexia, Multilingual Speakers and Otitis Media*. PhD Thesis: University of Sheffield.

Peer, L. (2009) Dyslexia and Glue Ear. In Reid, G. (ed.) (2009) *Routledge Companion to Dyslexia*. Abingdon: Routledge.

Pinker, S. (1994) *The Language Instinct*. London: Penguin Books.

Plomin, R., DeFries, J.C., McClearn, G.E. and McGuffin, P. (2001) *Behavioural Genetics* (4th edn). New York: Worth Publishers.

Reid, G. (2016) *Dyslexia: A Practitioner's Handbook* (5th edn). Chichester: Wiley.

Rice, M. and Brooks, G. (2004) *Developmental Dyslexia in Adults: A Research Review*. London: National Research and Development Centre for Adult Literacy and Numeracy.

Robinson, G. and Foreman, P. (1999) Scotopic Sensitivity/Irlen Syndrome and the use of Coloured Filters: A long term placebo-controlled and masked study of reading achievement and perception of ability. *Perceptual and Motor Skills* 88: 35–52.

Scerri, T., Morris, A., Buckingham, L., Newbury, D., Miller, L., Monaco, A., Bishop, D. and Paracchini, S. (2011) DCDC2, KIAA0319 and CMIP Are Associated with Reading-Related Traits. *Biological Psychiatry* 70(3): 237–245. Available online at: www.biologicalpsychiatryjournal.com/article/S0006–3223(11)00135–1/fulltext (accessed 01.08.17).

Shapleske, J., Rossell, S.L., Wooderuff, P.W.R. and David, A.S. (1999) The Planum Temporale: A systematic, quantitative review of its structural, functional and clinical significance. *Brain Research Reviews* 29 (1): 26–49.

Shaywitz, S. (2003) *Overcoming Dyslexia*. New York: Vintage.

Singleton, C. (2009) Visual Stress and Dyslexia. In Reid, G. (2009) (ed.) *The Routledge Companion to Dyslexia*. London: Routledge.

Singleton, C. and Henderson, L. (2007) Computerized Screening for Visual Stress in Children with Dyslexia. *Dyslexia: An International Journal of Research and Practice* 13 (2).

Snowling, M. (2000) *Dyslexia* (2nd edn). Oxford: Blackwell Publishers.

Snowling, M. and Hulme, C. (1994) The Development of Phonological Skills. *Philosophical Transactions of the Royal Society of London, series B – Biological Sciences* 29th Oct 1994 1315 (346): 21–27.

Stanovich, K. (1986) Matthew Effect in Reading: Some consequences of individual differences in the acquisition of reading. *Reading Research Quarterly* 21: 360–407.

Stein, J. (2012) *Developmental Dyslexia: Early Precursors, Neurobehavioural Markers, and Biological Substrates*. Baltimore: Brookes Publishing.

Stein, J., Talcott, J. and Witton, C. (2001) The Sensorimotor Basis of Developmental Dyslexia. In Fawcett, A. (2001) (ed.), *Dyslexia: Theory and Good Practice*. London: Whurr Publishers.

Taipale, M., Kamine, N., Nopola-Hemmi, J., Haltia, T., Myllyluoma, B., Lyytinen, H., Muller, K., Lindsberg, P., Hannula-Jouppi, K. and Kere, J. (2003) A Candidate Gene for Developmental Dyslexia Encodes a Nuclear Tetratricopeptide Repeat Domain Protein Dynamically Regulated in Brain. *Proceedings of the National Academy of Sciences of the USA*. Available online at: www.pnas.org/content/100/20/11553. vol. 100 (20) 11553–11558 (accessed 01.08.17).

Tarkar, A., Loges, N., Francis, R., Dougherty, G., Tamayo, J.V., Shook, B., Cantino, M., Schwartz, D., Jahnke, C., Olbrich, H., Werner, C., Raidt, J., Pennekamp, P., Abouhamed, M., Hjeij, R., Köhler, G., Griese, M., Li, Y., Lemke, K., Klena, N., Liu, X., Gabriel, G., Tobita, K., Jaspers, M.,

Morgan, L.C., Shapiro, A.J., Letteboer, S.J., Mans, D.A., Carson, J.L., Leigh, M.W., Wolf, W.E., Chen, S., Lucas, J.S., Onoufriadis, A., Plagnol, V., Schmidts, M., Boldt, K., UK10K, Roepman, R., Zariwala, M.A., Lo, C.W., Mitchison, H.M., Knowles, M.R., Burdine, R.D., Loturco, J.J. and Omran, H. (2013) DYX1C1 is Required for Axonemal Dynein Assembly and Ciliary Motility. *Nature Genetics* 45 (9): 995–1103.

Wadsworth, S., Corley, R., Hewitt, J. and DeFries, J. (2001) Stability of Genetic and Environmental Influences on Reading Performance at 7, 12 and 16 years of Age in the Colorado Adoption Project. *Behaviour Genetics*, 31: 353–359.

Wilkins, A. (1995) *Visual Stress*. Oxford: Oxford University Press.

Wolf, M. (2008) *Proust and the Squid: The Story and Science of the Reading Brain*. Cambridge: Icon Books.

# All the 'ologies . . . morphology, phonology and phenomenology

*That's one reason why [dyslexia] hasn't been eliminated from the gene pool, because for a long time, before human culture invented writing systems, you didn't need it.*
Usha Goswami, Professor of Cognitive Developmental Neuroscience, Fellow at St John's College Cambridge, and Director of the Centre for Neuroscience in Education, interview with Doughty for the *Daily Telegraph* 9 May 2015

## Introduction

In 1987, the actress Maureen Lipman hit our television screens as BT Beattie in the advert for British Telecom. Famously she tells her grandson, who has only passed exams in pottery and sociology, that he must be a scientist if he passed an 'ology! Somehow the addition of that suffix to a subject seems to produce legitimisation; suddenly it is academic, scientific, recognised, permissible and even well founded. However, the scientific and academic communities are sceptical, as well as culturally and educationally diverse. Science is not about a body of facts, rather it is about rational and critical analysis of beliefs, and reasons why others should also believe, set within a climate of doubt.

This chapter will attempt to explain some of the concepts and beliefs around the subject of dyslexia, and examine the most up to date research into the importance of phonological awareness, the advantages of teaching phonemic and morphological awareness to the young child and the importance of rhythm, rhyme and letter-sound training.

## Phonology

Phonology is the study of speech sounds used to make up language; phonological awareness is the ability to hear these sounds and know how to manipulate them to create language. Now try to pronounce the following word:

Pneumonoultramicroscopicsilicovolcanoconiosis

This is purportedly the longest phonetically consistent word in the English language, it refers to a type of lung disease. If you attempted to pronounce that word it is likely that you broke the word into manageable bits or phonemes. As it is unlikely that you have had to read that word before, it really is the only way that you could attempt it. This is exactly how we teach children to read, so whether you are trying to make sense of 'A cat sat on a mat' or wondering what on earth 'Pneumonoultramicroscopicsilicovolcanoconiosis' means, you will be using the same method. A phoneme is the smallest unit of sound in any language, it does not contribute any meaning to a word, so the phoneme 'H' does not contribute to the meaning of the word HAT, and on its own is likely to be entirely meaningless. As an example of this say aloud the following phonemes:

$$g - r - o - l$$

As a whole word 'grol' is entirely meaningless, but each individual phoneme can be sounded out to produce something that sounds like a word or a whole 'non-word'. So phonemes build towards meaningful elements of language:

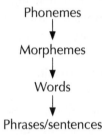

Phonemes
↓
Morphemes
↓
Words
↓
Phrases/sentences

> A division into independent discrete combinational systems, one combining meaningless sounds into meaningful morphemes, the others combining meaningful morphemes into meaningful words, phrases and sentences, is a fundamental design feature of human language.
>
> (Pinker, 1994: p. 163)

It is likely that you use phonics every day of your life; when you come across a word that you do not know, you process the word bit by bit, drawing on your existing knowledge to synthesise common letter patterns. Before learning to read it is thought that children need this tacit knowledge of how phonemes are strung together in their cultural language.

## Onset and rime

The consonant or group of consonants at the start of a word is called the onset.

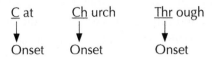

C at        Ch urch        Thr ough
↓           ↓              ↓
Onset       Onset          Onset

The vowel sounds, and any following consonants that come after the onset, are called the rime.

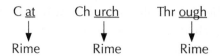

C at      Ch urch      Thr ough
↓          ↓          ↓
Rime      Rime      Rime

So words that rhyme often share a rime, and words that alliterate share an onset.

> The king with the bling had a ring made of string (rhyme)
> The cat called Casper caught a crafty crab (alliteration)

Language is a social and cultural experience with different languages spoken across the world, but all languages with an alphabetic orthography are made up of phonemes or sounds, and each language has phonological rules. Young children who have difficulty distinguishing phonemes in their spoken language are likely to find it hard to learn to read. Many researchers, such as Goswami (2016) and Nicholson (2016), believe that an impairment of phonological processing, particularly phonological decoding, is at the heart of the reading issues experienced by many people with dyslexia. This can be seen in the challenges that some have when reading:

- Short-term memory problems particularly phonological memory.
- Decoding words to phonemes – sounding out.
- Repeating long words.
- Difficulties with non-words (such as glin, drun, blyg etc.).
- Distinguishing colour, numbers and letters.
- Poor pronunciation.
- Limited ability to see stress patterns in rhymes.
- Poor understanding of syllables and phonemes.
- Poor understanding of rhyme.
- Poor rapid naming of number, pictures and colours.
- Difficulties playing word games such as rhyming, alliteration and nursery rhymes and story strings such as the *Little Gingerbread Boy* and *Rosie's Walk* (Pat Hutchins, 1968).

Some writers, such as Bryant and Bradley (1985) go so far as to say that phonological and phonemic awareness training with letter sound correlation and increased vocabulary can improve literacy and reduce the chances of literacy difficulties, such as that proposed by the Welsh Government in their National Literacy Programme (2012). Reid (2016) suggests that a lack of awareness of onset and rime is the strongest predictor of future reading difficulties and Bryant and Bradley (1985) showed that an awareness of rhyme by the age of three years was an excellent predictor of literacy by the age of six years. In 1980 a study by Lundberg et al., conducted in Sweden, showed that degrees of success in school could be calculated with high accuracy (over 70%) on the phonemic awareness of the children in the nursery. Such research results have been replicated many times since then, including Kirby et al. (2003), who showed that American kindergarten children with poor phonological awareness were more likely to develop problems with reading than those with good phonological awareness. However, a study by Krashen (2002) showed that phonological awareness training had only a limited impact on word reading and no effect on comprehension. Nicholson (2016) suggested that phoneme awareness training, whilst a good indicator of success, did need to be undertaken over a protracted period of time, and then it did appear to have a beneficial effect, particularly on spelling.

Most babies begin to learn the rhymes, rhythm and modulation of their native language when in the womb, as they listen to the muffled sounds of their mother talking. From birth onwards, there are not only auditory signals but also visual dynamics, as the familiar adults around them sing, clap, dance, drum the rhythms of their language, stressing the syllables through what Newport (1975) referred to as Motherese, or now more usually called Infant Directed Speech (IDS). IDS is the tendency of adults, around the world, across cultures and languages, to raise the pitch of their voice, exaggerate the intonation and include repetition when talking to babies and young children. Stern et al. (1982) showed that over 77% of the language that adults used with babies fell into this category of protoconversations, allowing pauses for response and comeback.

## Phonological awareness

Liberman and Whalen (2000) claimed that phonological awareness, whilst necessary for reading was not necessary for speech as phonemes are abstract, so they do not exist as part of acoustic language. It is interesting that as small children we recognise words and syllables first, so phonemic awareness is probably less to do with the sound that hits the eardrum and more to do with the perception of a concept in the brain. Liberman and Whalen (2000) suggested that at one level phonological awareness could be the cause, the symptom and the treatment for reading delay, requiring three component skills:

- Cognitive ability (thinking, reasoning, memory, recall, focus and attention).
- Short-term verbal memory (sometimes called language based memory – the ability to hold small amounts of verbal information and words in the mind for a short period of time).
- Speech perception (how highly variable language patterns are heard and mapped to a linguistic representation and understood).

So the development of phonological awareness becomes a cyclical process:

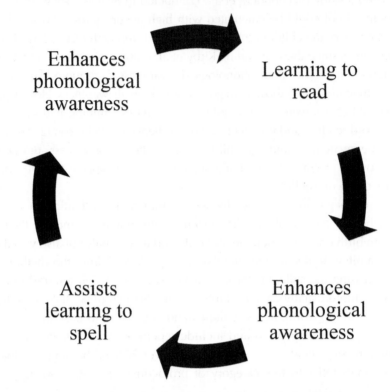

*Figure 4.1* The cycle of reading and phonological awareness

Phonological awareness can be recognised in the children in your care by their ability to:

- Appreciate rhyme – what rhymes with 'king'? Bring.
- Identify individual words within a sentence from the continuous stream of sound that forms general speech – segmentation.
- Blend sounds together to make up a word – c – a – t = cat
- Identify syllables within a word – how many syllables in the word 'elephant'?
- Delete a letter to make another word – say the word 'clog' without the 'c'.
- Delete a syllable to make another word – what is 'hedgehog' without the 'hog'?
- Recognise sounds within a word – what is the last letter of the word 'dog'? What other sounds can you hear in the word 'dog'?
- Competently blend syllables – ze + bra = zebra.
- Add sounds to make other words – add the word 'candle' to the word 'stick' to make a new word.
- Manipulate language – take the 'd' from 'dog' and replace it with an 'l'. What word is it?

All these can be made into great games to play with the children in your care, to encourage their phonemic awareness, but also as entertainment and great fun. Even small babies will enjoy playing pat-a-cake and clapping out rhymes. Books of rhyme and alliteration such as those by Dr Seuss, with great titles such as *Green Eggs and Ham* or *Cat in the Hat* and *I Can Read with my Eyes Shut* are fun to read repeatedly and accustom the child to sounds of rhyme. Traditional nursery rhymes are also important to practise with the under five-year-olds with Humpty Dumpty, Old King Cole and Mary, Mary Quite Contrary etc. However, according to research by the Governments Basic Skills Agency (2003) in Wales, teachers claimed that 61% of children who start school in Wales (at the age of four to five years) are unable to recite or sing the simplest nursery rhymes or songs in either English or Welsh. Learning nursery rhymes has traditionally been seen as an activity to do with parents and the first step to phonological awareness, but this research showed that parents themselves often had no knowledge of any songs or rhymes to play with their children. Interestingly, in this survey, the children in the Welsh medium schools were more aware of traditional rhymes than those in the English medium schools. The survey did however recognise that some children were picking up jingles and rhymes from the television and radio, rather than the traditional rhymes valued by the teachers, which it could be claimed does the same thing to familiarise children with the rhythm of their language.

Research into phonological awareness is relatively recent, probably only starting in the 1960s and 1970s with Russian psychologists Zhurova (1973) and Elkonin (1971). Although they worked in the 1960s this was not translated into English until a decade later, but showed that many pre-school Russian children were unaware that spoken language was made up of phonemes. They used counters with the children to show them the sounds in the words.

$$l - o - g \qquad c - ow$$
◎ ◎ ◎ ◎ ◎
3 counters     2 counters

In America, Liberman et al. (1974) showed that only one fifth of pre-school children could tap out the phonemes in a simple word such as:

$$i - ce$$

Bruce (1964) showed that English children aged five to seven found it hard to delete and substitute phonemes:

Say 'best' without the 's' . . . bet
Add a 'c' to 'lay' . . . clay

# Morphology

In linguistics, morphology is the study of how words are formed or the units of language that carry meaning. These could be base words, roots, combining forms, prefixes, inflectional endings or suffixes and these are particularly important for spelling. Morphemes are the smallest grammatical units in language.

- Base word: this is a word that can stand alone, so 'happy' is the base word for unhappy and unhappily and 'read' is the base word for reread and rereading.
- A root: this requires a suffix or prefix to be understood.

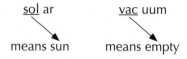

- Prefix: A letter or group of letters that precede a root or base word to make another word.

un – sure, multi – cultural, in – visible

- Suffix: A letter or group of letters that follow a root or base word.

child – ish, like – able, large – ly

- Inflectional ending: This can be added to a root or base word to change the verb tense but not to alter the form.

play, play – ed, play – ing
jump, jump – ed, jump – ing

- Combining forms: this is the glue sticking words together to form new words.

tooth + brush = toothbrush
lawn + mower = lawnmower

So, in a word like 'reaction' there is a prefix, base word and suffix.

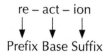

However, morphology can also have a biological interpretation, as the study of forms and structures of plants and animals – their physical appearance and the relationships between these structures both at a gross and microscopic level.

To understand language, you need to process information at two levels:

1) Semantic information: that is information that carries meaning, this may require context, for example:

'The dog was barking' depending upon what context this is said, could be a good thing (he alerted his owner to the burglar), or it could be a bad thing (he was annoying the neighbours).

2) Syntactic information: that is the rules of language or the grammatical relationship between the words – tense, plurality, aspect etc. For example:

'The boy bites the dog'
'The dog bites the boy'

This sort of information is conveyed through morphemes. When morphemes are assembled together they convey the necessary semantic and syntactic information to ensure meaning. These can occur as phonologically separate, so in words like 'cat' and 'cow' the word and the morpheme are the same. However, with more complex words they may be a combination of different morphemes, some of which are unlikely to appear as words in their own right, but only in combination with a root, such as:

cat – s (2 morphemes)
dark – ness (2 morphemes)

It is important that you understand how significant morphological skills are when learning to read. Reading at speed with pace and flow allows for comprehension of the text, try reading the following piece out loud.

You can calculate molecular geometrics, rates and equilibria, spectra, and other physical properties with the tools of computational chemistry. Molecular mechanics ab initio, semi empirical and density functional methods, and molecular dynamics.

(Lewars, 2016: p. 1)

You probably found that you had to slow down whilst you sounded out several of the words, this will have slowed down your reading speed and interrupted the flow, at a guess you got to the end with very little comprehension of what you had read. This is what it is like for children with reading difficulties. You may want to try this with a reading learner; allow them to read a page, most will do this quite slowly, then ask them what they have read about. Many will have read every word on the page, focusing carefully upon each word, but will be unable to put those words together to allow comprehension, so speed is important. Children with good morphological skills and awareness of the structure of language will become aware of the type of words that are likely to come next in a sentence, making for quick and efficient reading. You have already read in Chapter 3, that an efficient reader does not read every word on the page, and a lot of reading is about guesswork and comprehension. If the sentence seems to make sense you continue to read, if it does not you will retrace and read it again. If the word seems right you will progress, especially if it also fits syntactically and visually; knowledge of syntax and semantics dictate what the following sentences say:

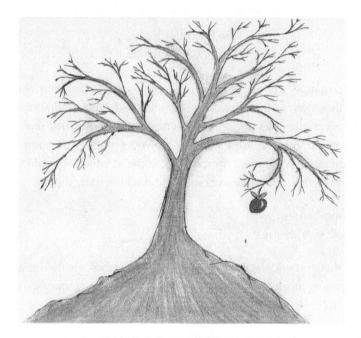

*Figure 4.2* Syntax and semantics

An apple grew on the tree.
An apple grew on the tray.
An apple is growing on the tree.
An apple is grew on the tree.

Morphological skills in this case refer to the grammatical functions of the word endings. Peer and Reid (2016) suggest that people with dyslexia often have poor syntactical or morphological skills, and accuracy and speed of reading are also affected by the complexity of the morphological structure (Schiff and Raveh, 2007).

Morphemic awareness is particularly important in languages such as English, which is classed as an opaque language, which is one that does not always follow a consistent phonology or includes irregular words.

caught cat

eye I aye

However, transparent languages such as Welsh are always phonetically regular:

ff always sounds like 'f'

(fforc = fork)

f always sounds like 'v'

(fan = van)

Developmental dyslexia and morphological awareness have been studied much less than phonological awareness. The few studies that there are appear to show that children with a familial risk of dyslexia show poor inflectional morphology at an early age, and in their language development in general (Lyytinen and Lyytinen, 2004). Schiff and Raveh (2007) undertook research on undergraduate students who were identified as dyslexic but who were seen as compensated readers.

> The major question we addressed was whether well compensated undergraduate students with dyslexia use morphological procedures during lexical access similar to those of normal readers. We found in sharp contrast to the strong morphological priming [that is where a word is identified by prior presentation of a morphologically related word – jump/jumpy, secret/secretary] found for the normal readers none of the dyslexic subgroups showed morphological priming.
>
> (Schiff and Raveh, 2007: p. 123)

It is possible that this impaired morphology is due to a difficulty in segmenting words into root morphemes, which may not be adequately represented in the lexicon of readers with dyslexia. Schiff and Raveh (2007) also observed the morphological disparity in the early stages of reading acquisition. So, word recognition processing is qualitatively very different in the child at risk of dyslexia, relying on whole word recognition; this means that each new word that the child comes across has to be learned as a whole, so rather than the ability to know the root and add the appropriate prefix or suffix, this renders it necessary to learn completely different units each time, making the reading process slow and laboured. An example of such morphological priming might be with the root word 'jump'.

*Table 4.1*

| **Jump** | Jumps | Jumpy | Jumping |
|---|---|---|---|
| Jumped | Jumper | Jumpers | Jumpier |
| Jumpily | Jump-off | Jump-jet | Jumped-up |
| Jumpsuit | Jumpiness | Show-jump | Long-jump |
| Outjump | Ski-jump | Base-jump | Long-jumping |

Once you can recognise the word 'jump', the variations upon it become much easier to identify and commit to your lexicon.

## Socio-economic disadvantage

Particularly low levels of phonological awareness have been observed in children from socio-economically disadvantaged homes compared to children from more financially secure homes. Nittrouer (2002) suggested that this was unlikely to be the result of innate learning difficulties, and more to do with an impoverished language environment in the early years. Such children may not be exposed to the true acoustics of language, with limited exposure to rhymes and limited range of vocabulary. Whilst this may indeed be true, it is also likely that poor phonological awareness in children from low socio-economic backgrounds could have multiple explanations related to both environmental and biological features. This may be particularly so of children at risk of dyslexia, thereby producing a double deficit theory.

It does appear that increasing numbers of children are arriving at nursery with such poor spoken language skills that they find the skills needed for reading and writing very difficult (Locke et al., 2002). A study conducted by Locke et al. (2002) showed that more than half of the children tested at nurseries in areas of financial poverty were found to be language delayed. Interestingly, in this study, the girls appeared to be less affected linguistically than the boys, but Locke et al. (2002) gave no satisfactory explanation for this.

By eight months of age, babies start to make canonical sounds (that is word-like sounds in the style of their native language). They start to distinguish sounds that they hear most frequently, this period is often referred to as the 'Critical Period'. It is possible that achieving a good ear for phonetic discrimination at this early stage could enable later language learning. From approximately one year of age, vocabulary and syntax begin to develop, from this point forward they learn to recognise similarities in words such as rhyme and alliteration, by manipulating phonemes and morphemes. All this suggests that normative development provides a foundation for reading and that deficits in development during the pre-school years can have serious and possibly far-reaching consequences. It is possible that any disturbance of the normative sequence of phonological awareness could also manifest itself in areas such as visual processing, general information processing and dyslexia.

There is no suggestion here that the socio-economic status of a child (which is correlated with parental occupation and education levels) is causal of dyslexia, but it is possible that this exacerbates further the difficulties already experienced by a child with dyslexia. It does appear that the opportunities and volume of language interactions between adults and children can influence a child's language skills at all levels. Bowey (1995) showed that parents, already stressed by a low socio-economic environment, find these interactions difficult to engage with; this was compounded by a lack of understanding of their importance.

---

**CASE STUDY**

The following are some extracts from a conversation with a mother coming to terms with the differences in her own children and the effects upon her family.

Jenny is the mother of two children with dyslexia. John is aged 11 years and Lizzie is aged seven years. John is in Year 6 and due to transfer to the secondary school later in the year.

Jenny is an intelligent and highly educated parent and had no contact with dyslexia until John's school alerted her to a problem with his reading and writing, when he was seven years of age. He was given an assessment through the local authority and was identified as having dyslexia. Interestingly Jenny's partner and John's father began to see parallels with his own life and realised that he had been struggling with the condition all his life. An investigation into the family history found a niece who was also dyslexic.

As an intellectual, Jenny has undertaken her own research, and reflected on her own attitudes and understanding. She says:

> I feel that it has made me a better, more tolerant person and opened my eyes to other ways of achieving in education. I have seen that education is so much more than the system currently allows.

> He [John] tries so hard but we have already been told that he will not pass his SATs because his handwriting is so bad. He is so bright and articulate but cannot translate what is in his head to paper. It is heart breaking to see, but I feel that every day I am fighting the system.

> At the moment, I have a good relationship with the primary school and they do try to put into place support for John, but I am afraid that when he goes to secondary school we will lose that contact and because the systems appear to be so inflexible, we will be unable to help him.

> The teachers are very well intentioned but often this does not translate to action.

Reflect on the statements made by Jenny.

- Do you think that they may be typical of families coping with dyslexia?
- How would you respond to a parent of a child in your care suggesting that they had concerns that their child may be dyslexic?
- Would that advice change if that same parent told you that they were themselves dyslexic?

---

# Phenomenology

Phenomenology is a philosophical and holistic approach to what we experience; in this context it examines how people with dyslexia experience the world and interpret the literature-rich environment in which they live. Phenomenology is the science of experience, it attempts to study and understand how the world appears to a person with dyslexia without considering causation, and therefore how someone with dyslexia constructs meaning. That means not looking at the concept of treatment or remediation, but inwards to the perceived experiences of the dyslexic person. Maurice Merleau-Ponty was the twentieth century philosopher who dedicated himself to the philosophical question 'What is seeing?' and his influential work *Phenomenology of Perception*, completed in 1945, shaped this movement and the phenomenological style of research.

It could be claimed that when you see a child with dyslexia you are only aware of it through your own senses, you see the child making reading errors or experiencing physical difficulties or hear them struggle with phonology and articulation, but you do not necessarily consider what else is going on inside that child, the bit that you cannot see or hear. You know that there are hidden facets to the child, but this is largely down to belief and you can believe in a world that embraces all these differing aspects, even when you cannot see them with your physiological senses. So, dyslexia can be a physical phenomenon, but you can also imagine what it is like to be embraced by it, and know that other people will imagine this differently, due to their different physiological, psychological and intellectual experiences.

> Dyslexia is not just a disturbance of someone's cognitive functioning; it is a way of relating to the world in which perceptual ambiguity is heightened, and the experience of space and time is distorted.
>
> (Widdershoven, 1998: p. 29)

Tanner (2010) showed that an inability to achieve socially acceptable levels of literacy (whatever that may be), ensured that people with dyslexia encountered a world where others often see them as of poor intellectual capacity.

> Failure to achieve expected levels of literacy was a sign of weakness, incompetence and low intelligence.
>
> (Tanner, 2010: p. 241)

This is potentially further exacerbated, according to Tanner (2010), by primary and secondary school sectors that do not always adequately cater for the individual needs of the children in their care. She complains that the current educational establishment is based on a paradigm of education which does not always account for these children, an economic climate which does not factor these needs into the sums and a social control climate that does not lend itself to their prerequisites and manifestations.

Philpott (1998) suggested that the behaviour commonly seen in people with dyslexia, such as difficulties with spoken language and short-term memory problems, could reflect the way that experiences are organised in the brains of people with dyslexia. Such phenomenological insights are probably largely responsible for those working in the field, shifting their language about dyslexia from discussions of a difficulty to the concept of a difference, hence possibly changing their own perceptions of the condition. Philpott's (1998) ideas emphasised that children with dyslexia have different ways of learning and that many of their difficulties could be exacerbated by well-intentioned attempts to make them learn in non-dyslexic ways. He equates this to the well-meaning way in which teachers in the 1950s and 1960s 'forced' left handed children to write with their right hand, reportedly tying their left hand behind their back and punishing and smacking children when they 'relapsed'. *The Prevention and Correction of Left-Handedness in Children* was a leaflet produced by J.W. Conway and published in 1935, a subtitle to this leaflet was *Curing the Disability and Disease of Left-Handedness*, which really indicates how this difference from the norm was viewed at this time. Left-handedness is a difference now fully accepted and supported by the law, so that facilities are in place to enable the left-handed child, but in 1935 this was seen as a handicap and even a disease, which was a deterrent to succeeding in the newly industrialised world. This certainly equates to some uninformed views of dyslexia.

Philpott (1998) believed that once dyslexia was accepted as a difference, or as he called it, an 'existential variant', and not a deficit, then different approaches to teaching and education could be developed to build upon the many strengths of dyslexia. He compared what people with dyslexia said that it was like to experience life from a dyslexic perspective with the understanding of how conventional experimental psychology and the mechanics of dyslexia might produce such perceptions. Philpott (1998) suggested that people with dyslexia find it difficult to perform tasks which require reflection, such as spelling or solving abstract problems, as they lose the rhythm of the activity, and how that activity is arranged in time and space. However, Widdershoven (1998) criticises Philpott for looking at what is different about the meaning making of the dyslexic individual and not at what is similar to the non-dyslexic meaning maker – in other words, not at where the dyslexic person fails, but at where they succeed. Widdershoven (1998) wants you to look at the potential as well as the limitations. By making connections with empirical data and life experiences, phenomenology helps you to identify the most effective ways to support development in the dyslexic child.

**CASE STUDY CONTINUED**

John [not his real name] is an articulate 11-year-old with an extensive spoken vocabulary. According to his mother Jenny, he started to talk very early and walked at 12 months of age. However, it soon became apparent that he had some co-ordination problems, which makes it almost impossible for him to swim or to undertake complex physical tasks such as forward rolls etc. His ability to form letters is a problem in school, and his handwriting is also extremely untidy. John has problems with his maths lessons, being unable to hold numbers in his head. He also suffers from difficulties with his short-term memory.

Interviewer:  Hi John, can you tell me what it feels like to be dyslexic?

John:  I don't know really . . . (pause) . . . it is just something in my head which makes things difficult. It does make me upset sometimes.

Interviewer:  Do you have any other friends who are dyslexic?

John:  Not really, there may be someone in my class . . . but I am not sure.

Interviewer:  So what do your friends think about you . . . do they understand?

John:  They don't really talk about it, they seem to understand . . . they leave me alone.

Interviewer:  What about your teachers?

John:  Most of them understand, but some of them do not. This makes me very upset sometimes.

Interviewer:  Why do you think they do not understand?

John:  They are rude.

Interviewer:  What do they do?

John:  They put on a disappointed face and say that I can do better. They are short tempered and shout sometimes. They say they cannot understand my handwriting.

Interviewer:  What things do you find really hard?

John:  Maths, times tables, handwriting and reading out loud but I don't like sport . . . I like science and history.

Considering what John has to say, what challenges do you think a child in your setting would face?

• How dyslexia friendly do you think your setting is? How could it improve?
• What do you think would help John to better come to terms with his dyslexia and achieve success?

**Reflect on this**

Consider the following statement:

What is good practice for dyslexic children is good practice for all children.

- Do you agree with this statement and why?
- Reflect on this statement in the light of your setting and the staff that you work with.

The next chapter will examine the apparently co-morbid conditions that surround dyslexia, and how these either exist alongside or as part of the same condition, manifesting in a variety of ways.

**Chapter reflections**

Dyslexia is often described as an unexpected failure to acquire language and written skills and in particular spelling and reading, but it is only unexpected if the first that is known of it is when a child fails to read at the same level as their peers. If these children had been identified at a much earlier stage, then the unexpectedness of this particular manifestation of the condition would cease to be unexpected.

Whatever dyslexia is or is not, it is clear that there does exist a group of people for whom day-to-day living in a literacy based society presents unique challenges.

(Tanner, 2010: p. iv)

Fluency is probably the most important characteristic of a skilled reader, and it is certainly a key assessment indicator looked for by teachers. However, the non-fluent reader (sometimes called dysfluent) is frequently incorrectly considered by peers, teachers and practitioners, to be of poor intellectual capacity, likely to be a danger to themselves and others, no-hopers and of low status. It is possible that a deficit in phonological awareness and a deficit in morphological awareness are completely separate conditions or sub-groups of dyslexia, but it is also possible that there is a double deficit, producing an automatisation deficit and thereby a lack of fluency and accuracy in reading. It is also possible that there is a relationship between phonological and morphological processing, but more research would need to be conducted to demonstrate this. Further research is also needed to understand the developmental sequence of phonological awareness in the first years of life. This could also have a significant impact upon the potential to identify dyslexia in children and to implement timely early support and remediation.

A lack of proper awareness of this condition, by those around a child with dyslexia, and a lack of awareness of what a child with dyslexia may be experiencing and feeling and their interaction with the world, could be at the heart of many of the difficulties that children with dyslexia experience. If only teachers, practitioners, parents and all those who come into contact with the person with dyslexia could see the world through the eyes of those experiencing it, it would then be possible to see how each individual creates meaning within their world. Perhaps then the child with dyslexia would not need to struggle so much with their emotions and feelings of vulnerability in daily life. For those working with children this means engaging with critically reflective practice to create supportive relationships and compassionate connections.

# Further reading

Hall, K. (ed.) (2010) *Interdisciplinary Perspectives on Learning to Read*. Abingdon: Routledge.

This is a skilfully edited book which has brought together the best of the experts on reading, such as Usha Goswami, Jackie Marsh, Kathy Hall, Vivienne Smith and many more. It covers the topic from a range of differing perspectives, with authors who often have very divergent views. Whilst this book does concern itself with reading and pedagogy in schools, the information has much to say to the practitioner in the nursery, including the particular issues facing children in Wales.

# References

Bowey, J.A. (1995) Socio-economic Status Difference in Pre-school Phonological Sensitivity and First Grade Reading Achievement. *Journal of Educational Psychology* 87 (3): 476–487.

Bruce, D. (1964) The Analysis of Word Sounds. *British Journal of Educational Psychology* 34: 158–170.

Bryant, P. and Bradley, L. (1985) *Children's Reading Problems*. Oxford: Blackwell.

Conway, J.W. (1945) *Curing the Disability and Disease of Left Handedness*. Available online at: www.anythinglefthanded.co.uk (accessed 09.08.17).

Elkonin, D. (1971) Development of Speech. In Zaporozhets, A. and Elkonin, D. (eds) *The Psychology of Pre-School Children*. Cambridge USA: MIT Press.

Goswami, U. (2015) Interview with Eleanor Doughty. *Daily Telegraph* 9 May 2015. Available online at: www.telegraph.co.uk/education/educationnews/11592620/The-last-word-ondyslexia.html (accessed 14.08.17).

Goswami, U. (2016) *Phonology and Dyslexia: A Sensory/Neural Perspective*. Keynote speech: British Dyslexia Association 10th International Conference, 12 March 2016.

Hall, K. (2010) (ed.) *Interdisciplinary Perspectives on Learning to Read*. Abingdon: Routledge.

Hutchins, P. (1968) *Rosie's Walk*. London: Red Fox.

Kirby, J.R., Parrila, R.K. and Pfeiffer, S. (2003) Naming Speed and Phonological Awareness as Predictors of Reading Development. *Journal of Educational Psychology* 95 (3): 453–464.

Krashen, S. (2002) The NRP Comparison of Whole Language and Phonics: Ignore the crucial variable in reading. *Talking Points* 13 (3): 22–28.

Lewars, E.G. (2016) *Computational Chemistry: Introduction to the Theory and Application of Molecular and Quantum Mechanics* (3rd edn). Switzerland: Springer International Publishing.

Liberman, I., Shankweiler, D., Fisher, F. and Carter, B. (1974) Explicit Syllable and Phoneme Segmentation in the Young Child. *Journal of Experimental Child Psychology* 18: 201–212.

Liberman, A.M. and Whalen, D.H. (2000) On the Relation of Speech to Language. *Trends in Cognitive Sciences* 4 (5): 187–196.

Locke, A., Ginsborg, J. and Peers, I. (2002) Development and Disadvantage: Implications for early years and beyond. *International Journal of Language and Communication Disorders* 37 (1): 3–5.

Lundberg, T., Olofsson, A. and Wall, S. (1980) Reading and Spelling Skills in the First School Years Predicted from Phonological Awareness Skills in Kindergarten. *Scandinavian Journal of Psychology* 21 (1): 159–173.

Lyytinen, P. and Lyytinen, H. (2004) Growth and Predictive Relations of Vocabulary and Inflectional Morphology in Children with and without Familial Risk for Dyslexia. *Applied Psycholinguistics* 25: 397–441.

Merleau-Ponty, M. (1945) *The Phenomenology of Perception*. Translated from French by Colin Smith. Delhi: Motilal Banarsidass.

Newport, E. (1975) *Motherese: A Study of the Speech of Mothers to Young Children*. PhD Dissertation: University Pennsylvania. Available online at: http://onlinelibrary.wiley.com/doi/10.1002/j.2333-8504.1975.tb01077.x/pdfhttp://onlinelibrary.wiley.com/doi/10.1002/j.2333-8504.1975.tb01077.x/pdf (accessed 14.08.17).

Nicholson, T. (2016) *Phonological Awareness and Reading Difficulties*. Keynote speech: British Dyslexia Association 10th International Conference, 10 March 2016.

Nittrouer S. (2002) Learning to Perceive Speech: How fricative perception changes, and how it stays the same. *Journal of the Acoustical Society of America* 112: 711–719.

Peer, L. and Reid, G. (2016) (2nd edn) *Multilingualism, Literacy and Dyslexia: Breaking Down Barriers for Education*. Abingdon: Routledge.

Philpott, M.J. (1998) A Phenomenology of Dyslexia: The lived-body, ambiguity and the breakdown of expression. *Philosophy, Psychiatry and Psychology* 5 (1): 1–19.

Pinker, S. (1994) *The Language Instinct*. London: Penguin Books.

Reid, G. (2016) *Dyslexia: A Practitioner's Handbook* (5th edn). Chichester: Wiley.

Schiff, R. and Raveh, M. (2007) Deficient Morphological Processing in Adults with Developmental Dyslexia: Another barrier to efficient word recognition? *Dyslexia: An International Journal of Research and Practice* 13 (2): 110–129.

Stern, D.N., Spieker, S. and MacKain, K. (1982). Intonation Contours as Signals in Maternal Speech to Prelinguistic Infants. *Developmental Psychology* 18: 727–735.

Tanner, K. (2010) *The Lived Experience of Adults with Dyslexia: An exploration of the perceptions of their educational experience*. Available online at: www.researchrepository.murdoch.edu.au/4128 (accessed 20.11.16).

The Basic Skills Agency/Yr Asiantaeth Sigiliau Sylfaenol (2003) *Summary Report of Survey into Young Children's Skills on Entry to Education*. London: Welsh Assembly Government.

Widdershoven, G. (1998) Commentary on 'A Phenomenology of Dyslexia'. *Philosophy, Psychiatry and Psychology* 5 (1): 29–31.

Zhurova, L. (1973) The Development of Analysis of Words into their Sounds by Pre-School Children. In Ferguson, C. and Slobin, D. (eds) *Studies of Child Language Development*. New York: Holt Rinehart and Winston.

# Strange bedfellows . . . co-morbid conditions

*Legg'd like a man! And his fins like arms! Warm, o'my troth I do now let loose my opinion,*
*hold it no longer: This is no fish, but an islander, that hath lately suffer'd by a thunderbolt.*
*[Thunder] Alas the storm has come again! My best way is to creep under his gabardine:*
*There is no shelter hereabout: misery acquaints a man with strange bedfellows. I will here*
*shroud till the dregs of the storm be past*

Shakespeare, *The Tempest* 2:2

## Introduction

Shakespeare first coined this phrase 'strange bedfellows' but what has it come to mean?
In this context, I have taken it to mean that two or more unexpected partner conditions
can be connected but different and can often be separate and individual. At first glance
these may appear to have very little in common, but perhaps they are not so strange and
only appear that way to the unthinking eye.

Way back in 1970 a real pioneer of the study of dyslexia was Emeritus Professor Tim
Miles. His theory of dyslexia was that it was not just a problem with reading, but was
in fact an 'anomaly of development', characterised by a range of symptoms including
speech production difficulties, short-term memory limitations, sequencing and number
difficulties, temporal processing difficulties, motor control and automatisation confusion etc. Since this, several researchers in the field have suggested that it is not possible
to see dyslexia as a completely separate and distinct condition as this quotation from
Richardson (2001) shows:

> Despite their separate diagnostic labels, the clinical overlap between dyslexia,
> dyspraxia, ADHD and ASD is very high, and 'pure' cases are the exception, not
> the rule. Thus around half of any dyslexic population is likely to be dyspraxic and

vice versa, and the mutual overlap between ADHD and dyspraxia is also around 50%. Dyslexia and ADHD co-occur in 30–50% of cases, although this association is stronger for inattention than for hyperactivity-impulsivity. All of these conditions also show some overlap with the autistic spectrum, although in severe cases, the autism diagnosis always takes precedence.

(Richardson, 2001: p. 19)

Richardson (2001) calls these differing conditions simply descriptive labels for 'particular constellations' of difficulties, in other words groupings of difficulties that often occur together. The trouble with this, as Richardson recognised, is that these difficulties are not uncommon in the general population, and in the early years they form part of 'normal' development, for example no one expects a two-year-old to read, or a child of 18 months to run and kick a ball accurately.

To view these conditions as categorical 'disease entities' is thus rather misleading, because in milder form, their core characteristics all exist as perfectly normal individual differences in behaviour and cognition.

(Richardson, 2001: p. 20)

# Co-morbidity

Put succinctly, and at a very basic level, co-morbidity means the common co-occurrence, in one person, of two or more conditions. When co-morbidity does occur, it presents certain problems for researchers, they must consider whether they are different and distinct conditions or just different manifestations of one condition. To understand co-morbidity, you need to understand the aetiology and pathogenic mechanisms that underlie the manifestations. However, as you have already read in Chapters 1 and 2 of this book, this is not always easy or even possible with any clarity. One important aspect of co-morbidity is that where two or more conditions exist in one person, one condition may influence the other in its trajectory, intervention and remediation.

It would appear rare that dyslexia exists in isolation, and difficulties with reading are also identified in children with other conditions such as:

Attention deficit disorder
Attention deficit and hyperactivity disorder
Asperger's syndrome
Autism
Developmental co-ordination disorder (DCD) or dyspraxia
Dyscalculia
Dysgraphia

Dysmapia
Specific language impairment and probably many others

Stein et al. (2001) suggest, perhaps a little cynically, that the label that the child is finally given probably relates to the research interest of the specialist that they are first referred to! So if the child has reading difficulties and co-ordination problems, and they are referred to a specialist in reading, s/he is likely to be labelled dyslexic with co-morbid DCD, if they are referred to someone with an interest in physical co-ordination development, they are more likely to be labelled DCD with co-morbid dyslexia. There do appear to be several overlapping conditions which seem like 'strange bedfellows' (see Figure 5.1). If the focus of dyslexia is purely upon difficulties with reading, then the development of research in this area is only going to focus on reading problems. However, if you reclassify this condition as an 'anomaly of development', as suggested by Miles (1970), or as I am suggesting as an Information Processing Disorder (IPD), then the research can be expanded and extended to a more co-ordinated approach, with potentially a more beneficial impact on remediation, rather than developing increasing numbers of subtypes of dyslexia related conditions.

Whether this is the case or not, there are certainly considerable overlaps between conditions which have been demonstrated repeatedly by researchers such as Badian (1983), White et al. (1992) and Lyytinen et al. (1994). Van de Leij (2001) even went so far as to say that up to 54% of those with dyslexia can also be identified with ADHD/ADD and Iverson et al. (2005) showed that approximately 60% of children with dyslexia

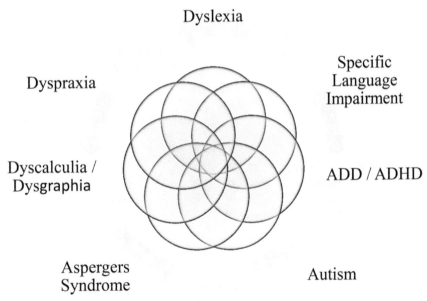

Figure 5.1 Overlapping co-morbid conditions (Information Processing Disorder)

also have manifestations of Developmental Coordination Disorder (dyspraxia). A large study in Finland by Viholainen et al. (2006) suggested that motor skills difficulties in the early years were highly predictive of a later manifestation of dyslexia and Fawcett (2012) suggests that the co-occurrence of specific language impairment and dyslexia may be as high as 90%.

With so much research providing evidence of co-occurring conditions it is perhaps reasonable to ask whether these conditions are a direct consequence of dyslexia or separate conditions appearing in parallel. If it is the latter you must also ask why two or more conditions should occur together so often, after all, if you are born with a visual impairment it is highly unlikely (though not impossible), that you will also have a hearing impairment. It is even more unlikely that two-thirds of those born with visual impairment should also have a hearing impairment. This raises the question as to whether the conditions that appear to co-occur with dyslexia are truly co-morbid or the development of one disorder as a consequence of another.

## Sensori-information affecting co-morbid conditions

Even when you are asleep, you are constantly surrounded by information bombarding you from your environment. This information is taken in by the nervous system with specific sensory organs for touch, taste, smell, sight and hearing, vestibular (balance/movement) and proprioceptors (detecting the movement of our bodies in relation to the space around us). This information is transmitted to the brain, which in turn sends

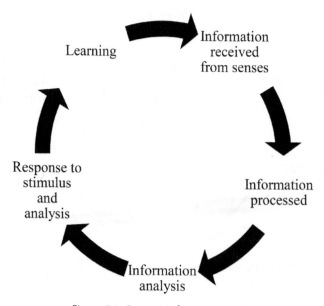

*Figure 5.2* Sensori-information cycle

information to your nerves and muscle groups to stimulate an automatised reaction. Often this is a complicated interaction of sensory information from the sensory receptors, neural pathways and parts of the brain involved in sensory perception. Systems need to be in place for this information processing to take place and any interruption in this cycle will probably cause a difficulty or delay in learning.

---

**CASE STUDY**

Aarav has just started to learn to walk; he must use the information from his senses to estimate the distance to be walked to reach some biscuits on a table (visual sense) in front of him. He must calculate whether he can fit between the chairs that are in the way, and how robust the chairs are to lean on to help him get into a standing position. He hears the biscuits being put on the plate (auditory/visual sense) and needs his sense of balance (vestibular sense) to help to keep his body upright and assess the gradient of the floor to be navigated. Nerve endings in his limbs (proprioceptors) allow him to estimate his posture, and his tactile sense helps him to grasp the chairs to aid his balance. A kinaesthetic sense and proprioceptors give him information about where his body parts are in relation to each other and the space around him. All this information needs to be fully co-ordinated to enable Aarav to navigate his way across the floor to the table of biscuits, considering any obstacles in the way or unevenness of the ground. He also needs a degree of technical skill and a level of intellectual ability to understand what must be done.

1. How can you support Aarav in his physical and sensory development?
2. Difficulty learning to walk is a normal part of development for children of nine to eighteen months; at what point do you think that additional support needs to be implemented?
3. What signs do you think you need to be aware of to ascertain whether Aarav may be at risk of an information processing disorder?

---

No doubt you, like me, were told in school that there were five senses, taste, touch, smell, sight and hearing, but in fact there are more than that and I will examine some of these a little further.

## Vestibular sense

This is the body's ability to remain balanced and steady. Imagine that a toddler like Aarav is walking along an uneven path with differing inclinations, it is vital that he can make appropriate adjustments to his posture to remain upright. However, the vestibular sense also helps you to maintain not only balance and movement, but also hearing and vision. Overstimulation of the vestibular system can cause giddiness and instability; imagine that you are on the big dipper at the fairground or spinning round and round on a roundabout. Such difficulties could result in:

- Poor spatial awareness
- Poor directional information
- Disorientation
- Difficulties with sudden changes of speed or direction
- General balance problems

The vestibular sense enables the child to interact safely with their environment and is closely associated with the movement of fluid in the inner ear. A severe disruption to the vestibular system will be very apparent, with symptoms of dizziness and vertigo; mild disturbance can go unnoticed, but can cause developmental delays, especially to reading and writing.

## Auditory sense

Tiny babies very soon learn to interpret the sounds in the world around them. Recognition of their mother tongue may even be taking place whilst they are in the womb, as they listen to the sound of their mother talking. They quickly learn to anticipate the sound of food preparation, the bath running and the arrival of different people to the home. They will also listen to the continuous stream of language as they lie in their cots, getting used to the rhythm and intonation of their mother tongue. Soon they start to engage with that language, not necessarily with recognisable words, but with sounds, turn taking and babbling. Gradually they learn, through games, stories, rhymes and close interaction, to use language to their own advantage – to summon help, attract attention and engage. Clearly any form of auditory impairment, whether temporary, such as glue ear, or permanent, will interrupt the auditory information processed by the brain. This will affect their phonology, their ability to hear rhyme, recognise vowels and consonants, and ultimately to spell (if you are unable to distinguish sounds such as 'ch', 'sh' and 'th' writing words becomes difficult). This is certainly something that you will see in the dyslexic child.

A further difficulty with an impairment of the auditory sense is auditory distractibility. This is the ability of the brain to select sounds of importance and ignore the general background noise. For some children being surrounded with noise and distraction is not a problem, and children based in a busy nursery are likely to have a constant barrage of background noise to filter, chairs scraping, children squealing, music playing, staff talking to other children etc. The sort of active and collaborative learning undertaken in an average nursery or key stage one classroom, results inevitably in a noisy environment. If the child is unable to filter these noises they may well find it hard to concentrate and over stimulating, they may exhibit behaviour consistent with attention deficit and hyperactivity – always getting up to see what others are doing, listening difficulties, lack of attention to a task, unable to follow instructions or to hold a sequence of instructions in their mind. This is particularly so for children in their early years, when they are still learning to listen. This is not so much a problem of a child being unable to hear, but more about them hearing too much. Children with ADD find this particularly troublesome, being distracted from the continuity of their thought processes. This is compounded when children are also hyperactive (ADHD), when their desire to move and fidget is also difficult to control. Macintyre and Deponio (2003) suggest that children with DCD are particularly prone to this restless behaviour. Understandably this can lead to a child either withdrawing from the confusion of noise, or alternatively becoming angry with it, resulting in short temper and potentially aggressive behaviour.

## Kinesthetic sense

One of the first senses to emerge in the foetus is the sense of touch, and in utero they will react to tactile stimuli. This is the sense that distinguishes:

- Different types and levels of pain
- Changes of temperature
- Increasing levels of pressure on the body
- Spatial positioning of the body
- Awareness of direction and laterality
- Awareness of weight carried
- Dimension in space

Clearly these are all aspects crucial to movement and travel, and to negotiate the world without bumping into or falling off things. They are also crucial to being able to write, knowing how tightly to hold the writing implement, how hard to press on the paper and how to enable the hand to flow and glide across the page. Macintyre and Deponio (2003) suggested that it could also be responsible for the child who becomes 'overly tactile defensive', that is the child who is unable to deal with cuddles and close physical contact, such as holding your hand or giving hugs, as seen in children on the autistic spectrum. Equally the reverse may be applicable, with the child who hugs too much and inappropriately with strangers.

# Proprioceptors

Proprioceptors deal with your position in the world in relation to your other body parts; they exist all over the body in muscles, skin, tendons and joints. These allow you to assess the depth of a pavement edge or a step, without having to take specific note, or to adjust posture when sitting or standing. These allow you to do things without looking, so putting food into your mouth or walking down stairs without checking each step. This is a sense of self and provides information to the brain about joint angle, muscle length and tension. It is easy to see that any interruption of that information to the brain, could result in behaviour that appears clumsy and slow, such as that seen in children with Developmental Co-ordination Disorder.

# Visual discrimination

Being able to see clearly is vital for reading (except in braille), without clear and focused vision the information conveyed by the eyes to the brain makes letter confusion inevitable. Blurred images also result in letter and word reversals (Miles, 1991). Impairment of visual discrimination is also likely to affect a child's ability to track along a line of print, and to estimate distance and direction. Children with dyslexia often complain that it is this tracking process that makes them slow and less fluent than their peers when reading. This inability to follow a line of print is likely to impact all their learning, including handwriting.

Following the trajectory of a ball or flying object may also be difficult for children with visual discriminatory difficulties, as can issues of balance as the visual sense is closely aligned to the vestibular system, hence the giddiness that occurs when spinning around.

Although each of these senses has been described separately, in fact they are inter-dependent and inter-reliant upon each other. Any change in one will almost certainly affect the efficiency of the others, causing a range of manifestations in the child.

# Neurologically based processing disorders

Children experiencing more than one information processing disorder is probably the norm rather than the exception, with one condition overlapping upon another and possibly another. Many researchers in the field such as Reid (2016) and Snowling (2008) describe this as a spectrum of disorders, a continuum of conditions, one merging into and emerging from another. As has been implied earlier, it is possible that they all have common underlying cognitive impairments, as their co-morbidity would appear to be too common to ignore, or to attempt to clarify as a range of distinctive and separate disorders. Examples of this may be the co-morbidity of dyslexia with ADHD, which has been shown to be as high as 40% (Pennington and Olson, 2005); Bohl and Hoult (2016) give figures for the co-morbidity of dyslexia and dyspraxia as 52% and dyslexia and visual stress at 30%; Stein and Walsh (1997) suggested that two-thirds of children with dyslexia also have visual processing deficits and Butterworth (2003) showed that over 40% of children with dyslexia also have dyscalculia. Macintyre (2015) puts the figure for children with ADD/ADHD and a co-existing condition at two-thirds, interestingly she also notes that another co-existing condition for ADD/ADHD is Tourette's Syndrome, resulting in frequent uncontrolled noises and tics. One study by Pauc (2005) – which considered dyslexia, dyspraxia, ADD, ADHD, obsessive compulsive disorder and Tourette's syndrome – showed that a clear pattern of co-morbidity emerged at a rate of up to 95%. Such high incidence of co-occurrence can surely not be by chance alone.

It is possible that what you are seeing is one fundamental information processing disorder, exhibiting a range of differing indicators. So, the identification of children with these difficulties under separate titles is problematic, and even attempting to cluster the conditions is perhaps not helpful. Neurological scans, such as PET (positron emission tomography) and MRI (magnetic resonance imaging), show that children with these conditions process information in the brain differently to children without. So perhaps it would be more helpful to their support and intervention to consider these conditions under one umbrella, as a single underlying impairment with a range of manifestations, rather than a series of discrete conditions which eventually only confuses the management of them, especially when they rarely occur alone. Discrete identifications could potentially lead to incorrect or incomplete determination of the condition, in turn resulting in delayed, or even no, appropriate support being put in place, just because no definitive label can be established. Perhaps a more holistic view of assessment should be considered, rather than looking for co-morbidity or co-occurrence of distinctive and separate conditions. Examining each condition as distinct may result in imposing artificial boundaries on that condition which could result in a 'preoccupation with increased specialisation' (Reid, 2016: p. 335). In an attempt to move away from the concept of separate conditions, Reid (2016) suggests that children with neurobiological processing disorders tend to share certain similar characteristics, he identifies these as:

- Attentional difficulties
- Memory problems
- Organisational difficulties
- Processing speed difficulties

However, even if it is possible to group these conditions under one title, the practitioner will still need to assess the particular difficulties of the individual child, if appropriate and effective intervention is to be established; for example, the child with attentional problems will almost certainly require different support to one with language impairments. However, this is no different to assessing the individual needs of any child with a special or particular need.

# Specific procedural learning theory

An interesting line of research into co-morbidity comes from Fawcett (2012), which she calls the Specific Procedural Learning Deficit hypothesis. She claims that skill development is something that takes time to achieve, this she refers to as 'procedural learning'. However, she describes a further type of learning based on language, called 'declarative learning', and this happens very quickly. Procedural learning might be something like Aarav (see case study above) learning to walk, taking time for the senses and motor movement to become automatised – he is unaware that he is in a learning process. Declarative learning is more conscious learning – it is how you learn facts, it is the school based learning approach. Fawcett (2012) suggests that whilst both systems can be affected by developmental difficulties, it depends upon which is more affected as to how they will manifest.

> For dyslexia we think it is the language-based procedural learning system, but it may also involve the motor procedural learning system. The declarative learning system can be intact or even over-achieving, and this is why dyslexic children can have a wealth of information about dinosaurs, football or motorbikes (and a really high IQ!) although they may have difficulty learning how to do things like riding a bike or tying shoe laces.
>
> (Fawcett, 2012: p. 18)

A problem in one learning system, in one brain region, can therefore lead to combinations of difficulties, depending upon which regions are most affected. This may also account for why there may be both strengths and weaknesses in children with dyslexia, as deficits in procedural learning can be combined with strengths in declarative learning.

Fawcett does stress that this hypothesis is in its infancy, and more research needs to be conducted. However, for that research to take place, intense collaboration will be needed across many specialist fields to achieve the consensus and co-operation needed, to consider co-morbidity across such a wide number of disorders and manifestations.

**Reflect on this**

- Work with a colleague to consider what the advantages and disadvantages are of considering different manifestations of an information processing disorder as distinct and separate, or as differing displays of the one condition.
- What are the challenges and rewards of working with children with an information processing disorder, and how can this shape your practice and that of your setting?
- Given the prevalence of co-occurring conditions, if you suspect a child in your care to be at risk of dyslexia, how could you also assess their possible risk of a co-occurring condition?

The next section of this chapter briefly defines some of these more common conditions at the symptom level, and describes some of the issues that surround these conditions.

## Attention Deficit Disorder/Attention Deficit and Hyperactivity Disorder

The definitions for ADD and ADHD have undergone numerous changes over the years. It is important that you understand that they are not the same condition. Whilst they are both concerned with the child's ability to focus and pay attention, the condition of ADHD is also compounded by an inability to remain still and a tendency to impulsivity, which in some cases can lead to aggression. Like dyslexia, ADD/ADHD have been identified as familial, with genetic influences probably accounting for as much as 75% (Broada et al., 2012). According to Macintyre (2015), under scanning procedures some structural brain differences have been observed in children with these conditions, including a smaller total brain volume and cerebellar hemispheres; there are also often differences in the frontal lobe of the brain. This is an area of the brain that inhibits behaviour and sustains attention, thereby controlling emotions, motivation and memory functions. It must be remembered that children with these conditions are not just 'badly behaved', but have very complex needs, which are often hampered by the potential for disruption that they often cause in a group setting such as a nursery or classroom. This results in adults, who struggle to understand the conditions, constantly reproving them, telling them that they are 'naughty' and not nice to be with. This potentially has the impact of the 'self-fulfilling prophecy', that is, the more you are told that you are 'naughty', the more you are likely to live up to those expectations, thereby exacerbating the situation.

Another way of looking at this is described by Parvey (2016), who suggests that rather than considering these children as being unable to focus, it is more likely that these children are trying to focus on too much, being unable to filter out the distractions and concentrate on one issue at a time.

Due to the variable nature of the manifestations of these conditions, assessment is extremely difficult and a definitive identification can only be made by a psychologist or medical professional. However, knowing what manifestations to look for in children in the early years may enable you to highlight children at risk of ADD/ADHD. Reid (2016) identifies this in the following ways:

Attention Deficit Disorder:

- A child who finds it difficult to focus attention on ALL activities, both at home and in the setting.
- A child who often does not appear to listen.
- A child who finds it difficult to follow instructions, or to sequence these and follow through.
- A child with organisational difficulties with tasks involving clothing and possessions.
- A child who constantly loses things and comes to activities without the appropriate equipment.
- A child who is forgetful and unfocused.
- A child who is easily distracted from an activity.

Children with Attention Deficit and Hyperactivity Disorder will probably have many of the traits described above but will also be likely to be:

- A child who is unable to sit still, is restless, fidgets and squirms in the seat.
- A child who jumps up impulsively when everyone else is sitting quietly.
- A child who is noisy and loud during play.
- A child who talks constantly, blurting out answers inappropriately.
- A child who is constantly active and moving, twiddling things and spinning things.
- A child who is unable to take turns, interrupting conversations.
- A child who is easily bored and lets you know about it!

O'Regan (2012) divides these two conditions into three subtypes which he calls:

1. Predominantly hyperactive impulsive type (ADHD).
2. Predominantly inattentive type (ADD).
3. Combined type (which is the most common). O'Regan (2012) suggests that this may in fact be a separate disorder with unfocused attention, with the child hypoactive (that is a child that is sluggish and slow to process information).

Children and young people with ADHD are characterised by 'consistent inconsistency'. Some days they can produce great work unassisted and within the allotted time; at other times, they struggle to stay on task and even with close supervision may not accomplish much. Their erratic performance perplexes teachers and parents and can create the impression of laziness.

(O'Regan, 2012: p. 73)

In certain extreme cases medication can be prescribed for these children, to ameliorate the impact of these conditions. Despite their often 'bad press', sometimes described as the 'chemical cosh', such medication can, in the right circumstances, be very helpful, allowing children and their families to live more enjoyable and satisfying lives.

# Developmental Co-ordination Disorder (dyspraxia)

DCD is a motor co-ordination disorder affecting both gross and fine motor control. In the past, this was called 'the clumsy child syndrome', but may also impact the muscles of the lips, tongue and larynx, thereby causing difficulties with speech and articulation. The terms DCD and dyspraxia are often used interchangeably, but according to Movement Matters (an organisation representing the major UK groups concerned with DCD/dyspraxia), the term dyspraxia does not appear in the Diagnostic and Statistical Manual of Mental Disorders (DSM-5), which is an internationally recognised text, which describes a wide range of mental disorders, unlike DCD, which is recorded. Interestingly an additional term appears in this manual, that of Verbal Dyspraxia, as a separate and distinct condition.

In the early years it is very easy to dismiss this condition as just an immaturity of movement, as it is quite normal for very young children to find difficulty with the co-ordination needed for walking, running, grasping etc. Put into simple terms Ripley et al. (1997) describe this as '[g]etting our bodies to do what we want when we want them to do it' (p. 3). Such concealment can result in children not getting the help that they need as early as possible.

Some of the effects of DCD may be that the child finds difficulty in some or all of the following activities:

- Eating with cutlery
- Speaking clearly
- Dressing and undressing
- Fastening and unfastening zips and buttons
- Riding a trike/bike/scooter

- Ball skills, such as kicking, catching, throwing etc.
- Handwriting and drawing, grasping a pencil

It must be emphasised that this is a condition that involves voluntary or planned movement and does not affect reflexes and reflex movement.

Wide variance of the age at which young children achieve development goals is perfectly natural and can be impacted by the learning opportunities that have been afforded to them. For example, a child of four years may be unable to pedal a trike, but if they have not had the opportunity to ride a trike and to practice, then it is highly unlikely that they will be able to ride it proficiently, and is certainly not necessarily an indicator of a child at risk of DCD. It is probably also true that some children will naturally have better co-ordination than others; after all we cannot all be Andy Murray or Darcey Bussell.

> Professional sports people have very good all-round co-ordination regardless of the sports skills they have learned. Some children, therefore, are going to find handwriting easier to learn than others because of their neuro/biology.
>
> (Ripley et al., 1997: p. 10)

Reid (2016) also notes that in addition to the difficulties mentioned above, these children also often exhibit problems with working memory, making it hard for them to remember instructions, and deadlines or to organise their time. He suggests a further range of indicators for practitioners to be aware of in the at-risk child:

*Table 5.1*

| | |
|---|---|
| Poor social skills | Poor spatial awareness |
| Attentional difficulties | Poor fine motor control |
| Visual motor skill difficulties | Poor balance and co-ordination |
| Automatisation | Speech difficulties |
| Hypotonic (poor muscle tone) | Poor gross motor skills |
| Difficulties with eye movements | Poor and delayed toileting |
| Slouching . . . affecting breathing and digestion | |

Reid also notes that crawling with a cross lateral pattern (that is left knee and right hand – right knee, left hand) may be poor or missed out entirely as in bottom shufflers. Reid (2016) suggests that although there are likely to be genetic indicators for DCD, there may also be a connection between DCD and pre-term births or stressful birth circumstances, but this will require more detailed research in the future.

# Dysgraphia

Children with DCD often find the co-ordination required for handwriting difficult and at its most extreme it can be seen as a separate condition referred to as dysgraphia. Typically, the child with dysgraphia will have poor fine motor skills; however, according to Macintyre (2015) 80% of children with handwriting difficulties did not crawl, possibly because they were unable to master the cross lateral pattern of one hand with opposing knee.

In the early years, before handwriting would usually have developed, some of the indicators of risk for dysgraphia could be:

- Confusion with hand dominance.
- How the child grips a pencil – too slack and the pencil falls away, or the lines are too spidery, too tight and they are unable to sustain a flow with the pencil pressure on the paper and they tear the paper as they push too hard.
- Poor posture at the table.
- Wrist movements are limited resulting in sore and cramped hands.
- Very slow to complete any drawing.
- Easily tires at a task.
- Poor shape discrimination.
- Finds it hard to stay on a line, reproduce a shape, trace a shape or colour within the lines.
- Difficulties tying laces and fastening buttons.
- Using scissors is very difficult.
- Using a keyboard or texting is a problem.
- Often adopts an awkward grip on a pencil.

By school age other difficulties may also become apparent:

- Illegible hand writing.
- Visuo-spatial difficulties
- Language processing problems – unable to commit thoughts to paper.
- Attentional problems
- Finds it hard to follow the rules of a game.
- Spelling issues – often spelling the same word in different ways within one sentence.
- Confuses upper- and lower-case letters.
- Grammar and punctuation issues.
- Difficulties organising written language.

# Dyscalculia

Learning and using abstract symbols and written calculations is challenging for all children, but none more so than those who have dyscalculia. Many people in this country claim to be poor at mathematical understanding, and it even seems to be acceptable to say 'I can't do maths' in a way that it would not be acceptable to say 'I can't read'. Montague-Smith and Price (2012) attribute many of our negative feelings towards maths to poor teaching, often in the early years with negative feelings from adults being passed on to children. However, dyscalculia, which is a difficulty with mathematical learning, is far more than a catching of negative thoughts. Wynn (1998) suggests that babies as young as four or five months can tell the difference between numbers of objects presented to them (within the range of zero to three), suggesting that this is not simply a learned behaviour. These babies cannot yet count but do appear to have an awareness of quantity. Wynn (1998) claims that the same part of the brain which is used for these skills is also used for processing symbolic number. Montague-Smith and Price (2012) point out that some researchers claim that, like Chomsky's theory of a 'Language Acquisition Device' for language learning, there may also be an equivalent, an 'accumulator model' by which children learn to count and understand number. Interestingly the overlap between dyscalculia, attention deficit and dyslexia is very common, making the reading of numbers a real challenge.

> They do not have the images if visual clusters of numbers in their minds and the related number relationships (decomposition/recomposition). They also depend much more on immature and inefficient strategies such as sequential counting to solve problems that most children know by heart.
>
> (Sharma, 2012: p. 125)

Indicators for at risk children in the early years might be:

- Difficulties with understanding one to one correspondence (matching one object to one other, so one fork to one knife, or one bead to one number etc.).
- Problems of sequencing (as in stories, a beginning, a middle and an end). Poor ability to estimate size or magnitude of number.
- General size visualisation.
- Number fact recall (this is particularly apparent in the older child learning tables).
- Poor counting and number comparison.
- Finding the estimation of distance and speed difficult.
- Time estimates are poor.

Many of these issues can lead to what Montague-Smith and Price (2012) call 'maths anxiety' which can impact social skills, with children avoiding playing games that involve number, such as hide and seek, 'What's the time Mr Wolf?', cooking, shopping and games which involve keeping score. This can affect their ability to make friends and have age appropriate experiences.

# Autism, Asperger Syndrome and PDD-nos

Autism, Asperger Syndrome and PDD-nos are related conditions on what is referred to as the autistic spectrum, and can all range from mild to severe. Russell (2012) claims that an autistic spectrum disorder, which affects how a child sees the world, must display a triad of behaviours from all three of the different behavioural domains, which are restricted or repetitive:

1) Social interaction impairments – that is eye contact, facial expression, body posture, gesture, and difficulties developing friendships and relationships.
2) Communication impairments – that is delays in spoken language, where language is often stereotypical or idiosyncratic, or no spoken language develops.
3) Imagination impairments – that is repetitive patterns of behaviour, pre-occupation with certain activities or resources.

The children on the autistic spectrum may find it hard to filter out extraneous noise and the general disturbance of a busy classroom or nursery, so they focus on one aspect at a time, blocking out the rest. They can therefore be either hyposensitive to the environmental noise – that is, an unusually low sensitivity to noise – or hypersensitive – that is, overly sensitive to noise. They can also be affected by bright lights, vivid colour and commotion.

Asperger Syndrome, first identified by Hans Asperger in Germany in 1944, is often referred to as high functioning autism, but this may not be entirely correct as there are some fundamental differences between autism and Asperger Syndrome. Children with Asperger Syndrome are likely to exhibit some of the following manifestations:

- The child finds it hard to empathise, to understand another person's thoughts and feelings.
- They may be unable to distinguish between different facial expressions and tones of voice. This can lead to a very literal approach to their world, for example the child told to 'hold on a minute' may be found looking for something to hold on to.
- These children find it difficult to accept change, so any reconfiguration of the furniture in the nursery can really distress them. This in turn can result in them adhering to rigid routines and patterns of life.
- Misunderstanding the social rules of society can lead them to violate other people's personal space, engage in inappropriate touching or even the withdrawal of all physical contact.
- There will often be perceptual and sensory difficulties.
- Pre-occupation with a very narrow set of interests and obsession with order and sequence. You say see them lining up the farm animals or the cars, in a set manner every day and becoming extremely distressed when they are moved.

- They will often refer to themselves in the third person, as though they were not present in the conversation.
- You may see a difference in their play, with toys used mainly to whirl, or flap repetitively rather than true pretend play or substitute play. Play will usually be solitary.
- There may also be physical developmental difficulties as they move in a distinctive manner, not swinging their arms and leaning forward on tip toes when they are walking.

You will be aware of films such as *Rainman* with Dustin Hoffmann, *Forest Gump* with Tom Hanks, *My Name is Khan* with Shah Rukh, and even books such as *The Curious Incident of the Dog in the Night Time* by Mark Haddon, which all heighten the awareness of autistic spectrum disorders. They usually focus on strengths of the condition, such as superior technology and maths skills, heightened aesthetic awareness or artistic skills, musical and other strengths. These depictions of autistic spectrum disorders encourage the general public to believe that these are a common feature of the conditions. In fact, Russell (2012) estimates that only 1–10% of those with autistic spectrum conditions have exceptional abilities, and these are more likely to be at the Asperger's and higher functioning end of the spectrum. Far more are likely to have 'mild to profound mental retardation' (Russell, 2012: p. 121). According to Baron-Cohen (2008) children

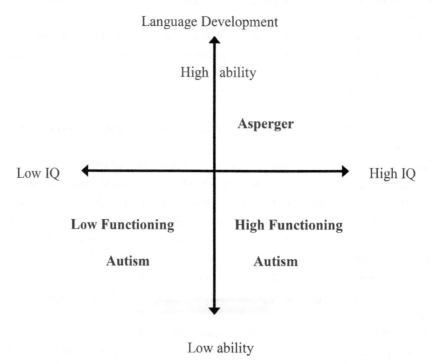

*Figure 5.3* Language development and IQ relationship with autism and Asperger Syndrome (adapted from Baron-Cohen, 2008: p. 13)

with Asperger Syndrome have an IQ which is at least average and language is develop-ing. Children with autism may have an IQ across the entire range, but there will almost certainly be a language delay (Figure 5.3).

Children with Pervasive Developmental Disorder-not otherwise specified (PDD-nos), are likely to have some traits common to autism and Asperger Syndrome, but where they exist they are likely to be mild (that is not to say that they are not incapacitating). The indicators for this condition are likely to be: a difficulty with the conventions of social interaction; difficulties with both verbal and non-verbal communication; and a tendency to repetition and highly focused interests. Some researchers feel that the man-ifestations of PDD-nos are too mild to be classed as autism or Asperger Syndrome, but these children do have an abnormally high number of autistic traits.

Researchers are still at odds about whether autism, Asperger Syndrome and PDD-nos should be distinct categories, or whether they are simply sub-categories of autism. Frith (1991) describes Asperger Syndrome as a 'type of autism', but what we do know, is that these conditions are largely developmental, although they can, rarely, be induced by disease or injury. This implies that the manifestations are likely to vary with age and ability, making it sometimes very difficult to identify. Indications are likely to be there in the first year of life, but will be difficult to differentiate from other more general developmental delays. Frith (1991) claims that one of the first indicators is a lack of pointing and wanting to share interactions with the people around them, but a true identification is very difficult before the child is two to three years of age. At this stage language would normally be developing well, but in the child with autistic spectrum disorders it is often a cause for concern, and practitioners will frequently query whether the child has a hearing impairment. Frith (1991) suggests that it is not until after the age of five years that the subgroups of autism begin to emerge and be identified, depending very much on the severity of the indicators, whether the child has language, their general intellectual ability and their levels of egocentrism and isolation.

In all these autistic spectrum disorders, social and imaginative play will be almost completely absent, and the child will often focus exclusively on one activity or resource to the exclusion of all others, with obsessive behaviour frequently exhibited. Commonly children with autistic spectrum disorders will be completely fazed by any change in routine, becoming abnormally aggressive and explosive when routine is disrupted.

> Today ASD [Autistic Spectrum Disorder] is conceived as a true spectrum, where autistic traits have a normal distribution in the general population, and an arbi-trary cut off point determines who is considered to be on the spectrum and who is not . . . as with dyslexia, there is no sharp line separating severity in those with a diagnosis, from less severe traits in those without.
>
> (Russell, 2012: p. 95)

# Specific Language Impairment

Specific Language Impairment was in the past referred to as dysphasia or even verbal dyspraxia but can be applied when speech, grammar, syntax or tense are impaired. A genetic twin study by Bishop et al. (1995) showed a significant heritability factor for SLI and according to Grist et al. (2012) it impacts approximately 7% of all five-year-olds. In the early stages, it is very difficult to identify because at the beginning of a child's speech development it is quite normal for them to mispronounce words, and in fact adults often find this rather endearing:

gog for dog
tar for car
pop for shop
bed for bread

Where these continue, and the child shows no indications of deafness (even temporary as in glue ear), low intellectual capacity, cleft palate or other physical difficulty, they need to be investigated. Of course, not all children in the early years with delayed speech will have Specific Language Impairment, for most their language skills will improve as they mature, and as they are exposed to richer veins of language and vocabulary. According to Parvey (2016):

it is the persistence and intractability of the problems in the face of regular, effective teaching that alerts practitioners to the possible presence of specific language difficulty.

(Parvey, 2016: p. 72)

Some children may be identified as having a language development delay, when speech develops more slowly than would be expected, but develops in the same order and trajectory as would normally be anticipated, but it is likely that this child, with the appropriate support and exposure to language, will eventually 'catch up'. In the case of SLI the language development is irregular and problematic to the point where all communication can be affected, it may even be that they do not talk at all, and this in turn impacts other areas of learning.

According to Taylor (2012), one of the most important pre-requisites for speech and language is good auditory memory. Firstly, you need to be able to adequately hear what is being said to you, but then to be able to store that information before an appropriate response can be formulated. Of course, words alone are not enough for communication, and knowledge of rhythm, stress pattern and intonation are vital to understanding. Consider for a moment the implications of the following simple statements to your responses:

*I* like your hat – implying that only you like the hat.

I *like* your hat – implying warm praise of your choice of hat.

I like *your* hat – implying that you do not like the other people's hats.

I like your *hat* – implying that the hat is the only thing she is wearing that she likes.

You can see how the emphasis upon a particular word adds a range of meaning to a sentence and would indicate your response. These problems are further exacerbated for the child with SLI by living in a society that expects children of a certain age to be able to talk and understand language. It often does not occur to some people that this child may not be able to do that.

For the early years practitioner, the hardest question is whether this is a lasting problem or an immaturity which will eventually right itself; there are a number of indicators which you will need to consider, although not all will be present all of the time:

- The child does understand what is being said but cannot articulate a suitable response. This could result in the child 'giving up' and refusing to speak.
- The child does not understand what is being said and has a very limited vocabulary.
- The child speaks clearly but does not respond appropriately.
- The child speaks in single words or disjointed sentences.
- The child struggles to learn new words.
- The child relies on routines to understand what is being said, so can get very upset when the routines are changed.
- The child finds it difficult to take turns in a conversation.
- Pragmatic language difficulties (understanding that you do not talk to the vicar in the way that you talk to your friend, or to the teacher in the way that you talk to your mum etc.).

These sorts of communication difficulties can be very frustrating for the child, and this in turn can cause problems with behaviour; this will inevitably impact their overall learning, and therefore their academic potential.

---

### CASE STUDY

Chloé is three years of age, bright and intelligent. She has attended Bluebells nursery for two and a half years and is a great favourite with the staff. However, her key worker, John, is becoming increasingly concerned about her language development. Often Chloé will only use single words when her peers are using simple sentences. John is pretty certain that Chloé can hear normally, but when she wants to play with a toy she just uses a single word, 'doll', 'paint', 'house' and cannot be persuaded to put these into a sentence, despite John modelling language:

Chloé:  Doll!

John:   Oh! Do you want to play with the doll? Why don't we both play with the doll?

Chloé plays with the children that she knows but finds it hard to communicate with children new to the setting. John is also concerned that some of the children do not want to engage with Chloé in play, as she often fails to respond to their language. She is now increasingly playing with activities that do not require a response, like sand and water, and more and more she is found engaged in solitary play.

- How and when should John inform Chloé's parents of his concerns?
- What support do you think Chloé needs?
- How will John's observations contribute to Chloé's support from the other practitioners?
- How will John distinguish whether Chloé is at risk of SLI or has a developmental language delay?

## Chapter reflections

This chapter reminds us that a difference in one sensory processing area can impact others, as the way that you make sense of the world relies on the coming together of all your senses. A child who is either hypersensitive or hyposensitive to a particular sense can therefore distort their overall perception of the information processed by the brain. However, if this is the way that you have always seen the world, you probably regard it as 'normal', and because that information processing difference cannot be readily seen by others, particularly not in the early years, in the way that a physiological condition might be seen, then neither the child with the condition nor those around them might easily recognise the difficulties that they are experiencing. Clearly the more overt or extreme the condition, the more likely that it will be investigated, understood and supported. So, a lack of concentration, such as might be seen in ADD or ADHD may be difficult to detect, and the child only understands this as 'normal' feelings. It is only when children find it difficult to experience the world and behave in an unexpected manner that alarm bells begin to ring, and this is compounded by differences of severity in these conditions. This could reflect the age at which the child might be identified with an information processing disorder, because although present from birth it may not become apparent until much later. For example, autism is typically identified at approximately two to four years of age but dyslexia six to eight years of age, by which time untold damage could have been done to the self-esteem, confidence and emotional development of the child. Potentially this could even result in a complete shutdown of communication and social interaction, as can often be seen in SLI children who refuse to speak.

As with many of the information processing disorders discussed above, they may appear to get better over time, but rather than this being 'cured', it is probably more to do with the adolescent and adult getting more skilful at understanding what society expects, the way that social skills and language are put together, and how to avoid and avert situations in which they feel vulnerable. All these conditions are life-long conditions, from birth to grave, but as most dyslexic children do eventually learn to read, to a rudimentary level and with some difficulty, so do children with the apparently co-morbid conditions learn to cope better at masking their difficulties.

Whether these are separate and distinct conditions is clearly debatable, but one advantage to keeping them separate could be for research, where greater homogeneity can be established when selecting research samples. This could increase the chance of finding specific cognitive and genetic factors that relate to the conditions. The problem with research into these information processing disorders is that no two children are exactly alike, with the same indicators and manifestations, but these are certainly profound and potentially very distressing conditions.

# Further reading

Reid, G. (2016) *Dyslexia: A Practitioner's Handbook* (5th edn). Chichester: John Wiley and Sons Ltd.

Gavin Reid is one of the foremost experts in the multifaceted field of dyslexia, but he writes succinctly and accessibly, allowing even the most complex aspects of the subject to be understood by the non-specialist. His practical experience of working with children with dyslexia shines through in this comprehensive text, always considering practice suggestions for those supporting children at risk of dyslexia. From the first chapter 'Defining Dyslexia' to the last which considers the positive aspects of the condition, this book is a must for any practitioners wanting to know more about the subject.

# References

Badian, N. (1983) Dyscalculia and Non-verbal Disorders of Learning. In Myklebust, H.R. (1983) (ed.) *Progress in Learning Disabilities* Vol. 5, 235–264. New York: Grune Stratton.

Baron-Cohen, S. (2008) *Autism and Asperger Syndrome*. Oxford: Oxford University Press.

Bishop, D., North, T. and Donlan, C. (1995) Genetic Basis for Specific Language Impairment: evidenced from a twin study. Available online at: http://onlinelibrary.wiley.com/doi/10.1111/j.1469–8749.1995.tb11932.x/full (accessed 20.01.17).

Bohl, H. and Hoult, S. (2016) *Supporting Children with Dyslexia*. Abingdon: Routledge.

Broada, R., Willcutt, E.G. and Pennington, B. (2012) Understanding the Co-morbidity Between Dyslexia and Attention-Deficit/Hyperactivity Disorder. *Top Language Disorders* 32 (3): 246–284.

Butterworth, B. (2003) *Dyscalculia Screener*. London: NFER Nelson.

Fawcett, A. (2012) Introduction – An Overview of Dyslexia and Co-occurring Difficulties. In Stein, J. (ed.) *Dyslexia and Co-Occurring Difficulties*. Bracknell: BDA.

Frith, U. (1991) *Autism and Asperger Syndrome*. Cambridge: Cambridge University Press.

Grist, M., Knowles, L., Lascelles, L. and Hunels, A. (2012) *The SLI Handbook*. London: ICAN/Afasic.

Iversen, S., Berg, K., Ellertsen, B. and Tonnessen, F. (2005) Motor Co-ordination Difficulties in Municipality Group and in Clinical Sample of Poor Readers. *Dyslexia* 11: 217–231.

Lyytinen, H., Ahonen, T. and Räsän, P. (1994) Dyslexia and Dyscalculia in Children – Risks, Early Precursors, Bottlenecks and Cognitive Mechanisms. *Acta Paedopsychiatrica: Special Issue* 56 (1): 179–192.

Macintyre, C. (2015) *Understanding Children's Development in the Early Years: Questions Practitioners Frequently Ask* (2nd edn). Abingdon: Routledge.

Macintyre, C. and Deponio, P. (2003) *Identifying and Supporting Children with Specific Learning Difficulties: Looking Beyond the Label to Assess the Whole Child*. London: Routledge Falmer.

Miles, E. (1991) Auditory Dyslexia. In Snowling, M. and Thomson, M. (eds) *Dyslexia, Integrating Theory and Practice*. London: Whurr.

Miles, T. (1970) *On Helping the Dyslexic Child*. London: Methuen.

Montague-Smith, A. and Price, A.J. (2012) *Mathematics: In Early Years Education*. London: David Fulton.

O'Regan, F. (2012) Attention Deficit and Hyperactivity Disorder. In Stein, J. (ed.) *Dyslexia and Co-occurring Difficulties*. Bracknell: BDA.

Parvey, B. (2016) *Dyslexia and Early Childhood: An Essential Guide to Theory and Practice*. Abingdon: Routledge.

Pauc, R. (2005) Comorbidity of Dyslexia, Dyspraxia, Attention Deficit Disorder (ADD) Attention Deficit Hyperactivity Disorder (ADHD), Obsessive Compulsive Disorder and Tourette's Syndrome in Children: A prospectus epidemiological study. *Clinical Chiropractic* 8 (4): 189–198.

Pennington, B.F. and Olson, R.K. (2005) Genetics of Dyslexia. In Snowling, M. and Hulmes, C. (eds) *The Science of Reading: A Handbook*. London: Blackwell.

Reid, G. (2016) *Dyslexia: A Practitioner's Handbook* (5th edn). Chichester: John Wiley and Sons Ltd.

Richardson, A. (2001) Fatty Acids in Dyslexia, Dyspraxia, ADHD and the Autistic Spectrum. *Nutrition Practitioner* 3 (3): 18–24.

Ripley, K., Daines, B. and Barrett, J. (1997) *Dyspraxia: A Guide for Teachers and Parents*. London: David Fulton.

Russell, G. (2012) Autism and Asperger's Syndrome. In Stein, J. (ed.) *Dyslexia and Co-occurring Difficulties*. Bracknell: BDA.

Sharma, M.C. (2012) Dyscalculia, Dyslexia and other Mathematical Difficulties and Disabilities. In Stein, J. (ed.) *Dyslexia and Co-occurring Difficulties*. Bracknell: BDA.

Shakespeare, W. (1978) *The Tempest. The Complete Works of Shakespeare*. London: Abbey Library.

Snowling, M. (2008) Specific Disorders and Broader Phenotypes: The case of dyslexia. *Quarterly Journal of Experimental Psychology* 61: 142–156.

Stein, J. and Walsh, V. (1997) To See but not to Read. The magnocellular theory of dyslexia. *Trends in Neuroscience* 20: 147–152.

Stein, J., Talcott, J. and Witten, C. (2001) The Sensorimotor Basis of Developmental Dyslexia. In Fawcett, A. (ed.) *Dyslexia: Theory and Good Practice*. London: Whurr Publishers.

Taylor, E. (2012) Speech, Language and Communication. In Stein, J. *Dyslexia and Co-occurring Difficulties*. Bracknell: BDA.

Van de Leij, A., Lyytinen, H. and Zwarts, F. (2001) The Study of Infant Cognitive Processes in Dyslexia. In Fawcett, A. (ed.) *Dyslexia: Theory and Good Practice*. London: Whurr Publishers.

Viholainen, H., Ahonen, T., Lyytinen, H. and Maki, N. (2006) Early Motor Development and Later Language and Reading Skills in Children at Risk of Familial Dyslexia. *Developmental Medicine and Child Neurology* 48: 367–373.

White, J., Moffit, T. and Silva, P. (1992) Neuropsychological and Socio-emotional Correlates of Specific-arithmetic Disability. *Archives of Clinical Neuropsychology* 7: 1–16.

Wynn, K. (1998) Numerical Competence in Infants. In Donlan, C. (ed.) *The Development of Mathematical Skills*. Hove: Psychology Press.

# Waiting to fail

*Being told I was thick and stupid made me angry, a bit like the Incredible Hulk, but I turned anger, pain and hatred of the education system into my ammunition to succeed against the odds; enough was enough! I was not thick, I wasn't stupid, I am me, I have a soul, I am human, I am here alive, roaring like a tiger. I am fearless, free and for the first time I am not afraid anymore!*

Milton, 2016: 66

## Introduction

Comments such as that in the quotation by Milton (2016) above are not uncommon among those experiencing dyslexia, and only go to illustrate that despite all the knowledge and research that we now have about this and other specific learning difficulties, our current education system is still not getting it right. It certainly appears that it is producing distressed and anxious young people and adults, who feel resentful that their differences have not been taken into proper account, and appropriate support has not been forthcoming.

As with anything, 'prevention is better than cure'. Whilst dyslexia is not a disease and therefore not curable, intervention at an early stage could potentially avert some of the 'at risk' children developing social and emotional difficulties, resentment of our education system and feelings of failure, that so often accompany those who are identified at a later stage. So often the intervention and remediation put in place by schools is already 'too little too late', as in the child's eyes, they are already failures. This chapter will examine a range of intervention strategies including alternative therapies that parents and dyslexic individuals can turn to for help.

# Brain plasticity – neuro-plasticity

Brain plasticity is the capacity for the brain to change and mould according to life experience. It is the brain's capacity to form new connections between the neurons and to reorganise the neural pathways. This is particularly prevalent in the early years, but does continue throughout life.

Imagine the newborn baby as s/he emerges from the womb, their brain is flooded with new experiences, light, sound, cold, touch, starting to breathe etc. This new information needs to be transmitted from the nerve receptors in the senses to the brain. These electrical impulses need to create a pathway through particular areas of the brain, for example, the nerve cells in the retina need to transmit to the visual areas of the brain (occipital lobe), and not to a language or emotion detecting area. It is a little like walking through a field of grass that has not been walked on before. To get from one side of the field to the other you may need to wander a bit through the grass until finally you find the quickest pathway through. As this route becomes well used, the pathway across the field becomes worn and distinct, a new pathway is forged which is then always used.

In the early years the brain grows rapidly with lots of new neural pathways appearing, and by eight months a baby may have as many as 1,000 trillion synapses in the brain (Hawley and Gunner, 2000). According to Hawley and Gunner (2000), no new neurons form after birth, but the brain continues to wire and rewire the connections between the existing neurons. The synapses that are used are retained, but those that are not used are pruned away. This probably accounts for the reason why Asian children who are born with the ability to articulate a full range of sounds, find it so hard to make the 'r' sound at a later stage, which is never used in their mother tongue. They find that as they age the ability to make that sound disappears. The brain works on a 'use it or lose it' basis so connections can be lost if the child does not have the expected experiences in the early years. An example of this may be the child who does not hear language in the early years, who will find it harder to learn language as they age. Hawley and Gunner (2000) talk about 'windows of opportunity' for learning certain tasks. Such windows not only occur in human beings, we know that puppies need to be securely socialised within the first twelve weeks of life, or their ability to deal with life experiences could be severely compromised. However, more modern research with fMRI scans has shown that although the plasticity of the brain is more visible in the early years it is possible to create new connections and new learning throughout life. This concept of brain plasticity is largely behind all of the alternative therapies discussed in this chapter, with the idea that the brain can be 'cured and healed'.

## CASE STUDY

In 1970, in California, USA, a 13-year-old girl was discovered tied to a potty chair. Genie, as she was known, had been locked away from the world and from human contact and language for her entire life. When she was found, she had very limited verbal language and communicated her needs through primitive signs.

This very unusual case drew the attention of the world's press, and of language experts internationally. Every effort was made to rehabilitate her and to help her to learn language, however, it was unsuccessful, although her vocabulary grew, her ability to use grammar did not. She learned to put two or three words together, but was unable to arrange words in a truly meaningful way.

Of course, it is possible that Genie was born with some form of undiagnosed learning difficulty, or the years of abuse could have caused her cognitive deficits. However, evidence from other feral children – such as Oxana Malaya, who lived with dogs and was found in Ukraine in 1991 and Shamdeo, found in the forest of Musafirkhana in 1972 living with wolves – would suggest that unless language is learned within a certain window of opportunity, it is difficult to successfully learn language.

1. Use the internet to research these and other cases of feral children.
2. What similarities and differences do you see in them?
3. Why do you think that they were unable to learn language? Reflect on a range of possibilities.

# Assessment for dyslexia

A full and definitive assessment for dyslexia in the UK can only be attempted by an educational psychologist or a specialist teacher for dyslexia which is completely appropriate, given their broad and specialist knowledge and understanding of what you have already seen is a highly complex and multifaceted condition. However, often referral to the educational psychologist or specialist teacher comes a long way into the child's life as a child with dyslexia, and has usually been preceded by parents, families, nursery practitioners and teachers struggling to understand the problems, urging the child to 'buck up', 'work harder' and 'pay attention!'. They are often reluctant to consider that there may be a more fundamental difference in the child's learning, for fear of labelling and instilling an expectation of failure and underachievement.

## CASE STUDY

Melanie was five years old and in Year 1 of her primary school. She always struggled with school, finding it hard to concentrate, and as all the other children
were reading, she fell further and further behind. She became more scared, afraid,
confused and bored. She just could not make sense of the marks on the page. She
tried so hard and got so upset, when every day she was met by the adults in her
life telling her that she needed to try harder. Some nights she would try to read a
book in bed, with a torch, under the covers, but no matter what she did it still did
not make any sense. This would often result in her crying herself to sleep.

In school her teacher was convinced that Melanie had general learning difficulties and was at a loss as to what to do with Melanie, after all she was a girl
and that surely did not fit the classical profile of a specific learning difference. So
Melanie began to withdraw and spent most of her day daydreaming, colouring
and undertaking unchallenging tasks which created boredom in this bright and
intelligent child.

My mother used to tell me that 'boredom created work for idle hands!' and
in this case it was true. Melanie devised her own entertainment, which did not
fit well with the expectations of the teacher. She fidgeted, she flicked things, she
talked incessantly and the teacher was 'forced' to be constantly disapproving
and eventually separated her from the rest of the children that she was disturbing. What started as mild disruptive behaviour escalated quickly into more serious misconduct of shouting out, throwing things across the room and clowning
behaviour, which made the other children laugh or gasp in horror. Melanie was
achieving a level of notoriety among teachers and children, which, for the first
time in her life, got her noticed, increased her self-esteem and achieved a level of
peer group admiration that she had not experienced before. She liked the feeling
that it gave her.

- With a colleague, reflect on the interrelationship between dyslexia and
  self-confidence.

The British Psychological Society (BPS) reported in 1999 from a working party which
concluded that educational psychologists should

work more closely with schools to develop effective school based assessment,
intervention and monitoring, and within that context, also carry out detailed psychological assessment and programme planning.

(British Psychological Society, 1999a: p. 69)

It is clear from this quotation that even in the BPS, there is a recognition that presenting a child to a so called 'expert' for a single assessment is not sufficient, and that information from the home, staff in the nursery and the school setting is potentially a major contributing factor. However, in order for this to happen, those working with young children and babies need to be aware of their potential role in the identification and assessment of dyslexia and specific learning difficulties. That is, not to 'diagnose' such a condition but to highlight 'at risk' children who may be displaying early signs of learning differences through their language, motor co-ordination and social and emotional development. Reid (2016) understands that there is no one point at which dyslexia should or even could be identified, this is a continuous process, a continuum of assessment and risk identification.

> If someone asks [when should early identification take place] then I would suggest that they have misunderstood the whole concept of early identification.
>
> (Reid, 2016: p. 58)

The importance of that early awareness is that difficulties can be highlighted, and therefore closely observed and monitored over a period of time. All practitioners working in early years know the importance of observation and assessment to planning, but in my experience as an Ofsted inspector and a lecturer in early years, observations undertaken in schools and nurseries are frequently poorly prepared and inadequately understood. Detailed factual information, through observation, could be crucial to an early warning of difficulties. Simply waiting for children to mature, to 'grow out of it' or to 'wait and see' should not be an option. Each setting now has a designated Special Educational Needs Co-ordinator (SENCO), who should have experience of what to look for, and the signs of delayed progress and development. These issues could be used to support and plan the best outcomes for the child, rather than condemning them. A 'wait and see' attitude could potentially lead to children with information processing disorders being overlooked until they are much older, by which time the difficulties experienced by the child will be much greater. Why wait for failure when vigilance could ensure that early intervention is in place, in the same way as any child with physical disabilities would expect. In that way, parents and practitioners can work to minimise the impact that dyslexia can potentially have on a child's social and emotional development and in turn on their cognitive and language development.

The difficulties, often encountered by those who are aware of their responsibilities in this area, are that children's holistic development in the early years can vary enormously from child to child; it could be that, at this stage, it naturally varies more than at any other period in their lives. Developmental rates will also be significantly impacted by their experiences; culture, mother tongue, family expectations and exposure to a rich learning environment will all have a part to play. Two children with similar manifestations of a learning difference will need repeated observations over a period of time, in different environments and preferably by different observers, to identify information processing disorders and maturational delays. These observations can create an ongoing portfolio for the child that will accompany them as they progress through the system. These should contain samples of the child's work, observations, both formal and informal, benchmark checklists and curriculum evaluations. The portfolio could contain multiple sources of information from which to draw conclusions and predictors of risk, including comments from parents and carers. Probably the greatest challenge in early years is to ensure the reliability and validity of such observations. This is only possible when practitioners have a clear understanding of the concepts and skills that are appropriate to the developmental stage of the child, and are meaningful to the whole process of screening. When considering identification of dyslexia at a very early stage of development there are possibly two key aspects to consider, first, the research into the isolation of potential gene variants which could be a contributory factor to dyslexia, and the possibility of new biological therapeutic interventions (gene manipulation) to be developed in the future. Second, identification through early universal screening could also bring benefits of early remediation. However, as Lundberg and Hoien (2001) point out, there are two questions that need to be considered before either aspect is implemented:

1.  Can anything be done if dyslexia is identified?
2.  What happens to children who are identified as 'at risk' but do not go on to show signs of dyslexia (the false positives)?

I would add a third question to this:

3.  What happens to the children who could slip through the net (the false negatives)?

Lundberg and Hoien (2001) 'advise caution' for universal screening, because the manner in which testing is currently undertaken is very imprecise, and there is currently no fool proof method of testing that is statistically reliable, or even a definitive checklist for observations. Add to this that very young children are notoriously difficult to engage with any task that they are not immediately interested in, their attention and stamina for a task is often limited and can vary on a daily and even hourly basis. It is also not always possible to know whether they really understand the instructions for any given task, or are too young to have language. A lack of accuracy in identification could also mean large variants in detection rates and Alexander-Passe (2015) warns that specialists currently diagnose according to different criteria, making prevalence rates almost impossible to compare nationally.

In truth, a universal screening programme for dyslexia in the early years is probably not a possibility, although it is a tempting concept. This is unlike medical screening for conditions such as breast cancer and bowel cancer, which identifies pre-symptomatic stages of an illness to enable medical intervention and appropriate choices to be made; it is unlikely to be as helpful as it may at first seem. The probability of false positives and false negatives is likely to be high, potentially causing unnecessary anxiety in some cases, and unfounded complacency in others. Looking further to the future this also has the potential to increase incidents of litigation.

## Is there a cure?

A cure implies that by undertaking either drug treatment, surgery or behavioural treatment, that condition no longer exists in a person. It is usually referred to in the case of disease, if you have a cough you can use medication to help it to go away. According to the *Concise Oxford Dictionary*, a cure is:

> To make healthy again after suffering from disease or medical condition. To end [a disease, condition or problem] by treatment or remedial action.

The problem with this definition, with regard to dyslexia, is the word 'end', what we do know about dyslexia is that it is a life-long condition and although 'remedial actions' can be put in place to allow the person with dyslexia to integrate well into society, and use their skills and talents to good effect, they will always have to work harder to achieve what the rest of society automatically expects of its members.

The concept of a 'cure' for dyslexia frequently appears in sensationalised headlines in newspapers and other social media. Claims of cures through dietary supplements, massage, exercise programmes, neurolinguistic programming, reorientation of the brain and others abound, and although it is not possible in this book to do a scientific examination of the efficacy of these ideas, I will identify some of those most talked about. The media clamour for a 'cure' is not helpful to the scientific and research community, as members of the public and employers are frequently looking to them for 'answers'. As this is a life-long condition, such answers are probably not possible to give, and artificially raising the hopes of people with dyslexia and their families is both cruel and unfounded.

> Although dyslexia cannot be cured, its severity can be ameliorated by early intervention targeted to address the specific difficulties which the student encounters.
> (Knight et al., 2009: p. 67)

## Alternative interventions

For parents of children with dyslexia the array of approaches and theories is confusing and bewildering. What they know is that they have a child who needs help. Parents are supposed to be there for their children, and they have always been there to pick them up when they fall, dry their tears and make them feel better. They have done all the things that they are told make 'good' parents, talking to their child, listening, reading with them and giving them experiences, but despite all their best efforts, that have often worked with their other children in the same family, this child is different. This child is experiencing emotional pain and distress that the parents feel unable to deal with. They possibly turn to the internet or to books, and find that unlike when their child had chicken pox there is no convenient list of symptoms which can lead to a diagnosis, and even when they do identify the wide range of manifestations as dyslexia, there is no agreement from the so called experts as to where it has come from, and most importantly what to do about it. They are, of course, looking for a 'cure', a short-term remedy to take away the pain and distress from their child and to get learning back onto a familiar trajectory. However, as you have seen in this book so far, even this cannot be agreed by the 'experts' and even the phonologically based interventions, which were mooted as the way forward by the Government and the Rose Review (2006), have not always demonstrated the levels of success with all children that they purported to (National Reading Panel, 2000). Fawcett and Reid (2009) cite results from the US National Reading Panel (2001) which showed that the mainstream interventions often only offer partial improvements in reading. So interventions that are based on phonological training may improve phonology, but are not always generalised to improve reading overall. However, it should be noted that the evaluation of the interventions is extremely difficult to administer, usually very expensive and frequently unpopular, often beset with huge ethical implications. To undertake such an audit would normally require a double-blind placebo study, which is when the research is undertaken with one or more groups that have an intervention programme allocated and one or more that have not. Children are allocated to a group in a completely randomised manner and no one involved (researcher, parent, child, practitioner) knows which group each child is allocated to. This, as you can imagine, is fine in the laboratory but less easy to administer in a busy nursery or classroom. The other difficulty is one of size effect, as results of research undertaken on a small manageable number of children are always at risk of having occurred by chance alone. Undertaking large scale research on children is frequently not viable, usually very expensive, and beset with huge ethical dilemmas. The other difficulty is how any improvement can be measured and on what scale, for example, how much of an improvement is significant and how comparable would one intervention be against another. It is also important to estimate whether that improvement would have to be long lasting, for example, would it still be measurable in two to three years' time?

Parents often turn to the practitioners and teachers who are working with their child for support, but as can be seen by the evidence of the small-scale research conducted for this publication (Chapter 9), most practitioners have no firm training or understanding of the issues involved, and therefore they are often unhelpful and frustrating for a parent.

For many parents this is the point at which they start to trawl the internet for alternative therapies, many making wildly exaggerated claims of cures and remediation. However, as Reid (2016) points out, not all are without their merit, but most have not undergone peer reviewed clinical trials and verification in double blind placebo controlled studies, which is so important to ensure their robust nature and likely success of the intervention.

The uncertainty and disagreement of definition and identification has almost certainly contributed to the rise in the number of alternative therapies. Parents, teachers, practitioners, employers and individuals with dyslexia all want to believe in a cure, or at the very least a quick fix amelioration of the manifestations of dyslexia. This rise has often been without the stringent research to support the claims made, but this is certainly not to dismiss any one of them outright. Research in the future may well validate any one, or all of them, as contributory factors, especially when the well evaluated mainstream interventions have been brought into question by more detailed research (Fawcett and Reid, 2009).

The fear is that there might be charlatans out there waiting to prey on the vulnerable and susceptible, charging large sums of money for the 'cure-all'. With all these caveats in place I have attempted to briefly discuss and identify some of the better known alternative therapies.

# Dietary supplements and fatty acids

Research by Stein (2000) sparked a debate about the addition of polyunsaturated essential fatty acids to the diet of children with dyslexia. He claimed that the deficiency of these in modern diets could inhibit the development of magnocellular neurons in the brain, or be a consequence of immunological attack.

Reid (2016) cites a study by Richardson (2001), which suggested that essential fatty acids (EFA) such as linoleic acid (omega 6 series) and alpha-linoleic acid (omega 3 series) should be added to the diet, either through supplements or from increased consumption of oily fish, to convert the essential fatty acids to highly unsaturated fatty acids (HUFA). She claimed that the brain needed these for learning, certainly these oils are essential because they probably make up 20% of the brain's overall weight, but the body cannot produce them for themselves, so must rely on dietary intake. They are especially important for the developing brain of the foetus and the under two-year-old, particularly if the child has been pre-term at birth. Reid (2016) claims that Richardson (2001) warned that an excess of processed foods, deficiencies in certain minerals and vitamins, plus over-consumption of stimulants such as coffee, alcohol and smoking, could deplete the advantages of supplementary EFAs.

A dietary approach to dyslexia intervention is certainly very appealing, add this or that to the diet, remove such and such and hey presto improvements occur, and usually cheaply. It is also possible to see that this sort of approach could be easily implemented in a nursery or school, along with parental consent. However, it is likely that just a healthy balanced diet would have a beneficial impact upon all children, although it is always wise to consult a GP before considering any major changes of diet. In 2006, the Government of the day even considered giving fish oil supplements to all children in school. After all it was not so long ago that every school aged child received a third of a pint of milk each day at school (introduced in 1946 with the Free Milk Act; repealed by Margaret Thatcher in 1971). During the second world war, even during rationing, all children under five years of age and pregnant women were issued with a weekly spoonful of cod liver oil, which most remembered many years later as a hated ritual, but the importance of fish oil supplements was clearly recognised, even at that time. Some researchers were even calling for EFAs to be added to all baby foods. However, in 2006 the Food Standards Agency conducted a review of research into omega 3 and 6 supplements on children's learning and behaviour and concluded that research findings were mixed and inconclusive. So despite some sensational claims for EFAs the evidence for them helping children with dyslexia is still very unclear.

## Exercise (balance training)

The most prominent proponent of using exercise and balance training to improve dyslexia was the Dore programme, named after its founder, a businessman called Wynford Dore. This programme was previously known as DDAT (dyslexia, dyspraxia and attention deficit treatment). The programme, which has since closed due to financial difficulties, was based on the idea that the cerebellum, which is the area of the brain responsible for balance and automatisation, was 'incorrectly wired'. Describing automatisation (the ability to do more than one thing at a time), Fawcett and Nicholson (2004) use the analogy of being able to drive a car in a country that drives on the right hand side – you can do it, but it requires supreme concentration and is very tiring. Dore (2006) believed that the wiring of the brain could be reconfigured by using balance exercises to form new neural connections. The exercises included spinning on the spot on one leg, eye focusing drills, tracking light patterns, catching bean bags, threading and balancing on wobble boards etc.

The programme was financially very costly for parents but, according to Reid (2016), had very little reliable evidence to substantiate the claims that Dore made for his course. However, it did receive a great deal of media attention, which was probably more down to great publicity than to concrete results. Reid (2016) suggests that there is no direct evidence that improved balance would directly improve reading performance, despite the fact that the circuits of the brain responsible for balance are located in the cerebellum, they are likely to be different from those areas involved in literacy based activities.

# Inhibition of primitive reflexes

The Institute for Neuro-Physiological Psychology (INPP) was set up in Chester by Peter Blythe for the assessment and treatment of what he called Neuro-Developmental Delay (NDD). The rationale behind this programme is that all full-term babies are born with a set of primitive reflexes which should disappear as the child develops but may, in some children, be retained into adulthood. Primitive reflexes are motor movement actions centred within the nervous system, they are involuntary responses to a given stimulus; you know what it is like when the doctor asks you to cross your legs and then knocks just below your knee with a medical hammer. No matter how much you attempt to stop it your leg involuntarily kicks out. Other examples of such reflexes that may be seen in the very young baby are:

- Morro reflex or startle reflex (if the baby is moved suddenly they will throw out their arms and arch their back).
- Rooting reflex (when baby is touched on the cheek they turn towards the touch).
- Sucking reflex (newborn babies will suck on anything that is placed in their mouth and swallow; they will even suck on a lemon!).
- Palmer grasp reflex (as the palms of the hands and feet are touched they curl and grasp tightly).
- Stepping reflex (when baby is held above a surface the feet move as if to walk).
- Swimming reflex (placed face down in water the baby makes co-ordinated swimming movements).
- Asymmetrical Tonic Neck Reflex (ATNR) (sometimes called the 'fencer's pose' where the baby forms fists with both hands and turns the head to the right).
- Tonic Labyrinthine Reflex (TLR) (the head tilts back, the back arches and the legs straighten).

Blythe (1992) explains that these are controlled by centres in the brain which also determine when these reflexes will 'switch off', or no longer remain active. This is usually within the first 12–24 months of the baby's life. Blythe (1992) suggests that in some children such reflexes remain active long after the time when they should have extinguished, and although these reflexes are survival actions for a young baby, when they remain they can seriously interfere with the activities of balance, co-ordination (both gross and fine motor), and even perceptual skills. Blythe's approach requires a daily exercise programme for each child.

Once again, fully validated, longitudinal, peer reviewed research evaluating the effectiveness of this system is hard to find.

# Brain Gym (Kinesiology)

Brain Gym has been used extensively in many schools in England and Wales and is often referred to as Educational Kinesiology. It is based in the USA, and a quick trawl through the available research indicates that there is very little scientific evidence to support the extravagant claims for Brain Gym. Like Dore and the INPP this is a commercial venture which appears, in my opinion, to be based on very flimsy evidence. There is a range of research relating to Brain Gym, but mostly this has been conducted by the Brain Gym Corporation. Brain Gym is based on 26 movements, co-ordinating eyes, hands and whole-body crawling, drawing, air tracing, yawning and drinking. It was devised in 2010 by Paul and Gail Dennison.

Clearly exercise is vital to the holistic health and development of all children, enabling them to move fluently and confidently. It also helps with social development, as being able to run, ride bikes and play games enables children to interact with each other, find friends and have common interests. It also enables children to have greater independence and to have experiences to talk about, hence improving vocabulary and articulation. Emotional learning is also helped when making friends and forming relationships, taking part in teams and abiding by rules. This increased confidence and self-esteem can clearly be transferred to other aspects of learning. However, evidence for specific programmes to help with dyslexia does appear to be slight at best, apart from the research undertaken by the proponents of the various programmes.

# Coloured filters

The use of coloured overlays to assist dyslexia has had wide appeal. The concept is based on an individual's sensitivity to certain wavelengths of light, which could cause distortions of the print when reading black on white. Helen Irlen's book *Reading by the Colors* (1991) was thought at the time to be quite a breakthrough, and so simple. All you had to do was to cover the text with a coloured overlay or gel, to help with reading fluency. Some children wear glasses with coloured lenses, thereby enabling them to see writing on a white board or to write with the colour shielding the glare. The difficulty is that there appears to be no universal colour, which seems to help, and Irlen used a photospectrometer to measure the characteristics of each colour; she called this condition Scotopic Sensitivity Syndrome. Selection of the appropriate coloured overlay or lens needs to be done by a specialist, trained optometrist on an Intuitive Colorimeter machine, which can show over 100,000 colour combinations, but this can be expensive for parents and no financial help is available.

Irlen claimed that this was a condition whereby there was insufficient contrast between the black letters and a white background, to the point where the background overpowers the black letters, making them difficult to read. She suggested that a contrast of colour causes hyper excitability of the visual cortex and hence visual stress. The theory is that the coloured overlays limit these perceptual difficulties by redistributing and reducing the hyper excitability. However, research from Albon et al. (2008) showed

> Meta-analysis of the quantitative assessment of eight included RCTs [random controlled trials] did not show that the use of coloured filters led to a clear improvement in reading ability in subjects with reading disability . . . it remains a possibility that there exists a subgroup of people who may experience an improvement in reading through the use of coloured filters, while others find that there is no beneficial effect.
>
> (Albon et al., 2008: p. 7)

In 2009, research by the American Academy of Pediatrics also concluded that there was no demonstrable effect on reading with coloured overlays. Interestingly the British Dyslexia Association still recommends their use for children with dyslexia and the International Institute of Colorimetry has a list of research papers supporting their use, including a double-blind placebo controlled trial by Wilkins et al. (1994), that suggests that the benefit of colour is not simply down to a placebo effect. So the research evidence on coloured overlays is definitely very mixed and the 'jury is out' on the efficacy of this intervention

## Binocular instability (eye wobble) and ocular dominance

Binocular instability refers to the dominance of one eye over the other, or the ability to bring the eyes together in a coordinated way. The work completed by Evans (1996) talked about the importance of a stable eye reference or dominant eye. To determine your dominant eye, consider which eye you would use to look through a telescope. However, Evans concluded that there were at least three types of eye dominance:

1. Sight
2. Motion
3. Sensory

As you have already read in Chapter 3, when reading the eyes travel quickly over the text jumping from word to word (saccades and fixations), but to enable you to see the word the eyes need to remain steady, or the text will appear blurred. Stein

(2012) suggests that the visual magnocellular system could be mildly impaired in some dyslexic children, giving a lower sensitivity to contrast and flicker, weaker and slower visual attention and reduced visual motion sensitivity, or unstable eye control (oscillopsia). Stein and Fowler (1985) believed that through exercise it could be possible to change a child's dominant eye, or improve convergence, by giving the children a pair of glasses with one eye temporarily covered or blurred and undertaking eye exercises to stabilise binocular fixation, and the use of blue or yellow overlays/lenses to improve reading. This implies that the uncovered eye has to work harder, and gains more control of the muscles to be able to fixate more accurately.

Back in 1981, Pavlidis and Miles suggested that children with dyslexia have poor control over their eye tracking and this influenced their ability to read. The back tracking, or right to left movements made during reading (in Roman text), are called regressions; these are essential to understanding text. As you have already read, you only actually fixate upon a percentage of the words in a line of print and 'skip' others; you are usually happy with this if the meaning of the sentence is clear. The faster you read the more skilled at reading you become, the larger the gaps or saccades. However, if the meaning is compromised you back track and this is a regression; in other words, you return to the previous text, to re-examine and read again to confirm meaning. This is a perfectly normal development of reading, but relies upon your comprehension of the text; so not with a difficulty of reading but with a difficulty of understanding meaning. This accounts for why when you are reading a difficult passage, one that you have poor understanding of (unfamiliar content perhaps), it takes so much longer to read than the 'trashy' novel that you take with you on holiday, as there need to be more fixations and more regressions. Pavlidis and Miles (1981) believed that the younger the child the more regressions can be observed, and this has a direct correlation to the rate of information processing. They concluded that in children with dyslexia there was an erratic nature to these eye movements in the number, size and position of the regressions, but in normal readers and developmentally delayed readers this was not apparent.

There has been considerable criticism of Pavlidis' work within the dyslexia research community, and Olson et al. (1983) suggest that there are other explanations for the findings of Pavlidis and Miles. One explanation could be the possibility that the group of dyslexic children made more regressions due to the oculomotor sequencing problems, rather than general oculomotor deficits. They claim that attempts to replicate this research have been limited, finding no difference between dyslexic and non-dyslexic readers.

## Accommodation dysfunction

Accommodation dysfunction is a difficulty sustaining prolonged focus or focusing stamina, being able to change focus quickly from long-sight to near vision. It must be emphasised that this is not a problem of vision but of the muscles that enable the change of focus from close to long sight and binocular convergence. Accommodation dysfunction is seen when the eyes do not function together effectively. Children with normal vision can use either each eye separately or both together to focus on an object, but the child with accommodation dysfunction finds this more difficult. Because these children often struggle with reading and writing they are often misdiagnosed as dyslexic. It is possible that a child with dyslexia also has accommodation dysfunction, but research by Evans et al. (1994) concluded that it was not a cause of dyslexia, but could correlate with it. Eye exercises are traditionally prescribed for children with this condition but I could find no credible evidence that this sort of vision therapy could improve dyslexia.

## Magno visual dysfunction

Although there is a heavy emphasis from the Government on children learning to read through a phonological approach (Rose, 2006), undoubtedly the first step to reading is a visual one (except perhaps in the visually impaired use of braille, where you could claim that it was tactile). The ability to visualise and analyse correctly what is seen is essential to reading. Stein (2012) points out that letters or characters must first be recognised. This is a process for the small neurons in the brain, the parvocellular neurons (P neurons). These neurons are able to recognise fine detail and colour, but it is equally important to be able to sequence letters in the right order. This is reminiscent of the famous sketch in 1971 by the comedians Morecambe and Wise, with the concert pianist Andre Previn. Eric Morecambe protests that he is playing all the right notes, just not necessarily in the right order! Stein (2012) believes that children with dyslexia are

> less accurate and slower at sequencing letters than they are at identifying each letter individually.
>
> (Stein, 2012: p. 32)

This sequencing process relies on the magnocellular system or the M neurons. They also help to guide and co-ordinate visual attention, eye and limb movements. The rate at which M cells project signals to the brain is, according to Stein (2012), approximately ten milliseconds, before the slower P cells. Therefore, he claims that if the magnocellular system is deficient,

> [f]ocusing attention and fixation of the eyes will be unstable and the process of sequencing letters will be slower and less accurate.
>
> (Stein, 2012: p. 33)

This magnocellular deficiency could be the reason why many children with dyslexia complain of visual stress, blurring, moving letters etc. Stein (2012) claims that up to 50% of the children with dyslexia that present to his clinic have visual stress problems due to magnocellular deficiencies.

Stein (2012) also claims that there is an auditory processing equivalent of the visual magnocellular theory. To understand speech, it is necessary to order a sequence of sounds, and be able to distinguish subtle changes of frequency and amplitude. Stein (2012) believes that poor visual magnocellular function often accompanies poor auditory temporal processing.

> I have suggested, therefore, that all the features of developmental dyslexia . . . visual, auditory, linguistic and motor . . . may be accounted for by improved development of CAT301 type magnocellular neurons throughout the brain. The differing degree of expression of this impairment in different systems could explain the large individual differences seen among people with dyslexia. . . . Some being mainly visual, others auditory, others uncoordinated, others more purely linguistic.
>
> (Stein, 2012: p. 38).

There has been much criticism of Stein's magnocellular theory, such as that by Skottun (2000), who whilst agreeing that visual disturbance is common to people with dyslexia, disputes that this is a result of visual magnocellular processing. Skottun (2000) reviewed 22 research studies into magnocellular deficits and found that only four of these were in agreement with it, 11 provided results which conflicted (at least in part) and seven were inconclusive.

---

### Reflect on this

It is important to take a cautious and critically analytical approach to alternative concepts.

Reflect on one alternative approach that you are aware of, either included in this chapter or from your own experience:

- Do you find it convincing?
- Why have you taken this view?
- What peer reviewed research can you find to back this up? The internet may help you here.

## Chapter reflections

Returning to the title of this chapter, 'Waiting to Fail' cannot offer a positive scenario for the child with dyslexia, but unaddressed and unidentified dyslexia in the young baby is doing just that. Children should not have to demonstrate continuous, abject failure before interventions are made available. In this way failure becomes a mandatory element of identification. Alexander-Passe (2015) reminds us that this is failure on many levels:

- Public failure, resulting in humiliation and even bullying.
- Family failure, where children feel that they have let down their parents and creating competition between siblings that causes conflict.
- Personal failure, probably the hardest to combat, often causing life-long self-denial, with an adverse reaction to risk taking and new challenges.

Our youngest children should not have to experience the levels of helplessness and depression that so often accompany dyslexia, when they are trapped in a misconception of their own abilities.

This chapter has very briefly examined a range of the interventions which have been available to individuals with dyslexia; there are of course many more, and claims from sectors such as homeopathy, chiropractic and acupuncture also exist. What is important is for you to understand the need for evidence based criteria to any claims, and however persuasive at first sight, nothing replaces critical scrutiny, even for the most well established and currently accepted interventions. Only then will you be able to make correctly informed decisions about the best fit intervention for a child in your care, and this is not necessarily a 'one size fits all' scenario.

As you have already read, these children are dyslexic and will always remain dyslexic so developing resilience to their condition is vital. This resilience will enable them to cope with adversity and as Alexander-Passe (2015) suggests:

See that failure is a vital cog in the development of mastery and that they are a mixture of areas of strengths and weaknesses, as are their friends, family and peers.

(Alexander-Passe, 2015: p. 21)

When considering any of these alternative approaches it is always wise to maintain an open mind and to use your common sense. Good old-fashioned teaching methods have stood the test of time, and in the absence of an off the shelf 'quick fix' they may be what you are left with.

In the case of dyslexia, often low self-esteem is the major factor in how a child feels about themselves and how they view their world, and many of these alternative therapies do work to alleviate this poor self-concept, anxiety and even depression with massage, aromatherapy, movement, diet and even various sound therapies, but 'let the buyer beware'!

# Further reading

Rose, J. (2006) *Independent Review of the Teaching of Early Reading*. Nottingham: Department of Education and Skills Publications.

The Rose review was commissioned by the Labour government of the day to make recommendations on the teaching of reading in schools. Rose was particularly concerned about the identification and teaching of children with dyslexia.

Although the review was not taken up by subsequent governments, this was a key document which has been influential to the introduction of systematic synthetic phonics into all state schools and nurseries in England. Rose emphasised the importance of consistency and regularity to good teaching and most experts in the field see this as a seminal document.

# References

Albon, E., Adi, Y. and Hyde, C. (2008) *The Effectiveness and Cost Effectiveness of Coloured Filters for Reading Disability: A Systematic Review*. University of Birmingham: Dept of Public Health and Epidemiology.

Alexander-Passe, N. (2015) *Dyslexia and Mental Health*. London: Jessica Kingsley Publishers.

American Academy of Pediatrics (2009) Joint Statement: Learning disabilities, dyslexia and vision. *Pediatrics* 124: 837–844.

Blythe, P. (1992) *A Physical Approach to Resolving Specific Learning Difficulties*. Chester: Neuro-Physiological Psychology.

British Psychological Society (1999) *Dyslexia, Literacy and Psychological Assessment*. Leicester: BPS.

Dennison, P.E. and Dennison, G.E. (2010) *Brain Gym*. GB: Edu Kinesthetics.

Dore, W. (2006) *Dyslexia: The Miracle Cure*. London: John Blake Publishing.

Evans, B.J.W. (1996) Assessment of Visual Problems in Reading. In Beech, J. and Singleton C. (eds) *Problems in Reading*. London: Routledge.

Evans, B.J.W., Dasdo, N. and Richards, I.L. (1994) Investigation of Accommodative and Binocular Function in Dyslexia. *OPO* 14 (1): 5–19.

Fawcett, A. and Nicholson, R. (2004) Dyslexia: The role of the cerebellum. In Reid, G. and Fawcett, A. (eds.) *Dyslexia in Context: Research Policy and Practice*. London: Whurr Publications.

Fawcett, A. and Reid, G. (2009) Dyslexia and Alternative Interventions for Dyslexia: A critical commentary. In Reid, G. (ed.) *The Routledge Companion to Dyslexia*. Abingdon: Routledge.

Food Standards Agency (2006) *Protecting the Interests of Consumers: Annual Report*. London: Crown.

Hawley, T. and Gunner, M. (2000) *Starting Smart: How Early Experiences Affect Brain Development* (2nd edn). New York: Zero to Three/The Ounce of Prevention Fund.

Irlen, H. (1991) *Reading by the Colors: Overcoming Dyslexia and Other Reading Disabilities through the Irlen Method*. New York: Perigee.

Knight, D.F., Day, K. and Patten-Terry, N. (2009) Preventing and Identifying Reading Difficulties in Young Children. In Reid G. (ed.) *The Routledge Companion to Dyslexia*. Abingdon: Routledge.

Lundberg, I. and Hoien, T. (2001) Dyslexia and Phonology. In Fawcett, A. (ed.) *Dyslexia: Theory and Good Practice*. London: Whurr Publications.

Milton, P. (2016) Fearless and Free. In Van Daal, V. and Tomalin, P. (eds) *The Dyslexia Handbook 2016: I am Dyslexic*. Bracknell: BDA.

National Reading Panel (2000) *Teaching Children to Read: An evidence based assessment of the scientific research literature on reading and its implications for reading instruction*. Washington DC: US Dept of Health and Human Services, Public Health Services, National Institute of Health, National Institute of Child Health and Human Development. Available online at: www.nichd.nih.gov/publications/pubs/nrp/Documents/report.pdf (accessed 14.08.17).

Olson, R.K., Kliegl, R. and Davidson, J. (1983) Dyslexic and Normal Readers' Eye Movements. *Journal of Experimental Psychology: Human Perception and Performance* 9: 816–825.

Pavlidis, G.Th. and Miles, T.R. (1981) *Dyslexia Research and its Applications to Education*. Chichester: John Wiley and Sons.

Reid, G. (2016) *Dyslexia: A Practitioner's Handbook* (5th edn). Chichester: Wiley.

Richardson, A. (2001) Fatty Acids in Dyslexia, Dyspraxia, ADHD and the Autistic Spectrum. *Nutrition Practitioner* 3 (3): 18–24.

Rose, J. (2006) *Independent Review of the Teaching of Early Reading*. Nottingham: Department of Education and Skills Publications.

Skottun, B.C. (2000) The Magnocellular Deficit Theory of Dyslexia: the evidence from contrast sensitivity. *Vision Research* 40 (1): 111–127.

Stein, J. (2000) The Neurobiology of Reading Difficulties. *Prostaglandins, Leukotrienes and Essential Fatty Acids (PLEFA)* 63 (1–2): 109–116.

Stein, J. (2012) The Magnocellular Theory of Dyslexia. In Benasich, A. and Fitch, H. (eds) *Developmental Dyslexia: Precursors, Neurobehavioral Markers and Biological Substrates*. Baltimore: Paul Brookes Publishing.

Stein, J. and Fowler, S. (1985) Effect of Monocular Occlusion on Visuomotor Perception and Reading in Dyslexic Children. *The Lancet* 13: 69–73.

Wilkins, A., Evans, B.J.W., Brown, J.A., Busby, A.E., Wingfield, A.E., Jeans, R.J. and Bald, J. (1994) Double-masked placebo-controlled trial of precision filters in children who use coloured overlays. *Ophthalmic and Physiological Optics* 14: 365–370. Available online at: www.colorimetryinstitute.org/research-papers#2 (accessed 14.08.17).

# Catch 'em young . . . planning and assessment

*Dyslexia is more than just an academic difficulty, but one that impacts the whole neural system*

Goswami, 2015. Available online at: www.telegraph.co.uk/
education/educationnews/11592620/the-last-word-
ondyslexia (accessed 24.11.17).

## Introduction

It would seem logical to assume that the earlier a difficulty is identified the better, enabling focused intervention to be put in place before a child experiences failure and low self-esteem. However, this is not always as easy as it sounds, particularly at a stage in a child's life when development rates vary enormously. Developmental sequence rarely changes, so the child cannot walk before they stand, cannot stand before they sit and so on; however, the ages at which these occur can vary wildly, meaning a huge diversity in learning needs. The exponential increase in the numbers of children attending early years provision in recent years, reflecting the increase in numbers of women in the workplace, means that most children now come into daily contact with a trained early years professional, which a few years ago would not have been the case. According to DfE statistics (2017a), there are currently 14,100 full day care providers in England and Wales, and an enormous increase came between 2001 and 2009 of over 81%. This, in theory, should mean that the chance of identifying developmental difficulties at an early age should be greater.

It is also a requirement of the SEND Code of Practice (DfE/DoH, 2015) that between the ages of two and three years, practitioners must assess a child's progress (see Figure 7.1) and communicate this assessment to the parents. You are required to outline the intervention strategies that you intend to put in place to help the child 'at risk' of developmental delay or potential special needs.

It is particularly important in the early years that there is no delay in making any necessary special educational provision. Delay at this stage can give rise to learning difficulties and subsequently to loss of self-esteem, frustration in learning and to behavioural difficulties. Early action to address identified needs is critical to future progress and improved outcomes that are essential in helping the child to prepare for adult life.

(DfE, 2014: p. 14)

## Observation

Research by Snowling (2012) showed that observations undertaken for the Early Years Foundation Stage Profile indicated a strong correlation between the predictors from the observation and language and literacy performance over two years later. If this is correct, this could provide strong and valid evidence for the use of observational assessments on very young children. Snowling (2012) concludes that the observations undertaken for the EYFS profile were likely to be a

good predictor of later literacy attainments.

(Snowling, 2012: p. 4)

Therefore, they could potentially be a good indicator for children at risk of dyslexia and other educational difficulties.

Screening children for the risk of dyslexia is a very appealing idea, but is perhaps not as easy as it at first sounds. The Welsh Government, Llywodraeth Cymru (2012), suggest that any screening procedure needs to be quick and low cost and able to be administered by 'trained, but not specialist, personnel' (p. 31), certainly focused and targeted observations would fall under that definition. However, before you can begin to contemplate identifying children at risk of dyslexia you need to have confidence not only in your own ability to observe, but also in the validity and reliability of the whole process of observation. In other words, whether the assessment observation measures what you think it measures, and whether the results can be replicated, even by another observer.

Hurst (1991) described observation as 'the foundation of education in the early years' (p. 70). As a skilled and effective practitioner, you should be assessing children all of the time, whether formally or informally. Observation must be 'up there' with safety, protection and care as one of the most important roles of an early years worker. Learning to observe children closely is a key part of all practitioners' training programmes, and most will have written many observations before they leave their initial training. However, often the key to a 'good' observation is not necessarily how to observe, but why to observe, or even what to observe, but a question often not asked is 'What do I look for?' This question is really important to a practitioner caring for a child who may be at risk of dyslexia.

No one is suggesting that you could, or even should, be making a formal identification of dyslexia in babies and very young children in early years settings. Formal identification can only be undertaken by a dedicated educational psychologist or a specialist teacher trained in dyslexia assessment and recognition. In this case the child is likely to be put through a series of commercially produced, norm based tests, which yield a series of number based scores, enabling comparison between individuals and an examination of the standard deviation from the norm. It is highly unlikely, or even desirable, that children of such tender years will be subjected to such a battery.

However, before a child reaches that point, much information can be gained by a skilled and observant practitioner. Unfortunately, in my experience of working with practitioners, many do not have enough confidence in their own abilities, and fear that their concerns will not be taken seriously, or that they will be dismissed as subjective opinion seeing only what they 'want' to see. Human nature will always play a part in your interpretation of what you see, but you need to be mindful that your interpretation is only one viewpoint, and other competing perspectives from other observers need to be taken into account, producing not one observation but a portfolio of evidence.

> The range of variance in the observer interpretation is largely dependent on the instrument used and the extent to which the observer is concerned with 'low inference' or 'high inference' factors, as well as the purpose of the observation. These terms are best seen as part of a continuum rather than as polar opposites. Typically a high inference observation requires a significant degree of subjective judgement by the observer. In contrast a low inference observation concerns factors that are considered transparent and as such interpretations are less likely to vary widely from one observer to another.
>
> (O'Leary, 2014: p. 64)

Practitioners often underestimate their potential to gather a wide range of important information, obtained in natural settings, through observation and interview techniques. Yet observation is a statutory requirement for those of you working within the Early Years Foundation Stage. Practitioners are also often unaware of the power of observation, and their ability to systematically direct that to areas of the child's development that appear not to be progressing as expected. Parvey (2016) does point out that there are disadvantages to observation such as the tendency to provide information only about the 'what' and not 'why'. Observations must be factual and objective, recording in considerable detail what a child is able to do or not do, however, evaluations of such an observation can creep into the territory of speculation, subjectivity and jumping to conclusions. Consideration needs to be taken to match the appropriate type of observational method to the nature of the activity, the temperament of the child, their age and stage of development. However, observations can also create ethical dilemmas about issues of consent, intrusion and confidentiality and these need to be carefully addressed within the policies of the setting.

## Ethical issues

Any process of assessment and identification must be characterised by ethical considerations which Palaiologou (2012) claims must begin with the careful consideration of three things:

1. Why the assessment is necessary.
2. How the records will be kept secure and confidential.
3. How, if and when, to share that information.

The key to this is probably parental involvement, as they can provide corroborating evidence for what is observed in the early years setting, if they are kept up to date and informed throughout the process. It is also part of the SEND Code of Practice (DfE/DoH, 2015) that the views of children, parents and carers are taken into consideration. Children can also be involved in the process even from a very young age, as they can role play, draw, engage with stories and demonstrate co-ordination and memory skills when requested.

So, from an ethical perspective, it is vital to consider whether the assessments are:

- In the best interests of the child.
- Used to aid planning and devise appropriate intervention strategies.
- Likely to cause distress or promote unsafe practices.
- Confidentiality and security is maintained at all times.
- Kept and undertaken purely to see what the child can do, in order to plan an appropriate way forward – next steps.

Practitioners are often concerned about the hazards of highlighting a child as 'at risk' when perhaps they are not, in other words a false positive. Certainly, identification could lead to intervention and more intensive teaching and support being put in place that strictly may not be needed, but such intervention is only ever going to be of value to a child, even if they do not subsequently prove to be dyslexic. Therefore, this should not produce an ethical dilemma. It is surely better to give support now, rather than wait for potential failure to occur. However assessment is undertaken, even by the most expert assessor in the land, there will always be a potential for false positives and false negatives. Clearly what is important to assessment is recognition of the balance between these two.

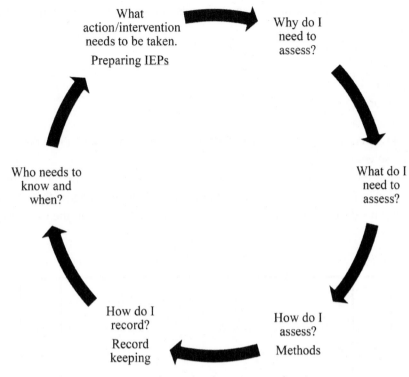

*Figure 7.1* The cycle of assessment planning

---

**Reflect on this**

Badian (1988) undertook a series of assessments on pre-school children using a wide range of potential predictors and claimed that he was able to accurately predict 14 out of 15 subsequent poor readers. However, a number of false positives went on to develop as normal readers.

1. How acceptable do you feel this is?

2. Do you believe that these children were at any disadvantage having an 'at risk' label?

3. How might they have benefited from the intervention which was put in place, which could have positively affected their eventual reading scores?

---

In a bid to understand the complex and differing theoretical positions of dyslexia and how best to assess children with this condition Morton and Frith (1995) put forward an argument that there are three levels of description which intimately interact to produce the condition and assessment needs to take account of each of these. The three levels they describe are:

1. Biological
2. Cognitive
3. Behavioural

Each of these in turn will be influenced by the environmental context in which the child finds themselves (Figure 7.2).

At the top there is the biological element, the concept that dyslexia is genetic and neurological in origin so is likely to be familial. This would suggest that any assessment would need to start with a sensitively taken family history. On the next level there

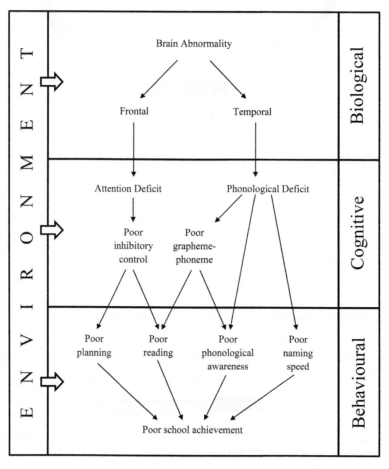

*Figure 7.2* Causal model of dyslexia (Hayes 2016, p. 118: adapted from Frith in Reid and Wearmouth, 2002, p. 58)

needs to be a cognitive or information processing part of assessment and finally the behaviour that can be observed, such as poor reading, difficulties with phonology, co-ordination etc. However, alongside all this is the influence of the environment, family, attitudes, culture etc.

# Birth date

In 1993, Livingston et al. undertook a study to determine whether there was a correlation between birth date and dyslexia. They examined 558 males in schools and did indeed find a relationship between those born in May, June and July and their risk of dyslexia. They hypothesised that it was possible that the incidents of flu like viral infections in mothers in the second trimester of their pregnancy might be the cause of this finding. Livingston et al. (1993) went so far as to suggest that all women of child bearing age should receive flu vaccine. Whilst this is the only study that I could find that came to these same conclusions, a number of other studies in the past have linked autism and flu symptoms in mothers. Johnson et al. (2001) suggested that it could be another indicator to add to the child's profile and yet another question to sensitively ask a parent on admission to the setting. So, Johnson et al. (2001) concluded that the most powerful indicators of an at-risk child would be:

1.  A genetic (familial) disposition
2.  A summer birth date
3.  Difficulties with speech and language development

Peer (2001) also showed a correlation between a summer birth date and dyslexia but it must be remembered that these children are only likely to have one term in a school reception class. This means that by the end of Key Stage 1 these very young children will have experienced considerably less teaching time than those who started school one or two terms earlier.

# Avoidance behaviour

Often it is what the child does not do that is interesting to observe, more than what they do attempt. Johnson et al. (2001) observed what they call avoidance behaviour in children with dyslexia. These children attempt to relieve the pressure of the overwhelming literacy based tasks in their school environment, by undertaking alternative activities. It is entirely possible that such behaviours could be observed in much younger children, but such behaviour could easily be overlooked. This suggests that one area of observation that needs to be undertaken is a detailed review of what activities a child engages with, as well as how they play. Perhaps, to a skilled observer, what they do not play with may give a better insight into that child's potential risk factors.

# Norm based assessment and identification

A number of norm based tests have been developed to assist with the identification of children at risk in the early years. The following is a brief description of just four of these, but there are others available. These are usually commercially produced and sometimes costly and long winded to execute, and it must be remembered that these are screening tests for at risk children and NOT a diagnostic instrument, as a consequence as with all screening programmes, they are never going to be 100% accurate.

### DEST

This is the Dyslexia Early Screening Test devised by Nicolson and Fawcett (1996) and is designed to be administered to children aged 4.6–6.6 years of age, in under 30 minutes. DEST consists of a number of subtests such as:

- Rapid naming of 40 outline pictures.
- Blindfolded bead threading, in a strict time limit.
- Phonological discrimination, where the child is able to detect slight differences in the spoken word such as 'sing' and 'sling'.
- Postural stability, looking at dual task balance activities.
- Rhyme and alliteration, when the child must identify first letter sounds, such as 'king' and 'kick', and rhyming words, such as 'king' and 'ring'.
- Forward digit span, which is a working memory test recalling a series of numbers in order.
- Digit naming and their knowledge of number.
- Letter naming and their knowledge of letters.
- Sound order, requiring the child to identify which sound comes first in a word when the space between them decreases.
- Shape copying.
- Vocabulary.

This is a test that examines not only phonology and memory but also physical skills and speed of processing. It is designed to be administered and interpreted by teachers or specialist classroom assistants, and provides a broad profile of the child to inform the production of an individual education plan (IEP). After examining the research into dyslexia screening tests, the Welsh Government, Llywodraeth Cymru (2012), claimed that DEST gave the best accuracy predictor results of them all at 88% accuracy, and took only 30 minutes to conduct. It is to be noted that there is also a Welsh language version of this screening procedure DEST-W. It is important to emphasise that a child who is identified 'at risk' with the DEST or DEST-W now needs further investigation to take place, and possibly further testing and assessment.

### Nessy Dyslexia Screening Test

This is a computerised programme suggested by the British Dyslexia Association for children aged five to seven years of age. It must be remembered that this is not a standardised test, but is designed for use by teachers, practitioners and parents, to identify 'at risk' children, it does not replace a full dyslexia screening test undertaken by a trained professional.

This test is intended to be fun for the children to undertake and consists of six different levels, with the child 'climbing' Yeti Mountain. It is expected that they complete this within twenty minutes and is very low cost. The aspects that are screened are:

- Visual word memory
- Auditory sequencing memory
- Visual sequencing memory
- Processing speed
- Phonological awareness
- Working memory

It is interesting to note that no physical, social or emotional aspects are screened for, and it was difficult to find any objective, independent evaluation of the screening programme other than that sponsored by the developing company. However, the company concerned does claim to have identification results that closely equate to other more closely researched screening procedures.

### CoPS

The Cognitive Profiling System, devised by Singleton (1995), was first launched by LUCID in 1996 and is a computer-based assessment programme for all children four to eight years of age. It comprises nine tests of cognitive skills presented as games designed to take no more than five minutes each. It is intended for use by classroom teachers and according to the manufacturer it provides standardised and age equivalent scores on areas including:

- Phonological awareness
- Phoneme discrimination
- Auditory short-term memory

- Visual short-term memory
- Visual and verbal sequencing

It should be noted that there are no assessments with this screening programme for physical skills, co-ordination or social-emotional factors.

According to Marks and Burden (2007) there are few independent studies to back up the manufacturers claims that CoPS can predict the cognitive profile of a child. Marks and Burden (2007) tested 66 children at the start of their school career (4–5.6 years), and compared their scores with the results of the children's Standard Assessment Task (SATs) scores at the end of Key Stage 1. Whilst they did find some correlation, they also showed that there needed to be extreme caution regarding the strength of the predictive validity of the tests.

There are clearly advantages to a computerised system, which reduces the pressure on teachers and practitioners, but some have claimed that by not administering the screening themselves they could miss out on identifying more subtle aspects, which a computer cannot 'read'.

### MiST

This is the Middleton Screening Test; the biggest disadvantage to this school-based programme is that it tends to be very long winded, which is difficult with such young children. This test includes the assessment of the child's ability to:

- Follow instructions
- Repeat two sentences verbatim
- Understand digit span
- Play Kim's game
- Sequence – number and letters
- Engage with developmentally appropriate activities using fine and gross motor skills
- Draw and colour appropriately
- Engage with psychomotor skills and the links to writing
- Copy simple shapes
- Undertake rapid naming tasks
- Understand rhyme

Clearly all these tests differ in their theoretical basis, but each presents its own strengths and weaknesses. No screening test is ever going to be 100% accurate, and according to the Welsh Government, Llywodraeth Cymru (2012), literature review of dyslexia research, a more realistic target for predictive accuracy would be 85%. They claim that on average screening tests only ever achieve 75% accuracy, and should identify strengths as well as weaknesses, meaning that results from any screening test need to be viewed with extreme caution. With such young children to screen it is vital to the accuracy of the test that it is quick, but this in turn probably reduces the accuracy of the test. When used across a range of children it also needs to be low cost, and must never replace a full assessment with a qualified psychologist or specialist trained teacher.

Such commercially produced materials do need to be used with great care. Reid (2017) suggests that the results can be heavily influenced by the context of the setting, the approach of the staff and the materials used. Any results, Reid (2017) says, probably only contribute in part to the overall profile of a child, which should include observations and close contact with the family.

It is also important to note that none of the commercially produced assessments relate to children under four years of age, and they are likely to be only snapshot assessments of the child at a particular time in their lives. There are no screening tools that are perfect, and no programme of intervention will benefit every child, which is why ongoing observation and monitoring will be essential to prevent false positive and false negative predictions. This implies that continuous formative assessment, obtained through detailed observation, is likely to be more accurate and informative in the long run. Such good quality, evidence-based observation is also likely to be less costly and does not run the risk of financial implications skewing the data.

# Identification

The following lists some possible characteristic identifiers of dyslexia in the early years, the most important and influential of which is probably the familial aspect of this condition. This is not to say that all children with dyslexia will have a family member who has been identified as dyslexic, or that having a family member who is dyslexic will inevitably mean that a child will be dyslexic. However, it does suggest that perhaps this is a question that could be sensitively asked of parents when they present their child to the nursery, when the staff are attempting to build a profile of the new arrival.

The following is not intended to be a definitive list of identifiers, neither is it intended to be a check list, and as each child is different the indicators for that particular child may also be different. However, in my review of the research and literature surrounding dyslexia these are the most commonly recognised indicators, and where there are clusters of these, it would be advisable to consider that child to be at risk, and for further observations and assessments to be undertaken.

- Family members have been identified as dyslexic or have a specific learning difficulty.
- Speech is often delayed with the child not saying first words until after fifteen months or not speaking in sentences until after two years.

- Baby talk persists for longer than expected (beyond 12–15 months), with difficulties pronouncing words and generally poor articulation – for example, 'jamies' for 'pyjamas' and 'dink' for 'drink'.
- The child often has a very literal interpretation of language – 'Hold on a minute' gets the response 'Hold on to what?'
- The child does not appear to appreciate rhyme – Humpty Dumpty, Mary, Mary Quite Contrary etc.
- Finds it hard to clap or tap a rhythm.
- General difficulties with language and phonology – segmentation weaknesses, blending, recognising the first and last sound in a word.
- Poor application of syntax – the rules of language and grammar.
- Unusual word choices when speaking, and generally a poor vocabulary with short and simple sentences.
- Substitutes words in speech – goalkeeper for goalpost etc.
- The child has difficulties making links between graphemes and phonemes – sound-letter correspondence.
- A visual sensitivity to light flicker is not uncommon.
- Visual stress – resulting in headaches, sore eyes, and even nausea and dizziness.
- The child complains that the letters move on the page, or are muddled up or blurred.
- Finds it difficult to fixate on a word, with associated eye movement difficulties.
- Really enjoys being read to, but has no interest in picking up books to look at on their own. Often deliberately avoids literacy based activities.
- The child constantly changes position in front of the page and rubs their eyes excessively.
- Tires very quickly, especially with a literacy activity, due to the increased concentration and effort required to undertake the task.
- Limited attention span, especially for literacy based activities.
- Short-term memory and sequential problems, so they cannot remember instructions, especially multiple instructions or directions such as 'stand up, pick up the Lego and put it in the box before you sit down on the mat'.
- The child struggles to remember the names of familiar things – rapid automatised naming tasks (RAN tests); these test the child's ability to rapidly name aloud a series of familiar items, such as letters, numbers, colours or objects, to assess processing speed.
- Struggles to learn linear sequence – the alphabet, the order of numbers, tables etc.
- Finds colour concepts hard to establish.
- Has difficulty telling the time and sequencing past, present and future, days of the week, seasons etc.
- Finds difficulty retelling a story in the right sequence.
- Personal organisation difficulties – never where s/he is supposed to be at an allocated time, always losing their possessions etc.
- Unable to easily recognise shapes traced onto the skin with a finger.
- Cannot reliably recognise letters in their own name.

- Slow speed of general information processing.
- Becomes confused when attempting to identify right and left.
- Difficulties with activities that involve spatial awareness such as jigsaws, nesting boxes etc.
- Difficulties with gross motor control such as leg balance, walking backwards etc.
- Often walks without crawling first (the bottom shuffler or tummy wriggler).
- Generally has poor co-ordination, often referred to as the 'clumsy' child.
- Difficulties with specific co-ordination such as catching a ball, kicking, throwing, hopping, skipping etc.
- Finds it difficult to dress and undress, and often cannot remember the sequence of clothing. This is the child who puts a vest over their shirt or consistently puts shoes on the wrong feet etc.
- Difficulties with fine motor skills such as grasping a pencil, using scissors, copying a pattern, drawing, manipulating buttons and tying shoe laces, etc.
- Often appears to be 'not trying' or 'not trying hard enough' – the 'dreamer' who does not appear to be listening.
- The child often has a poor self-image and lacks confidence in their abilities.
- Low birthweight babies (less than 2,500 grams).
- Has been exposed to drugs or alcohol prior to birth.
- Experiences good and bad days for no apparent reason.

A skilled observer will see many of these issues reflected at Frith's behavioural level (Figure 7.2) in a variety of ways during a child's play, if the observer is aware of what to look for.

---

### Reflect on this

1. How are observations used in your setting?

2. Do observations inform your practice?

3. Read the Code of Practice (DfE/DoH, 2015) pages 84–87. Does this offer a good and helpful basis for the work in your setting?

---

April Benasich is a professor of neuroscience, working in the USA. In 2014 she and her team used highly sensitive electroencephalogram brain mapping techniques (EEG) to examine the brains of young babies. They believe that it is possible to identify subtle changes in the brains of these babies (four to seven months) and map them to different components of language, in particular phoneme recognition. They suggest that they can predict, with 90% accuracy, the babies who will eventually have language problems and potentially dyslexia, by the age of three years. Benasich et al. (2014) suggest that if these babies can be highlighted, then appropriate intervention can be put in place from a very early stage to help to prevent failure for the child. They examined primary research undertaken on rats which appeared to show that it was possible to set up more effective language maps in the brain by re-programming their responses to non-speech acoustics. They devised a robot which they called AABY, designed to be used with babies as young as four months. The robot contains an eye tracking device and flashing LED lights to attract the baby's attention. A variety of sounds are played and as the sounds vary a short video clip starts as reinforcement. Benasich suggests that this intervention training can boost sound processing by up to 18 months.

Clearly on the surface, these are exciting results of very different interventions but these are very early results and the concept of our babies surrounded by a collection of high tech gizmos and gimmicks does perhaps not sit well with the classical ideas of Pinker (1994) that learning language is a natural process which human babies are well equipped to do.

## EHC plans/the graduated response

The now repealed Education Act (1993) gave parents of children of any age the right to request that their child be assessed for special needs. This is reinforced by the SEND Code of Practice (DfE/DoH, 2015), emphasising that parents and children must be involved in that assessment. It is incumbent upon you as a practitioner to take account of a child's thoughts, views and wishes, even with the very youngest children, and to devise age and stage appropriate ways to achieve this.

Under the SEND Code (DfE/DoH, 2015), settings must provide appropriate special educational needs support for any child suspected of learning needs. This should take a graduated approach with four key elements (see Figure 7.3):

1. Assessment (identification)
2. Planning (including preparation for transition)
3. Do (implementing an agreed policy)
4. Review (continuous reflection)

These may also require the involvement of other specialist workers, such as health visitors, speech and language therapists, educational psychologist, settings, area special educational needs co-ordinators (SENCO) and the team around the child. This may also lead to the preparation of an Education, Health and Care plan (EHC). An EHC plan replaces the old statements of special educational need and learning assessments, Early Years Action/School Action/Action Plus; like the old statements it is legally enforceable and sets out what support and intervention a child with special needs requires for equality of access, to enable progress within education and to achieve to their potential.

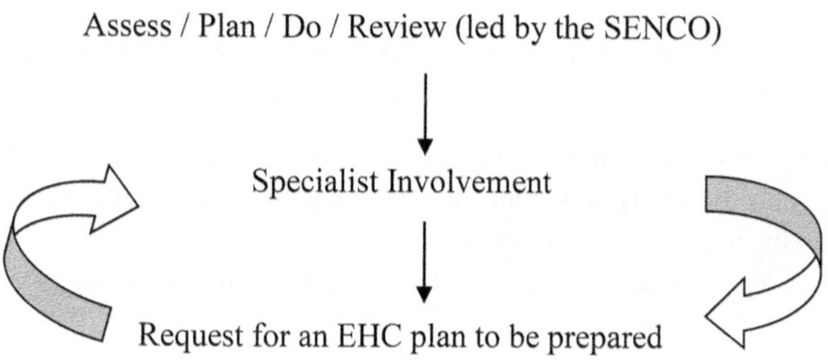

Assess / Plan / Do / Review (led by the SENCO)

Specialist Involvement

Request for an EHC plan to be prepared

*Figure 7.3* Graduated response

Each child referred will go through a needs assessment, and the local authority will use this to decide whether to issue an Education, Health and Care plan. The local authority then has a legal responsibility to fulfil the requirements of the plan and to review that plan at least annually. An EHC plan can be issued for any child or young person aged 0–25 years of age.

The EHC plan is usually developed by the Local Authority with parental support, although they may request that the setting lead this assessment on their behalf, and they require that this is totally child centred to ensure that the child's needs and interests are taken into account. According to the Code of Practice (DfE/DoH, 2015), the assessment is likely to focus on four areas of need:

1. Communication and interaction
2. Cognition and learning
3. Social, emotional and mental health
4. Sensory or physical needs

The Early Years Foundation Stage framework (DfE, 2017b) also deals with issues of Special Educational Need and Disability (SEND), and ensures that every registered childcare setting has an identified SENCO and each child has a named Key Worker. This also requires that the statutory two-year-old checks are maintained, and that as the child transitions to reception class, an EYFS Profile is completed detailing their strengths and weaknesses.

## CASE STUDY

Pamela Phelps was 22 years of age when she went to court to claim that her school had appropriately identified that she was experiencing difficulties, but subsequently failed to put appropriate intervention in place. As a consequence, she left school with no qualifications, poor self-esteem and generally had bad memories of her school days. This, she claimed, severely impeded her ability to gain employment as an adult. This true case brought the legal status of dyslexia to the fore. Eventually after a number of appeals, she awarded £45,650 in damages by the High Court.

1. Do you think that Pamela Phelps was right to sue the local authority and why?
2. Consider the legal phrase 'duty of care'; what do you think this means for you working in the early years sector?
3. Consider the moral and legal implications of the Phelps' ruling.

The Code of Practice (DfE/DoH, 2015) sets out quite strict statutory requirements for the timing and sequence for the writing and instigation of an Education, Health and Care plan as can be seen in the diagram below:

Statutory timescales for EHC needs assessment and EHC plan Development

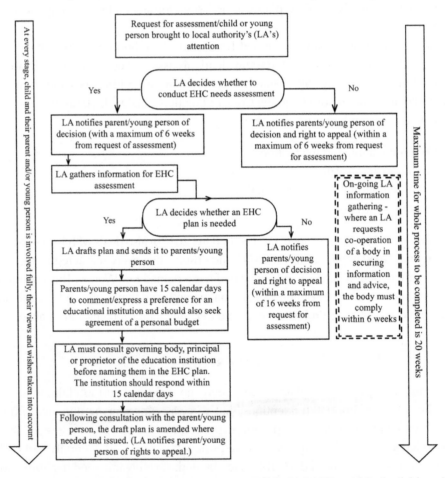

Figure 7.4 Statutory timescales for EHC assessments (DfE/DoH (2015) p. 154). Available online at: www.nationalarchives.gov.uk/doc/open-government-licence/version/2/

The Code of Practice (2015) demands that all people and institutions associated with the child be involved with the preparation of an EHC plan:

- Parents, carers and family – reviewing what happens in the home learning environment, communication, interaction, language, culture, interests and aspirations.
- Child – even the youngest child needs to be involved, this may be through observations, film clips, photographs or by asking them about their interests, friends, likes, dislikes etc.
- SENCO – this person is likely to take responsibility for leading and informing other practitioners, they will coordinate parent/child/professional roles.
- Key person – will build relationships between children, families and the setting. The key person will be particularly important in supporting the child's social and emotional well-being.
- Practitioners/teachers – they will have knowledge of the day to day contact with the child and will notice nuances and changes in the child's behaviour and developmental progress.
- Other professionals – this could be a health visitor, speech and language therapist, general practitioner, educational psychologist etc.

However, coordinating this number of people and consultations, and encouraging them to attend transition and planning meetings will never be an easy task. Each individual local authority is responsible for the process of compiling an EHC, so there are inevitably different processes in each authority, with different paperwork and official procedure. This means that any transfer between local authorities could be difficult, and it could be argued that the EHCs do not have the 'teeth' to appropriately provide for SEND learners in the way that was originally intended, leaving authorities open to legal challenge and case or tribunal law.

## Individual Education Plan

Whilst an Individual Education Plan (IEP) is no longer a legally binding document, or a requirement under the new Code of Practice (DfE/DoH, 2015), it is seen in many quarters as being good practice (see Figure 7.5), and can either stand alone or run alongside the EHC plan if one has been devised.

The main reason for writing an IEP is to inform practice, both in the long and short term, so the importance of accurate, achievable and measurable goal setting cannot be over-emphasised. An IEP needs to start from where the child is now, and allow multiple professionals, practitioners, parents/carers to see, at a glance, how and when progress is anticipated and achieved. For this reason, the objectives need to be both context specific and measurable.

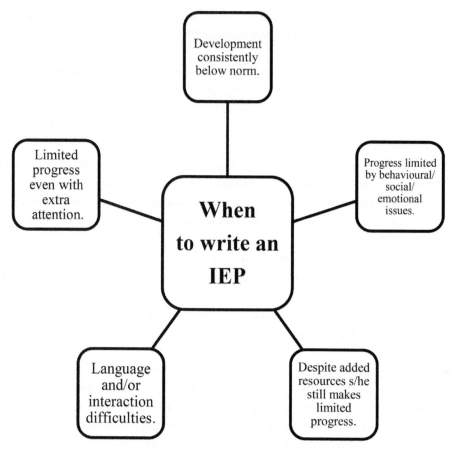

*Figure 7.5* Writing an Individual Education Plan

**Reflect on this**

Examine an IEP for a child with a disability in your setting.

1. Explain how the writer has prepared specific, measurable and achievable targets?

2. Who has contributed to writing this? In your opinion who else should have been involved and why?

3. Explain why it is important for this to have clear time constraints?

4. How accessible is this document for appropriate members of staff?

5. What was the last review date? Why is this important?

6. What security is in place for this document?

Poorly written objectives may look like these:

1. 'Rasha understands the stories read this week by the practitioner.'
   [How do you know that he understands? – you cannot see understanding.]
2. 'Rasha listens to the practitioner's explanation of the activities.'
   [How do you know that he is listening? – you cannot see listening.]
3. 'Rasha's social and emotional skills are developing.'
   [This is an enormous and lifetime objective. Developing in what way and how quickly? This is too broad and cannot be measured or readily observed.]

Better objectives might be:

1. 'Rasha can tell the practitioners three things about each of the stories read this week.'
2. 'Rasha undertakes each activity this week in a behaviourally appropriate manner and without prompting.'
3. 'Rasha can be seen interacting appropriately with at least one other child at play time each day this week.'

The whole concept of an IEP then becomes about the end goals and not necessarily how they will be achieved – the outcomes rather than the process.

# Interventions

Whilst identification of at risk children is an important first step, the significance of preparing well informed intervention programmes is vital. The case of Pamela Phelps in 1997 (seen in the case study earlier in this chapter) illustrates the moral and legal implications of ignoring an assessment when identification has been made. This case also highlights the importance of not only assessment, but of putting in place a well-structured intervention to tackle the particular issues experienced by the child.

Before an effective intervention process can be devised, certain key features need to be considered. Firstly, the way that the child processes and retains information, in other words their short-term memory and retrieval skills, as this will impact upon their understanding and upon how they organise and sequence their learning. In turn this will need to be reflected in the way that potential learning is presented to the child. Reid (2017) talks of three aspects to consider when assessing and screening the 'at risk' child which should influence intervention:

1. Input: this refers to the information that you want the child to learn and how this is presented to them. Careful consideration needs to be made of the pace of learning, breakdown and chunking, thereby encouraging motivation and repetition, and allowing the child to experience success.

2. Cognition (processing): the way in which new knowledge and understanding is organised to ensure ease of retrieval, developing concepts and acquiring and fostering schemas, to enable new knowledge to relate to existing insights.
3. Output: this relates to the way in which the child exhibits mastery of that new learning.

Another consideration must be their attentional capacity. Very young children notoriously have relatively limited attention spans, particularly for things that they find difficult and of no immediate interest, so observing activities with which they do engage will be vital to ensuring concentration and motivation. Older children and adults can defer gratification, often for long periods, consider the undergraduate who embarks on a three-year pilgrimage to achieve a degree, often enduring hours and even days of lectures and reading that they find tedious, but will keep going until the end to achieve their aims. However, children in the early years demand instant gratification, it must be interesting *now* or they will not engage. This level of motivation will be closely bound with self-concept and self-esteem – whether the child believes in themselves enough to believe that they can achieve. For the child with dyslexia, it is likely that self-belief will diminish rapidly if they are presented with more and more activities which they feel unable to achieve. Self-motivation is probably the most powerful learning tool, and encouraging children to learn in an independent and self-motivating manner is a valuable skill to direct their learning throughout life. This independence of learning can, I believe, only be achieved in an open and self-regulated learning environment, so there needs to be an atmosphere where the child feels safe and supported, and encouragement is readily available from uncritical families, practitioners and teachers. A skilled learning supporter will know the importance of deciding when to step in and when to withdraw. This highlights the importance of the child's home learning environment, as well as the nature of the setting. In turn this means a close relationship between settings and parents and carers, with help, advice and guidance readily available to them.

Careful thought needs to go into working with the child who is 'at risk', and in particular the importance of ensuring that they feel that they can achieve success. That means that any new information needs to be presented in small bite sized chunks, which will likely involve breaking down an activity into component parts. An example of this might be the child who finds learning to use scissors difficult, clearly just more of the same is unlikely to work, and will cause frustration and demotivation, but you might consider the following breakdown of using scissors to strengthen hand muscles and be able to hold them correctly, with activities such as:

- Playdough.
- Tearing and screwing up paper into tight balls – first with both hands and then with individual hands independently.

- Squeezing spray bottles in the water play or squeezing sponges.
- Improving pincer grip by picking up money to post into a money box or beads in a container.
- Drawing and scribbling.
- Climbing and grasping, and thereby improving shoulder and arm muscles and co-ordination.
- Snipping pieces of card or coloured paper into random shapes to make mosaics and collages.

It is too easy to overload a child and reduce the motivation to learn; there is an old adage that 'practice makes perfect' and this is probably as true today as it ever was. This inevitably means repetition, repetition, repetition, but all too frequently this results in boredom and 'turn off'. Consider some of the things that you learned at school and what made them boring; I have a theory that says that there are no boring subjects only boring teachers! You have already read that short spells of learning are better than tedium, but presenting material in a number of different, imaginative ways, context driven and relevant to the child will enable repetition to be in place without the child being aware of it. There are so many ways in which creative and imaginative pedagogy can enable the child to learn through repetition without becoming bored and demotivated, using all their senses and a range of positive learning strategies. Only when the child starts to experience success, achieves praise for their efforts and experiences pride in their attainments, can they build trust with you and confidence in your ability to lead their learning and understanding.

When considering an appropriate pedagogy there are some things to take into consideration:

- Teach one thing at a time, combining the small steps into a graduated response.
- Try to analyse the subskills involved in any activity (see above when using scissors).
- Small achievable targets will increase confidence and motivation to continue and progress.
- Allow the child to understand the end targets that are expected.
- Use visual images, concrete experiences and associations with pictorial and diagrammatic ways of recording information.
- Use rhythm, pace and tempo to reinforce learning and recall.
- Support their short-term memory with lists, charts, mnemonics (the funnier the better!), spellcheckers, technology, interactive medium etc.
- Engage the children actively in drama, role play and rehearsal.
- Use jokes, fun and humour to good effect.
- Praise achievements readily in innovative and creative ways.

Technology, if used well, can allow children some control of the pace of their own learning, with access to an immense range of multisensory resources. Technology can also allow children to be proactive in their own learning, and less affected by their immediate environment so that they can continue their learning even when not in the setting

Some writers talk about the importance of adapting interventions to the learning styles of the child (Reid, 2017), that each child has a particular learning style (often referred to as visual, auditory and kinaesthetic [VAK]). I believe that you need to engage with a range of learning styles, as all children need to learn how to learn in a variety of ways, and to suit the management of learning to the nature of the task, rather than attempting to fit tasks into a particular learning style, which may not be appropriate. So the child learning to cook needs to be hands on (kinaesthetic) but listening to a story requires auditory learning and multi-media learning requires visual skills etc.

The range of activities that can be put in place to develop a suitably targeted intervention programme in the early years is endless, and is probably only constrained by your own imagination and resourcefulness. Some suggestions are made below which remain multisensory and can build upon the child's own strengths and interests.

- Learning nursery rhymes and poems, particularly those with actions, such as 'Insey Winsey Spider', 'Wheels on the Bus', 'Miss Polly had a Dolly' etc. These combine working memory, auditory discrimination and physical co-ordination.
- Sequential songs, rhymes and stories such as: 'One, two, three, four, five' or 'The Gingerbread Man' etc.
- Clapping and stamping games, requiring the child to follow a regular beat or use a drum to accompany a song.
- Improving auditory acuity by listening for and identifying sounds from behind a screen, or going on a sound walk around the nursery.
- Singing well-known songs with nonsense words inserted ('If you're happy and you know it clap your "drogs"'). The children can be encouraged to identify the non-word and to make up their own non-words in songs.
- Viewing sequential pictures of everyday activities and putting them in order (getting dressed or having a wash). The children can have fun considering what might happen if they get things in the wrong order – their underwear on the outside of their clothes, shoes on their head etc.
- Matching activities such as jigsaws, nesting boxes, snap and other card games. Snap games can be made with pictures of themselves doing various activities.
- I Spy, using the first letter sounds and later using the last letter sounds ('I Spy with my little eye something ending with T' – cat).
- Scribbling, drawing and colouring, including air drawings and guessing games – draw a number in the air. What is it?

- Tearing and scrunching up paper – scissors.
- Kim's Game.
- Pelmanism and sorting activities.
- Physical skills such as throwing, catching, hopping, skipping etc.
- Telling and retelling stories or 'news' events.
- Picking up objects with tweezers and putting in a jar (this can be timed to make it a game) small sweets, raisins, beads etc.
- Bead threading and making jewellery.
- Mazes to follow using both fine and gross motor skills.
- Dancing and rhythm activities using the whole body.

There are so many commercially produced intervention approaches that it is not possible to critique them all within the confines of this book, most however are aimed at reading and improving reading skills, rather than targeting the at risk, pre-reading child. To be effective it is likely that they will be multi-sensory and sequential, incorporating repetition in a creative and imaginative format, broken down into small and achievable sub-skills. Reading programmes are likely to be highly structured, systematic and include phonics and phonemic awareness elements. Whatever the programme claims to do, it needs to be relevant to the child and to their experiences.

---

### Chapter reflections

Surely there can be no excuse for waiting until a child experiences failure, humiliation and degradation, before appropriate intervention takes place that could prevent that. Goswami (2015) suggested that training phonological awareness in babies and young children could promote literacy development and may help to ameliorate the emergence of literacy difficulties later on in some children. It is very likely that there are large numbers of pre-school children who need to be identified as at risk of dyslexia and then offered the appropriate interventions, yet there appears to be almost nothing done in the UK to work with either this group of young children or those who work with them. Access to support for special needs in England comes through the procedures detailed in the Code of Practice (DfE/DoH, 2015) yet there is very little related to the identification of dyslexia in the early years in this document.

This chapter has demonstrated that successful intervention requires a truly reflective practitioner who is able to think creatively and empathetically about their practice and the impact that this practice has upon the children in their care.

## Further reading

Hayes, C. (2016) *Language, Literacy and the Early Years: A Critical Foundation*. Northwich: Critical Publishing.

This is a basic down to earth book explaining the fundamentals of children learning to speak, listen, read and write. It breaks down some really complex areas into manageable 'chunks' but finally draws it together into a holistic and readable text. There is a balanced approach to theory and research, examining the usual trajectory of language development and some of the deviations along that line. This book gives a firm understanding of the development and observation of language in the early years child.

# References

Badian, N. (1988) Predicting Dyslexia in a Pre-school Population. In Masland, R.L. and Masland, M. (eds) *Pre-school Prevention of Reading Failure*. New York: York Press.

Benasich, A., Choudhury, N.A., Realpe-Bonilla, T. and Roesler C. (2014) Plasticity in Developing Brain: Active auditory exposure impacts pre-linguistic acoustic mapping. *Journal of Neuroscience* 34 (40). Available online at: www.jneurosci.org/content/34/40/13349.full (accessed 20.08.17).

Department for Education (2014) *Early Years: Guide to the 0–25 SEND Code of Practice: Advice for Early Years Providers that are Funded by the Local Authority*. Available online at: www.gov.uk/government/uploads/system/uploads/attachment_data/file/350685/Early_Years_Guide_to_SEND_Code_of_Practice_-_02Sept14.pdf (accessed 18.08.17).

Department for Education (2017a) *Statistics: Childcare and Early Years*. Available online at: www.gov.uk/government/collections/statistics-childcare-and-early-years accessed 03.03.17.

Department for Education (2017b) *Statutory Framework for the Early Years Foundation Stage Setting the Standards for Learning, Development and Care for Children Birth to Five*. London: Crown.

Department for Education/Department of Health (2015) *Special educational needs and disability code of practice: 0 to 25 years*. Available online at: www.gov.uk/government/uploads/system/uploads/attachment_data/file/398815/SEND_Code_of_Practice_January_2015.pdf (accessed 20.08.17).

Education Act (1993) London: HMSO. Available online at: www.legislation.gov.uk/ukpga/1993/35/pdfs/ukpga_19930035_en.pdf (accessed 20.08.17).

Goswami, U. (2015) The Last Word on Dyslexia [Interview with Eleanor Doughty]. *Daily Telegraph* 9 May.

Hayes, C. (2016) *Language, Literacy and the Early Years: A Critical Foundation*. Northwich: Critical Publishing.

Hurst, V. (1991) *Planning for Early Learning*. London: Paul Chapman Publishing.

Johnson, M., Peer, L. and Lee, R. (2001) Pre-school Children and Dyslexia: policy identification and intervention. In Fawcett, A. (ed.) *Dyslexia: Theory and Good Practice*. London: Whurr.

Livingston, R., Balkozar, S.A. and Brach, H.S. (1993) Season of Birth and Neurodevelopmental Disorders: Summer birth is associated with dyslexia. *Journal of American Academy of Child and Adolescent Psychiatry* 32: 612–616.

Marks, A. and Burden, B. (2007) How Useful are Computerised Screening Systems for Predicting Subsequent Learning Difficulties in Young Children? An exploration of the strengths and weaknesses of the Cognitive Profiling System (CoPS1). *Educational Psychology in Practice* 21 (4): 327–342.

Morton, J. and Frith, U. (1995) Causal modeling: Structural approaches to developmental psychopathology. In Cicchetti, D. and Cohen, D. (eds) *Developmental Psychopathology*. New York: Wiley.

Milton, P. (2016) Fearless and Free. In Van Daal, V. and Tomalin, P. (eds) *The Dyslexia Handbook 2016: I am Dyslexic*. Bracknell: BDA.

Nicholson, R. and Fawcett, A. (1996) *Dyslexia Early Screening Test* (2nd edn). London: Harcourt Assessment: Pearson.

O'Leary, M. (2014) *Classroom Observation: A Guide to the Effective Observation of Teaching and Learning*. Abingdon: Routledge.

Palaiologou, I. (2012) *Child Observation for the Early Years* (2nd edn). London: Learning Matters.

Parvey, B. (2016) *Dyslexia and Early Childhood: An Essential Guide to Theory and Practice*. Abingdon: Routledge.

Peer, L. (2001) Dyslexia and its Manifestations in Secondary School. In Peer, L. and Reid, G. *Dyslexia: Successful Inclusion in the Secondary School*. Abingdon: David Fulton Publications.

Pinker, S. (1994) *The Language Instinct*. London: Penguin Books Ltd.

Reid, G. (2017) *Dyslexia and the Early Years: A Handbook for Practice*. London: Jessica Kingsley Publishers.

Reid, G. and Wearmouth, J. (eds) (2002) *Dyslexia and Literacy: Theory and Practice*. Chichester: John Wiley and Sons Ltd.

Singleton, C.H. (1995) *Cognitive profiling system CoPS-1*. Newark, Notts.: Chameleon Assessment Techniques Ltd.

Snowling, M. (2012) Early Identification and Interventions for Dyslexia: A contemporary view. *Journal of Research in Special Educational Needs* 13 (1): 7–14.

Welsh Government – LLywodraeth Cymru (2012) *Research into Dyslexia Provision in Wales: Literature Review on the State of Research for Children with Dyslexia*. Cardiff: Crown.

# English as an additional language

*To learn a language is to have one more window from which to look at the world.*

Old Chinese proverb

## Introduction

It is estimated that 60–75% of the world's population is bilingual/multilingual, so monolingual people like me are in the minority across the globe. According to the National Association for Language Development in the Curriculum (2015), there are one in six primary school children in England who do not have English as their first language; this has more than doubled since 1997. If you include secondary schools, special schools and pupil referral units, that is over one million children. With this number of children involved, it is inevitable that some will have dyslexic tendencies, and will perhaps need additional consideration.

> In the first months infants can discriminate a wide range of sounds, but over time, just by listening to their native language, their receptive language becomes tuned to their native language. The process involved is called 'statistical learning' that tunes up infants' neural networks between 6–12 months to commit to their native language. Children who are multilingual have an extended period where they are able to benefit from receiving this broader range of sounds. This means that their neural commitment is naturally delayed, which brings both costs and benefits.
>
> (Fawcett, 2016: p. 12)

Changes on the world stage have vastly increased the diversity of languages and cultures in our society in recent years, and it is no longer unusual for a setting to admit a child and family for whom English is an additional language. In some settings the numbers of children speaking languages other than English as their first language, exceed the number of English first language speakers, according to Martin (2016), this has come to be known as 'superdiversity'. However, your first language is likely to be full of fruitful vocabulary, idiom, light and shade with history, culture and heritage defining your identity and place in the world in a way that second and subsequent languages may not be. This has been described by many as your 'tool of thought', enabling reflection and problem solving to take place.

## Bilingualism and multilingualism

The type of bilingualism and multilingualism that you have no doubt encountered is likely to be varied, and certainly does not come as one package. There are, for example, children who have been monolingual from birth and come to this country, such as refugee children from places such as Syria and Afghanistan. These children need to learn English from scratch and are immersed in a culture which is very different from their own. Many of these children come from monolingual families proficient in their native tongue only, and therefore do not have home learning immersion in their second language, they still need to communicate with family and friends in their mother tongue; these children often become translators from a very early age.

However, some children are born into bilingual/multilingual homes and will be proficient in two or more languages when they arrive at your setting. One three-year-old that I met had a French father and a Finnish mother, but the parents spoke to her in English; she was able to switch her language code easily and effectively, readily understanding who understood which language. These parents had also enrolled her into a Welsh medium nursery, conscious of the advantages of being able to speak Welsh for employment in Wales at a later stage. Despite already being proficient in three languages she was immersed into a fourth. It is quite common in Wales for English monolinguals to send their children to Welsh medium schools and nurseries, to immerse them into the language, believing it to be advantageous. A similar situation occurs in Canada, where parents elect to send their children to French medium schools, for similar reasons.

The Foundation Phase is the statutory curriculum framework in Wales (Llywodraeth Cymru/Welsh Government, 2015), and is applicable to all maintained and non-maintained settings in Wales catering for children aged three to seven years. The Welsh language development area of learning is a key element of that framework, being one of seven areas of learning (AoL).

> Language skills learned in one language should support the development of knowledge and skills in another.
>
> (Llywodraeth Cymru, 2015: p. 36)

> Children should appreciate the different languages . . . and gain a sense of belonging to Wales and understand the Welsh language, literature and arts as well as the language.
>
> (Welsh Assembly Government, 2008: p. 39)

It is therefore imperative that children should not be regarded as having a learning difficulty solely because their mother tongue is different from the language in which they will be educated.

## Language transparency

Dyslexia appears to be present in all languages, including those which use a non-alphabetic or character based orthography, such as Chinese or Japanese, although the manifestations of the condition may not always be the same. English is a very irregular language, making it difficult to learn as an additional language. English is often referred to as an opaque language or a deep orthography, along with Polish and French, that is, learning all the 'rules' and all the sounds does not guarantee that you can say all the words. Look at the following examples:

| 'f' sound | 'c' sound |
|-----------|-----------|
| eno<u>ugh</u> | ti<u>ck</u>le |
| tele<u>ph</u>one | <u>c</u>igarette |
| <u>f</u>ish | <u>ch</u>ur<u>ch</u> |
| cli<u>ff</u> | <u>c</u>at |
| gira<u>ff</u>e | <u>ch</u>rysalis |

Can you read the following word – ghoti?
Would it surprise you to know that this says fish?

gh as in laugh – 'f'
o as in women – 'i'
ti as in nation – 'sh'

This demonstrates some of the irregularities of the English sound system, which has no consistently direct relationship between grapheme and phoneme. However, some languages are more transparent, consistent and regular, such as Spanish, Welsh, Italian, German, Greek and Hungarian; in these languages once you have established and learned the rules they usually remain the same, except in instances where words are imported from other languages. Such regularity of a language allows readers to use an alphabetic-phonetic strategy for reading and spelling. This can be very effective, especially in the initial stages of language learning. For example, in Welsh, once you know that a single 'f' makes the sound of a 'v' and 'ff' makes the softer 'f' sound, it remains that way throughout the language whenever you see that letter in combination:

hoffi – like                     ofni – afraid
ffatri – factory                 dafad – sheep

Strangely this transparency of orthography may in fact make it harder to identify the children at risk of dyslexia, as it is possible that they will cope better with the complexities of their language learning than the children coping with an opaque language.

Despite the complexity of English, it is overwhelmingly the primary international language being used in most forms of communication between nations. All air traffic control is conducted in English, as is naval and military communication; it is also the diplomatic language of choice and most web pages on the internet are written in English. Therefore, the value to children and adults of learning English for employment and in commercial contexts is enormous. English is taught in almost every country in the world and spoken by 300 million people as their native language; over 2 billion people worldwide speak English as an additional language.

# Advantages of bilingualism

In this country we often take a deficit view of bilingualism, that is, some believe that it is a barrier to learning and therefore a problem. Fawcett (2016) suggests that children learning more than one language at a time are usually slower to achieve literacy in both languages than monolingual children, logically this is probably not surprising. Children identified as 'at risk' of an information processing difference are often encouraged to concentrate upon learning one language effectively but, in some families, this may cause additional stress. These families may find themselves having to choose between their home language and the majority language. In some households the parents speak different languages, which could be different again to the majority language. My experience of talking to parents of children attending Welsh/English bilingual schools clearly reflects their concern that encouraging their children to learn two languages simultaneously will cause confusion, and may impede their learning. However, Fawcett (2016) shows that whilst these children may have delayed English skills when they start school, this is more than compensated for by an improvement in executive skills, improved memory, becoming more creative and versatile in their thinking, enhanced cognitive control, better conceptual transfer, greater metalinguistic awareness and an increased attention span. Conkbayir (2017) also showed that learning more than one language could enhance a child's overall cognitive abilities, with bilingual children often out-performing their monolingual peers in the executive function skills. Conkbayir (2017) describes these executive skills as mental skills that enable you to control your thoughts, emotions and actions. These help you to plan and organise, focus attention, remember instructions and multi-task (such as walking and talking at the same time). Fawcett (2016) fully supports the concept of bilingualism, and suggests that multilingualism allows children to enter a world of enriched language, which not only allows improvement in their intellectual ability, but is also likely to improve the child's awareness of how languages work in general. She even suggests that there could be more lifelong advantages to this increase in executive skills:

> These advantages persist throughout life and protect them from the potential depredations of dementia.
>
> (Fawcett, 2016: p. 18)

However, Fawcett (2016) also warns that:

> In terms of education, by the end of reception the chances of showing a good level of development in EAL children is 10% lower than in their peers but this gap decreases with age, with greater progress between the ages of 7 and 16.
>
> (Fawcett, 2016: p. 12)

Spencer and Hanley (2003), in a small-scale study of five- to six-year-old Welsh language bilingual readers, showed that they were more skilled at phoneme awareness and at reading both real and nonsense words, than the monolingual English speakers. They attributed this to the transparency of the language and orthography of 29 letters, some of which are diagraphs, such as 'ff', 'll' and 'rh'. Siegel (2016) showed that bilingual children often exhibited an enhanced visual memory and Cummins (2012) talks about the advantages of the cross-linguistic transfer, which appears to improve the flexibility of metalinguistics, cognition and phonology.

Cummins (2012) engaged in neuro-imaging research which appears to show that there is an impact on the neural circuitry of the brain when children are bilingual and learning to read. This research was reinforced by Kovelman et al. (2016), who showed that there was greater activity in the left superior temporal region of the brain and less activity in the left inferior frontal regions in bilingual readers than in monolingual readers. They suggested that because dyslexia is often associated with a difference of activity in the left posterior temporal region, that there is a possibility that encouraging early bilingualism could increase the plasticity of these areas in children with dyslexia, which could be particularly helpful in improving their phonological skills. This implies that rather than restricting the child with dyslexia to learning one language, perhaps you should be encouraging them to engage with more than one language.

Conkbayir (2017) talks of two particularly common occurrences in bilingual children: code switching (shifting between two languages, often in the same sentence), and the silent period (this is a well-recognised early stage of second language learning when the child observes and takes account of their new surroundings and the sounds and rhythms of the new language). She suggests that what appears at first to be the child's confusion with two languages is in fact the child trying to decide the most appropriate words to express their needs in the most appropriate language. She claims that this happens particularly when the parents each speak a different language to the child, this she suggests is also what the parents do when they speak with each other and bilingual friends and relations. During the silent period (Conkbayir, 2017), it may appear that there is delayed verbal language development, although gestures and actions indicate understanding. She finds that this is particularly common when the child first starts at school or nursery, when they realise that the setting does not understand their home language. However, rather than being a non-productive period this can be a time of watching, learning, reflection and familiarisation; the child needs encouragement and confidence building to start to create language in the unfamiliar tongue.

## Challenges

Despite the advantages of bilingualism, it is also clear that there are many challenges, particularly so for those with an information processing difference. It is likely that you learned your first language apparently effortlessly and with no formal instruction, and if a very young child is immersed in two or more languages they too will usually learn them simultaneously and incidentally. However, the size of that task is immense and should not be underestimated. They have to learn not only the vocabulary of a language, but also the complex rules and grammar in languages that often have very different syntax, morphology and phonology.

Whilst children, for whom English is not their first language, may have difficulties with language development, children with dyslexia are likely to have additional problems, including difficulties in their first language. It could be suggested that for these children there is also a moral dilemma for practitioners, of which language to base the support around, and whether that matters as these problems are likely to be the same in both languages.

> This suggests that the same underlying cognitive and linguistic component skills that are crucial for learning literacy skills in monolingual or first language pupils (e.g. phonetic awareness, speed of processing, visual processes), contribute across diverse languages and writing systems.
>
> (Reid, 2017: p. 21)

Of course, the difficulties experienced by a child learning a new language could mask the child's risk of dyslexia, and the difficulties that they exhibit could be incorrectly attributed to their second language status.

> Is a child struggling with text simply because the language is unfamiliar, or do they have more deep seated learning difficulties?
>
> (Cline, 2002: p. 206)

Cline (2002) believes that the only way to answer this question is for their carers to have a firm understanding of a child's community, culture, family life, individual characteristics and educational experiences. This needs to be someone who is with that child regularly and consistently, getting to know that child as a person and an individual first and foremost.

According to Palti (2016) the most challenging issues for EAL children who are also at risk of dyslexia are likely to be:

- Phoneme awareness.
- Understanding structures of language such as possessives, plurals, tenses, suffixes etc.
- Understanding that the correct grammatical order of words may change according to the language.
- Rapid retrieval of words.
- Being able to identify the key words in a text to enable skim reading.

---

**Reflect on this**

1. What particular issues are there for bilingual/multilingual children in your setting?
2. What steps could you put in place to address these issues?
3. How could you encourage parent participation with parents who may not speak your mother tongue?
4. What difference do you think that reaching out to non-English speaking parents will make to the children in your care?

---

According to Robertson (2000), a small study by Kim et al. in 1997 used fMRI scanning to show that age was a significant factor when learning a different language. When the second language was acquired after the first language had become habituated, significantly different areas of the brain were engaged, but when both languages were learned simultaneously during early childhood, there was a sharing of activity in the Broca's area of the brain, not apparent when the second language was acquired later. Robertson (2000) concluded that

> the infant brain which is capable of discriminating phonetically relevant differences may modify the perceptual acoustic space based on early and repeated exposure to the native language. These cortical areas would not be as responsive when the second language is learnt, therefore making it necessary for L2 to utilise adjacent cortical areas.
>
> (Robertson, 2000: p. 207)

The social status of a language may also impact societal attitudes towards it, and some communities will attribute more positive values to some languages than another. Lambert (1977) suggests that if the second language has low status, then learning that second language will not be detrimental to the first. However, when the new language is more socially prestigious (as can be the perception of learning English to the first language Welsh speaker), then there is a danger that the first language can be phased out to avoid possible isolation, rejection, low self-esteem, psychological and social problems, making language acquisition more difficult. I am aware of many people who started life as a first language Welsh speaker, who as an adult will say that they are no longer able to speak the language fluently. External cultural and societal factors such as this, combined with internal factors such as dyslexia, will interlink in a highly complex and intricate manner to make literacy acquisition very difficult for the child.

## Culture-fair assessment

Mortimore et al. (2012) emphasise that the first language spoken by a person is often fundamental to their whole cultural identity. However, one of the major difficulties for children who have EAL and also dyslexia is that most norm referenced diagnostic tests and formal screening procedures have been developed in English, making any identification of 'at risk' much harder. This also means that the tests are likely to have a cultural bias to an English monolingual population. The worry is that the confusion caused by this for the child will lead to false positive identification of the risk of dyslexia. In Wales, approximately 25% of primary school children are educated entirely through the medium of Welsh (Fawcett, 2016), and there have been numerous representations to the Welsh Assembly Government to develop an all Wales, Welsh Language screening test. However, a further complication is that Welsh is not a monogamous language, and usage in North and South Wales is often significantly different, sometimes referred to as the 'north/south dialect divide'. The differences are not only in pronunciation but in structure, word format and graphics, for example:

*Table 8.1*

| English | North Wales | South Wales |
| --- | --- | --- |
| Boy | Bachgen | Hogyn |
| Milk | Llaeth | Llefrith |
| Now | Nawr | Rawn |

Professors Angela Fawcett and Rod Nicholson developed the Dyslexia Screening Test (1996), which is now internationally renowned and translated into several different languages. The DST-W is the Welsh version of this test. As you have seen the difference between North and South Walian Welsh is considerable, and in an attempt to address this DST-W is targeted at South Walian Welsh speakers, as Fawcett and Nicholson claim that there is a higher percentage of settings in South Wales, and almost three-quarters of the population in Wales live in the South. Clearly this does not help the Welsh language speaking children living in North Wales. It is likely that all languages differ in their written and spoken formats, and even in their colloquial forms and dialects, there is for example a huge difference between a Scouse accent, spoken by some in Liverpool and a Geordie accent, spoken by some in the North East of England, and this presents a conundrum for anyone devising assessment methods. For example:

Geordie:   Get up the dancers man, it's time for bed (up the stairs).

Scouse:   Going down the ozzy, mate, think I've broken me finger (hospital).

Should you for example adopt the spoken language presentation that the children may be more familiar with, or the more formal literary form, or should you, like Fawcett and Nicholson, opt for the majority vernacular.

Translating a test, word for word, into another language is clearly unacceptable; for example, a refugee child from Syria is unlikely to be familiar with a double decker bus or an acorn from an oak tree. A child familiar with the Kurdish language or Arabic will be more used to reading from right to left, and this can produce left-right confusion. Tests which include reference to alliteration and rhyme are also not likely to translate well from one language to another. So a culture-fair assessment needs to be one that is designed without reliance upon knowledge specific to a particular cultural group, to ensure that those taking the test are not disadvantaged. Peer and Reid (2012) give the example of the Wechsler Intelligence Scale for Children which asks the child what they should do if they find a wallet or a purse on the street, in the UK you would probably expect an answer such as 'take it to the police', but imagine that you were a child from a war-torn country such as Afghanistan or Syria who may indicate that they would leave it alone, for fear that it might be booby trapped and explode in their hands!

Reid (2017) suggests that for children for whom English is not their first language it may be helpful to assess their non-verbal intelligence and the Wechsler Nonverbal Scale of Ability (WNV) compiled by Wechsler and Nalieri in 2006 (also available in Spanish, German, Dutch, Chinese and French) may be a useful measure. This pictorial test can be used with children from the age of four years and is largely language free and culture-fair. It is possible with WNV to gain a measure of intelligence which would not be possible in a language based test, and whilst not designed to assess risk of dyslexia, it may give an indication of a child's overall ability which may be masked by the language barriers. However, even with a pictorial test such as this a child originating from a different societal culture may still have difficulty 'reading' the word, understanding the picture and relating the picture to their own frame of reference.

Reid (2016) refers to two elements that are essential for a truly culture-fair assessment:

1. Materials available to the child (in the language being taught) must have a strong visual component.
2. Materials need to be available in the child's first and most competent language, to ascertain whether dyslexia is present.

Sunderland et al. (1999) developed an assessment procedure, specifically for a bilingual child, which has a face to face interview as the major component. The interview involves assessment of both the child's visual and motor skills but also takes account of the child's language history, previous schooling experiences, language-listening, map reading and the ability to follow directions. However, face to face interviews come with their own in-built difficulties relating to the relationship between the interviewer and interviewee. This can be a particular problem with very young children who may feel pressurised and intimidated, unable to talk openly and freely, by such a procedure.

# Equality of opportunity

It is incumbent upon all settings to ensure that they regularly examine and re-examine their practice and policies to ensure that no child, family or member of staff is placed at a disadvantage because of ethnicity, culture, religion, home language, background, disability, gender or ability. This is particularly stark when related to special educational needs such as dyslexia, and to those for whom English is an additional language. Such reviews must take account of the involvement and participation of local neighbourhoods, communities and the families that live within them. This may require reconfiguration and restructuring of the policies of the setting to ensure full diversity and inclusivity of the pedagogy, curricular framework and experiences of the children and their families.

# Pedagogy and intervention

One difficulty that practitioners often encounter is that having identified that a child could be 'at risk' of an information processing difference, they are uncertain of the appropriate intervention strategies and this is particularly so when the child has English as an additional language. It is important to ensure that a child's first language, whatever that may be, is always respected and practitioners need to be reassured that success in one language is likely to support the success in a second or subsequent language. Pavey (2016) suggests that a pedagogy which does not take sufficient account of a child's first language (concentrating only on assimilating the second language) could not only cause resentment, but could also be an additional barrier to further learning. Cummins (1986) claimed that the whole issue of multilingualism needed to be seen as the responsibility of the whole setting, and that the outcomes for EAL children depend on the setting's ability to adapt to the cultural aspects of the children by embedding them into the day to day running of the setting. This holistic approach to the pedagogy, assessment, and social and emotional learning needs to involve parents, the community and the curriculum framework (Cummins, 1986).

The challenges that this change in the culture of the pedagogy engenders cannot be overemphasised, particularly when many settings are faced with numerous languages being spoken throughout the setting. According to the 2013 school census, analysed by the National Association for Language Development in the Curriculum (NALDIC, 2015), nearly three hundred different languages are recorded as spoken in English schools, the most frequently spoken are Punjabi, Polish, Urdu and Arabic. In places such as Tower Hamlets and Newham in London 75–76% of the settings have a majority of children who are bilingual. Just putting 'Welcome' in 40 different languages on the nursery door, which I often see, does not really address the complexities of this level of diversity.

---

**CASE STUDY**

Nadya is four years old and goes to a predominantly English-speaking nursery. Her home language is Urdu and when she came to the nursery last year, she had no effective English communication. At home Nadya uses only Urdu to her family who do not speak English. Slowly her understanding of English has emerged, but her spoken language is developing much more slowly and her social and emotional development is now giving rise for concern.

The staff in the setting find it hard to communicate with the family when they come to collect Nadya.

---

- Are Nadya's difficulties the result of her bilingual background or could they be demonstrating a risk of an information processing disorder?
- How could you tell?
- Does Nadya's first language matter when trying to assess her difficulties?
- What holistic impact do you think her cultural and linguistic background can have on her? Consider this from both positive and negative aspects.
- What resources do you think would be helpful to assess Nadya, and to implement an effective intervention programme?

The case of Nadya also brings up the issue of how the home learning environment values the learning of English. Whether the families really do support the bilingual learning, or whether they regard this as a low priority issue. Hartas (2006) warns that learning English for these children could be influenced by social, cultural and political factors which are wider ranging and more complex than the setting may be able to address. Hartas (2006) talks of a continuum process on three levels, as shown in Figure 8.1. Hartas (2006) claims that a lack of support, on any one of these levels, is likely to have a negative effect on the child and their ability to learn another language.

The importance of children in the early years developing sound oral skills cannot be over emphasised. This is particularly so for children for whom English is an additional language and is even more significant in their first language, where they come to understand that association between sound/word and object or action. Hartas (2006) rightly points out that good oral skills are an essential precursor to reading and literacy, so

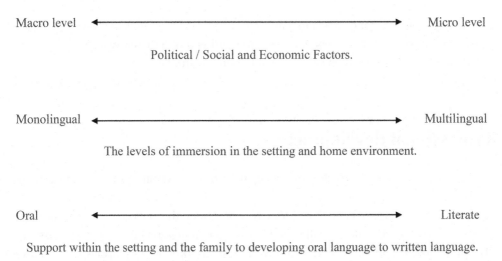

Figure 8.1 Continuum of support

within the nursery setting the importance of developing good listening skills is crucial. Listening clearly involves hearing but listening is far more than this. The children need to be able to distinguish different sounds and differentiate between them, different sounds in the two languages being attributed to a similar object or action (Hayes, 2016). This needs to be sustained over a period of time, enough to understand different rhythms of the languages, different rhymes etc. Listening also demands the ability to concentrate and to filter out distractions and erroneous sounds. Activities which enhance these skills need to be incorporated into the day to day activities of the child such as:

| | | |
|---|---|---|
| Stories | Rhymes and jingles | Listening to and creating music |
| Stop-go games | Audio equipment, recording and listening | Listening to others' news |
| Quiet times to listen to environmental noises | Puppets | Telephones |
| Listening guessing games | Tapping rhythms | Role play |
| I Spy | | |

A study by Moll et al. (2016) showed that pre-school children with oral language difficulties were at high risk of dyslexia, although that relationship was not fully understood. What they found was that early language skills predict code ability with related skills, that is phoneme awareness, letter knowledge and rapid automatised naming. These in turn are highly predictive of later literacy difficulties.

> Findings suggest that dyslexia in Slavic languages has its origins in early language deficits, and the children who succumb to reading problems show impaired code related skills before the onset of formal reading instruction.
>
> (Moll et al., 2016: p. 120)

## Professional development

Considering the rapid expansion of immigration to this country within the last twenty years, it is vital that greater attention is given to ensuring that multilingual education allows all children to succeed in our society. Compound this with the near certainty that a proportion of these children will have information processing differences, it is essential that practitioners and teachers working with these children receive appropriate training with a firm understanding of how linguistics, culture, family and socio-economics can influence their educational potential. Most training providers do not currently offer specific initial training about teaching children with specific learning difficulties, and most do not offer training in teaching children for whom English is not their first language. When both challenges combine in a child, staff are often at a loss as to how to cope, and often there is no knowledgeable and specialist support available. The demographics of our society are very different today compared to even twenty years ago and initial training of teachers and practitioners needs to reflect this, alongside in-service professional development. Unfortunately, it is possible that the trainers themselves have little or no training for working with children for whom English is an additional language and who may also have SpLDs. Therefore, policies need to be reviewed to include bilingualism and information processing differences, alongside rigorous professional development, to ensure that all staff working with children are approaching them with greater knowledge and understanding of the possible issues involved.

## Chapter reflections

This chapter has shown that when working with children at risk of dyslexia who are also bilingual/multilingual, the child's academic, social, emotional and cultural development all need to be carefully considered. Without a level of understanding and sensitivity these children can easily struggle academically, socially and emotionally through their lack of self-belief and then feelings of failure can easily spiral out of control.

There are so many challenges facing practitioners working with young children and each will come with financial constraints, training and identification issues and need to be prioritised accordingly. However, with the explosion in numbers of English as additional language children attending schools and nursery settings, the imperative is to cater for the particular needs of these children. By the law of averages a small number of these children will also be dyslexic, compounding their difficulties further and potentially causing distress and anxiety for both them and their families.

As this is a world-wide problem it is vital that we liberally share research internationally as only then can we develop appropriate, culture-fair tests and assessment methods in a range of languages and dialects. It is also vital that those working with these children have a greater awareness of how children acquire language, and the particular issues which surround children with dyslexia. This is likely to mean better initial training of both teachers and practitioners to ensure that they have the most up to date and advanced knowledge upon which to base the development of their practice and pedagogy.

Movement between nations and cultures has brought about globalisation and rapid language diversity to traditionally monolingual cultures, which has brought with it demands which perhaps our research, thinking and pedagogy have not yet managed to catch up with. This must be a key challenge for educationalists of the future.

# Further reading

Peer, L. and Reid, G. (2016) *Multilingualism, Literacy and Dyslexia: Breaking Down the Barriers for Educators* (2nd edn). Abingdon: Routledge.

This is the most comprehensive text that I could find on this subject area, written by two leading experts in the field. Understanding the difference between literacy difficulties caused by additional languages and dyslexia is difficult for anyone and particularly the practitioner in the setting trying to help children in their care. This book helps to guide you through the complexities and the manifestations of dyslexia that could be masked by an inexperienced user of a language. This is certainly an authoritative text for teachers, practitioners and SENCOs.

# References

Cline, T. (2002) Issues in the Assessment of Children Learning English as an Additional Language. In Reid, G. and Wearmouth, J. (2002) *Dyslexia and Literacy: Theory and Practice*. Chichester: John Wiley and Sons.

Conkbayir, M. (2017) *Early Childhood and Neuroscience: Theory, Research and Implications for Practice*. London: Bloomsbury.

Cummins, J. (1986) Empowering Minority Students: A framework for intervention. *Harvard Educational Review* 56 (1): 18–36.

Cummins, J. (2012) The Intersection of Cognitive and Sociocultural Factors in the Development of Reading Comprehension among Immigrant Students. *Reading and Writing* 25 (8): 1973–1990.

Fawcett, A. (2016) Dyslexia and Learning: Theory into practice. In Peer, L. and Reid, G. (eds) *Multilingualism, Literacy and Dyslexia: Breaking Down the Barriers for Educators* (2nd edn). Abingdon: Routledge.

Fawcett, A. and Nicolson, R. (1996) *Dyslexia Screening Test*. London: The Psychological Corporation.

Hartas, D. (2006) *Dyslexia in the Early Years: A Practical Guide for Teaching and Learning*. Abingdon: Routledge.

Hayes, C. (2016) *Language, Literacy and Communication in the Early Years*. Northwich: Critical Publishing.

Kim, K.H.S., Relkin, N.R., Lee, K.-M. and Hirsch, J. (1997) Distinct Cortical Areas Associated with Native and Second Languages. *Nature* 388: 171–174.

Kovelman, I., Bisconti, S. and Hoeft, F. (2016) *Literacy and Dyslexia Revealed Through Bilingual Brain Development*. International Dyslexia Association. Available online at: https://dyslexiaida.org/literacy-dyslexia-revealed-through-bilingual-brain-development/ (accessed 20.08.17).

Lambert, W.E. (1977) Effects of Bilingualism on the Individual. In Hornby, P.A. (ed.) *Bilingualism: Psychological, Social and Educational Implications*. New York: Academic Press.

Llywodraeth Cymru/Welsh Assembly Government (2008) *Learning and Teaching Pedagogy*. Cardiff: WAG.

Llywodraeth Cymru/Welsh Government (2015) *Curriculum for Wales: Foundation Phase Framework*. Available online at: http://gov.wales/docs/dcells/publications/150803-fp-framework-en.pdf (accessed 20.08.17).

Malaguzzi, L. (1920–1994) (Translated by Lella Gandini) *No way. The hundred is there*. Available online at: www.reggiochildren.it (accessed 21.08.17).

Martin, D. (2016) Multilingualism and Dyslexia: A critical perspective. In Peer, L. and Reid, G. (eds) *Multilingualism, Literacy and Dyslexia: Breaking Down the Barriers for Educators* (2nd edn). Abingdon: Routledge.

Moll, K., Thompson, P.A., Mikulajova, M., Jagercikova, K., Kucharska, A., Franke, H., Hulme, C. and Snowling, M. (2016) Precursors of Reading Difficulties in Czech and Slovak Children at Risk of Dyslexia. In Talcott, J. (ed.) *Dyslexia an International Journal of Research and Practice* 22 (2).

Mortimore, T., Hanson, L., Hutchings, M., Northcote, A., Fernando, J., Horobin, L., Sanders, K. and Everett, J. (2012) *Dyslexia and Multiculturalism: Identifying and Supporting Bilingual Learners who might be at Risk of Developing SpLD/Dyslexia*. Bath: BDA.

National Association for Language Development in the Curriculum (2015) *EAL pupils in schools: The latest statistics about EAL learners in our schools*. Available online at: www.naldic.org.uk/research-and-information/eal-statistics/eal-pupils/ (accessed 21.08.17).

Palti, G. (2016) Approaching Dyslexia and Multiple Languages. In Peer, L. and Reid, G. (eds) *Multilingualism, Literacy and Dyslexia: Breaking Down the Barriers for Educators* (2nd edn). Abingdon: Routledge.

Pavey, B. (2016) *Dyslexia and Early Childhood: An Essential Guide to Theory and Practice*. Abingdon: David Fulton.

Peer, L. and Reid, G. (eds) *Multilingualism, Literacy and Dyslexia: Breaking Down the Barriers for Educators* (2nd edn). Abingdon: Routledge.

Reid, G. (2017) *Dyslexia in the Early Years: A Handbook for Practitioners*. London: Jessica Kingsley.

Robertson, J. (2000) The Neuropsychology of Modern Foreign Language Learning. In Peer, L. and Reid, G. (eds) *Multilingualism, Literacy and Dyslexia: Breaking Down the Barriers for Educators* (2nd edn). Abingdon: Routledge.

Siegel, L. (2016) Bilingualism and Dyslexia: The case of children learning English as an additional language. In Peer, L. and Reid, G. (eds) *Multilingualism, Literacy and Dyslexia: Breaking Down the Barriers for Educators* (2nd edn). Abingdon: Routledge.

Spencer, L.H. and Hanley, J.R. (2003) Effects of Orthographic Transparency on Reading and Phoneme Awareness in Children Learning to Read in Wales. *British Journal of Psychology* 94 (1): 1–28.

Sunderland, H., Klein, C., Savinson, R. and Partridge, T. (1999) *Dyslexia and the Bilingual Learner: Assessing and Teaching Young People who speak English as an Additional Language*. London: Borough of Southwark Language and Literacy Unit.

Wechsler, D. and Nalieri, J.A. (2006) *Wechsler Non-verbal Scale of Ability*. London: Pearson Educational.

# Is my setting dyslexia friendly?

*If a child can't learn the way we teach maybe we should teach them the way they learn.*
Accredited to Ignacio Estrada, grants administrator at the Gordon
and Betty Moore Foundation, San Francisco

## Introduction

What is a dyslexia friendly setting? The initial idea for the concept was suggested by Neil MacKay, as he worked as a SENCO teacher in a comprehensive school in North Wales and then adopted by the British Dyslexia Association (BDA), who developed their Dyslexia Friendly Quality Mark. This quality assurance mark is awarded to schools, further education and higher education centres that, in their opinion, provide an environment where children and young people with dyslexia can thrive and excel.

> Holding the BDA Dyslexia Friendly Quality Mark is a very positive statement that tells learners, parents, staff and stakeholders that your school is a safe place for dyslexic individuals.
>
> (Cochrane et al., 2012: p. 7)

There is no equivalent quality mark for settings outside the schools arena, but it could have a trickledown effect as it is based around four basic standards:

- Leadership and management
- Learning and intervention
- Environment
- Parent partnership (and other interested parties)

The philosophy behind the BDA Quality Mark is that the sort of practice required to assist children with dyslexia is probably good practice for all children, and should therefore be incorporated into all settings for the benefit of all.

A Dyslexia Friendly setting is also going to value parental contributions; it understands that parents are likely to be concerned and anxious about their child. A child at risk of dyslexia in your setting is actually a family at risk of dyslexia, and the consequences of the condition are likely to radiate out into both the nuclear and extended family. A Dyslexia Friendly setting is very aware, not only of the familial nature of dyslexia but also the family involvement, and this will be explored throughout this chapter.

## Dyslexia Friendly

MacKay (2005) observed that the education of children with dyslexia, in most mainstream settings, focused almost entirely upon their weaknesses and deficits; as a consequence there was an emphasis on remediation and special needs provision. He was really the first person to attempt to progress the concept of dyslexia from a difficulty to a difference. MacKay started from the premise that dyslexia was about strengths as well as weaknesses, and that settings that successfully work with children with dyslexia, are able to build upon these strengths.

> Dyslexic learners are often imaginative and creative lateral thinkers who develop original solutions to problems. They may be skilled in design and construction, IT etc., often seeming to 'know' how things work without reading instructions, manuals etc.
>
> (MacKay, 2005: p. 6)

MacKay (2005) claims that the specific difference only becomes a difficulty when the dyslexic child is required to learn in a manner that places unnecessary emphasis on accurate language and literacy as an end product. His starting point is that Dyslexia Friendly is not about special needs, nor should it be solely within the domain of the SENCO, but it is more to do with the busy, non-specialist teacher/practitioner, meeting the needs of all the children in their care. MacKay (2005) also stresses that to be successful this needs to be a policy for the whole setting, and is about inclusion, differentiation and general good practice, thereby enhancing the education and well-being of all the children in that setting. His concept of Dyslexia Friendly is in fact 'learning friendly' or 'mind friendly', when applied to all children.

One key factor in a Dyslexia Friendly setting is the 'feel-good factor', the ability to ensure that learners have high self-esteem, clearly secure in their own understanding of their strengths and weaknesses, knowing that they can build on these in the way that we all acknowledge our various strengths and weaknesses. This means that teachers and practitioners must know how and when to give appropriate support to any vulnerable learners. MacKay (2005) believes that fear, stress and anxiety are the key factors in academic failure, and settings that generate that anxiety cannot hope to get the best from their children. I am sure that you can remember instances in your life when an adult/teacher/bully has created the sort of anxiety that has paralysed your ability to think straight and act logically and intelligently. In my school the maths teacher ruled the class with a combination of fear and physical violence; despite my anxiety about her reactions to me, I was unable to learn and came last each year in her form tests and assessments. Her shouting and admonishments, far from encouraging me to concentrate and learn more, had the opposite effect, and lying in bed at night afraid of the next day's teaching is not the way to learn effectively.

MacKay (2005) claims that 80% of learning difficulties for children at risk of dyslexia are due to this type of stress; he suggests that a Dyslexia Friendly setting is supportive, non-judgemental and empowering, and this is achieved through the use of positive language and expectation. He cautions the use of language such as 'Must try harder' to be replaced with 'Yes, it can be hard in places, but I can help you with some of it'. This implies that they are trying their hardest but we all need help at times. MacKay (2005) describes this as 'the language of success' building confidence and self-esteem.

---

**Reflect on this**

Reflect upon how comfortable you think children identified as at risk of dyslexia, are in your setting.

- Do they have the resources needed to ensure that their health and wellbeing (both mental and physical) is well catered for?
- How does your setting show that they respect every child, their backgrounds, abilities, cultures and family structures?
- How are the developmental needs of the children in your setting met, to ensure equality of learning opportunity?
- How does your setting involve parents and other professionals in a collaborative and inclusive manner?

---

# Fear, stress and anxiety

Alexander-Passe (2015) believes that it is important to understand the difference between fear, stress and anxiety, as often these are grouped together as the same thing. He describes these as:

- Fear: a normal response to a definite and imminent threat (such as confronting a burglar in your house).

- Stress: what is caused by an existing stressor or daily pressures and can be long term (you may have experienced this at work when preparing for an Ofsted inspection).
- Anxiety: worrying about what could potentially happen. This can be a result of stress.

When an individual is highly motivated towards a particular objective (in the case of dyslexia, literacy and reading), they are unlikely to accept any alternative. When this happens frustration occurs, which often results in aggression directed outwards towards the person or thing believed to be the instigator of the frustration, and/or inwards to the self, with feelings of anxiety and guilt. Such traumatic inner emotional states often result in feelings of failure and low self-esteem. Fear of social disapproval, of letting people down can trigger anxiety and possibly even more importantly self-disapproval and loathing for failure. Eventually the child fears performing activities, or engaging in situations in which they feel that they are exposing their incompetence and personal inadequacy to social disapproval.

This avoidance behaviour results in attempts to evade situations where this will occur, and will tend towards easier and less challenging tasks that involve only a moderate degree of risk. This often results in children sticking to tasks that they find familiar, less challenging and perhaps no longer age appropriate. Tasks which are perceived as difficult are liable to deteriorate due to lack of practice and use, thereby negatively impacting learning, but in the child's eyes it is an attempt to protect themself from further psychological harm.

High levels of anxiety can produce increased levels of adrenaline, which cause a rise in heart and breathing rates, increased blood pressure, higher body temperature, excessive sweating and the child can become tense, fidgety and restless. Butterflies in the stomach make it hard to think, and confusion sets in, making it difficult to make well founded choices. For some children this can also result in physiological problems with sleep disruption, nightmares, nail biting, uncontrolled crying or laughing, sickness and diarrhoea, even stammering and oral language difficulties.

Some stress and anxiety is good and perfectly normal, it 'keeps you on your toes'. If you are faced with a threat, such as a herd of cows running towards you on a dog walk, your flight/fight response, quite properly, materialises and allows you to react quickly and appropriately to the challenge. However, when this state of anxiety remains after the initial trigger is removed, the body can act in a very different way and can cause a 'freeze' or 'shut down' (Alexander-Passe, 2015). These emotional states are particularly likely in the early years, when the child may be aware that they are struggling to do things that others appear to do easily, but it is unlikely that dyslexia or an information processing disorder will have been identified, so they do not understand why these problems occur and how it can impact their learning, so they and their families understandably conclude that they are 'just thick'.

# Risk taking

It is important to understand that what may be stressful to one child could be quite normal to another and Alexander-Passe (2015) emphasises that stress is normal, and can work to the good. No doubt you consider it your role to protect children from harm, but it is not always possible to remove all stress, and may not even be desirable. Emotional development can be enhanced through risk, although often when that overprotection is first removed it can be a big shock.

Defining risk is more problematic, especially in today's risk averse society, because acceptable risk will vary depending on a range of conditions, such as the age of the child, prior experience, special needs and context, so what may be acceptable risk for one child in one context may not be for another. So risk refers to probability, likelihood or chance of an adverse reaction; it is a value judgement about the likely outcomes (Ball et al., 2013).

Clearly when you consider risk for your children you need to take a balanced approach between risk and safety. All life contains risk from the moment that you get up in the morning – walking downstairs, cooking breakfast, driving the car to work etc. – so risk is at the very heart of being alive, and without it you would not learn anything new. Think about babies learning to walk, they certainly risk taking a tumble and hurting themselves, but unless they pull themselves up on the furniture for the first time they will never learn to walk and be mobile. So risk is about being prepared to 'have a go' and if you prevent this, for fear of injury and harm, they will never progress; in fact I would go so far as to say that, in some circumstances, preventing children from risk taking is abuse.

Risk taking is something that is frequently associated with physical development, as in the examples above; however, all new learning carries risk, the risk of not succeeding. Imagine the child on their first day at nursery, if they are going to make friends they have to break into other friendship groups, they have to risk social rejection when they go over to another child and ask them to play. In the same way when you go to a party where you know very few people, remember how hard it is to approach strangers talking in a group, and have the courage to join in with the conversation – this is social risk taking. What are you risking? You are risking humiliation when the group turns away or looks at you in a disapproving manner; you risk embarrassment about what others may think of you and how this might influence the future, maybe a job or a relationship, so social risk taking can be high stakes.

Risk taking is associated with all learning, such as learning to talk and learning to read. In the early years children are learning new words at an amazing rate, some estimate as many as nine new words a day. This means not only that they recognise these words or even understand their meaning, but they are able to use these words in the appropriate context. Of course, sometimes there are mistakes, and you have all experienced trying to maintain your composure when a child uses a word in an inappropriate context. A sensitive adult will understand that children need to practise their language acquisition, and will allow for a number of mistakes to be made before ultimate success – 'practice makes perfect'.

As a Welsh language learner, I know how hard it is to create language, however good your receptive language and understanding is. I often know what I want to say, and think that I have the correct syntax and pronunciation, but I frequently lose courage when faced with a fluent Welsh speaker in a shop, and take the 'coward's' way out by asking for the item in English rather than Welsh. Why am I so reluctant to use the language that I know that I have? I am risking the shop keeper laughing at me for my efforts, belittling my attempts, ignoring me, or even refusing to take the time to listen carefully to my rather slow and laboured sentences. In the early years when the child is learning their mother tongue, or even more than one language simultaneously, they must feel very like this, but unless they are prepared to take the risk and use, and practise, the language that they have, it is unlikely to progress their language learning and for some children this results in the 'silent period' that you have already read about in the last chapter, or even selective mutism.

Similar risk taking is required to learn to read. I have often observed young children sitting beside an adult, painfully sounding out word after word in their reading book, with a look on their face that implies distress and anxiety, worried about taking the risk and saying a word for fear of the adult's reaction.

However, unsuccessful attempts at new learning in all areas of development, can be an important part of the learning process, depending upon how they are managed and whether the children perceive this as a positive or negative experience. Statistically the more the child speaks the more likely they are to expose themselves to the risk of failure, however they need to challenge themselves, to take academic risks, to try out their language, to practise, to enable them to build confidence and independence of thought.

> Over emphasis on safety creates the biggest risk of all – that of creating a generation of children who may become either reckless in their pursuit of thrills and excitement, or risk averse, lacking the confidence and skill to be safe and also lacking the disposition to be adventurous, creative and innovative in their thinking.
>
> (Tovey, 2014: p. 24)

## Social and medical models of dyslexia

The whole concept of Dyslexia Friendly appears to be based largely on a social model of disability, which is an assumption in Norwich's words, that:

> Disabled people are disabled by prejudice and discrimination.
>
> (Norwich 2009: p. 182)

Norwich (2009) describes this as a social model of disability, implying that simply by providing an inclusive environment or encompassing society, free of discrimination, these children will be aided to achieve their potential. Norwich (2009) argues that this is a very one-sided view of disability which is more to do with our 'blame culture', our insistence, in modern society, that someone or something is to blame for all the difficulties experienced – blame an individual for not trying hard enough, or blame society for not providing an appropriate environment.

> Although the social model is not explicitly presented as about responsibility attributions, advocates of the social model seem to assume that it is because it diverts moral blame away from those with difficulties. And in focusing blame on those in authority this provides the basis for political action. However, it is also relevant that the concept of 'dyslexia' has functioned to divert blame from individual children who struggle with literacy learning.
>
> (Norwich, 2009: p. 184)

However, this is not to ignore a medical model of dyslexia, and looking back at Chapter 3, you can see the strength of research into the genetic origins for dyslexia, meaning that there are physiological and neurological roots within the individual beyond their control. An understanding of these opposing models must contain a balance between these two explanations, and the way in which the environment impacts upon what we are born with, the epigenesis between the two (Figure 9.1).

An example of this might be a child born to tall parents, who may grow to be over two meters tall and become a top-flight basketball player, a route not considered by the relatively diminutive 1.6 metre jockey. The height difference did not make them take these very different roles, but society, culture and their environment acted upon their

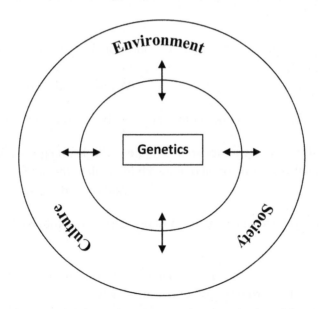

*Figure 9.1* Epigenesis between social and medical models

biology to steer them along a particular path, implying an interaction of social, psychological and biological factors.

# Inclusion

Whilst I am sure that you are all familiar with the term 'inclusion' and the emphasis placed on it by the Government, Ofsted and other inspection and regulatory bodies, it is likely that you will find defining the term much more difficult. You will probably be able to say what it is not quite easily. It is certainly not about treating all children the same. It is not about physical proximity. It is not about integration, with adaptations made for the child, but then expecting them to fit into the existing structures.

After researching this section extensively, I am still not really sure what is meant by inclusion. If it means putting all the children into one mainstream setting and 'doing your best' to supply their needs, is this enough? It could mean providing specialist help, with targeted resources in the mainstream setting, but is this exclusionary if the child is taken aside for the specialist help, often missing important play sessions or physical activity etc.? Could it even mean providing for their needs in a specialist unit or separate setting, where staff have expert knowledge and training in the particular needs of these children to achieve their potential? What is clear is that inclusion has economic, sociological, political and educational implications so needs to be seen in a more global perspective than just one setting or one group of individuals.

Warnock and Norwich (2010) suggested that inclusion was not about a setting or a physical place but about a process. They talk about inclusion in terms of a common curriculum.

> Including all children in the common educational enterprise of learning, wherever they learn best.
>
> (Warnock and Norwich, 2010: p. 14)

Perhaps you should also consider the statement by Waldron and McLeskey (1998):

> While inclusion may work for some children with learning disabilities some of the time, it will not work for all of these children all of the time.
>
> (Waldron and McLeskey, 1998: p. 37)

The definition which I found to be the most persuasive was from Nutbrown et al. (2013) which was:

> The unified drive towards maximal participation in and minimal exclusion from early years settings, from schools and from society.
>
> (Nutbrown et al., 2013: p. 8)

Nutbrown et al. (2013) do point out that there are almost as many definitions of inclusion as there are settings, and the potentially exclusionary elements that could be considered within this category can be extensive, for example:

*Table 9.1* Potentially exclusionary elements

| | |
|---|---|
| Age (of child or parent) | Behaviour |
| Disaffection | Emotional and behavioural difficulties |
| Parental employment | Gender |
| Housing | Language |
| Mental health | Body weight and physical appearance |
| Physical impairment | Poverty |
| Race / ethnicity / nationality | Religion |
| Sexual orientation | Social class |
| Special educational need | |

(List adapted from Nutbrown et al., 2013).

A discussion of 'rights' has to be central to any debate on inclusion, and for this you could revisit the United Nations Convention on the Rights of the Child (UNESCO, 1992). However, it must be remembered that with 'rights' come 'responsibilities'. These responsibilities apply to parents/carers and practitioners, to ensure that all children are able to achieve to their potential and any barriers to that achievement are opened up and drawn aside.

> Inclusion is always a 'state of becoming'. There can be no such thing as a fully inclusive 'arrived-at' institution or society.
>
> (Nutbrown et al., 2013: p. 3)

## Reflect on this

1. Consider your own setting, how inclusive do you think that it is?
2. Compile a list of reasons for your answer to question one, or highlight specific incidents of inclusive practice, which you have observed in your setting.
3. How could your setting improve on its levels of inclusivity?
4. How inclusive do you think your setting is for the staff who work there?
5. What workplace accommodations can be put in place to ensure inclusivity for any staff members with dyslexia?

# Is Dyslexia Friendly the panacea?

MacKay (2001) talks about empowering learners, but to do this Dyslexia Friendly needs to transcend the setting. One practitioner interested in the ideals of Dyslexia Friendly, no matter how knowledgeable and persuasive, cannot constitute a Dyslexia Friendly setting, although they may prove to be the instigators of change. A Dyslexia Friendly setting means that the whole setting must be on board and this probably results not only in a Dyslexia Friendly setting but a whole special educational needs friendly setting with a broad and inclusive culture where inclusion is for all children whether at risk or vulnerable.

However, Norwich (2009) describes a tension between all-encompassing inclusivity and specific kinds of inclusivity. He claims that this emphasis on all vulnerable and at-risk children could compromise the specific needs of particular groups of children, such as those with dyslexia, ADD/ADHD, autism etc. Norwich (2009) expresses concern that the broader view of individuality and diversity could work against the specific interests of such groups, when there may be specific elements which relate to dyslexia, which may not be covered, or are overlooked by concern for general inclusivity. Norwich (2009) also suggests that the concept of Dyslexia Friendly is too narrow, and will not be wide ranging enough to change policy and practice.

Considering the very word 'friendly' is possibly not as helpful as it may at first seem, implying a warm and cosy feel. The Oxford English Dictionary describes a friend as a 'person joined by affection and intimacy to another' and also 'a person who is not hostile or enemy to another'. If friendly is used in the sense of environmentally friendly, then the dictionary describes it as 'not harmful to the environment', but is this really the intention of the term Dyslexia Friendly? Surely the child at risk does not need affection and intimacy, but wants more than an environment which is not harmful or hostile to them. What they do need is a safe environment where they can grow and progress, but also to accept that there will be compromises for them. They need to understand and be comfortable with the idea that there will always be activities that they find more difficult than others, but also to be able to value themselves as individuals, different in some ways to others but also the same as others in their differences. For this you do not need a friend, but a far more complex and contradictory relationship which is provocative but also nurturing and challenging. Whilst formal support structures do need to be in place, flexibility is also required to meet the evolving individuality of interests and learning.

This relationship between the children and families at risk of dyslexia and their settings need to be founded not on friendship but on mutual respect and trust, ensuring that support will be non-judgmental and treated with confidence and open-mindedness. For this to happen the staff in the setting need to be:

- Aware: cognisant of their own strengths and weaknesses, but also confident in their own abilities. They need to be realistic with the boundaries of their own professionalism, recognising where they need additional support and knowledge, and when to refer on to other professionals.

- Adaptable: to be flexible in their approach, to suit the individual needs and interests of the child to be supported.
- Empathetic: able to relate to the children and their families in their care, aware of the language/s that they use and what values and priorities these families place on their children's education and potential.
- Inspirational: motivational, showing a genuine desire to ensure that each child feels secure enough to make mistakes, without feeling a failure. It is vital to encourage the child to take some responsibility for their own learning by constructing their own knowledge and understanding through positive and dynamic interactions with the activities they are encouraged to embark upon. Staff must recognise that there is a critical balance between support and challenge.
- Communicative: aware of the nature of the communication between the setting and the children, their families and outside agencies, to strengthen the relationship of critical equality and mutual respect.
- Time aware: to facilitate these complex relationships will take time, and this will not be easy in a busy setting, so needs to be factored into the day and rigorously planned for:
  - Time to listen to other people's ideas.
  - Time to share information.
  - Time to be honest with each other.
  - Time to put forward ideas and accept challenge and argument.
  - Time to think and change your mind.

## Learning styles

This is a very controversial and unscientifically supported concept concerned with how we learn and whether there are different ways to learn effectively. Certainly it appears that there are many different ways to learn; take for example the difference between how you would learn about a philosophical question such as 'What makes you you?' and learning to change a lightbulb, or learning the sort of aesthetic awareness to appreciate the Mona Lisa. The argument goes (Honey and Mumford, 1982) that you all have learning style preferences and you learn better when the activity matches your learning style. This brings with it an implication that you who work with children in education need to be identifying learning styles, and adapting your pedagogy to match the styles of individual learners.

> Research has questioned the validity of notions of discrete learning styles, and studies have also failed to find conclusive links between gender and learning style.
>
> (DCSF, 2009: online)

Reading the available research concerning learning styles shows that there are literally thousands of papers written about this, but also shows that reliable and valid, peer reviewed research is in very short supply. What you will find is a wealth of commercial companies willing to sell you their latest, expensive version of the idea. Each has different names for the so-called learning styles, and the bewildering number can range from two to over 70! Jarrett (2015) says with tongue in cheek that,

> if we view each learning style as dichotomous (e.g. visual vs. verbal) that means that there are 2 to the power of 71 combinations of learning styles – more than the number of people alive on the earth!

> (Jarrett, 2015: p. 208)

The controversy surrounding learning styles is great and often focused upon how static a learning style is – it could be a genetic given, or perhaps it can be shaped and changed; in other words is it nature or nurture? If it does exist, and perhaps it can be shaped and moulded, then maybe it needs to be done in the early years when the plasticity of the brain is at its most malleable, or perhaps it can be fashioned throughout life, changing with maturity and experience. If there are learning style preferences, are they set within you, and therefore you learn all new things best in this way, or more likely is it task specific, so that you use different styles to achieve different types of learning?

Mortimore (2003) and other writers believe that learners need to be aware of their predominant learning style to enable them to use their learning strengths to their best advantage, however, this could mean that individuals stick rigidly to a particular approach, their 'Comfort Zone' as Mackay (2005) calls it, regardless of the nature of the task or the method of delivery. For practitioners working with children in the early years, discovering a child's learning style could be difficult, and even with close observation, could be time consuming for very little reward. After examining the research in this area, it is highly likely that different people do learn in different ways, and it seems, on the surface, to be logical that if the style of presentation of learning matches their particular way of learning, they will learn best. However, even if this is so, the feasibility of dealing with a group of children in a class or nursey and differentiating the learning so specifically is doubtful, and its overall worth is probably also doubtful. It does seem unlikely that you would only have one learning style and it is probably more likely that it is an eclectic mix and a unique blend of styles.

If you accept that there are different ways to learn different tasks, then the important thing to ensure is that you do not persistently use one style to teach that task, or even expect the same response to the task from every child. Perhaps you should be stretching children to use less preferred learning styles, so that they better understand where they are experiencing difficulties. If you continually teach in the way the children find easy, and therefore always succeed, they may never 'test' themselves and learn things that require a different way of learning. Providing a wide-ranging pedagogy will ensure that no child is disadvantaged and all children are exposed to a full range of learning styles, thereby enabling them to have the confidence to tackle different tasks in the future, with the ability to adapt their ways of learning to the task, even when outside their comfort zone.

It is likely that children will naturally come to understand the way they learn best, and do not need artificial labels to classify what they feel, or to put them under one umbrella, which could lead them to believe that they cannot learn under any other label and become reluctant to challenge themselves.

# Learning strategies

What is probably more important for the child at risk of dyslexia than ascertaining their learning style is to develop an arsenal of learning strategies which can be applied to a range of different tasks. Learning strategies are not fixed or apparently innate, but can be taught and trained by exposing children to as many of them as possible, which could increase their ability to process information and commit to memory. There is a wealth of such strategies, too many to list here but some examples follow:

- Mind maps and concept maps.
- Visual imagery.
- Mnemonics – such as spelling the word 'rhythm': Rhythm Helps Your Two Hips Move.
- Mental modelling and frameworks.
- Singing, music and rhythm – such as singing the times tables or the letters of the alphabet.
- Talking aloud.
- Drawing.
- Developing schemas.
- Repetition and rehearsal.
- Active listening.
- Touch and kinaesthetic – such as feeling wooden letters in a velvet bag.
- Bridge building from existing knowledge to new understanding.
- Prediction – 'I had t_ _ _ _ and marmalade for breakfast this morning'.
- Highlighting key words/ideas.
- Chunking and labelling – a string of letters such as xhastoastforhistea is hard to recall, but when chunked together 'X has toast for his tea' is easier to remember. Hooks to hang further learning.
- Matching and sorting.
- Story Boards.

- Flow charts – Pick up the toys ⟶ Put in the toy box ⟶ Close the lid
- Quizzes.
- Time lines, cycles and sequential boxes – for example, birthdays in the group:

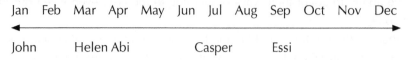

Jan  Feb  Mar  Apr  May  Jun  Jul  Aug  Sep  Oct  Nov  Dec

◀————————————————————————————▶

John        Helen Abi        Casper        Essi

- Turn taking and question and answer.
- Humour and cartoons.
- Lists and word columns.
- Visual hierarchies:

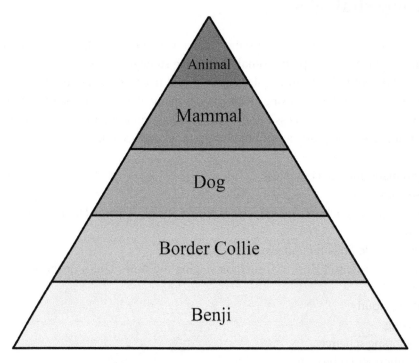

Animal

Mammal

Dog

Border Collie

Benji

*Figure 9.2* Example of visual hierarchy

- Paired teaching – one child teaches another.
- Imagery and mental 'movies'.
- Colour associations – colour coding characters/letters/numbers.
- Role play and drama.
- Technology – tape recordings, Dictaphones, text to word software, voice activated systems, e-books etc.

What is generally agreed by researchers is that we all learn differently, we have different talents, abilities, interests, experiences and backgrounds. Each of us is an individual and we probably all learn in different ways, but this once again highlights the impossibility of teaching to a particular learning style for every member of your group or class. You might even question whether this is desirable or not; surely we all need to have a range of ways of learning in our arsenal, to enable us to learn things as diverse as maths, changing a light bulb, philosophy, the creative arts etc. If we are not particularly adept at one, perhaps we should be trying to practise this and improve.

## Professional development

> The provision of specialist resources, which are available in abundance, is not the key to success. The key is informed understanding and this stems from effective training!
>
> (Reid, 2013: p. 3)

The Dyslexia Friendly Quality Mark places great emphasis on employing knowledgeable and appropriately trained staff, who offer an understanding and sensitive approach to their practice. Understanding that all children bring with them a set of strengths and weaknesses, whether they are dyslexic or not, should always be the starting point for learning. Staff who are eager to identify those individual strengths and weaknesses are therefore vital to a Dyslexia Friendly setting. As you have already read, one of the biggest difficulties that children at risk of dyslexia face is that of low self-esteem, so staff that go the extra mile to play to those strengths and help to raise self-esteem, are crucial to enabling the child to develop to their potential. This requires a knowledgeable and reflective practitioner, one who is open to new ideas and new thinking, one who seeks to keep up to date with research and its implications for practice, but is also willing to ask for help and share their successes and failures with colleagues.

To ensure that we have a workforce appropriately trained to work with children at risk of dyslexia it is vital that, even in the initial training of teachers and practitioners, some element of theory and practice is devoted to this area. In a small-scale piece of research, conducted for this book, it would appear that currently this is not the case, and teachers and practitioners are identifying for themselves that they have not been adequately equipped to deal with an issue, which is so widespread that it will certainly be frequently met during their careers.

A group of 32 primary teachers were asked 'How much information did you receive about dyslexia during your initial training?' The response that none felt that they had had a satisfactory degree of information is really disturbing, particularly as the majority had had no information (Figure 9.3).

A slightly larger group of practitioners (76 in total) were asked the same question, and the responses showed an even greater disparity, with 60 practitioners claiming that no mention was made during initial training of the special skills needed to work with these children (Figure 9.4).

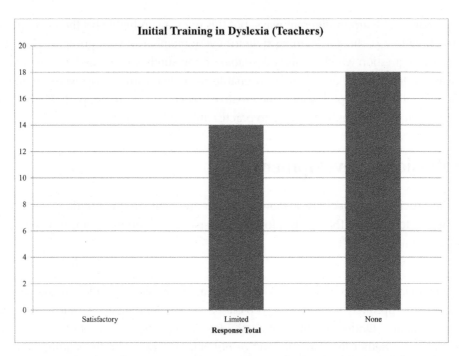

*Figure 9.3* Graph to show responses from teachers to the levels of dyslexia information received during their initial training programmes

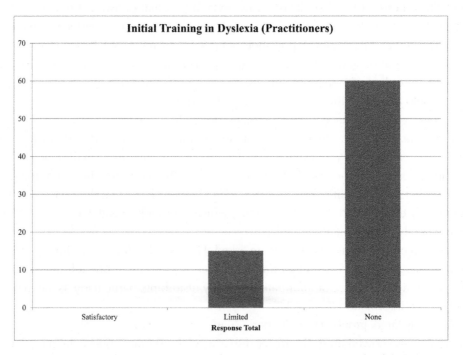

*Figure 9.4* Graph to show responses from practitioners to the levels of dyslexia information received during their initial training programmes

Finally the teachers and practitioners were asked 'Do you feel *confident* that you could identify a child in your group who may be at risk of dyslexia?' They were only offered a yes/no answer as the word 'confident' had been deliberately emphasised. It would appear unlikely that these teachers and practitioners had undertaken extensive training in this area, following initial training, so it was disturbing to find that so many did feel confident to identify children who were at risk of dyslexia (Figure 9.5).

Professional development for practitioners and teachers does appear, from this small-scale piece of primary research, to be a major issue, and the qualitative responses received showed that most of the respondents did not feel adequately prepared or equipped to work with children at risk of dyslexia.

I have had no training throughout my course about dyslexia (practitioner).

No training was given on dyslexia nor was dyslexia discussed at my setting even though I have been there for a year (practitioner).

The topic of dyslexia has not been brought up since starting in the setting; no child has been diagnosed with dyslexia or to be at risk of dyslexia (teacher).

I completed school based teacher training and dyslexia and other forms of SEN did not form any part of my training. After nine years of teaching a bit more training would be very useful (teacher).

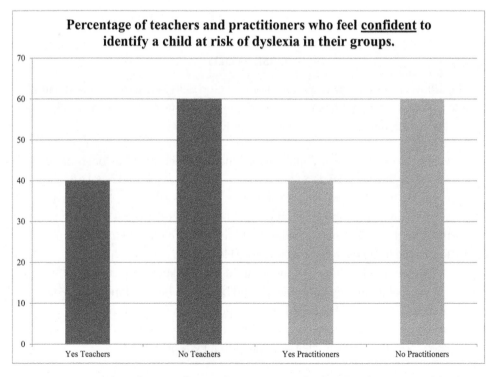

*Figure 9.5* Graph to show teachers and practitioners who feel that they can confidently identify children in their group at risk of dyslexia

The qualitative comments suggested that most of their knowledge was gained 'on the job' and in informal discussions with other more experienced colleagues. However, one of the major criteria for a Dyslexia Friendly setting is that staff are appropriately trained. Possibly only when all staff are appropriately trained and have sufficient understanding, will dyslexia receive the recognition within the setting and only then will the children receive the high quality of education and inclusion that they need to prepare them for life. The children at risk of dyslexia need to be taught the strategies they require to cope with a condition that they are likely to struggle with for the rest of their lives and they need to overcome the difficulties that could actually prevent them from achieving their potential.

Mackay (2005) and the BDAs Dyslexia Friendly concept advocate that there is a trained member of staff in every setting, but this is probably not a tenable position, especially with staff turnover and promotion, so there needs to be a shift within the whole profession to ensure that every member of staff that comes into contact with the child is trained to be aware of the possibility of dyslexia. This ambitious ideal can only be achieved with the co-operation of the colleges and universities, which may require a financial commitment from Government. This also is dependent upon the teacher and practitioner trainers also having the appropriate expertise and willingness to carry this through.

---

### CASE STUDY

The following case study is part of a conversation with Sylvia (not her real name), a teaching assistant, who had her own dyslexia identified when she was 32 years of age and starting a part-time degree at university.

When I look back at my life I realise that so much of it has been determined by dyslexia. I was a very anxious child; I wet the bed regularly and even had accidents in school sometimes. I felt so ashamed. I just did not seem to be able to absorb what was said in class and I found it hard to remember things. My little brother could read before me, in fact he seemed to be able to do everything before me. He used to tease me about it.

I was bullied in the playground and I did not know how to stop it, so I never really had any good friends and became a bit of a loner. It worked both ways really as because I was not popular I wanted to be alone and became very introverted and closed myself off. My teachers did not really know how to cope and clearly thought that I was just 'thick'!

I had a lot of time off school with illness as I had frequent headaches, stomach-aches and unexplained rashes. My mum just thought that I was a sickly child.

Consider the case study interview above.

- Sylvia says a lot about what happened to her, but not a lot about how it made her feel. What do you think she would say if asked?
- Explain why teachers/practitioners/parents/carers need to be more aware of what they can do to help.
- In what way do you think that this anxiety and experience influenced the rest of Sylvia's life?

# Scaffolding and turn taking

The concept of scaffolding builds upon Vygotsky's (1978) theory of the Zone of Proximal Development (ZPD), which is a term that he coined for the range of tasks which children find difficult to master alone, but with the help of adults or more able peers, can be achieved. Vygotsky called these the 'buds' or 'flowers' of development, rather than the 'fruits' which are the end products. Scaffolding was a term probably first used by Bruner in the 1950s but discussed in his later work (1986), and he used it to describe the changing levels of support given by that adult or more knowledgeable peer. The 'teacher' adjusts the amount of guidance according to the learner's current performance level, so that as the learner progresses the level of support is reduced. The important aspect of this type of support is timing the level of interactions to engage the child in turn taking; allowing the child greater and greater levels of responsibility for their own learning as their confidence and ability progresses. Clearly this does not imply a rigid teaching structure, but rather more fluid and flexible methodology, suiting the needs of the individual at the time. This fits well into Bruner's ideas of a social constructivist theory of learning.

The term scaffolding is a metaphor, a skilful piece of imagery to describe a temporary structure, which is not meant to remain for long, but supports the building work whilst in construction. In this context it is a temporary framework built through adult and child interaction, to motivate and encourage a child to use their own ideas and resourcefulness (Reid, 2017), before eventually the scaffolding is dismantled and the child 'goes it alone'. The defining skill of the 'teacher' is to understand when and how much support to offer and when it is 'safe' to withdraw.

Mortimore (2003) calls this a three-stage process:

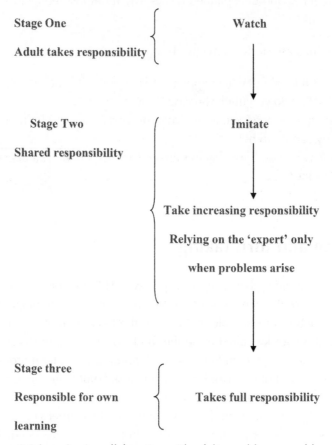

*Figure 9.6* Learning in collaboration with adults or older more able peers

# Parent partnerships

The BDA Dyslexia Friendly Quality Mark demands that good relationships with parents can be demonstrated before a setting can be granted the coveted quality award. The Effective Provision of Pre-school Education project (EPPE) (Sylva et al., 2004) showed emphatically that where there were positive relationships with parents, settings were able to provide a better quality of learning environment for all children.

Partnerships are always built on trust but this can be a very fragile concept. Trust, according to the *Shorter Oxford Dictionary* (5th edn), is

Faith or confidence in the loyalty, strength, veracity etc., of a person or thing; reliance on the truth of a statement etc. without examination.

(p. 3367)

This is clearly a very 'tall order' to achieve in the relationship between parents/carers and settings. One advantage to working in early years is that you are likely to have much closer contact with parents/carers than those working with children over the age of eight years, enabling those partnerships to be developed. Parents will bring and collect their children each day, allowing opportunities to engage with them and share information, Rodd (2013) suggests that this information sharing is essential for ensuring a high-quality learning environment for the child, and at the heart of that is the ability to maintain confidentiality.

> Research continues to show that, when families are involved positively in their children's early learning and education, their children demonstrate higher levels of achievement, better attendance and display more positive attitudes and behaviour.
>
> (Rodd, 2013: p. 221)

---

**Reflect on this**

Partnerships however, can be very varied in their nature, and the strength of the relationship from at one end of a continuum a tokenistic approach, to the other end a genuine and enduring sharing of responsibility and advocacy. For this to be achieved the professionals need to work with and be supportive of families' lives, their cultures, educational levels and expectations. This requires the professionals to understand that parents are the experts in their own children and can, if appropriately engaged, provide equal, but very different, contributions to their child's care and education.

1. Reflect on the policies of parent partnership in your setting. Indicate where on the following continuum your setting falls:

**Tokenistic**                                    **Full and accountable**

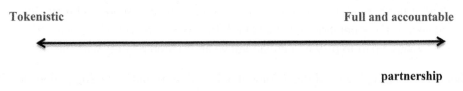

                                               **partnership**

*Figure 9.7* Partnership continuum

2. How does your concept of partnership fare if parents have alternative perspectives on child rearing practices to those of you or your setting?
3. Is there a fine line between an empowering partnership of equals and parents dictating practice? Reflect, with a colleague, on how this could be resolved.

Time and again when talking to parents of children who have been identified as dyslexic, I hear of the struggle that many of them have had to highlight the issues with practitioners and teachers, only to be dismissed as 'fussy parents' or 'over anxious'. Unless that pathway between settings and parents remains open, there are always going to be those reluctant to talk to the staff in the setting about the difficulties that they see in their child, perhaps concerned about labelling or even having to admit to themselves that their child may be experiencing a lack of progress. Parents, if allowed to, have a key role to play in the identification of the 'at-risk' child, particularly in the early years, and communication is the key word.

Settings need to work with parents/carers to focus on how they can best support the child. In order to do this, it is vital that professionals are aware of the power relationship between parents and settings. Dale (1996) identified a number of issues within that power debate:

- The 'Expert Model': he describes this as one that I am sure you are familiar with, not only as a practitioner, but also perhaps as a parent yourself. The experts are seen as the professionals and the parent is expected to defer to their superior knowledge and expertise. This removes the power from the parent to the practitioner/teacher, as the professional finds it hard to value the parental contribution.
- The 'Transplant Model': this is an extension of the 'expert model', as the professional is expected to instruct the parent and transfer skills and knowledge to them, that they can use to work with their child. The power to control what happens to the child remains with the professional.
- The 'Empowerment Model': this implies that the professional has empowered the parent to meet their child's needs and to make decisions about those needs.

I would add a further model to Dale's power debate, which I will call the 'Egalitarian Model':

- This model sees all those who work with the child or have the best interests of the child at heart, work in equal measures to communicate, share and make informed judgments in cooperation with that child. This model recognises that each person or agency has a part to play in a collaborative and shared process with the child.

There is no one right way of developing that partnership, but some suggestions to help could be:

- Parents being invited to work with staff in settings.
- Staff and parents engaging with home visits.
- Parents encouraged to become governors or join management committees.
- Parents encouraged to attend workshops and courses with staff.
- Parents running services within the setting such as book libraries, toy libraries etc.
- Staff and parents engaged in fund raising activities.

- Parents and staff sharing observations.
- Registration booklets available detailing the benefits of parent partnerships.
- Brochures, diaries, photos, videos involving parents, staff and children.
- Sharing expertise such as cooking, knitting, gardening, art and creative crafts etc.
- Parents and staff cooperating on concerts, parties and celebrations.
- Parents and staff cooperating on outings.
- Open days and open evenings with reciprocal passing of information.

It is however, important to see partnerships from both sides. There are not many parents who do not want to see the very best for their children, but there are obstacles which can get in the way, such as a lack of time, pressures of work, no child care facilities for younger children, lack of a shared language or even the parents' own emotional experiences of education when they were young, both positive and negative, which can all influence the ability to make a success of that partnership. Repeatedly in this book I have reiterated that a familial link is probably the most important when identifying the children at risk of dyslexia; if that is the case, then it is likely that some of the children at risk will also have one or both parents that may be struggling with reading and literacy, and they may also have very poor memories of their educational experience. These parents may have difficulties using the partnership diaries and home/setting link books, they may find it hard to read letters home or to maintain an organised existence. Such parents may also be fearful of their own spelling and grammar, and so reluctant to commit any ideas to paper. A knowledgeable and sensitive setting will be aware of this, and as with some of the other obstacles to partnership, that are listed above, they need considerable thought and understanding to overcome with creative solutions, to reassure parents and support them in their parenting by balancing the needs of the parent with the needs of the child.

Practitioners and teachers and parents should all have one thing in common, that is that they all want the very best for that child, however their roles are very different but can be complementary. This is a professional relationship and not a friendship. You do not have to like someone to have a professional relationship with them and professional boundaries must always be maintained.

Being friendly is not the same as being a friend.

## Chapter reflections

What this chapter has tried to show is that Dyslexia Friendly is certainly not a magic bullet and the children will not be helped by an overemphasis on positive images and opportunities without recourse to the practicalities. You need to consider three things: first, who will identify the children in your care who may be at risk of an information processing difference; second, how you intend to meet their needs within the setting; and, third, who will deliver this. It is surely madness to consider that these children can be further disadvantaged by either an unsuitable physical environment or the behaviour of the teachers and/or practitioners who are supposed to be caring for them.

There will inevitably be similarities in the way that children learn and process information, but for as many similarities there will be many individual differences that require a holistic appreciation of the child's learning abilities and a multi-sourced, multisensory graduated approach to teaching.

## Further reading

Nutbrown, C., Clough, P. and Atherton, F. (2013) *Inclusion in the Early Years* (2nd edn). London: Sage.

This book takes a highly critical and sensible approach to inclusion in the early years, seeing inclusion in the broadest sense. These highly experienced and well renowned authors argue the case for inclusion as a far-reaching political issue which influences policy, curriculum, pedagogy and society. This is an insightful text that will really make you reflect on your own practice and inform your own critical thinking.

# References

Alexander-Passe, N. (2015) *Dyslexia and Mental Health*. London: Jessica Kingsley Publishers.

Ball, D., Gill, T. and Spiegal, B. (2013) *Managing Risk in Play Provision: Implementation Guide*. London: Play England on behalf of Play Safety Forum by NCB.

Bruner, J. (1986) *Actual Minds. Possible Worlds*. Cambridge, MA: Harvard University Press.

Cochrane, K., Gregory, J. and Saunders, K. (2012) (eds) *Dyslexia Friendly Schools Good Practice Guide: Abridged Version*. Bracknell: BDA.

Dale, N. (1996) *Working with Families of Children with Special Needs: Partnership and Practice*. London: Routledge.

Department for Children, Schools and Families (DCSF) (2009) *Gender and Education . . . Mythbusters*. Available online at: http://webarchive.nationalarchives.gov.uk/20130401151715/www.education.gov.uk/publications/eOrderingDownload/00599–2009BKT-EN.pdf (accessed 28.08.17).

Honey, P. and Mumford, A. (1982) *Manual of Learning Styles*. London: P. Honey.

Jarrett, C. (2015) *Great Myths of the Brain*. Chichester: Wiley-Blackwell.

MacKay, N. (2005) *Removing Dyslexia as a Barrier to Achievement: The Dyslexia Friendly Schools Toolkit*. Wakefield: SEN Marketing.

Mortimore, T. (2003) *Dyslexia and Learning Styles: A Practitioner's Handbook*. London: Whurr.

Norwich, B. (2009) Dyslexia and Inclusive Education. In Reid, G. (ed.) *The Routledge Companion to Dyslexia*. Abingdon: Routledge.

Nutbrown, C., Clough, P. and Atherton, F. (2013) *Inclusion in the Early Years* (2nd edn). London: Sage.

Reid, G. (2016) *Dyslexia: A Practitioner's Handbook* (5th edn). Chichester: Wiley.

Rodd, J. (2006) *Leadership in Early Childhood: The Pathway to Professionalism* (4th edn). London: OUP.

Sylva, K., Melhuish, E., Sammons, P., Siraj-Blatchford, I. and Taggart, B. (2004) *The Effective Provision of Pre-school Education (EPPE) Project*: Technical paper 12 –The final report: Effective Pre-school Education. London: The Institute of Education, University of London.

Tovey, H. (2014) All about Risk. *Nursery World* 13–26: 21–24.

UNESCO (1992) *United Nations Convention on the Rights of the Child*. Paris: UNESCO.

Vygotsky, L. (1978) *Mind in Society*. Cambridge, MA: Harvard University Press.

Warnock, M. and Norwich, B. (2010) *Special Educational Needs: A New Look*. London: Continuum International Publishing Group.

Waldron, N. and McLeskey, J. (1998) The Effects of an Inclusive Education Program on Students with Mild and Severe Learning Disabilities. *Exceptional Children* 64 (3): 395–405.

# 10 | Not all bad news! Rewards and challenges

*The moment you doubt whether you can fly you cease for ever to be able to do it.*

Barrie, J.M. 2015, Chapter 14

## Introduction

This chapter aims to take a very different perspective on dyslexia, moving away from a deficit theory, that is the perception of disadvantage and remediation, and towards a concept of advantage, talents and gifts. Working to enhance these advantages can be beneficial not only to the child, but also to society as a whole. Eide and Eide (2011) describe this as the importance of learning to become better at 'being dyslexic'.

## Success: what does it look like?

The list in Table 10.1 is an example of people who are all highly successful in their own fields; I am quite sure that you will recognise some, if not all of them. All those on this list have identified themselves as being dyslexic, and what this shows is the immense diversity of special skills and talents that can be found with people at the very top of their 'game', who have often struggled with traditional methods of education.

Such lists appear in most books concerned with dyslexia and are undoubtedly listed to 'give hope' to those children and their families who are diagnosed with dyslexia. However, I could equally have listed numerous wealthy and famous people who are not dyslexic, so that in itself is not the issue. The important point to make is that this list (and others like it) is made up of a variety of people who have succeeded in their field because of their dyslexia and not despite it. I know of no one with dyslexia who will

*Table 10.1*

| | |
|---|---|
| Sir Richard Branson | Entrepreneur and businessman |
| Sir Alan Sugar | Entrepreneur, businessman and TV personality |
| Duncan Goodhew MBE | Olympic swimming medallist |
| Sir Jackie Stewart | Motor racing world champion |
| Sir Steve Redgrave | Olympic rowing medallist |
| Mohammed Ali | World heavy weight boxing champion |
| Ben Fogle | TV presenter, author and adventurer |
| Eddie Izzard | Comedian and TV personality |
| Henry Winkler | Actor (the Fonz) and children's author |
| Tom Cruise | Actor |
| Sir Winston Churchill | Prime Minister and First Sea Lord |
| Sir Norman Foster | Architect |
| Pablo Picasso | Artist |
| Lynda La Plante | Author and screen writer |
| Jamie Oliver | Chef, TV host, writer and campaigner |
| Benjamin Zephaniah | Poet |
| Ozzie Osbourne | Musician |

not recount tales of upset, educational failure, distress, often bullying, low self-esteem, feelings of depression and even thoughts of suicide. Although I have not had the privilege to talk to any of the people on the list, I would be highly surprised if any one of them could not relate to at least some of these feelings, yet they were still able to drive forward and make a great success of their lives, influencing not only themselves but also those around them. For every one of the rich and famous on the list there will be thousands of other individuals who have to be grateful to their dyslexia for allowing them to succeed.

You have already read in this book that I regard dyslexia not as a learning disability but a learning difference. Individuals with dyslexia process the information from their senses in a very different way to those who are not dyslexic. That is in no way to diminish the many challenges that these children and adults face, and the hardships that many of them endure by being asked to 'fit in' with the system of education and society which has a 'one size fits all' attitude and expects everyone to comply with this. However advantageous these talents might appear to be, they are often not valued in schools and universities in the mainstream of education, but are often highly valued in employment.

Logan (2009) examined the incidence of dyslexia in entrepreneurs in both the USA and UK, compared to the general population, and showed a significantly higher incidence of dyslexia in the sample of entrepreneurs than in the control group. The research showed that 35% of the entrepreneurs from the USA had traits of dyslexia, with 22% shown to be highly or extremely dyslexic. In the UK the proportions were lower at 19% with traits of dyslexia, but nevertheless a higher proportion than would be expected compared to the likely prevalence in the general population. Interestingly it was also shown that entrepreneurs with dyslexia employed more staff per business than non-dyslexic entrepreneurs. Logan (2009) explained this by suggesting that one coping strategy employed by individuals with dyslexia is to delegate tasks that they find difficult, and to trust others to do the tasks that may contribute to their ability to grow their businesses. Logan (2009) surmised that delegation is essential to good management, but non-dyslexics often find it difficult to delegate and to transition from control to delegation.

Logan (2009) also showed that the incidence of risk taking (which is essential to an entrepreneur investing in setting up a new venture) was higher in entrepreneurs with dyslexia. They were often also better oral communicators than the non-dyslexic business people, which could possibly be attributed to their difficulties with written material.

> Communication skills are an essential business tool. Those who can communicate well can inspire those around them to achieve a vision; they can network to build resources around an opportunity and motivate others to act; therefore, having enhanced communication skills would provide an entrepreneur or a manager with a definite business advantage.
>
> (Logan, 2009: online)

## Thinking differently

In evolutionary terms reading and literacy are very new skills for the human species; even 200 years ago most people could not read, go back 1,000 years and the number of readers was very small indeed. It is then possible to understand that the literacy skills, which you now regard as essential, involve a very new and particular way to use your brain. This is possibly the reason why in the past dyslexia was unheard of, and certainly was not seen as a disability. It is highly unlikely that it did not exist, only that it was not apparent as a problem. If you reflect on a non-reading culture it is possible to see how advantageous it was to think differently, to be able to think 'outside the box'. It could even be claimed that that was what, in evolutionary terms, brought us to where we are now, leading to new inventions, technologies and life enhancing and life extending agriculture and medicine. Individuals who were capable of doing this sort of thinking would probably have been prized, admired and respected.

# Dyslexia advantages

To consider what these different ways of thinking may involve requires you to suspend what is possibly your current concept of dyslexia, and to see it not in negative terms but as liberating and advantageous. A number of researchers in the field, such as Davis (1997), Eide and Eide (2011) and Nicholson (2015), have tried to analyse what this different way of thinking might look like and have identified a particular number of positive characteristics that some dyslexic individuals use to process information. It is important to realise that they are not saying that all individuals with dyslexia have all these characteristics or even any, but there are statistical trends which indicate that these are features common to more people with dyslexia than would be expected in the general population. The following list is an amalgam of the ideas put forward by a range of researchers:

- An ability to manipulate visual material in the mind and see things from a range of differing perspectives – enhanced visual conceptualisation (Nicolson, 2015; Davis, 1997; Eide and Eide, 2011).
- An ability to 'see' in a 3-dimensional manner with increased spatial awareness – seeing different levels and angles (Vail, 1990; Eide and Eide, 2011).
- An enhanced ability with mechanical systems (West, 2005).
- An ability to detect unusual relationships, patterns and connections between things – their similarities and differences in data sets and systems (Vail, 1990).
- An ability to think in metaphor and analogy (Davis, 1997).
- An ability to understand abstract information in concrete terms (Eide and Eide, 2011; Davis, 1997).
- An ability to remember episodes played out like dramatic scenes in their head – what is often called episodic memory (Eide and Eide, 2011; Davis, 1997; Vail, 1990).
- An ability to associate colour, touch and emotion with events – the 'imaginer', the daydreamer and creative inventor (Eide and Eide, 2011; Davis, 1997).
- An ability to bring together seemingly unrelated ideas, designs and concepts into a whole representation – a 'big picture' view of the world (Nicolson, 2015; West, 2005).
- A sensitivity to empathy and teamwork (Nicholson, 2005; Davis, 1997).
- An enhanced ability to communicate (Nicholson, 2005).
- A predisposition to resilience, proactivity and flexibility (Nicholson, 2005).
- A heightened level of curiosity (Vail, 1990; Davis, 1997).
- An ability to have divergent thinking, intuition and insight (Vail, 1990; Davis, 1997).

West (2005), who has written extensively about the advantages of dyslexia, believes that recognition of these talents in the early years could aid final identification of appropriate support for children with dyslexia. He believes that we could learn more about these learning differences if research focused more on the strengths rather than the weaknesses of the condition, and thereby understand better how to nurture the talents where they exist, and support the weaknesses from a position of strength.

> Perhaps it is time to recognise that many of the problems that dyslexics have are, in reality, artefacts of an old print-based technological culture whose prime is past. Perhaps it is time to recognise that many of the talents that many dyslexics exhibit are, in reality, strikingly appropriate for a new image based technological culture whose prime is yet to come.
>
> (West, 2005: p. 156)

Gardner (1984), famed for his theory of multiple intelligences, also suggests that the present system of education really only values and rewards abilities in linguistic and logical mathematical intelligences. He believes that these forms of intelligence are what define what psychologists call IQ, which until very recently was the most important feature of an assessment for dyslexia. Even today the deficit between IQ and achievement is seen by some as the main criterion for identification. There are understandably many critics of Gardner's theory of multiple intelligences, such as White (2005) who feels that the theory has no empirical evidence to back it up and is too subjective, but whether you agree with it or not, it does make you think more seriously about the way that certain talents are recognised by society, to the point that those who cannot excel in these areas are written off as failures.

> We may find that the conditions that give rise to dyslexia are in fact located in the deeper structures of the education system or society as a whole and that the current approaches that are taken to alleviate dyslexia-related difficulties are rather more superficial in their scope and impact than we would care to admit.
>
> (Amesbury, 2006: online)

## A glass half full

One of the reasons for these advantages, according to Nicolson and Fawcett (2007), is perversely because of a disadvantage. Children with dyslexia often have poor procedural learning ability, which is to know 'how' to learn something and to automatise that learning so that you no longer have to think about it. Davis (1997) refers to this as the 'gift of mastery', where conscious thought is no longer required. Observe a young child of 12 months of age learning how to stand and walk – it is something that they find very hard, with problems of stability, co-ordination, balance and sensory awareness, which involves deep concentration. However, five years on this highly complex and sensory task has become completely automatised and now the child can walk efficiently and accurately whilst at the same time the brain is able to multi-task and talk at the same time as they walk, whilst unwrapping a chocolate bar or performing other functions.

Walking no longer needs to be consciously thought about, the learning is so embedded. A difficulty with automatisation probably makes learning any new task very difficult and will take so much longer, but precisely because it is difficult the child with procedural learning challenges must work harder at it, they may need to think through different ways to achieve the end goal. Eide and Eide (2011) describe this as 'mindfulness' or 'task awareness'. This greater focus on tasks that most people learn easily and accept in the way they are taught, without question, means that the children with dyslexia need to be more inventive, more creative and analytical, with the most basic tasks, from the earliest stage of their lives. Nicolson and Fawcett (2007) suggest that it could be they become accustomed to that logical and resourceful manner of thinking, which is then applied to all tasks throughout life, giving them the ability to 'see' new things in activities that the rest of the population takes for granted, so these tasks are never examined or questioned.

This sort of thinking really does require you to turn things completely on their head and to look at things from more than one perspective. My husband, who in his youth was a parachutist, tells me that if when you are sitting alongside the wing of the aircraft,

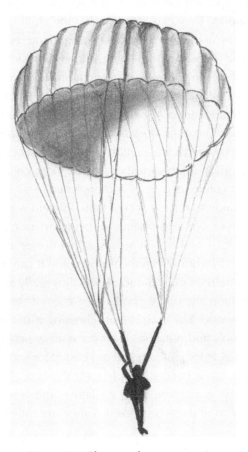

*Figure 10.1* The parachute perspective

waiting to jump out, you view this moment of adrenaline rush with fear, dread and horror, you will not jump; but if you can feel anticipation, excitement and exhilaration, then you leave the aircraft and go back the following day to jump again. It really is a matter of perspective.

## Recognising those strengths and resilience

Unless children recognise that they do have strengths and talents they can easily be persuaded along the route of 'I am thick', 'I cannot achieve'. This can easily become a self-fulfilling prophesy, whereby the child unknowingly allows themselves to have such low expectations of themselves that they cannot achieve. Of course, the opposite of this is what I will call the *Educating Rita* effect; you may remember the iconic film of 1983 (directed by Lewis Gilbert) when Rita, who has very poor self-esteem starts to achieve in higher education, due to the high expectations of her tutor who persuades her that she can achieve. The effect on her whole life is transformational.

Probably the most important elements to the recognition of strengths are families and their support networks. They can identify what the child is good at from an early age and allow them to use and develop these talents and interests, thereby enabling the child to feel that they can succeed at something, and instilling in them the confidence to value themselves. The things that they do succeed at may not necessarily be something within the confines of a traditional educational setting, or even something valued by those settings, but the boundaries of our curriculum are so narrow and there is so much learning to do 'out there'. The child does not have to have exceptional ability in their area of interest, but they do need a recognition of that interest or an aptitude that permits success and thereby motivation, this instils so much more confidence and feelings of self-worth than constant failure, negativity and powerlessness.

Helping children to understand and accept their different ways of learning and information processing allows them to get better at 'being dyslexic', by encouraging them to learn more about dyslexia and what it means to themselves and others. This can also enable feelings of positivity from within themselves, and it can start from a very young age by encouraging all children to be proud of who they really are, and to have honesty with themselves. Education should be challenging but not stressful, and it can never be a one size fits all scenario. The truth is that schooling is not education, and what is currently taught in schools and nurseries is a very narrow perspective on knowledge. Arguably this is not a best fit for children and not best fit for society.

Looking back at the list of famous people with dyslexia above, you will see that what all these people have in common is resilience and proactivity, enabling them to embrace their strengths and interests even if they are different to the mainstream of society.

**CASE STUDY**

Jackie Stewart OBE, is probably the most successful racing driver that has ever lived, being world champion three times and winning 27 Grand Prix races.

He had been very unhappy at school and found reading very difficult, he describes feelings of frustration and numerous physical illnesses that kept him away from school.

He believed that he had been given a 'gift', which was his ability to drive a car, and he had been enabled to channel that talent in a positive way without distractions. He often said that there were twenty-six drivers on the starting grid of a Grand Prix all with a fairly equal distribution of natural talent, but only one of these will have the mental adaptability to win.

He believed that dyslexia had had a positive impact on his life, giving him the determination and motivation to succeed by giving him mental flexibility.

(Interview with Jackie Stewart with Susan Hampshire 1990).

Jackie Stewart 'found' his talent and was able to capitalise upon it to change his life.

- How can you help the children in your care to 'find' their own talents, even when they may not relate to the mainstream of education?
- How can you encourage children to explore their interests and talents?
- How does this relate to the child-led programmes that you are encouraged to develop in early years?

Jackie Stewart clearly had resilience in bucket loads, which is the ability to 'bounce back' from adversity and setbacks. For this he recognised that he needed the help and support of his family and other key adults. With this kind of support children can learn to see a way forward and have the confidence in their strengths to carry them through, to develop self-esteem and a feeling of control over their lives.

# Two mind theory

You have already read in Chapter 3 that the brain is divided into two roughly equal parts called hemispheres – the right hemisphere and the left hemisphere. Research under-taken by neurologists such as Sperry (1968) has indicated that these two hemispheres process information received from the senses in subtly different ways. The left hemisphere is thought to process the fine detail and the right hemisphere processes the bigger features of an object or idea. Eide and Eide (2011) use the analogy of a forest, one side 'sees' the forest as a whole and the other 'sees' the individual trees that make up the whole.

To be able to appreciate a holistic view of something requires both hemispheres to work together with information passing between the two hemispheres through the Corpus Callosum, which is a bundle of nerve cells which carry electrical impulses from one side of the brain to the other to facilitate communication between the two sides. Of course, this is a very basic analysis of an extremely complex picture of brain function, and clearly the brain functioning of left and right hemispheres does not always run in parallel. For example, Faglioni et al. (1969) showed that although language, both spoken and print based, is largely a domain of the left side of the brain, the stress, rhythm and intonation of spoken language is processed more by the right side, and written language, if the letters are ornate and decorated, is also the preserve of the right. They showed that whilst the left hemisphere largely deals with language, the right hemisphere deals with functions which are not easily translated to language, such as spatial awareness, music, emotion etc. Mortimore (2008) emphasises that there is probably considerable adaptability of the brain from one hemisphere to the other.

Interesting research by Robertson and Bakker (2002) showed that age could be a factor in hemisphere dominance. When attempting to learn English as a second language before the age of three years, the left hemisphere appears to be dominant, but when learning English after the age of six years, both hemispheres appear to be used. This research only goes to show how complex this area is, and how incomplete our knowledge concerning information processing and brain structure still is.

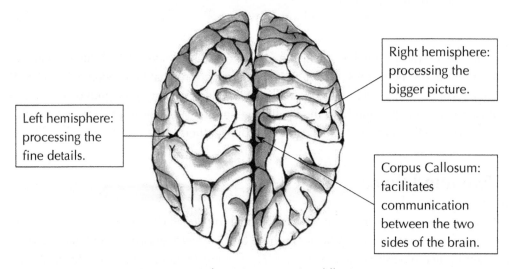

*Figure 10.2* Information processing differences

The important aspect of this research shows that information needs to move effort-lessly from one side of the brain to the other, and the two hemispheres need to be mutu-ally supportive. However, Eide and Eide (2011) suggest that in individuals with dyslexia this is not the case, and the dyslexic individual is more right brained than left brained. If this is so, and the right hemisphere is better at looking at the 'big picture', it is likely that it will follow that individuals with dyslexia are better at inference, intuitive guessing and of 'filling in the gaps'. This is sometimes referred to as the 'two mind theory'.

Inevitably there are critics of the 'two mind theory', such as Zenhausern (1982), cited by Mortimore (2008), who hypothesised that the contributions of both hemispheres to information processing were so great that it is impossible to differentiate between the two. Eide and Eide (2011) and Mortimore (2003) both point out that there are many individuals who are not dyslexic that appear to have enhanced visual-spatial skills, and many with dyslexia who do not have heightened visual-spatial skills. However, they suggest that there does appear to be a higher proportion than would be expected in the general population of individuals with dyslexia working in areas where increased visual-spatial skills are required, such as the arts, creativity and architecture, builders, mechanics, engineers, surgeons etc.

> dyslexic brains function differently from non-dyslexic ones, not because they are defective but because they're organised to display different kinds of strengths. These strengths are achieved at the cost of relative weaknesses in certain kinds of fine detail processing.
>
> (Eide and Eide, 2011: p. 43)

Mortimore (2003) asks why strength in one mode of processing should automatically come at the cost of any other. She cites research by Sperry and Gazzaniga in the 1970s where the connections between the two hemispheres have been severed, and showed that whilst the initial findings did support the two mind theory, later assessments showed that there is little evidence to back it up, and the individuality of the difference is of more importance as both sides of the brain are needed in an interconnecting manner to appropriately process information of any kind. Whilst language processing is almost certainly a result of that interconnectivity the left side does appear to be favoured, but that does not detract from the right hemisphere, which can also process language in the appropriate circumstances. What this shows is that while this incompatibility of the two hemispheres is an attractive theory, it is certainly not one accepted by all.

# Spatial reasoning

Spatial reasoning is a term used to describe the ability to visualise in the mind, and to remember, an entity from different angles and sides and to be able not only to 'see' the shapes and entities in the mind, but also to move them around, taking into account how they will look and react when they are realigned and rotated. This was referred to by Gardner (1984) as 3D reasoning. Someone with good spatial reasoning ability is likely to be able to see how objects interact and combine with other images and solve three-dimensional problems, such as navigating around unfamiliar places or buildings, packing boxes, understanding the interaction of parts of machinery or the ability to see a mirror image such as brushing your hair in the mirror or putting on your makeup. Such ability is also essential to mathematicians, engineers, astronomers, builders etc.

Eide and Eide (2011) note how young children at risk of dyslexia are drawn to games and toys that involve spatial awareness, such as Lego, building blocks, geometric shapes, ball games, gymnastics etc.

> Even when these children engaged in 2-D art projects like drawing, their art tended to have a more multi-dimensional and dynamic quality, featuring elements like foreshortening and perspective, moving figures, arrows indicating action or process and schematic elements like cutaway sections or multi-angle or multi-perspective blueprints.
>
> (Eide and Eide, 2011: p. 53)

Some years ago, we approached an architect to design a house to be built for us. After numerous attempts to get what we wanted from the designs that he offered I approached my son, who is dyslexic and at the time in his early teens. After a short conversation detailing roughly what we wanted, he promptly redesigned the blueprint which was then presented to the architect to follow (I do not think that he was very pleased!). My son had no formal training to do this but was able to use his enhanced visual-spatial awareness to use the space available to its best advantage. When I asked him later how he had done this he commented that 'I could just see it in my head'. Interestingly in the USA some architectural firms have even advertised for 'dyslexic architects', believing them to be more insightful and more creative in their thinking.

Of course, just because there are proportionally higher numbers of people with dyslexia in these sorts of occupations does not necessarily mean that they have special skills, but it could be that their poor literacy skills have drawn them to employment where literacy is not the overwhelming importance that it may be in other occupations.

## Interconnectivity

Lying on the grass on a beautiful sunny day, with my seven-year-old son who is dyslexic, I was enjoying the warmth of the sun on my face when he said, 'I can see a castle and a giant walking towards it'.

'What?' I responded.

I sat up and looked, but he was still lying down gazing up at the clouds. He then went on to recount a whole tale about what he could 'see' in the clouds and how they made meaning to him. It took me a long time and lots of direction before I could see anything but clouds, and he could not understand why I could not see what he could.

This is a great example of what Eide and Eide (2011) called interconnected reasoning. It is common to hear parents of children with this interconnected reasoning to talk about the way that their children see or hear things in a different and creative way.

> They tend to be highly creative, perceptive, interdisciplinary and recombinatory. No matter what they see or hear, it always reminds them of something else. One idea leads to another.
>
> (Eide and Eide, 2011: p. 83)

Some years ago, as part of a lecture on language use, I asked a group of undergraduate students to write down as many uses of a chair as possible. For most the answers were predictable – sit on it, stand on it, lean on it, fall asleep in it etc. However, two students, who had been previously identified as dyslexic, were notable in that their list was three times the length of the others and included such uses as:

Lion taming
A hat rack
A flower shelf
Firewood
A commode!

This is an example of that interconnective thinking. The ability to see connections between ideas and entities which at first sight appear to have no connection is often used to great advantage by the dyslexic individual, and this includes the ability to see links between words and word manipulation. It is therefore probably not unexpected that many of our top comedians, who are the masters of seeing unexpected connections, are dyslexic:

Ross Noble
Ruby Wax
John Bishop
Billy Connolly
Eddie Izzard
Whoopi Goldberg . . . to name but a few

This ability to make jokes and make us laugh, by seeing strange connections between the things that we do every day, and largely take for granted, has enabled these people to rise to the top of their profession. This is probably coupled with their need, as small children, to raise their self-esteem by becoming the 'class clown' when they realise that they can attract friends and achieve social status by making people laugh at themselves. As children, this may not have endeared them to their teachers, and almost all of those on the list above say that they had a 'hard time' at school. I remember being doubled over with laughter when Billy Connolly did a whole stand-up routine on hand washing – how can such a mundane subject, that I do several times a day, be so funny? His quirky way of thinking and amazing observational skills brought the house down. This ability to be sensitive to connections, similarities and differences between things, to see patterns and analogies and things that appear to be out of place, is clearly useful in so many other very different disciplines, such as science, medicine, technology and engineering where new problems and projects are posed every day, which require novel and creative solutions. Examples of this can be seen in many places, but notable is the Nobel Prize winner Carole Greider's research into the medicine behind cancer through chromosomes and molecular biology; she believes that this research would not have been possible but for her dyslexia, and her ability to see patterns and anomalies.

# The 'big picture'

Another advantage of the dyslexic way of thinking is the ability to see the 'big picture'. This is the ability to see the outline and interpret meaning, without the detail; Eide and Eide (2011) describe this as being able to see the forest without the individual trees within it, and they remind us that we all interpret language in this way. Language requires that you get the essence of a sentence for understanding to take place, you do not examine each word within that sentence in fine detail, word by word. The context of what you say will determine the recipients' understanding, and you use the cues in the sentence to make meaning. You do not even need all the words.

I had _____ on my toast for breakfast this morning.

The missing word is unlikely to be some random word such as 'rhinoceros' or 'geology'! The context and syntax will tell you what that word is likely to be, so you are using the cues in the sentence to guess the meaning. There are a limited number of answers that it could possibly be:

marmalade, Marmite, butter, peanut butter, jam etc.

The child who has language difficulties needs, more than anyone, to be making these connections and making meaning of what s/he hears and reads. There are many words in the English language that have more than one meaning which is another reason why English is such a difficult language to learn. These words can even be spelt the same, but not always; these are called homophones and homographs. A homophone is a word that sounds the same but is spelt differently and a homograph is a word with the same spelling but a different meaning; of course some words sound the same and are spelt the same so are both homophones and homographs (see Table 10.2). Are you with me so far?

*Table 10.2*

### Homophones

| Rain | The rain is pouring down | Reign | The Queen reigns over us |
|------|--------------------------|-------|--------------------------|
| Here | Come over here | Hear | Can you hear the birds? |
| Be | Can this be true? | Bee | The honey bee is buzzing |
| Pear | This is a pear tree | Pair | This is a pair of socks |

### Homographs

| Left | She left the book behind | Left | On the left of the shelf |
|------|--------------------------|------|--------------------------|
| Bark | The tree had silver bark | Bark | The dog bark was loud |
| Bat | He hit the ball with the bat | Bat | The bat flew away |
| Can | The tin can was rusty | Can | Can I talk to you? |

### A Homophone and Homograph often called a Heteronym

| Tear | There was a tear in her eye | Tear | She had a tear in her dress |
|------|------------------------------|------|------------------------------|
| Lead | The dog lead was red | Lead | The lead mine was dark |
| Bass | A bass is a fish | Bass | The bass drum |
| Bow | She tied a bow in her shoe | Bow | He made a low bow |

This constant search for contextual cues is what Eide and Eide (2011) call 'peeling back the onion' (p. 93) as the dyslexic individual looks for deeper and deeper meaning in things that most of us take for granted. It is likely that it is just this search for meaning that is so advantageous to those problem-solving occupations already described. The disadvantage is that this type of thinking also makes learning very slow, as each layer of the onion is peeled and revealed. It can also cause confusion when they are searching for meaning in very simple routines and tasks.

## Episodic memory

Episodic memory is the ability to 'see' memories in context and to recall experiences in this way better than learning in non-contextual and abstract ways. Eide and Eide (2011) believe that this ability is more common in dyslexic individuals than in non-dyslexics. It is likely that those with an acute episodic memory will learn better by relating abstract ideas to structured concrete experiences in their lives, by turning them into a story; in this way they often stick in the memory better. Once again this can be a slow process as the learner needs to construct these stories in their head.

Some parts of language are clearly easier to picture than others, probably nouns are the easiest to visualise. Think of the word 'dog' and you will have one in mind, but dogs come in all sorts of shapes, sizes and colours, and picturing a Chihuahua is very different to a Great Dane! Verbs can be conceptualised as most have experienced them, consider the word 'run' and most people have experienced running. However, conjunctions can be hard to conceptualise, words such as 'but', 'the', or, 'because', are particularly difficult. However, these words can become more apparent when the over-all gist of a sentence is understood. Very young babies have to learn language with lots of gaps and blank spaces which are difficult to fill:

The _____ in the swimming pool is really cold.

This is really easy to 'guess' and to use the cues but now try:

This house _____ _____ _____ white, with windows _____ _____ side.

This just causes confusion and frustration. Davis (1997) claimed that there are more than 200 very common English words that are particularly difficult for those with dys-lexia to visualise. Often these words appear to be the simplest words in the language, and the most often recurring, words such as 'a', 'and', 'the' etc. Unfortunately, these are also the words that are used most frequently in the beginner readers given to four- and five-year-old children as they start school. In the 1960s the Ladybird readers with Peter and Jane were in almost every school, they were famously based on 'one hundred key words'. These were words that were thought to be the most frequently occurring in English and included words such as:

| A | and | I | in | is | it | of | the | he |
|------|------|------|------|------|------|------|------|------|
| was | all | want | well | will | you | come | call | can |

Clearly these are all words which are very difficult to visualise, but they are vital to understanding the English language.

Davis (1997) suggests that one of the greatest advantages of dyslexia is this ability to think in pictures, which he suggests allows thought processes to be quicker than when thinking in words. He reminds us of the saying 'a picture is worth a thousand words' – the ability to see in your mind a picture of a concept is quicker than having to describe it in probably hundreds or even thousands of words. Davis (1997) claims that picture think-ing is 200–2,000 times faster, deeper and more complex than verbal thinking.

## Curiosity

The difference between attention and concentration is discussed by Davis (1997) in which he says that paying attention to something is a wide-ranging state requiring the individual to take in all around them, focused but aware. Concentration on the other hand, is focused attention, which is so intense that there is no awareness of anything else around them. Davis (1997) believed that because children with dyslexia are so curious and aware of their surroundings, it causes them to shift their attention constantly, rarely achieving a state of concentration. Clearly curiosity can be a great asset to any child encouraging new ideas and learning, but it can also cause distractions if something is not of interest to them and they can become easily bored unless there are immediate rewards.

---

**Reflect on this**

Scarlet is three years old and the staff in her nursery describe her as 'easily distractible'. She will start an activity but rarely finishes it, as she sees something else of more interest to her and has sparked her curiosity, in another area of the nursery. Staff are concerned that she could have some form of attentional disorder.

- How can staff use her driving curiosity to encourage her to stay on task?
- I have a maxim that 'there are no boring subjects, only boring teachers'. Do you think that this is true and if so why?
- What does this maxim say about the way we work with children in education?

---

All children are naturally curious about the world around them and anyone who has spent time with young children will know the dreaded 'Why?' word! For many children, as they learn to read, they are able to answer their own questions through books and internet connections. For anyone who has difficulties with reading this is not available to them, and this can lead to frustration which in turn can lead to further exploration and be a powerful driver for creativity and innovation.

This cycle of curiosity (Figure 10.3) means that for the child with dyslexia every day can be full of surprises as they find things of beauty that others have not really looked at, they find the unusual in the usual. This often leads to alternative ways of regarding things and makes many hungry for knowledge. This sort of curiosity can also extend to being curious about people and their existence, wanting to understand their lives and feelings, leading to sensitivity and empathy.

Curiosity combined with creativity allows you to conceive of things that do not currently exist, it is about invention and innovation, and it could be that it produces a higher level of thinking and learning with the ability to reason and critically evaluate.

> Curiosity is more important than knowledge: it is the root of knowledge. Without it there would be no such thing as knowledge.
>
> (Davis, 1997: p. 108)

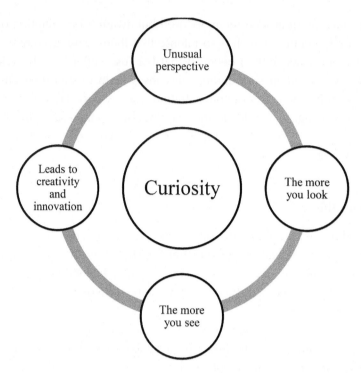

*Figure 10.3* The curiosity cycle

## Creativity

The idea that individuals with dyslexia are likely to be more creative than those without is written about in numerous texts on dyslexia, such as Eide and Eide (2011) and Nicolson (2015), but it has not always been accepted by research papers. Creative thinking combined with curiosity and interconnectivity is the ability to take novel, innovative and imaginative ideas and produce reality. It is often spontaneous, unpredictable and free flowing, but it is centred on the ability to see the 'big picture', to visualise, and the ability to manipulate 2- and 3-D images. The essential element of creativity is an end product, this could be a story, poem, sculpture, art work, business plan, musical composition, dance choreography, a technological invention or creation, and the list can go on and can apply to all areas of interest, only inhibited by the boundaries of human imagination. However, it is important to understand that creativity is probably not a static process but it is about potential, and needs to be trained, enhanced and nurtured if it is to be brought into the open.

A study by Cancer et al. (2016) looked at a group of Italian students who were identified as dyslexic. The research acknowledged that creativity is a broad and multifaceted construct which is difficult to identify, but identified three basic skills of creative thinking:

1. Divergent thinking – the ability to adapt existing ideas and generate new ones from them.
2. Connectivity – the ability to interconnect ideas and to achieve new and original solutions.
3. Reorganisation – the ability to consider things from a different perspective, thereby manipulating data into new conceptual organisations.

The study found a link between dyslexia and creativity, with a statistically significant relationship occurring on one aspect in particular, that of connectivity. They speculated that because people with dyslexia are constantly facing difficulties with other everyday tasks, particularly reading, they are used to coming up with novel alternative strategies for achieving the tasks. They give the example of a child who performs physical motor tasks well, whilst listening to rhythmical music, they find that they can speak aloud in a rhythmical way and can therefore transfer this to reading, also by using rhythm. Cancer et al. (2016) also acknowledged that this could be the result of atypical brain structures, as suggested by Schneps (2014).

## Why do some people with dyslexia have these strengths?

This is certainly a question with no credible answer at this time of writing, we only have theory and supposition. It could be that there is something inherent in the design and structure of the brain that produces these different ways of thinking. However, one theory (Schneps, 2014) examines the issue from a different aspect, the idea that because people with dyslexia read less these strengths are some form of compensation. Schneps (2014) suggests that the act of reading changes the structure of the brain. His research, which was conducted on adults learning to read for the first time, suggests that as they acquire the skills for reading they appear to lose their ability to process other visual information.

> This would suggest that the visual strengths in dyslexia are simply an artifact of differences in reading experience, a trade off that occurs as a consequence of poor reading in dyslexia.
>
> (Schneps, 2014: online)

Schneps (2014) believes that reading focuses the visual perceptual field to such a degree that you lose the ability to see the 'bigger picture'. He suggests that dyslexia is about attentional difficulties and in particular visual spatial attention. This is in line with Facoetti et al. (2010) who showed that the pre-school non-reader who has deficits in visual attention is likely to be more at risk of dyslexia.

Many of the occupations discussed in this chapter do appear to have an over-representation of individuals with dyslexia, but is that because they particularly attract people with dyslexic talents or do they have any special requirements in common which involve special abilities? West (2005) questions whether the sorts of tests and assessments required for some of these occupations, which are based on school based or societal, and government expected literacy skills, could be eliminating many with very valuable abilities from the employment pool.

---

### Chapter reflections

> Those crucial early years from kindergarten to mid adolescence, are when the battle to develop confidence, resilience, and a positive self-image is largely won or lost. If a student with dyslexia can reach the age of 14 or 15 with a healthy sense of self-esteem and a realistic acceptance of both personal strengths and weaknesses, that student is much more likely to enjoy a happy and successful life.
>
> (Eide and Eide, 2011: p. 206)

Dyslexia is seen by most people in terms of a deficit, a weakness to be 'fixed' and a problem requiring treatment, remediation and support. What I am trying to say in this chapter is that children and families with dyslexia need to show pride in their creative and innovative ways of thinking, rather than just focus upon the weaknesses. Not so many years ago their original way of thinking would have been prized and valued in society, as we did not try to force children into a framework for education which often does not allow for their differences in our modern, literate society. For the sake of future humanity, technology and innovation, these talents, where they exist, need to be nurtured and supported. Our current education systems are largely based on the concept of conditioning, where children learn reinforced behaviours, but this is a rudimentary way of learning which could be unsuited to the child with dyslexia, who processes information through pictures and visualisation.

Practitioners and teachers must work with children – all children, to their strengths and not their weaknesses – and the trick to this is to know how to identify those strengths through observation and to move forward from there. In this way you can create your pedagogy from their strengths, to give the children hope and ambition for a successful future. Perhaps our criteria for success need to change, as perhaps our present education system is getting in the way of progress into the new technologies and a more imaged based and visual-spatial based culture. This would certainly require further consideration of a way of thinking that until recently has been perceived as a problem.

Perhaps it is time for society to relook at the unconventional talents that young people with dyslexia can bring to the table, and realise that these visual and creative thinkers could be the answer to many of the current problems of the world, such as climate change, poverty, security, famine and water shortage, pollution, over population etc. Only by looking at these problems from a different perspective, the 'big picture', can they be overcome.

No-one will ever employ you because your reading has got less bad – they will employ you because of your strengths.

(Nicolson, 2015: p. 2)

# Further reading

Eide, B.L. and Eide, F.F. (2011) *The Dyslexia Advantage: Unlocking the Hidden Potential of the Dyslexic Brain*. London: Hay House Ltd.

This is an easy to access book dealing with some highly complex issues of neuroscience. The book is written to enable parents, teachers, practitioners and people with dyslexia to come to terms with the condition by changing the perspective from one of a deficit, with negative implications, to one of positivity and celebration. This book poses the question as to whether the dyslexic brain could paradoxically be seen as superior to the non-dyslexic brain. The book focuses upon what they call the MIND strengths (Material reasoning, Interconnected reasoning, Narrative reasoning and Dynamic reasoning), and is a great resource book for those looking to understand another perspective on dyslexia.

# References

Amesbury, L. (2006) *Dyslexia: A Holistic Review of the Strengths and Difficulties*. Available online at: www.wlv.openrepository.com (accessed 12.06.17).

Cancer, A., Manzoli, S. and Antonietti, A. (2016) The Alleged Links between Creativity and Dyslexia: Identifying the specific process in which dyslexic students excel. *Cogent Psychology* (3) 1190309. Available online at: www.cogentoa.com/article/10.1080/23311908.2016.1190309 (accessed 24.08.17).

Davis, R.D. (1997) *The Gift of Dyslexia: Why Some of the Brightest People Can't Read and How They Learn*. London: Souvenir Press.

Eide, B.L. and Eide, F.F. (2011) *The Dyslexia Advantage: Unlocking the Hidden Potential of the Dyslexic Brain*. London: Hay House Ltd.

Facoetti, A., Corradi, N., Ruffino, M., Gori, S. and Zorzi, M. (2010) Visual Spatial Attention and Speech Segmentation are both Impaired in Pre-schoolers at Familial Risk for Developmental Dyslexia. *Dyslexia* 16 (3): 226–239.

Faglioni, P., Scotti, G. and Spinnler, H. (1969) Impaired Recognition of Written Letters Following Unilateral Hemispheric Damage. *Cortex* 5: 120–133.

Gardner, H. (1984) *Frames of Mind: The Theory of Multiple Intelligences*. London: Fontana Press.

Hampshire, S. (1990) *Every Letter Counts: Winning in Life Despite Dyslexia*. London: Corgi Books.

Logan, J. (2009) Dyslexia Entrepreneurs: The incidence, their coping strategies and their business skills. *Dyslexia*. Available online at: www.ncbi.nlm.nih.gov/pubmed/19378286 (accessed 24.08.17).

Mortimore, T. (2008) *Dyslexia and Learning Style: A Practitioner's Handbook* (2nd edn). Chichester: John Wiley and Son.

Nicolson, R. (2015) *Positive Dyslexia*. Sheffield: Rodin Books.

Nicolson, R. and Fawcett, A. (2007) Procedural Learning Difficulties: Reuniting the developmental disorders? *Trends in Neurosciences* 30 (4): 135–141.

Robertson, J. and Bakker, D. (2002) The Balance Model of Reading and Dyslexia. In Reid and Wearmouth (eds) *Dyslexia and Literacy: Theory and Practice*. Chichester: Wiley and Sons.

Schneps, M. (2014) The Advantages of Dyslexia. *Scientific American*. Available online at: www.scientificamerican.com/article/the-advantages-of-dyslexia/ (accessed 24.08.17).

Sperry, R.W. (1968). Hemisphere Deconnection and Unity in Conscious Awareness. *American Psychologist* 23 (10): 723.

Vail, P. (1990) *About Dyslexia: Unravelling the Myth*. Cheltenham, Australia: Hawker Brownlow Education.

West, T.G. (2005) The Gifts of Dyslexia: Talents among dyslexics and their families. *Paediatrics* (10): 153–158.

White, J. (2005) *Howard Gardner: The Myth of Multiple Intelligences*. London: Institute of Education, University of London.

Zenhausern, I. (1982) Education and the Left Hemisphere. In Keefe, J.W. (ed) *Student Learning Styles and Brain Behaviour*. Learning Styles Network Conference.

# 11 The social and political spectrum

*And the beginning, as you know, is always the most important part, especially in dealing with anything young and tender. That is the time when the character is being moulded and easily takes any impress one may wish to stamp on it.*

Plato, 1941: p. 67

## Introduction

The purpose of the last chapter of a book is often to draw together the threads from the other chapters and cement the ideas that they have read into the readers' heads – this book is no exception. However, the intention of this chapter is also to broaden out the arguments and allow you to consider issues which may take you outside your comfort zone, to move outside the setting and to understand the external, national and global influences that can affect the provision of support for children with particular needs in your place of work.

Research into all areas of early years provision is often very contradictory, but certainly what we do know is that it is a crucial time for a child and their development, and the more research that is undertaken the more this message will be reinforced. These first years of a child's life are the foundation of his/her future being, and this makes it essential that we get it 'right' for the child, the family, the culture and society. This is even more important when the child is a little different to the norm, when they struggle to fit into the cultural, behavioural and educational world that we present to them. If these vulnerable children are to achieve their potential it is likely that they will need targeted, specialist support from well qualified, understanding professionals whose practice is founded on up to date and relevant research.

# Politics and policy

Politics and policy formation is vital to almost everything that we do. Perhaps this is a bold statement at a time when politicians are often vilified and criticised, but party politics and political stance aside, the decisions made by governments and the laws that they ratify will impact every one of you, and the children and families that you care so much for. Whether you believe that you are a 'political animal' or not, politics are key to whether a nation is at war or peace, whether there are laws concerning equality and discrimination, the distribution of wealth and economic funding, healthcare, education and generally who gets what, when and how.

Politics will therefore inevitably be implicated in the management of early years settings and their workforce, because of the importance of their work to the future of the country, to economics, social and cultural management and ideology. Political influence on children can also be seen in the provision of maternity services, health visitors, early years and education places (take for example the current issues around the funding of two-year-olds: DfE, 2017), school starting age, support for special needs etc. You are probably also well aware of the reductions in funding for early years, changes in local authority responsibilities and cutbacks in training opportunities for those working in the sector. The fears of some from the child care and education industry (Professional Association for Childcare and Early Years, 2016) are that it is likely to lead to a reduction in experience and knowledge for these workers, which will have a detrimental effect on children, particularly those with special needs where the training is very limited anyway (see Chapter 9).

Political and social involvement in terms of resources, values and priorities also heavily involve the legal system, as recent court cases involving disputes over dyslexia support, and remediation have shown. Examples of this can be seen in child 'C' in 2015, who had dyslexia and Irlen Syndrome, who claimed discrimination from a Leicester grammar school (Holmes, 2015); the Starbucks employee with dyslexia, who in 2016 successfully sued her employer for discrimination (Power, 2016); and the police chief superintendent who in 2007 took his employers to court for not accepting his dyslexia under the Disabilities Discrimination Act (DDA) 1995. (The DDA was replaced in 2010 by the Equality Act.)

The more you reflect upon the role of politics in early years the more that you realise that the whole concept of education has become a political issue, particularly since the 1970s. Prime Ministers Edward Heath, Harold Wilson, James Callaghan and even Margaret Thatcher put education high on their political agenda, recognising the importance of education to the economic growth of the country. This brought about a change in the whole concept of education, with Government involvement not only in why and what was taught, but also how it was taught and even when it was taught.

This was cemented with the introduction of the National Curriculum in 1988, and only two years later the standard assessment tasks (SATS), which were brought into state schools for all seven-year-olds, to check that the will of the Government was being achieved. In 1996 Prime Minister John Major introduced the 'Desirable Learning Outcomes' as a framework for learning for three- to four-year-olds, and this was followed in 2008 by the Early Years Foundation Stage (which has since been subject to a number of amendments).

In 1972 Margaret Thatcher's Government produced the white paper 'Education: A framework for expansion' (DfES, 1972) prioritising nursery education for all three- and four-year-olds who wanted it, and who can forget in 2001 Tony Blair's famous speech mantra 'Education, Education, Education' making Britain what he repeatedly called a 'Learning Society'.

---

### Reflect on this

Such a political stance to education brings about a whole debate on the nature of education, schools and their purpose. Does education have its own intrinsic value, undertaken for the fulfilment of the person, or do we send our children into education only as a preparation for adulthood, or is it more to do with the economic asset to society, providing the workforce of the future or perhaps a combination of these?

- Personal (self-fulfilment).
- Preparation for adulthood and the next generation.
- Economic and workforce asset.

If it is a combination of these, could there be any sort of hierarchy?

---

In Wales devolution in 1999 allowed the Welsh Assembly Government to determine its own policies for education and in 2008 the Early Years Foundation Phase was introduced as a framework for all children aged three to seven years of age. Thomas and Lewis (2016) calculate that this was at a cost of over one hundred million pounds, so 'big money' politics.

When you consider the politics of dyslexia, you need to distinguish between Politics and politics, in other words politics with a large 'P' and politics with a small 'p',

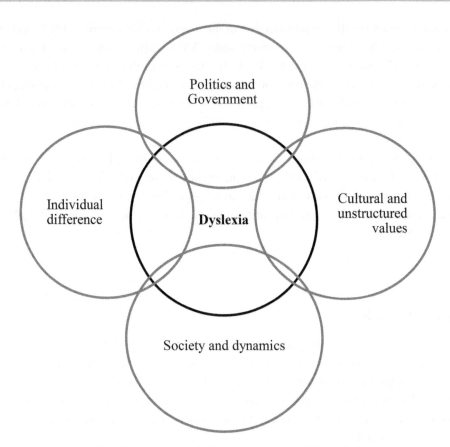

*Figure 11.1* The interaction between dyslexia and the global society

both refer to a system of power, but in very different ways. When you say the word politics, most people probably assume that you are talking about party politics, about voting, campaigning, electoral systems and what happens globally and nationally. Clearly this is something that will directly impact the individual with any form of special needs, determining funding streams, training routes, supply and demand. However, politics with a small 'p' is not in opposition with large 'P' politics but needs to run alongside. This is the way in which you organise everyday life, it is about personal power, your decisions about the clothes you wear, the food you buy and is about the passion you have for the work you do, wanting to help others and provide appropriate solutions to problems, it is about your own philosophy of life and that of your setting. As Aristotle is credited with saying, 'man is a political animal'. I have called these the political 'Ps':

*Table 11.1*

| Small 'p' politics | Large 'P' politics |
| --- | --- |
| Philosophy | Power |
| Passion | Policy making in Government |
| Providing solutions | Parties |
| Personal | Parliamentary |
| | Political leadership |

# Standards

In the pursuit of standards successive Governments have introduced testing, assessments and generally a heavy top-down approach to working with children; statutory programmes have been introduced and increasing levels of legislation. It is possible that a more bottom-up approach to policy now needs to be considered with Government really listening to the practitioners who are working at the 'coal face', day in, day out with children, informing policy with a shared understanding of pedagogy to support children. The current Children's Commissioner, Ann Longfield, recently commented in an interview with Adi Bloom in the *Times Educational Supplement* that children need to be at the centre of children's services and the services need to be shaped around the children and not children trying to fit a mould.

> I guess I'm a believer in the fact that if you shape services around what children need, you get better outcomes for kids.
>
> (Ann Longfield, interview in Bloom, 2017: p. 20)

Legislation such as the National Literacy Policy, introduced under the Blair Government in 1998, was called the Search-lights policy; this was later repealed in 2005, but is a classic example of this highly centralised system and interventionist approach to education. It consisted of four strategies:

1. Phonics
2. Contextual knowledge
3. Grammatical knowledge
4. Word recognition and graphical knowledge

The policy was so highly prescriptive it even required specific timings:

1. 15 minutes of whole class shared reading/writing
2. 15 minutes of whole class word level work
3. 20 minutes of group and independent guided work
4. 10 minutes of whole class plenary session

The National Literacy Strategy was thought to be the largest school improvement programme in the world, with 180 local authorities participating, and at least 18,500 schools with 200,000 teachers actively involved with implementation on over three million children (Mroz, 2017).

However, such highly prescriptive policies were seen by many to be a burden, despite a slight improvement in literacy rates at that time. These improvements were according to Mroz (2017) probably more to do with the focus that teachers placed on literacy rather than down to the inflexible strategy.

> it was due to an unremitting strategic focus combined with sheer hard work by teachers.
>
> (Mroz, 2017: p. 3)

Another area strongly regulated by national governments is the age of school entry, and this has become both controversial and divisive. The legally enforceable date for starting school in England and Wales is the beginning of the term following the child's fifth birthday, however most children are now in formal education by the age of four years, and some have only just had their fourth birthday. In Wales although they are still functioning within this regulatory framework the children are working within the Early Years Foundation Phase, which is based on a play-based philosophy for children aged three to seven years of age. Elliott (2016) discusses the concept of reading readiness and his belief that this should be more flexible to the needs of the child, believing that not all children are ready for formal reading instruction at the same time. Perhaps the same argument could be attributed to the school starting age; it is unlikely that all children are ready to attend formal schooling at the same time, and be able to achieve to their potential. It could be claimed that not all children will have the maturity of neural circuitry to cope with the complex experience of formal schooling, and with the multi-faceted understanding required for reading at the same time.

Longfield (Bloom, 2017) is keen to help the children that she considers fall through the gaps, and she stresses the importance of believing in children, of seeing potential and giving them the confidence to achieve that potential. She is insistent that anxiety, depression and the general mental health of children, at all levels, be addressed. In her role as Children's Commissioner, she recognises that this will require additional funding, and for the Government to prioritise this in their spending.

In lots of areas, actually, the amount spent on children's services has gone up. But that's because it is spent on crisis intervention when things are going wrong. And probably less so on early intervention, when of course it's more cost effective.

(Ann Longfield, interview in Bloom, 2017: p. 21)

---

**Reflect on this**

1. Which piece of legislation since the 1970s do you think has best facilitated the recognition and support for children with dyslexia and why?
2. Reflect on the concerns expressed by parents of children at risk of dyslexia in your care. Consider the legislation and policy on inclusion and the Code of Practice: how can you reassure them that they will be able to obtain the best possible support and guidance for their children and their future?

---

# Commodification

In the years since the introduction of the Early Years Foundation Stage and the Early Years Foundation Phase, accountability has become a key motivator for governments and the inspection process. It could be said that education has become commodified, that is reduced to a product that can be lifted off the shelf and bought and sold. Governments want to see results equal to the funding put into the system, 'prioritising efficiency' and 'customer satisfaction'. Schwartzman (2013) calls this the

> adoption of a market based, consumer-driven philosophy to guide education
>
> (Schwartzman, 2013: p. 1096)

This philosophy of education is likely to fail to ensure that each child is seen as an individual whose needs are unique. If children are going to maximise their opportunities to fulfil their potential, they deserve to have these needs met. Reid (2016) claims that this kind of political pressure on settings is not inclusive and can even be seen as discriminating towards children with special needs and conditions such as dyslexia. The private and market led nature of many early years settings could also unwittingly contribute to this concept of commodified education.

This brings into conflict a dilemma about whether early years education is principally a purveyor of education, or a business to be run along marketplace lines. This brings with it the danger that decisions made in the best interests of a child could be intruded upon by a business model of promoting the setting to best advantage. I am certainly not arguing that early years settings should not make money, after all they are employers who have to pay their employees, and the financial health of the setting is in the numbers of children they work with. However, it is vital that this 'tightrope' walking process does not become detrimental to the individual needs of the child, particularly the child who may be struggling with the system they find themselves in.

Certainly, there is no 'bottomless pit' to pay for the needs of children, but a preoccupation with economic policy over educational, social and cultural policy could potentially have a detrimental impact upon the children, and in turn upon society. Nicholson (2016) calls this a broken system with politics first and science second.

## Dyslexia: the cost to the country

If, as would seem likely, there are children and adults who are not achieving to their potential because of dyslexia, this must be having a detrimental effect upon our society as a whole. The frustrations caused by having poor literacy skills, yet living within a literate society, are potentially enormous and can, as you have read earlier, cause serious mental health problems and social and emotional difficulties. According to Driver (2016) pupils with low literacy skills have a school exclusion rate of up to five times that of their literate peers, and the charity, Every Child a Chance, reported in 2009 that by the age of 37 years each individual with low literacy had cost the taxpayer over £45,000 in criminal justice, special educational support, adult literacy classes, health care costs etc. Over a lifetime this could be as much as £64,000 per person, which potentially amounts to over £2.5 billion a year in total – what could the politicians do with that? This figure probably increases again if you take account of the cost of social services, social housing, possible drug and alcohol abuse, homelessness and loss of tax on pensionable income etc. These estimates were made in 2009, so it is highly likely that these figures will have increased again since then. While all of those with low literacy skills will not be dyslexic, it would be appropriate to say that many of those included in this research review probably were.

According to Rutter et al. (1975) there is a significant link between poor literacy and antisocial behaviour, with up to one-third of all ten-year-olds who have antisocial behaviour referrals having specific reading difficulties, and school exclusions were particularly high for these children. The research by the charity Every Child a Chance (2009) also showed that excluded children were far more likely to turn to crime, with over 63% in one sample having a criminal conviction for violence by the age of 24. This same research showed that suicide rates were almost nineteen times the national average, and people with low literacy skills were up to eight times more likely to be claiming unemployment benefits. Research in 2002 by Parsons and Bynner, linked poor literacy to smoking, alcohol abuse and obesity (2–3 times the national average), causing a possible further drain on an already overstretched health service. Every Child a Chance (2009) calculated that approximately 10% of women with average literacy skills experienced depression at some point in their lives, which required medication and attention from the health service, but in women with low literacy skills this increased to 36%. Parsons and Bynner (2002) estimated that on the costs at that time, there could be an average saving of between £55.2 million and £1.2 billion, if effective support for children were put in place before the age of seven. This is, of course, merely speculation, but it certainly gives food for thought. Parsons and Bynner (2002) also make the point that the costs at Key Stage 1 and 2 of the support required are likely to be less than at secondary level, meaning that at secondary level the cost probably outweighs the advantages, making it possible to see that such interventions would be better placed within the early years.

## Big money

The DfE budget for all special needs is probably more than £2.5 billion, with each individual assessment with an educational psychologist costing up to £750 – this is big money. So, dyslexia is 'big business', as pointed out by Nicholson (2005), and the rewards for devising a unique and effective instrument for remediation would be huge, given that although experts cannot agree on a definitive percentage of prevalence (estimates of anywhere from 5–25%), they do agree that it is the most common form of special need. It has been estimated that there are probably approximately six million people with dyslexia in the UK alone. However, no distinct status is accorded to dyslexia within the Code of Practice (2015), which treats all children with special educational need on an equal footing. The dyslexia 'industry' can potentially play upon the vulnerability of parents who are desperate to do the best for their children.

Whether this country is prepared to invest in these children depends upon the way in which society regards childhood in general. Piper (2008) suggested that society regards childhood as a period of preparation for an economically active adult, law abiding citizens making a positive contribution to society. In this view investment is only likely to be undertaken in anticipation of societal rewards. This is clearly in sharp contrast to an alternative view, which emphasises personal happiness and fulfilled adults.

## Criminal justice

Having positive self-esteem and feelings of self-worth are so important to us all in life, and no more so than when we are attempting to learn, attempting to do something difficult. In this circumstance it is so easy to give up, and it is only your inbuilt resilience that keeps you going. For those who have a poor sense of self-worth, possibly exacerbated by a lack of past achievement in things that the education system values, this sense of failure, probably first experienced at a very early age, can remain with you throughout life. Only when you find success in other fields, and you have others that believe in you, are you likely to regain your self-belief. The constant drip-drip of minor failures can result in criminal actions and illegal experimentation. Mortimore (2003) believes that unlike non-dyslexic individuals, who tend to blame failure on things that are outside of themselves, those with dyslexia tend to blame failure on themselves, and their lack of ability to achieve.

These links between dyslexia and the criminal justice system have been seen repeatedly in other research programmes starting with poor attendance in school and following down a brutal spiral of events (Figure 11.2).

Talbot (2008) undertook some extensive research for the Prison Reform Trust and estimated that there were from 20–30% of offenders with learning difficulties, compared with 2% in the general population. However, the Dyslexia Institute (2005) highlighted a study by probation officers in London, which showed that 52% of the inmates had dyslexic tendencies, but prisoners who were given appropriate support were less likely to reoffend, many going on to college or work at a level way above the average for ex-offenders. The Dyslexia Institute review (2005) of the literature also showed a number of disturbing statistics:

- 80% of those leaving prison did not have the literacy skills needed for 96% of the available jobs
- 50% were at or below level one in their literacy (the level expected of an 11-year-old)
- 67% were at or below level one in their numeracy
- 80% were at or below level one in their writing
- 30% had been school truants
- 49% of males had been excluded from school
- 58% re-offended within two years
- 80% had already served a prison sentence
- 52% of males and 71% females had no qualifications

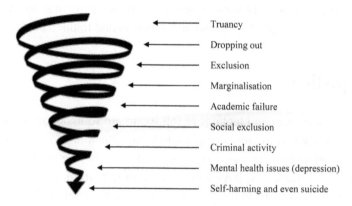

*Figure 11.2* The downward spiral of poor self-worth

The Dyslexia Institute (2005) estimates that 40% of those with low literacy skills in prison are dyslexic, a far higher proportion than would be expected in the general population. Of course, poor literacy and dyslexia are not the only reason for individuals ending up in the criminal justice system, and there is no reason to suppose that dyslexia of itself predisposes anyone to commit crime. There are in fact numerous, complex and multifaceted factors which contribute to the cycle of offending and re-offending, but poor literacy skills and low self-esteem are generally recognised as critical factors.

According to the Government's own statistics (Ministry of Justice, 2017), the total prison population in England and Wales in 2016 was 85,128. Each prisoner purportedly costs between £27,505 and £87,280 per annum, an average of £33,291 cost to you, the tax payer. From these figures it can be seen that there is an urgent social and economic argument for doing everything possible to preventing re-offending.

# Training

The Special Educational Needs and Disability Code of Practice (DfE and DoH, 2015) is a legally binding document of statutory status, which means that it is a legal requirement to abide by it. It also means that it has been through a Parliamentary process, which relates to the Children and Families Act 2014 (Gov.UK, 2014). It is interesting therefore that it is a legal requirement for all settings to ensure that all children gain the support that they need. This by its very nature implies that settings need to know what that support is, and that this has been identified and defined. For this to occur, staff in the settings need to have been appropriately trained to identify and assess that particular need. The importance of training is also mentioned in the Code of Practice (DfE and DoH, 2015), but unless there are an appropriate number of suitable training courses and suitably qualified trainers, this cannot be achieved.

It is vital for the outcomes of children that all initial training courses in this sphere consider critically, and as part of their mainstream curriculum, the issues involving different ways of processing information and thinking, that the practitioners will certainly encounter in their careers when working with children. They need to understand how to progress the child's development from their starting position, in a stress free and graduated manner. According to research by the Driver Youth Trust (Driver, 2016), over 50% of the teachers surveyed said that they had had no training related to dyslexia, and nine out of ten of the remainder had received less than half a day, and yet 84% said that they felt that it was important to be trained to teach children with dyslexia. The Teacher Standards (DfE, 2011), by which all teachers are assessed, require all teachers to be able to recognise the strengths and challenges for the children in their care, but with so little training and guidance in dyslexia it would appear to be unlikely that they would be able to do this for children with information processing differences.

Most teachers do not have a basic understanding of dyslexia.

(Driver, 2016: online)

Very worryingly in the same research, nine out of ten parents of children with dyslexia recognised that the teachers did not understand how to help their children. It is therefore highly unlikely that parents will have confidence in schools and nurseries to ensure the best outcomes for their vulnerable children.

Well trained staff are probably the critical aspect for achieving good outcomes for children; this was highlighted in the well-respected research the Effective Provision of Pre-school Education Project (EPPE) (Sylva et al., 2004):

Settings that have staff with higher qualifications have higher quality scores and the children make more progress.

(Sylva, 2004: p. 1)

As can be seen in the small-scale research for this book described in Chapter 9, staff training is woefully limited, particularly for those working with the under four-year-olds. The current training programmes for early years practitioners and teachers do not really prepare them for the multifaceted role of working with children at risk of dyslexia, which up to date research has identified. There are of course many challenges to ensuring that staff have the knowledge and skills required, not the least of which is finding higher and further education tutors that have that knowledge and skills themselves to pass on. In the short term it could also be seen as an additional financial burden to upskill and retain the existing workforce.

The research reviewed shows that literacy difficulties are linked to costly special educational needs provision, to truancy, exclusion from school, reduced employment opportunities, increased health risks and a greatly increased risk of involvement with the criminal justice system. These increased risks operate over and above those associated with social disadvantage in general, and those associated with lack of qualifications.

(Every Child a Chance, 2009: p. 5)

---

**Reflect on this**

Consider for a moment your own initial training and reflect on the following questions:

1. In what way do you think that it prepared you for your present role?
2. How could this have been improved upon?

---

If you were given the opportunity to help to design a new module for this course, which would encompass the knowledge and understanding of dyslexia, its support and remediation, what would be the five learning outcomes that you would propose?

At the end of this module the student will be able to:

1.
2.
3.
4.
5.

# Research for the future

Whilst difficulties with literacy are undoubtedly a very serious consequence of dyslexia, it is by no means the only one and, as you have already read, there is a range of difficulties experienced by the dyslexic individual in areas of organisation, physical acuity, memory etc. Therefore, it is possible that these are being overshadowed by the research concentration upon reading and language. Whilst not denying the potentially devastating effects of poor literacy skills upon the individual, this is only one manifestation in the enigma of this fascinating, multifaceted condition. It is possible that society is getting too 'hung up' on the reading and literacy manifestation of dyslexia, and ignoring the many others which are often more identifiable in the non-reading child in the early years, when dyslexia is clearly present, but not related to reading. Perhaps future research should focus on the early years child, to identify the characteristics of this information processing difference, without the clouding of poor reading capacity to infiltrate and direct the research into what could be a 'blind alley'.

> [T]he disorder seems to be the result of a subtle yet significant snarl in the brain's ability to process information about words . . . but why include 'about words'?
> (Underwood, 2013: p. 1158)

Perhaps researchers need to take a step back, to examine whether this is an abnormality, a snarl, a malfunction, deficit, disorder or whether it is a difference in the brain functioning commensurate with a normal distribution curve of human brain functioning, and whether such equivalence could be found in other intelligent animal species such as primates, dogs or birds.

# Recommendations

To conclude this book I have taken the liberty to compile a list of my recommendations for governments, early years policy makers and practitioners of the future:

- Nationally agreed standards and procedures should be agreed and implemented with all children.
- All staff working with children in the early years, including inspection teams, need to be dyslexia aware, and to be appropriately trained during their mandatory initial training programmes, to see the 'warning' signs and know how to act appropriately. Staff need to be aware of the devastatingly negative consequences of low self-esteem and lack of confidence.
- All settings should develop a policy statement and implement practices to ensure that children are assessed and identified as 'at risk' as soon as possible, with observations and screening methods used routinely and systematically.
- Where children are thought to be at risk, SENCOs and families need to be informed and made aware of the concerns.
- Individual action plans should be developed to support the practice of even the most junior members of staff.
- A multidisciplinary approach to support should be implemented, with access to appropriate specialist support if this is deemed necessary.
- Suitable training programmes for staff working with children need to be devised and implemented at a full range of levels from level one to level seven.
- Staff in higher and further education colleges/universities need appropriate awareness of the up to date research, to enable them to pass on this information to their initial students.
- Every setting should have at least one member of staff with additional training and responsibility for children at risk of dyslexia to lead policy and practice.
- Examples of good practice should be highlighted and disseminated to all settings.
- The value of parental concerns should be recognised and actioned upon as a close partnership between staff and parents is encouraged.
- There should be opportunities and funding for continuing professional development for those already in practice.
- Ofsted should monitor how children at risk of dyslexia are identified and supported.
- Searching and rigorous research needs to continue to understand more about this information processing difference in all its manifestations.

## Chapter reflections

This book has examined what I believe are the key issues which appear to impact the outcomes for young children at risk of dyslexia or information processing differences: a lack of informed knowledge by practitioners and teachers about the aetiology, identification and management, largely attributable to poor training and professional development. An information processing difference, and all its manifestations, is a complex amalgam of a range of indicators and, as has been shown in this book, there are no easy answers to identification, prevalence, and support, but there are also positive aspects to such a diverse way of thinking. Pumfrey (2001) describes dyslexia as being 'hydra-headed' as when one head is chopped off, or one question answered, another appears to replace it that needs to be addressed. Dyslexia International (2014) claim that if those working with these children were appropriately trained then 90% could be well educated within the mainstream system. Of course, there is no way to verify this claim, but it would appear logical that outcomes for children would be better. Dyslexia International (2014) also appeal to world leaders, experts and educationalists to convene a community of world sharing, to develop better policy and practice, and perhaps we do need a radical new vision of the concept of dyslexia, that better meets the needs of the children at risk. It is certainly true that there is more information now about dyslexia than ever before, perhaps too much information, to the point whereby it is less informative and more bewildering. This is compounded by huge ethical and moral dilemmas concerning economics and resourcing. However, perhaps the most troubling issue is whether the education systems in both England and Wales are fit for purpose, and whether the system as it stands can deal with the diversity of interests and abilities of the children it purports to educate. Hyman (2017) describes it as a

> [o]ne-dimensional education system in a multi-dimensional world.
>
> (Hyman, 2017: p. 26)

He believes that there needs to be a radical rethink within the care and education system, to ensure that it educates the whole child, and acknowledges children in all their glorious diversity, difference and individuality. This he suggests, can only be done by nurturing their abilities, without ignoring their challenges, valuing creativity and providing content that is of value beyond the current rigidity of the educational sphere.

## Further reading

Elliott, J. and Nicolson, R. (2016) *Dyslexia: Developing the Debate*. London: Bloomsbury.

This is an unusual and approachable text which brings together two of the world's leading experts in dyslexia, who take totally opposing views of the research as presented. This is a book which is a 'must-read' for anyone writing an assignment into the complexities of dyslexia and related conditions, enabling the reader to review different approaches and philosophies within one text. This book offers a very down to earth approach and recognises the need for a cost-effective stance led by government policy. The arguments are pulled together and critically evaluated in the final section by Andrew Davis who is the book's editor.

## References

Bloom, A. (2017) I would really love a dialogue with teachers about the issues they are facing. *Times Educational Supplement* 5254: p. 20.

DfE (2011) *Teachers Standards*. Available online at: www.gov.uk/government/publications/teachers-standards (accessed 27.08.17).

DfE (2014) *Children and Families Act 2014*. Norwich: Crown. The Stationery Office.

DfE (2017) *Will I qualify for 30 hours free childcare?* Available online at: www.gov.uk/government/uploads/system/uploads/attachment_data/file/615804/30_hours_free_childcare.pdf (accessed 27.08.17).

DfE and DoH (2015) *Special Educational Needs and Disability Code of Practice: 0–25 Years*. London: Crown.

DES (1972) *Education: Framework for Expansion* (White Paper). Available online at: www.educationengland.org.uk/documents/wp1972/framework-for-expansion.html (accessed 27.08.17).

Driver, S. (2016) *The Fish in the Tree: Why we are Failing Children with Dyslexia*. Available online at: www.driveryouthtrust.com/df/fish-in-the-tree-report-and-drive-for-literacy/ (accessed 27.08.17).

Dyslexia Institute (2005) *The Incidence of Hidden Disabilities in the Prison Population: Yorkshire and Humberside Research*. Surrey: The Dyslexia Institute.

Dyslexia International (2014) *Better Training, Better Teaching*. Available online at: www.dyslexia-international.org (accessed 27.08.17).

Elliott, J. (2016) Dyslexia: Beyond the debate. In Elliott, J. and Nicolson, R. (2016) *Dyslexia: Developing the Debate*. London: Bloomsbury.

Every Child a Chance Trust (2009) *The Long Term Costs of Literacy Difficulties* (2nd edn). Available online at: https://readingrecovery.org/images/pdfs/Reading_Recovery/Research_and_Evaluation/long_term_costs_of_literacy_difficulties_2nd_edition_2009.pdf (accessed 28.08.17).

Holmes, R. (2015) *Disability Discrimination Recent Cases*. Available online at: www.farrer.co.uk/Global/Briefings/14.%20School%20Briefing/Disability%20discrimination%20-%20recent%20cases%20.pdf (accessed 28. 08.17).

Hyman, P. (2017) A New Vision of Education: The head, the heart and the hand. *Times Educational Supplement*: 19 May 2017, pp. 26–27.

Legislation.gov.uk. (2014). *Children and Families Act 2014*. Available online at: www.legislation.gov.uk/ukpga/2014/6/contents/enacted (accessed 29.08.17).

Ministry of Justice (2017) *Criminal Justice Statistics Quarterly for England and Wales 2016*. Available online at: www.gov.uk/government/uploads/system/uploads/attachment_data/file/614414/criminal-justice-statistics-quarterly-december-2016.pdf (accessed 29.08.17).

Mortimore, T. (2008) *Dyslexia and Learning Style*. Chichester: John Wiley and Son.

Mroz, A. (2017) Harry Potter had a Major Effect on Pupils Literacy: siriusly? *Times Educational Supplement Editorial* 5254: p. 3.

Nicolson, R. (2016) Developmental Dyslexia: The bigger picture. In Elliott, J. and Nicolson, R. *Dyslexia: Developing the Debate*. London: Bloomsbury.

Parsons, S. and Bynner, J. (2002) *Basic Skills and Social Exclusion*. London: The Basic Skills Agency.

Piper, C. (2008) *Investing in Children: Policy Law and Practice in Context*. Devon: Willan Publishing.

Plato (1941) *The Republic of Plato*. Translated by Cornford, F. M. London: Oxford University Press.

Power, B. (2016) *Starbucks Dyslexia Case: Implications*. Available online at: www.springhouselaw.com/updates/starbucks-dyslexia-case-implications/ (accessed 27.08. 17).

Professional Association for Childcare and Early Years (PACEY) (2016) *Working in childcare: What's happened to CPD?* Available online at: www.pacey.org.uk/news-and-views/pacey-blog/2016/february-2016/working-in-childcare-whats-happened-to-cpd/ (accessed 28.08.17).

Pumfrey, P. (2001) Specific Developmental Dyslexia (SDD): 'Basics to back' in 2000 and beyond. In Hunter-Carsch (ed.) *Dyslexia: A Psychosocial Perspective*. London: Whurr Publishers.

Rutter, M., Cox, A., Tupling, C., Berger, M. and Yule, W. (1975) Attainment and Adjustment in Two Geographical Areas, 1: The prevalence of child psychiatric disorder. *British Journal of Psychiatry* 126: 493–509.

Schwartzman, R. (2013) Consequences of Commodifying Education. *Academic Exchange Quarterly* 17 (3): 1096–1453.

Sylva, K., Melhuish, E., Sammons, P., Siraj-Blatchford, I. & Taggart, B. (2004). *The Effective Provision of Pre-school Education (EPPE) Project: Findings from Pre-School to End of Key Stage 1*. Nottingham: Department for Education and Skills.

Talbot, J. (2008) *No One Knows*. The Prison Reform Trust. Available online at: www.prisonreformtrust.org.uk/Portals/0/Documents/No%20One%20Knows%20report-2.pdf (accessed 29.08.17).

Thomas, A. and Lewis, A. (2016) *An Introduction to the Foundation Phase: Early Years Curriculum in Wales*. London: Bloomsbury.

Underwood, E. (2013) Faulty Brain Connections in Dyslexia? *Science* 342 (6163): 1158.

# Further help

Whether you are a parent of a child at risk of dyslexia, professional working with children or a student studying in further or higher education, you may well find the following contacts useful to you and your studies.

**British Dyslexia Association (BDA)**
http://www.bdadyslexia.org.uk/
Tel: 0333 405 4555
The British Dyslexia Association, Unit 6a Bracknell Beeches, Old Bracknell Lane, Bracknell RG12 7BW

**Department for Education (DfE)**
https://www.gov.uk/government/organisations/department-for-education

**Department for Education Standards and Testing Agency**
https://www.gov.uk/government/organisations/standards-and-testing-agency

**Dyslexia Action**
http://www.dyslexiaaction.org.uk/get-help
Tel: 0203201 8000
Dyslexia Action Training and Guild, Centurion House, London Road, Staines-upon-Thames TW18 4AX

**Helen Arkle Centre**
https://www.helenarkell.org.uk/
Tel: 01252 792 400
Helen Arkell Dyslexia Centre, Arkell Lane, Frensham, Farnham, Surrey GU10 3BL

**Dyslexia-SpLD Trust**
http://www.thedyslexia-spldtrust.org.uk/

**Dyslexia Research Trust**

https://www.dyslexic.org.uk/

Tel: 0118 958 5950

Dyslexia Research Trust, 179A Oxford Road, Reading RG1 7UZ

**European Dyslexia Association**

http://www.eda-info.eu/

c/o Bureau Felix & Felix sprl, Chaussée de Tubize 135, B-1440 Braine Le Château, Belgium.

**International Dyslexia Association**

https://dyslexiaida.org/

Tel: (410) 296–0232

40 York Road, 4th Floor, Baltimore, MD 21204, USA.

**Listening Books**

https://www.listening-books.org.uk/

Tel: 020 7407 9417

Listening Books, 12 Lant Street, London SE1 1QH

**Professional Association of Teachers of Students with Specific Learning Difficulties (PATOSS)**

https://www.patoss-dyslexia.org/

Tel: 01386 712 650

Evesham College, Davies Road, Evesham, Worcestershire WR11 1LP

**Royal College of Speech and Language Therapists**

https://www.rcslt.org/

Tel: 020 7378 120

2, White Hart Yard, London SE1 1NX

**ICAN**

http://www.ican.org.uk/

Tel: 020 7843 2510 31

Angel Gate (Gate 5), Goswell Road, London EC1V 2PT

**Driver Youth Trust**

http://www.driveryouthtrust.com/

Tel: 020 3096 7711

CAN Mezzanine, 7–14 Great Dover Street, London SE1 4YR

# Glossary

**Automaticity**   The ability to do things without having to think about them – walking, talking, breathing etc.

**Autosomal dominant transmission**   This is a type of inheritance when a dominant gene for a particular disorder or trait will affect a person. This is usually a mutated gene and requires only one parent to carry it to pass on to the child.

**Binocular instability**   When one or both eyes drift from the point of focus, making it difficult to maintain a fixation.

**Canonical sounds**   Babbling sounds and sound combinations made by babies that are 'word like'.

**Ciliogenesis**   This is the formation of cilia or minute 'hairs' on the surface of cells which beat in rhythm to move fluids across the cells.

**Cluster**   A number of difficulties and/or abilities occurring together.

**Code switching**   Changing from one language to another in the course of one conversation.

**Continuum**   A change that occurs gradually with no distinctive dividing points.

**Contrast sensitivity**   The ability to distinguish between objects and their background. This is particularly important in situations of low light, fog and glare. This is frequently referred to by children with Scotopic Sensitivity Syndrome.

**Commodification**   To treat something or someone as a commodity or product.

**Cortical excitability**   This is the interaction of neurotransmitters and cellular receptors to determine the level of neuronal activity or inhibition.

**Dysfluency**   The inability to produce a smooth flow of speech sounds.

**Epistatic effects**   Usually related to genetics, when the effect of one gene is dependent upon the interaction with another.

**Executive skills**   These are neurological functions which enable a good working memory/recall, inhibition control and reflection, or the ability to consider something from more than one perspective.

**Genetic linkage analysis**   This is a method used to locate an abnormal gene on a chromosome – gene hunting or genetic testing.

**Grey matter**   The darker grey areas of the brain (sometimes yellowish/pinky), containing mostly neuronal cells.

**Inflectional morphology**   These usually refer to either number, tense, person, case or gender. They are different forms of the same word and add meaning to that word. For example: 'jump', 'jumps', 'jumped'.

**Iatrogenesis**   Inducing a condition unintentionally, leading to the self-fulfilling prophecy.

**Loci**   This is the plural of locus and refers to places or locations.

**Magnocells**   These are neurons in the brain that have large cell bodies. They are sometimes referred to as M-cells.

**Matthew effect**   Individual differences when learning to read, and the progressively widening gap between the good and poor readers. Good readers read more and become better at it, poor readers shun reading and continue to be poor readers.

**Morphological priming**   Readers are influenced by the morphological structure of the words they see. For example, the word 'garage', is more likely to be recognised when followed by the word 'car' than if followed by 'octopus'.

**Neural migration**   The manner in which neurons move from their place of origin to their final location during brain development.

**Norm based tests**   Also referred to as norm referenced tests, or standardised tests. Assesses how the participants compare to the hypothetical average for that test.

**Onset**   The initial sound unit of any word. For example, 'c' in cat and 'ch' in church.

**Ontogenetically**   The holistic development of an individual attributable to their interaction with their close environment.

**Orthography**   The conventional spelling system of a language and the representation of sounds of that language through a symbol based system.

**Parvocells**   Sometimes referred to as P-cells these are neurons within the brain with small cell bodies, compared with magnocells.

**Phoneme**   This is the smallest unit of sound in a language. For example, the 'f' sound in 'fat', 'telephone', 'gaffe', 'cough'.

**Phonological processing**   The ability to analyse and manipulate sounds into words, and to process those sounds and words into letters on a page.

**Phylogenetically**   Holistic development of an individual attributable to their genetic make-up.

**Polysemous**   Several meanings in a single word. For example, 'tear' (there was a tear in his eye/there was tear in her skirt), 'table' (he put a book on the table/she learned the multiplication table), 'play' (the children went out to play/we went to see a Shakespeare play).

**Profile**   A set of characteristics or distinctive features (strengths and/or weaknesses) that identify a particular person.

**Range**   A characteristic or behaviour with upper and lower limits identified.

**Rime**   This is the sound made by the letter or string of letters that follow the onset. For example, 'cat' = c (onset) at (rime), 'dog' = d (onset) og (rime). They help children to understand word families – 'king', 'ring', 'sing' etc.

**Silent period**   This usually refers to a stage when children who are learning a second language do not speak in that new language. They may have understanding, but are not confident with expressive language.

**Specific learning difficulties**   Difficulties or differences in particular aspects of learning, such as reading, number, movement etc. This is opposed to general learning difficulties/ differences when the ability to learn is globally well below the expected norms.

**Syndrome**   A collection of associated characteristics that vary in intensity from person to person.

**Vestibular**   Parts of the inner ear and brain that control balance, eye movement and spatial orientation.

**White matter**   This takes up the majority of the brain. It is paler than grey matter and consists mostly of nerve fibres.

# Index

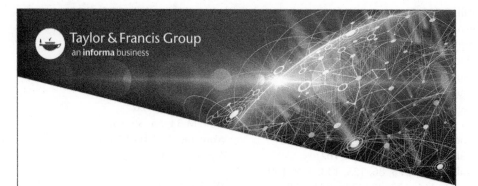

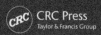

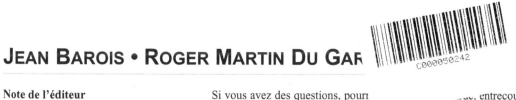

## Note de l'éditeur

Les descriptions du livre que nous demandons aux libraires de placer en évidence préviennent qu'il s'agit d'un livre historique contenant de nombreuses coquilles ou du texte manquant ; il n'est pas référencé ni illustré.

Le livre a été créé en recourant au logiciel de reconnaissance optique de caractères. Le logiciel est précis à 99 pour cent si le livre est en bon état. Toutefois, nous comprenons que même un pour cent peut représenter un nombre agaçant de coquilles ! Et, parfois, il peut manquer une partie d'une page voire une page entière dans notre copie du livre. Il peut aussi arriver que le papier ait été si décoloré avec le temps qu'il est difficile à lire. Nous présentons nos excuses pour ce désagrément et remercions avec gratitude l'assistance de Google.

Après avoir recomposé et reconçu un livre, les numéros de page sont modifiés et l'ancien index et l'ancienne table des matières ne correspondent plus. Pour cette raison, nous pouvons les supprimer ; sinon, ignorez-les.

Nous corrigeons attentivement les livres qui vendront suffisamment d'exemplaires pour payer le correcteur ; malheureusement, c'est rarement le cas. C'est pourquoi, nous essayons de laisser aux clients la possibilité de télécharger une copie gratuite du livre original sans coquilles. Entrez simplement le code barre de la quatrième de couverture du livre de poche dans le formulaire Livre gratuit sur www.RareBooksClub.com.

Vous pouvez également remplir les conditions pour adhérer gratuitement et à l'essai à notre club de livres pour télécharger quatre livres tout aussi gratuitement. Entrez simplement le code barre de la quatrième de couverture sur le formulaire d'adhésion qui se trouve sur notre page d'accueil. Le club de livres vous permet d'accéder à des millions de livres. Entrez simplement le titre, l'auteur ou le sujet dans le formulaire de recherche.

Si vous avez des questions, pour vous d'abord consulter la page de n. Foire Aux Questions sur www.Rare-BooksClub.com/faqs.cfm ? Vous pouvez également nous y contacter.

General Books LLC™, Memphis, USA, 2012. ISBN: 9781235128370.

⚜ ⚜ ⚜ ⚜ ⚜

IL A ÉTÉ RÉIMPOSÉ ET TIRÉ A PART

DE LA PREMIÈRE ÉDITION, 30 EXEMPLAIRES

SUR VERGÉ D'ARCHES NUMÉROTÉS DE I A 30

TOUS DROITS DE REPRODUCTION

ET DE TRADUCTION, RÉSERVÉS POUR

TOUS LES PAYS Y COMPRIS LA RUSSIE

« A M. MARCEL HÉBERT. -, *Votre sensibilité religieuse ne peut qu'être blessée par certaines tendances de ce livre. Je le sais; et je vous remercie d'autant plus d'en avoir accepté la dédicace. Votre nom, au seuil de ces pages, n'est pas seulement le témoignage du respectueux et vivace attachement que je vous porte depuis vingt ans. Je suis assuré qu'il me vaudra, de tous ceux qui connaissent la noblesse de votre pensée et le riche apport critique de votre œuvre, une attention plus grave, et comme un reflet de cette estime qui entoure l'éloquent renoncement de votre vie. R. M. G. (Octobre 1913 J*

## PREMIÈRE PARTIE
## GOUT DE VIVRE

La chambre de Mme Barois.

Pénombre. Derrière les rideaux, la lune strie de noir et de blanc les"persiennes. Sa lueur sur le parquet, met en relief un bas de robe, une bottine d'homme qui bat silencieusement la mesure. Deux respirations; deux êtres s'immobilisant dans une même attente'.

Par moments, dans la pièce voisine, le grincement d'un lit de fer; une voix

.ue, entrecoupant des mots .e rêve ou de délire. Dans l'entrebaîllement de la porte, un reflet mouvant de veilleuse.

Longue pause.

LE DOCTEUR (à voix basse). — Le bromure agit, la nuit va être plus calme.

Lourdement Mme Barois se lève et, sur la pointe des pieds, s'approche de la porte; appuyée au vantail, le masque inerte et douloureux, les paupières à demi baissées, elle regarde fixement dans la chambre éclairée.

Mme Barois: grande vieille femme, au ventre déformé, à la démarche pesante.

L'état cru de la veilleuse fouille impitoyablement son visage ravagé; la peau est Jaune, distendue; des ombres soulignent la bouffissure des yeux, la chute des joues, le gonflement des lèvres, le fanon.

Une bonté rigide, un peu bornée; une douceur têtue; de la réserve.

Quelques minutes. MADAME BAROIS (bas). — Il dort.

Elle ferme avec précaution la porte, allume une lampe et vient se rasseoir.

LE DOCTEUR (posant sa main sur celle de sa mère, et, par habitude, glissant les doigts jusqu'au pouls). — Vous aussi, Maman, ce voyage vous a épuisée.

Mme Barois secoue la tête.

Madame Barois (bas). — Je sens que tu m'en veux, Philippe, d'avoir.emmené Jean là-bas.

Il ne répond pas.

a, Le Docteur Barois: cinquante-six ans. Petit, alerte; gestes vifs et précis.

Le poil déjà gris. Un visage fin et comme aiguisé: l'arête du nez est coupante, la moustache darde deux bouts cirés, la barbe pointe; un demi-sourire, malicieux et bon, amincit les lèvres; l'œil mobile et perçant luit à feux brefs à travers le lorgnon.

MADAME BAROIS (après une pause). — Pourtant, ici, tous me l'ont conseillé... Et Jean, qui me tourmentait pour que je l'inscrive! Il avait le pressentiment, ce petit, qu'il reviendrait débarrassé de son mal. Pendant tout le voyage, il s'est fait répéter l'histoire de Bernadette...

Le docteur retire son lorgnon: regard myope, plein de tendresse. Mme Barois se tait. Leurs pensées se reconnaissent et se heurtent: tout un passé entre eux.

MADAME BAROIS (les yeux au ciel). — Oui, tu ne peux plus comprendre... Nous ne pouvons plus nous comprendre, toi et moi, mon fils et moi I Et voilà ce qu'ils ont fait de toi, à Paris, de l'enfant que tu étais...

LE Docteur. — Ma pauvre Maman, ne discutons pas... Je ne vous reproche rien. Rien, sinon de m'avoir averti lorsqu'il était trop tard pour que je dise non. Jean n'était pas capable de supporter un pareil voyage, dans un train omnibus, en troisième...

Madame BAROIS. — Est-ce que tu ne t'exagères pas son état, mon enfant? Tu l'as retrouvé ce soir, avec de la fièvre, avec du délire... Mais tu ne l'as pas vu tout cet hiver...

Le DOCTEUR (soucieux).. — Non je ne l'ai pas vu, tout cet hiver.

Madame BAROIS (enhardie). — Depuit cette bronchite, il n'a jamais repris sa mine, c'est certain... Il se plaignait d'un point, là... Mais enfin, il n'avait pas l'air d'un enfant malade, je t'assure... Souvent le soir, il était gai, trop gai même...

Le docteur remet soigneusement son lorgnon et se penche vers sa mère; il saisit sa main.

Le DOCTEUR. — Trop gai, le soir... Oui... (Secouant la tête.) Vous oubliez trop vite le passé, Maman.

MADAME BAROIS (têtue). — Là-dessus, mon enfant, tu sais ce que je pense. Jamais je n'ai voulu croire que ta chère femme ait été... ce que tu crois. C'est Paris qui te l'a tuée: comme tant d'autres!

Le docteur baisse la tête. Il écoute à peine. A la lueur de la lampe, il vient d'apercevoir cette main qu'il caressait machinalement: lourde main, usée et molle, tachée de rouille, aux doigts déformés. Il touche, avec un recul subit à sa petite enfance, cette alliance amincie, prête à rompre, que la jointure enflée tiendra prisonnière maintenant, jusqu'à la fin... Et spontanément, pour la première fois de sa vie peut-être, avec la tentation lâche de pleurer, de fuir, d'échapper à l'impitoyable, il porte à ses lèvres cette vieille main méconnaissable, qu'il ne confondrait pourtant avec aucune autre.

Mme Barois, gênée, retire sa main.

Madame BAROIS (avec âpreté). — Et d'abord, Jean est de notre côté, tout à fait... C'est ton portrait, voyons! Tout le monde le dit! Cet enfant-là n'a rien de sa mère...

Pause.

LE DOCTEUR (à lui-même, sombre). — J'ai été tellement occupé, tout cet hiver... (Il s'aperçoit qu'il n'a pas répondu à sa mère. Il se tourne affectueusement.) C'est dur, le métier, dans ces cas-là, Maman... Un fils malade, à quelques heures de Paris, et se laisser prendre son temps, tout son temps, heure par heure, pour d'autres... Chaque fois qu'on inscrit un rendez-vous nouveau, penser à cette feuille d'agenda qu'on ne peut garder blanche... Ah I si je pouvais quitter tout, m'installer là, près de lui, près de vous deux!... (Tranchant.) Mais je ne peux pas. C'est impossible.

Il soulève son pince-nez, l'essuie, réfléchit quelques instants, puis le replace avec décision. La parole devient brève, affirmative, — professionnelle.

LE DOCTEUR. — Il va falloir redoubler de surveillance, nuit et jour; combattre pied à pied le mal...

Mme Barois laisse échapper un geste d'incrédulité.

Le docteur s'arrête net, enveloppe sa mère d'un coup d'œil rapide. Une seconde de désarroi: ainsi, lorsqu'au cours d'une opération il doit brusquement renverser son plan. Puis l'œil s'aiguise, se fixe; une résolution nouvelle.

Long silence

II

Huit jours après, un dimanche matin.

LE DOCTEUR (entrant dans la chambre de Jean). — Bonjour, mon petit. Comment allons-nous, ce matin? La fenêtre fermée, par ce beau soleil?

Il prend les mains de l'enfant, et le place devant lui, face au joui,

LE DOCTEUR. — La langue... Bon. .. As-tu bien dormi, cette semaine? Pas trop? Tu t'agites toujours dans ton lit? Tu te réveilles parce que tu as trop chaud?Ah... (Une tape sur la joue.) Déshabille-toi que je t'ausculte.

/ Jean: un gamin de douze ans, pâlot. Des traits fins, sans caractère. Le regard est plus personnel: caressant, réfléchi, sans gaieté.uKS

Un torse malingre; des traînées mauves, sur la peau mince, soulignent les côtes.

LE DOCTEUR. — Voyons, maintenant... Appuie-toi, le dos au mur, comme l'autre jour; les bras pendants. .. Lève le menton, ouvre la bouche... C'est ça... (Il retire son lorgnon.) Respire profondément, régulièrement... Recommence...

Il écoute, le masque douloureux, l'œil clignotant, isolé du monde par sa myopie et son attention crispée.

L'angoisse du père. L'insouciance de 1 enfant qui bâille et. regarde le ciel.

Longue auscultation.

LE DOCTEUR (simplement). — C'est bien, mon petit, tu peux te rhabiller... (Sourire très tendre.) Maintenant, voici ce que je te propose: nous allons descendre au jardin, tous les deux, et causer tranquillement, au soleil, en attendant que ta grand'mère soit revenue de la messe. Quoi?

JEAN. — Grand'mère ne doit pas être partie... (Timide.) C'est la Pentecôte, papa... Jiaurais voulu...

LE Docteur (doucement). — Non, mon petit, ce ne serait pas prudent Il fait chaud en marchant, et l'église doit être très fraîche.

JEAN. — C'est si près...

LE DOCTEUR. — Et puis, il faut que je prenne le train de trois heures: une consultation, ce soir, à Paris.,. Je veux te voir un peu, tu comprends (Changeant de ton.) J'ai à te parler, Jean, sérieusement, très sérieusement... (Un temps.) Descendons.

LevrëuxlQgis_degBôa.«.fr4u sommet de_la ville. ' Le bâtiment du rond, adossé au clocher, "Haye l'église; les-deux ailes, basses, çopyertes en tuiles, avancent vers la rue; un mur de prison les relie, que ferme un large portail.

L espace ainsi clos est mi-cour, mi-jardin. Plusieurs fois par jour, le son des cloches s'engouffre dans ce puits sonore et l'emplit jusqu'à ébranler les murailles. *jjJ Èr* .

Le docteur emmène Jean sous le berceau de vignes vierges.

LE DOCTEUR (enjouement factice). — Allons, assieds-toi là... Nous sommes très bien, ici...

JEAN (prêt à pleurer sans savoir pourquoi). — Oui, papa.

Le docteur a son visage d'hôpital: le nez pincé, l'œil fureteur et grave.

LE DOCTEUR (fermement). — Voici ce que j'ai à te dire, Jean, en trois mots: « tu es malade »...

Pause. Jean ne bouge pas.

LE DOCTEUR. — Tu es malade, et plus que tu ne crois. (Nouvelle pause. Le docteur ne quitte pas l'enfant du regard.) J'ai voulu que tu le saches,, parce que, si tu ne te soignes pas toi-même, énergiquement, ça pourrait: devenir grave... tout à fait grave...

JEAN (retenant ses larmes). — Alors... Je ne vais pas mieux?

Le docteur secoue la tête.

JEAN.— Alors, ce qui s'est passé à Lourdes? (Il réfléchit une seconde.) Peut-être que ça ne se voit pas encore...

Le DOCTEUR. — Ce qui s'est passé là-bas, moi. je n'en sais rien. Je dis seulement ceci: aujourd'hui, tel que tu es là, devant moi tu es... très sérieusement atlféTnt.

JEAN (demi-sourire). — Qu'est-ce que j'ai?

LE DOCTEUR (fronçant les sourcils). — Tu as... (Longue hésitation.)

Laisse-moi t'expliquer, écoute-moi, et tâche de comprendre ce que je vais te dire. Ta mère... (Il retire son lorgnon, l'essuie, et tourne vers Jean son regard myope.) Tu ne te rappelles rien de ta maman?

Jean, confus, fait un signe négatif.

Le DOCTEUR. — Ta maman,jeune fille,vivait ici; à la campagne; elle se portait bien, mais elle n'était pas très robuste. Après notre mariage, il a fallu qu'elle vienne habiter Paris, à cause de moi. Ta naissance l'a beaucoup fatiguée... (Aspiration.) C'est à ce moment-là qu'eue a commencé à.être malade... (Insistant.) D'abord une bronchite infectieuse.-Tu sais ce que c'est?

JEAN. — Comme moi?

Le Docteur. —...Elle s'en est mal remise: elle passait de mauvaises nuits à se retourner dans son lit, avec de la fièvre... (Mouvement de l'enfant.) Elle sentait toujours un point douloureux, là. .. (Il se penche, résolument.) Tiens, là...

JEAN (angoissé). — Comme moi?

LE DOCTEUR. — Quand je me suis aperçu qu'elle était malade, j'ai voulu qu'elle se soigne. Je lui ai dit à peu près tout ce que je veux te dire aujourd'hui. Malheureusement, elle ne m'écoutait pas... (Une pause. Hésitant sur les mots, mais d'une voix très ferme.) Ta maman, vois-tu, était une femme très bonne, douce, dévouée... et que j'aimais profondément... Mais elle était beaucoup plus jeune que moi... excessivement pieuse... (Avec lassitude.) Je n'ai jamais pu prendre la moindre influence sur elle... Elle me voyait, tous les jours, conseiller, guérir des gens: pourtant, elle n avait pas confiance... Et puis, elle ne se sentait pas vraiment malade. Moi, je venais d'avoir mon service à l'hôpital, j'avais une vie très occupée, je ne pouvais pas la surveiller comme il aurait fallu. Je voulais l'installer ici, au bon air; elle refusait... La toux a commencé... Il y a eu des consultations... C'était trop tard...

(Une pause) Alors... ça a été très vite.. . L'été... l'automne... l'hiver... Au printemps elle n'était plus là...

Jean fond en larmes.

Le docteur l'enveloppe d'un regard attentif et froid, sans un geste: il attend, au chevet d'un malade, l'effet d'une piqûre.

Quelques minutes.

LE DOCTEUR. — Je ne te raconte pas ça pour t'attrister, mon petit. J'essaye de te parler comme à un homme, parce que c'est nécessaire... Tu _âyais hérité de ta mère une prédisposition à être malade *mmmp AU jjn"* prédisposition, tu comprends.? rien de plus. C'est-à-dire que, si tu te trouvais dans certaines conditions défavorables,"le même mal pouvait s'attaquer à toi.

Eh bien, tu en es là, exactement. Tu es, depuis cet automne, dans un état de. .. faiblesse générale, qu'il est urgent...

très urgent de...

Jean, épouvanté tout à coup, glisse du banc et se jette audevant de son père, qui le serre maladroitement contre lui.

LE DOCTEUR. — N'aie pas peur, mon petit, n'aie pas peur, je suis là...

JEAN (à travers ses sanglots).— Oh, je n'ai pas peur... J'ai déjà rêvé... que j'étais au ciel...

Le docteur l'écarte d'un geste brusque, et le plante devant lui.

LE Docteur (violemment). — Il ne s'agit pas de mourir, Jean, mais de 'vivre. Tu peux te défendre, défends-toi!

Le gamin, interloqué, cesse de pleurer. IleÇarde son père. Il aurait aimé à être pris sur les genoux, câliné Il se heurte à l'éclat froid d'un lorgnon. *(— V«*

Un sentiment nouveau: de la crainte, un peu de fancynè mais — l'ascendant de l'intelligence et de la force, — un con-/ fiance absolue, une foi,

LE DOCTEUR. —Tu ne sais pas.. . Un corps humain, ça nous paraît har monieux, ordonné?... Eh bien, ce n'est qu'un vaste champ de bataille... Il y a là des myriades de cellules qui se heurtent et s'entremangent... Je t'expliquerai ça.. . Sans cesse, des millions de petits êtres nuisibles nous assèiHeàt, et parmi eux, naturellement, la tuberculose, qui guette les prédisposés comme toi... Alors, c'est très simple: si l'organisme est fort, il repousse l'attaque; s'il est déprimé, il se laisse envahir...

(Saisissant le bras de Jean, et scandant les mots.) Il n'y a donc qu'un moyen, un seul: devenir fort, le plus vite possible, pour reprendre le dessus. La guérison est à ta portée, il suffit de la « vouloir »! Attelle-toi à cette besogne! C'est uniquement une question d'énergie, de persévérance... Comprends-tu?... L'existence tout entière est un combat; la vie, c'est de la victoire qui dure... Ah, comme tu t'en apercevrais bientôt, si tu « voulais vraiment!

D'instinct, l'enfant est revenu se blottir contre son père.

LE Docteur (l'entourant d'un bras). —Si je pouvais quitter mes malades, ma clinique, ma salle d'opération, et me consacrer à toi, mon petit, je te tirerais d'affaire, j'en réponds... (Avec force)

Eh bien, ce que je ne peux pas, ce que je n'ai pas le droit de faire, tu le peux, toi, guidé par.moi. (Au visage.) Veux-tu?

JEAN (dans un grand élan). — Ah, papa, je te promets... Je vais m'y mettre, va!...

Une pause.

Le docteur sourit.

JEAN (après réflexion, à mi-voix). — L'abbé Joziers va dire des messes pour moi...

LE DOCTEUR (avec douceur). — Si tu veux. Mais ça ne suffirait pas. Il y a plus pressé, pour l'instant.

Jean recule d'un pas.

LE DOCTEUR (lentement). — Comprends-moi, mon petit, et crois ce que je te dis... Je te répète que ta pauvre maman a succombé parce qu'elle n'avait pas eu confiance...

L'enfant se rapproche.

LE Docteur. — Tu penses bien que je n'ai pas cherché à te blesser. Je compte même beaucoup sur ta piété pour te soutenir dans cette lutte. Seulement, vois-tu, il y a un proverbe: « Aide-toi, le ciel t'aidera. » Prie de tout ton cœur, mon enfant, mais n'oublie jamais qu'il faut subordonner tout, — même tes prières, tu entends?— au traitement d'hygiène que je vais te donner. (Avec une fougue persuasive.) Et ce traitement-là, Jean, si tu veux guérir, il faudra le suivre, je ne dis pas seulement avec bonne volonté, ni avec suite, comprends-tu, mon chéri..
.

A pleines volées, toutes les cloches de la Pentecôte annon'l cent l'Elévation.

I i Le docteur est obligé de hausser la voix, de crier, dans le vacarme trépidant.

LE DOCTEUR. —...je ne dis pas seulement avec courage, mais avec une passion, une ténacité enragées! Avec la volonté farouche de remonter le courant, de conquérir des forces, de repousser le mal, de repousser la mort! Avec le goût frénétique de la vie! Vivre, Jean. .. Si seulement, une fois, tu avais tien compris ce que c'est I Rester vivant, aimer encore ce que tu aimes, voir longtemps encore ce soleil-là, sur la treille de ta vieille maison...' Longtemps encore être assourdi et grisé par ces cloches... Regarde un peu autour de toi,

cette lumière, ces arbres, le ciel, le clocher... (Il le secoue par les épaules.) Vivre, Jean!...

L'enfant, électrisé, frémissant, soulevé par une impulsion nouvelle, s'est dressé tout droit devant son père, le feu aux joues, les yeux étincelants.

Le docteur le toise longuement, gravement, et l'attire à lui.

Les cloches se taisent. Un instant encore leurs vibrations tourbillonnent dans la cour, avant de s'évanouir dans l'espace

Silence.

Le DOCTEUR (pesant ses mots). — Trois choses: la nourriture, l'air, le repos... Il faut bien retenir tout ce que je vais te dire...

III

A Buis, chez Mme Pasquelin, la marraine de Jean.

Une chambre. Pénombre. Aux vitres, crépuscule neigeux d'hiver.

Devant la cheminée, éclairé par la braise, un groupe silencieux:

Mme Pasquelin, debout, se penche vers Jean qui sanglote sur son épaule. La petite Cécile, haletante, le mouchoir sur les lèvres, incapable d'assister au chagrin de Jean, se serre contre les jupes de sa mère.
.

Sur le tapis, deux dépêches froissées:

« Pasquelin. Buis-la-Dame. Oise. « Mère très ébranlée par la traversée de Paris. Opération retardée par suite de complications imprévues. Suis inquiet.

Dr Barois. »

« Pasquelin. Buis-la-Dame. Oise. « Mère a succombé ce matin onze heures maison de santé sans avoir repris conscience. Intervention était devenue impossible. Prévenez Jean avec grands ménagements, évitez toute secousse.

Dr Barois. »

Trois ans plus tard.

Une cellule carrelée derrière la sacristie. Éclairage bas d'un jour de souffrance. Deux chaises, deux prie-dieu. Au mur, un christ.

Jahhp JnTi'pt-»; un visage jeune; le front haut, déjà découvert; des cheveux blonds, coupés courts et frisés. L'œil gai et pur: la paix d'une foi simple et active. La lèvre supérieure mince et grave; la

lèvre inférieure charnue, d'une ironie un peu provocante, mais cordiale.

Dans le regard, dans le sourire, le joyeux défi de ceux pour qui tout est définitivement éclairci en ce monde comme en 1 autre, et qui se sentent avec sérénité les seuls dépositaires du Vrai.

L'abbé Joziers clot soigneusement la porte et se tourne vers Jean, les deux mains tendues.

L'abbÉ. — Eh bien, l'ami Jean, qu'y a-t-il donc? (Gardant la main de Jean dans la sienne.) Asseyez-vous d'abord.

Jean Barois: quinze ans.

Grand, souple et charpenté. Le buste large; le cou dégagé et solide.

Une tête vigoureuse; un front carré, bordé de cheveux bruns, drus et durs. Entre les paupières courbes, légèrement plissées, qui marquent une attention vigilante, luit un regard vif et direct: le coup d'œil pénétrant de son père.

Le bas du visage est encore d'un enfant. La bouche, peu formée, mobile, change à tout instant; le menton au galbe rond, dissimule la lourdeur de la mâchoire.

Une volonté tranquille et tenace, résultat de cette lutte acharnée: quatre ans d'obstination méthodique vers la résurrection, quatre ans d'épouvantes et d'espoirs. La vie pour enjeu!

Mais la bataille est gagnée.

L'abbÉ. — Eh bien?

JEAN. — Monsieur l'abbé, j'ai beaucoup réfléchi, avant de me décider. Depuis longtemps j'en ai envie, et je remets cette visite... Voilà... (Un temps.) Il y a des questions que je me pose aujourd'hui, qui me troublent...

Un tas d'idée_S qm m vipnnpt à pr/?p«y» fle la religion."Surtout iTpTiis que je vais prendre ces répétitions à Beauvais... (Hésitant.) J'aurais besoin qu'on discute avec moi, qu'on m'explique...

L'abbé tourne son regard décidé vers Jean.

L'abbÉ. — Mais, rien n'est plus simple. Je me mets entièrement à votre disposition, mon enfant. Il y a des sujets qui vous embarrassent? Lesquels?

Le masque de Jean prend une gravité inattendue. Il renverse un peu le front. La tension des muscles fait tomber les coins de la lèvre, qu'ombre un duvet brun. Le regard est fiévreux.

L'abbÉ (souriant). — Allons...

JEAN. — Monsieur l'abbé, d'abord. .. Qu'est-ce que c'est au juste que les libres-penseurs?

L'abbé se redresse et répond tout de suite, sans une hésitation, avec un demi-sourire satisfait. Il s'exprime avec une énergie contenue, très particulière, les dents un peu serrées, en insistant longuement sur certains mots qu'il met exagérément en vedette.

L'abbÉ. — Les *libres-penseurs* ? Ce sont des naïfs le plus souvent, qui s'imaginent que nous pouvons *penser librement.* Penser librement! Mais les fous seuls pensent librement. (Riant.) Est-ce que je suis libre de penser que cinq et cinq font onze? Ou que l'article masculin se met devant le substantif féminin? Voyons? Il y a des règles partout, en grammaire, en mathématiques. — Les libres-penseurs croient pouvoir *se passer de règles;* mais aucun être vivant ne peut se développer, sans être attaché à quelque point solide! Pourrmarcher, il faut un sol ferme. Pour penser il fanages principes stablêsTcIes ventés contrôlées, — que *seule* la religion dfient/

JEAN (sombre). —Monsieur l'abbé, je crois que j'ai des tendances à devenir libre-penseur..

L'abbÉ (riant).— Ah, diable! (Affectueux.) Non, mon enfant, n'ayez pas peur: de cela, je réponds... Comment pouvez-vous faire une supposition pareille!

JEAN. — J'ai changé. Autrefois, j'avais une vie religieuse tranquille, jamais je n'aurais eu l'idée de réfléchir, de discuter. Maintenant, ça me prend, je cherche à m'expliquer tout ça, je n'y arrive pas, et alors, j'ai des espèces d'inquiétudes...

L'abbÉ (très calme). — Mais, mon enfant, c'est tout à fait normal. (Mouvement de Jean.) Vous êtes à l'âge où l'on entre vraiment dans l'existence, où l'on découvre *quantité* de choses que l'on ignorait. On arrive à la vie d'homme avec sa religion d'enfant; l'une n'est plus en rapport avec l'autre. (Le visage de Jean s'éclaire peu à peu.) Ce n'est

rien. Il s'agit de franchir vite ce passage difficile, *d'étayer* votre foi avec des raisonnements solides, de *l'adapter* à vos nouveaux besoins. Je vous aiderai.

JEAN (souriant). — Rien que de vous entendre, monsieur l'abbé, ça me fait du bien. (D'un ton plus alerte.) Autre question: un péché, par exemple, un péché habituel, qu'on connaît à fond, qu'on est fermement résolu à ne pas commettre... Bien... On prie, on prend la résolution: on croit pouvoir être rassuré. .. Et puis, on a beau faire,'l'habitude est plus forte que le bon Dieu!

L'abbé. — Mon enfant, c'est pour cela qu'il n'y a rien de plus dangereux pour la foi que le péché fréquent, *même véniel.* Ce sont ces secousses répétées sur la sensibilité religieuse qu'il faut éviter à tous prix.

JEAN. — Justement, monsieur l'abbé... Mais pourquoi donc est-il possible que je succombe?

L'abbé fait un geste amusé, que Jean, le regard tendu, ne remarque pas.

JEAN. — Je me demande pourquoi toutes ces tentations, pourquoi ces «preuves? Quand on est petit, on trouve tout naturel qu'il y ait des heureux et des malheureux, des bien portants et des malades... C'est comme ça, voilà tout. Mais, en réfléchissant, on est épouvanté de tant de choses, qui sont par trop injustes, par trop mauvaises... Si encore on pouvait affirmer que le malheur, c'est toujours un châtiment mérité!

Il faut bien que Dieu ait eu ses motifs pour créer le monde tel que nous le voyons; mais vraiment...

L'abbé (souriant).— D'abord Dieu n'a pas créé le monde *tel* qu'il est. C'est l'homme, oui, par sa désobéissance au premier ordre du Créateur, est responsable de ce dont il souffre depuis.

JEAN (tenace). — Mais si Adam avait été parfait, il n'aurait pas pu désobéir... Et puis, à l'origine du monde, Dieu avait bien créé le serpent?

L'abbé, devenu sérieux, avance la main pour couper court. Il enveloppe Jean d'un regard amical, où perce malgré lui la conscience de sa supériorité.

L'ABBÉ. — Vous pensez bien, Jean, que vous n'êtes pas le premier à être / frappé par ces contradictions appa-

rentes. C'est *tobjection du mal.* Ellè a "été réfutée, depuis longtemps, et de mille manières. Vous avez très bien fait de m'en parler. Puisque cette question vous préoccupe, je vous choisirai sur ce sujet des lectures qui vous tranquilliseront *définitivement.*

'.

Jean se tait, un peu déçu.

L'abbÉ. — Je ne voudrais pas toutefois méconnaître ce qu'il y a de bon dans votre indignation: c'est par la vision de la souffrance humaine que nous pouvons fortifier *en nous* l'instinct de charité, et, dans ce sens, on ne peut aller trop loin. (Lui prenant la main.) Pourtant, vous êtes à l'âge, Jean, où le cœur s'ouvre, tout neuf, plein de tendresse universelle, et où ces découvertes peuvent être si cruelles qu'il est bon d'être quelque peu prévenu. Méfiezvous, en ces matières, de votre sensibilité: il y a dans le monde *beaucoup moins de mal* qu'il ne vous paraît au premier abord T Réfléciïssêz âcela T si-brsomme des *maux* était supérieure, ou seulement équivalente à la somme des tiens, mais le désordre serait partout! Au contraire, que voyons-nous? Un ordre merveilleux, qui confond notre petitesse! Chaque" jour, tes nouvelles étapes des pionniers de la science; TrnnisHpêlïnettent d'approfondir davantage les perfections du plan divin. Qu'est-ce que les peines individuelles des pécheurs, auprès de *tant* de bonté? Et puis, les blessures humaines, — que je ne nie pas, hélas! puisque mon ministère est de les panser et si possible de les guérir, — ont bien leur prix, vous le reconnaîtrez vousmême un jour, puisque c'est *par elles seulement* que l'homme peut progresser dans le bien, et entrer plus avant dans la voie de son salut. Or, qu'est-ce qui importe? Est-ce la vie présente, ou l'autre?

JEAN. — Mais, il n'y a pas que l'homme... Et les animaux?

L'abbÉ. — La souffrance de toute créature est *voulue* par Dieu, mon enfant, comme une condition, comme *la condition même* de la vie: et cela doit suffire pour courber votre orgueil qui se révolte. L'existence de l'Etre. *Parfait,* infiniment bon et tout puissant, qui a fait *de rien* le ciel et la terre, et qui, chaque jour, nous donne mille preuves de ses sentiments paternels pour nous, est notre meilleure garantie de la nécessité du mal en ce monde, qu'Il a créé *au mieux* de nos besoins. Et quand bien même Ses raisons seraient impénétrables à nos facultés imparfaites, nous devrions nous incliner et vouloir avec Lui cette souffrance que nous ne comprenons pas, mais qu'il a voulue... « Fiat voluntas tua... K

Jean se tait, les sourcils froncés, cherchant à assimiler." Dans une cellule voisine, des voix grêles accompagnent un harmonium poussif.

L'abbe. —-Je vois en vous, Jean, une tendance *un peu trop* prononcée à la réflexion.'(Sôûrîânt.) Je ne veux pniTiirini-'iirr lr mrirr Hfnprnilatinnfl de l'-esprir. Mais, voyez-vous, plus je vais et plus je crois que l'intelligence n'a sa véritable valeur que lorsqu'elle vise un but *extérieur* à elle, lorsqu'elle cherche à s'appliquer *pratiquement*. L'intelligence doit vivifier l'action; sans elle l'action est vaine. Mais, sans l'action, comme"TînTetli-)( gence est stérile 1 C'est la lumière qui brûle à côté du phare et se consume 1) pour rien. (Avec émotion et recueillement.) Vous venez à moi, mpn"' enfant, en quête d'une direction. Eh bien, je vous pousserai toujours à ferff. plutôt qu'à philosopher J Cultivez votre intelligence, soit: c'est plus qu'un droit: un devoir. Mais que ce soit en vue cFunTésuItat *humain*. Si le Maître vous a confié un petit trésor, des facultés supérieures à la moyenne, faites-les fructifier; mais que la grande famille humaine en profite. Ne soyez pas celui qui a enterré son talent. Enrichissez-vous, mais pour partager. Soyez de ceux *qui se donnent.*

J'ai été comme vous: j'ai eu mon heure de spéculation théorique... Dieu a permis que je reconnaisse bientôt mon erreur. C'est *dans l'action,* dans le don de soi, dans l'abnégation et le dévouement, qu'on trouve la vraie récompense, la santé physique et morale, le véritable bonheur. Croyezmoi. Notre bonheur, que l'on va quelquefois chercher si loin, il est tout près de nous, dans quelques sentiments naturels, comme la fraterni-

té: et tout le reste n'est n'en!

Venez un de ces soirs à mon patronage. Je vous donnerai les livres dont je vous ai parlé. Et puis (le visage transfiguré d'entrain et de fierté) vous resterez un peu avec nous, vous verrez vite *quels cœurs* il y a là, et quel plaisir on a à se donner de la peine pour eux. (Se levant.) Allez, Jean! Il n'y a que ça de vrai: sentir qu'on fait un peu de bien autour de soi... (se frappant la poitrine, gaiement)...qu'on communique un peu de *cette chaleur* que le bon Dieu nous a mise... là...!

Le petit salon des Pasquelin.

Pièce au rez-de-chaussée, longue, étroite, encombrée de meubles démodés.

Cécile, seule. Ole range le désordre que sa mère a laissé en sortant.

Le jour baisse vite: octobre.

Un pas sur le pavé.

Vivement, elle court à la fenêtre et sourit: Jean traverse la rue, une serviette sous le bras.

Elle bondit gaiement au-devant de lui.

Cécile Pasquelin: seize ans.

Grande et frêle. Pas jolie: de la fraîcheur. Une souplesse élégante du cou et de la nuque. Des épaules étroites, sous une pèlerine de laine blanche.

Une tête petite, en boule; les cheveux bruns, frangés. Des yeux noirs, ronds, un peu saillants; le charme agaçant, à peine perceptible, d'une asymétrie dans le regard. La bouche: deux lèvres charnues, humides, bien rouges, très mobiles sur des dents courtes et luisantes. Sourire gai, superficiel.

Par instants, un léger zézayement, CÉCILE. — Tu n'es pas en avance!Viens, ton lait doit être froid.

Le goûter de Jean est préparé sur un plateau. Cécile s'assied en face de lui; les yeux brillants, elle le regarde croquer sa tartine.

Ils se dévisagent en riant; pour rien, par plaisir. JEAN. — Maintenant, au travail!

Il vide sur la table sa serviette de livres.

30 au feu, et approche sous l'abat-jour sa chaise basse. CÉCILE. — Qu'est-ce que c'est, ce soir? JEAN. — Une prépa-

ration grecque.

Le salon est tiède. Le ron-ron de la lampe, le ron-ron du feu. Le rythme de leurs deux souffles. Un froissement d'étoffe, un froissement de feuillet.

Au tournant d'une page, au bout d'une aiguillée, leurs regards se croisent.'

JEAN (d'une voix singulière). — Tiens, j'ai trouvé ce matin quelque chose... Dans Eschyle... Il parle d'Hélène, il dit: « Ame sereine comme le calme des mers... '» C'est beau, n'est-ce pas? (Il la regarde.) « Ame sereine comme le calme des mers... » peine... Dans les parties de cache-cache, quand on voit celui qui vous cherche s'approcher sans vous voir, vous frôler presque, et passer..r

Jean s'est remis au travail.

Une demi-heure plus tard.

Un talon de femme martelle le vestibule dallé. Irruption de Mme Pasquelin.

Mme Pasquelin: petite femme noiraude, au teint jaune, aux cheveux très noirs et frisés sur le front. De beaux yeux, légèrement asymétriques, comme ceux de Cécile; le regard caressant et gai; une bouche souriante, un peu pincée.

A été jolie et s'en souvient. *fzs*

Preste, remuante, bavarde. La voix aigue, l'accent rude des Picards. Toujours en mouvement, n'épargnant ni temps, ni peine, tranchant sur tout, surveillant, dirigeant, réformant toutes les œuvres catholiques de la ville.

Madame PASQUELIN. — Vous êtes sages, mes enfants? (Sans attendre la réponse.) Prends donc un fauteuil, Cécile, je déteste te voir pliée en deux sur cette chaise basse... (Elle va au coffre à bois.) Sans moi, vous laissiez éteindre le feu!

JEAN (voulant l'aider). — Attendez, Marraine.

MADAME PASQUELIN. — Non, tu n'en finirais pas.

En un instant, elle a jeté deux bûches dans le foyer, et baissé la trappe. Elle se relève; tout en parlant, elle dégrafe son mantelet, va à la fenêtre et tire les rideaux.

MADAME PASQUELIN. — Ah, mes enfants, j'ai cru que je ne rentrerais jamais! Je suis morte de fatigue. Rien ne marche, j'ai dû me fâcher toute la journée. Je suis furieuse après l'abbé Joziers. Il a obtenu de M. le Curé que le catéchisme des garçons soit à neuf heures et demie le jeudi! Juste à l'heure où se réunit le conseil de l'ouvroir! C'est ce que j'ai dit à M. le Curé: Je ne peux pourtant pas être en haut et en bas de la ville en même temps!

Jean, veux-tu relever la trappe... Merci.

Et puis, tu sais, il est six heures un quart. Si tu veux communier avec nous demain, tu n'as que le temps de courir te confesser; l'abbé quitte l'église à la demie... (Jean se lève.) Couvre-toi bien, il y a du vent ce soir...

Le lendemain, à la messe de sept heures.

Le moment de la communion.

Mme Pasquelin se lève et s'avance vers l'autel. Cécile et Jean la suivent. Côte à côte, les yeux à terre, ils gagnent, à pas recueillis, la table sainte.

L'abbé Joziers officie. Il élève vers la nef une hostie consacrée.

L'abbÉ Joziers (d'une voix contrite). — Domine, non sum dignus... Domine, non sum dignus... Domine, non sum dignus...

Cécile et Jean sont à genoux. Leurs coudes se touchent. Sows la nappe, leurs mains glacées voisinent.

Une même angoisse, maladive et délicieuse; une même attirance d'infini...

Le prêtre approche. L'un après l'autre ils tendent le front vers le ciel, entr'ouvrent les lèvres et frissonnent. Puis leurs paupières s'abaissent sur l'intensité de leur joie.

Fusion Deux âmes, déliées de toute adhérence humaine, s'élèvent sans effort jusqu'à la dernière cirrie de l'amour, s'étreignent subtilement en Dieu.

COMPROMIS SYMBOLISTE

*« Quand j'étais un petit enfant, je raisonnais comme un petit enfant; mais quand je suis devenu un homme, je me suis dépouillé de ce qui était de l'enfant.* » St Paul, I Cor. XIII. II.

« Paris, 11 janvier

« Cher Monsieur l'Abbé,

« Je voudrais mieux répondre à cette confiance que vous avez en moi. Mais, hélas, je ne puis vous donner sur mon moral les bonnes nouvelles que vous attendez. Ce premier trimestre n'a guère été satisfaisant. Je me sens toujours très dépaysé dans ce Paris où tout est nouveau pour moi.

« Cependant mon existence est définitivement organisée maintenant: outre les cours préparatoires à l'École de Médecine, j'ai pris des inscriptions à la Sorbonne, pour la licenciées-sciences naturelles; de sorte que, depuis quelques semaines, je vis davantage encore au quartier latin. (Que ces détails, cher Monsieur l'Abbé, ne vous inquiètent pas; et, à ce propos, les conseils affectueux de votre dernière lettre m'ont infiniment touché. Non, ne craignez rien à ce sujet: j'ai, grâce à Dieu, le cœur assez haut pour triompher des tentations auxquelles vous avez pensé; et puis, vous oubliez le sentiment profond et pur que j'ai emporté de Buis, le projet si cher, qui est toute ma raison de vivre, et ma sauvegarde).

« Ces études de sciences me font un emploi du temps très chargé; mais elles complètent celles de médecine et m'intéressent au delà de ce que je puis vous dire. D'ailleurs que ferais-je de plus de loisirs? Mon père, comme vous le savez peut-être, vient d'être nommé professeur; son cours complique encore une vie très occupée, où je n'ai guère de place.

« Vous serez certainement satisfait de savoir que j'ai fait la connaissance d'un jeune prêtre suisse, nommé Schertz, qui se destine à enseigner l'histoire naturelle dans son pays, et qui est venu prendre ses grades à Paris. C'est un passionné de biologie; nous sommes voisins de laboratoire, et sa collaboration m'est précieuse. Toutes ces études sont extrêmement attachantes; je ne peux pas encore analyser ce que je ressens, mais certains cours me transportent: je crois qu'il est impossible de ne pas éprouver une espèce de vertige, à ces premiers contacts avec la Science, lorsqu'on commence à distinguer, pour la première fois, quelques-unes de ces grandes lois qui ordonnent la complexité universelle!

« Je m'applique, sur vos conseils, à me pénétrer de cet ordre, et à y exalter la certitude de Dieu.__Mais votre optimisme communicatif me manque plus que vous ne pouvez croire. Peut-être l'amitié de l'abbé Schertz me sera-t-elle, à ce point de vue, de quelque profit? Sa gaieté naturelle, son entrain au travail, prouvent une foi robuste, dont l'appui peut venir en aide à mon déséquilibre moral. — Je le souhaite, car jjiL traverséces dernières semaines, des heures de dépression bien pénibles.

« Excusez-moi de vous attrister "une fois de plusà ce sujet, et croyez, cher Monsieur l'Abbé, à mes sentiments de respectueuse sympathie.

Jean Barois. »

II

Salle à manger du Dr Barois.
La fin du dîner.

LE DOCTEUR (se levant de table). — Vous m'excusez, monsieur Schertz? (L'abbé et Jean se sont levés.) Il faut que je sois à Passy à neuf heures, pour une consultation... Je regrette de ne pas prolonger cette soirée auprès de vous, j'ai été tout à fait heureux de faire votre connaissance. — Allons, bonsoir mon petit. Au plaisir de vous revoir, monsieur Schertz... (Souriant.) Et croyez moi, je tiens beaucoup à mon idée: il faut agir d'abord, et réfléchir ensuite; la jeunesse d'aujourd'hui, elle réfléchit trop, et, n'ayant pas agi, elle réfléchit mal...

La chambre de Jean.

L'abbé est assis dans un fauteuil bas, les jambes croisées, les coudes sur les bras du siège, les mains jointes sous le menton.

L'abbé Schertz: trente et un ans.

Un corps plat et long, gaîné dans la soutane. De grands bras musclés, aux gestes pleins de mesure.

Une tête osseuse et forte. Un teint blanchâtre. Un front fuyant, qu'exagère le port des cheveux noirs, plantés haut, et rejetés en arrière. Le visage, dénudé par le rasoir, est rendu plus glabre encore par la pauvreté des sourcils. Dans l'ombre, sous l'encorbellement rectiligne des arcades, une paire d'yeux clairs et précis; des prunelles vert-degris, entre des cils noirs. Le nez long, rattaché aux maxillaires par deux sillons mobiles. Les lèvres fines et gaies; par instants, blêmes et comme figées.

Gravité aimable, formaliste.

Un parler pesant, rude, un peu nasillard. Des phrases longues, des tournures peu usitées: il paraît traduire en français ce qu'il pense.

Jean, assis sur son bureau, fume en balançant les pieds / JEAN. — Vous me faites plaisir. J'aime beaucoup mon père... (Souriant.) Croiriez-vous qu'il m'a fait très peur, pendant longtemps?

SCHERTZ. — Est-il possible?

JEAN. — Il m'intimidait. Je ne le connais vraiment que depuis quelques mois, depuis que je vis avec lui... Ah, un métier comme le sien, hausse un homme!

SCHERTZ — Il n'y a pas seulement l'apport du métier dans une pareille richesse morale! Car, sans cela, tous les médecins...

JEAN. — Évidemment; j'admets qu'il y ait eU, chez mon père, prédisposition naturelle.

Je voulais dire... qu'il n'a pas l'appui de la religion.

SCHERTZ (subitement intéressé). — Ah?... J'en avais le doute.

JEAN. — Oui. La famille de mon père était d'un milieu catholique très pratiquant, et lui-même a reçu une éducation foncièrement religieuse. Pourtant, depuis longtemps je crois, mon père a cessé de pratiquer.

SCHERTZ. — Et aussi de croire?

JEAN. — Je le suppose. Jamais il ne s'en est expliqué avec moi... Mais il y a un je ne sais quoi qui ne trompe pas... D'ailleurs...

Jean se tait, réfléchit une seconde en fixant l'abbé; puis, sautant de la table, il traverse la pièce à pas incertains, allume une cigarette, et se laisse tomber sur un canapé de cuir, vis-à-vis de l'abbé.

SCHERTZ. — D'ailleurs?

J EAN (après une seconde d'hésitation). — Je voulais dire que la profession de mon père est, en somme, bien dangereuse pour la foi...

Schertz: geste d'étonnement.

JEAN. — A cause de l'hôpital... Songez à l'opinion que peut avoir celui qui, tous les jours de sa vie. du matin jusqu'au soir, n'a pas d'autre fonction que de se pencher sûr de la souffrance?

Quelle conception peut-il se Taire de Dieu?——

Schertz ne répond pas.

JEAN. — Je vous scandalise?

SCHERTZ, — En aucune manière. Vous m'intéressez. C'est la vieille objection du mal.

Jean. — Elle est formidable!

SCHERTZ (flegmatique). — Formidable.

JEAN. — Et, jusqu'à présent, nos théologiens ne l'ont, en somme, jamais réfutée...

SCHERTZ. — Jamais.

JEAN — Vous en convenez?

SCHERTZ (souriant). — Mais comment pourrais-je autrement?

Jean tire quelques bouffées en silence. Puis il jette brusquement sa cigarette et considère l'abbé bien en face.

Jean. — Vous êtes le premier prêtre à qui je l'entende dire...

SCHERTZ. — Avez-vous distinctement posé la question à quelqu'autrè?

JEAN. — Oh, souvent!

SCHERTZ. — Eh bien,?

JEAN. — On m'a fait toutes les répdnses possibles... Que j'étais trop sensible... Que j'étais un orgueilleux révolté... Que le mal est la condition du bien... Que 1 épreuve est nécessaire pour l'amélioration de l'homme... Que, depuis le péché originel, Dieu avait voulu le mal, et qu'il faut le vouloir avec lui...

Schertz (souriant). — Eh bien?

JEAN (haussant les épaules).— Des mots... Des apparences d'arguments...

Schertz: un regard aigu vers Jean; puis son masque change d'expression, s'aggrave. Il évite de relever les yeux.

JEAN. — Au fond des choses, on se heurte à un sophisme: on veut me prouver la puissance et la bonté de Dieu en faisant l'apologie de l'ordre universel £et dès que je veux faire remarquer combien cet ordre est imparfait, on me refuse le droit de pprter un jugement sur cet univers, justement parce qu'il est l'œuvre de DieuJ (Quelques pas; il élève la voix.) Si bien que jamais on ne m'a permis de concilier ces deux affirmations: d'une part, que Dieu est la somme de toutes les perfections; et, d'autre part, que ce monde imparfait est

son œuvre!

Il s'arrête devant l'abbé et cherche à rencontrer son regard. Mais Schertz détourne la tête. Un silence. Enfin leurs yeux se croisent; ceux de Jean voilés d'une expression anxieuse, qui questionne.

L'abbé ne peut pas se dérober entièrement.

SCHERTZ (sourire mal assuré.) — Ainsi, vous aussi, mon pauvre ami, vous voilà soucieux de ces grands problèmes. ..

JEAN (avec vivacité). — Qu'y puis-je? Je vous assure que je voudrais bien ne pas en être obsédé comme je le suis!

Il va et vient, les mains aux poches, secouant la tête comme s'il poursuivait intérieurement la discussion. Son visage énergique s'est encore durci: une émotion concentrée plisse le front et donne à la bouche un pli perplexe et têtu.

JEAN. — Tenez, mon cher, vous parliez tout à l'heure de mon père... Il y a une chose qui m'a toujours confusément choqué, même enfant: c'est Tju'on puisse, au nom de la religion, condamner un homme comme lui, uniquement parce qu'il ne fait pas ses pâques, et ne met jamais le pied dans une église! Là-bas, à Buis, on le jugeait très séyèrement...

SCHERTZ. — Parce qu'on ne le comprenait pas.

JEAN (interloqué). — Mais vous-même, en tant que prêtre, vous êtes bien obligé de le condamner aussi?

Geste réservé de Schertz.

JEAN (avec passion). — Quant à moi, je m'y suis toujours refusé, d'instinct! Une existence comme celle de mon père, c'est une aspiration ininter i rompue vers ce qui est noble et grand. Et on pourrait la flétrir, — et on devrait la flétrir — au nom de Dieu? Non, non.. . Des vies comme la sienne, vous savez, c'est autre chose, c'est au-dessus... (Il fait quelques pas et regarde l'abbé avec angoisse. Sur un ton morne). Et puis, le terrible, mon cher, c'est quand on réfléchit posément à ceci: Un_Jiamme comme mon père ne_ *croit pas*... Des hommes comme lui ne *croyent pas*... Ce ne sont pas des sauvages, pourtant? Us ont connu notre religion, ils l'ont même pratiquée, avec fervéufr Pourtant, un jour, délibérément, ils l'ont rejetée!... Hein? On se dit: « Je crois, *et eux, ils ne croyent pas...* Lequel a raison? » Et malgré soi, on ajoute: « C'est à voir... » De ce jour-là, on a perdu le repos! « C'est à voir... », voilà le seuil maudit, voilà la formule liminaire de l'athéisme!

SCHERTZ (gravement). — Ah, pardon... Vous abordez là un malentendu capital!De tels hommes n'acceptent pas le culte actuel de l'Église... Mais soyez certain que la force qui les fait grands est de même nature, exactement, que celle du meilleur prêtre, du meilleur!

JEAN. — Il y a donc deux façons d'être chrétiens?

SCHERTZ (poussé plus loin qu'il ne voudrait). — Cela est possible.

JEAN. — Cependant, au fond, il ne peut, il ne doit y en avoir qu'une!

SCHERTZ. — Sans doute... Mais à travers les divergences, qui sont plus apparentes que réelles, c'est toujours la même chose, le même élan de la conscience vers la bonté et la justice infinies...

Jean l'examine avec attention, en silence.

Longue pause.

SCHERTZ (gêné). — Tenez, l'odeur de votre tabac me tente: je vais faire une sortie à mon régime... Merci... (Voulant à tout prix dévier l'entretien.) Je vous ai apporté le cours préparatoire que vous m'avez demandé...

Jean prend les cahiers, et les feuillette d'un air distrait.

Quelques jours après.

Pension de famille, place Sairit-Sulpice.

La chambre de l'abbé.

SCHERTZ (se levant promptement). — Ach!une bonne visite!...

JEAN. — Je viens bavarder avec vous jusqu'à l'heure du cours.

L'abbé débarrasse le fauteuil.

Jean fait en souriant le tour de la chambre: Un petit bureau; une grande table à expériences; un arsenal de flacons, de porcelaines; un microscope. Sur les murs, un christ, une vue panoramique de Berne, un portrait de Pasteur, des planches anatomiques.

JEAN (riant). — Je me demande comment vous pouvez vivre dans cette atmosphère!

Schertz. — C'est mon acide sulfurique...

JEAN. — Non, je parle au figuré. Je me demande souvent comment un prêtre peut vivre dans cette atmosphère scientifique.

SCHERTZ (s'approchant de lui). — Mais pourquoi donc?

JEAN. — Parce que moi, — qui ne suis pas prêtre, pourtant, — j'y respire difficilement... et mal.

Sous le sourire, une souffrance contenue.

JEAN (s'asseyant). — Ah, j'aurais besoin, un jour, de causer longuement avec vous, de vider mon sac...

Schertz (rêveur). — Oui...

Son regard fait le tour de la pièce, se pose sur celui de Jean, et s'y enfonce brusquement. Puis il hésite, baisse les yeux, et réfléchit intensément quelques secondes.

SCHERTZ. — Vous le voulez?

Ils se regardent en silence, émus tous deux. Ils pressentent une de ces heures d'épanchement total, où deux âmes de jeunes hommes, préparées par l'amitié, s'étreignent spontanément et se pénètrent.

SCHERTZ (avec douceur). — Qu'y a-t-il donc?

JEAN (s'abandonnent). — Il y a que je suis dans un fichu état moral...

SCHERTZ. — Moral?

JEAN. — Religieux, plutôt.

SCHERTZ. — Depuis quand?

JEAN. — Ah, depuis longtemps, plus longtemps que je ne croyais! Il doit y avoir des années déjà, que, sans m'en rendre compte, je suis obligé de me débattre pour conserver la foi.

SCHERTZ (vivement). — Non pas la foi! Mais cette foi *réceptive* des enfants: ce n'est pas la même chose!

JEAN (tout à sa pensée). —. Je ne m'en suis aperçu vraiment cjue depuis quelques mois. Paris, peut-être... L'ambiance de Paris! L ambiance surtout de cette Sorbonne! Ces cours où l'on analyse toutes les grandes lois universelles, sans jamais prononcer le nom de Dieu...

SCH Ertz. — On ne le nomme pas, mais on parle de lui sans cesse.

JEAN (amèrement). — J'avais l'habitude d'en parler plus nettement.

SCHERTZ (avec un sourire encourageant). — Il faut seulement s'entendre. (Hésitant.) Je pourrais peut-être vous aider, cher ami;mais je suis retenu par le peu que je sais de votre vie religieuse... Où en êtes-vous réellement?

JEAN (découragé). — Je n'en sais rien moi-même. Mais ça ne va plus, plus du tout...

L'abbé s'est assis, les jambes croisées, le buste penché en avant, le menton sur ses doigts entrelacés.

JEAN. — Je suis partagé entre des tendances qui se contredisent. Un déséquilibre atroce, d'autant plus douloureux que j'ai connu le calme, la foi sereine, le bon feu intérieur... Je vous jure que je n'ai rien fait pour en arriver là: au contraire. Longtemps j'ai refusé à ma raison le droit de s'attacher à ces questions. Mais maintenant je ne peux plus. Les objections s'amoncellent autour de moi; presque chaque jour j'en rencontre une nouvelle! J'ai bien dû m'apercevoir, bon gré, mal gré, qu'il n'y a pas un seul point de la doctrine catholique qui ne soulève aujourd'hui d'innombrables contradictions... (Tirant de sa poche un fascicule de revue.) Tenez, connaissez-vous ça? Un article de Brunois: « *Les rapports de la raison et de la foi* » (Geste négatif de Schertz.) Ça m'est tombé sous les yeux, par hasard, il n'y a pas bien longtemps. Je n'avais jusque-là aucune idée de ce que pouvait être l'exégèse moderne, je ne soupçonnais pas ce qu'étaient les attaques de la critique historique... Quelle révélation!

C'est là-dedans que j'ai appris, pour la première fois des choses comme ceci: Que les Évangiles ont été rédigés entre les années 65 et 100 après Jésus-Christ, et que, par conséquent, l'Église s'est fondée, a existé, pourrait exister sans eux... Plus de soixante ans après le Christ! Comme si, de nos jours, sans un seul document écrit, à l'aide de souvenirs et de vagues témoignages, on voulait consigner les actes et les paroles de Napoléon... Et voilà le livre fondamental, dont l'exactitude ne doit être mise en doute par aucun catholique!

(Tournant des pages.) Que Jésus ne s'est jamais cru Dieu, ni prophète, ni fondateur de religion, si ce n'est à la fin de sa vie, grisé par la crédulité de ses disciples...

Qu'on a été très long à édifier et à préciser le dogme de la Trinité, et qu'il a fallu plusieurs réunions de conciles pour fixer la double nature du Christ, faire la part de son humanité et de sa divinité... Bref: qu'il a fallu des années de controverses pour constituer ce dogme et le rattacher avec quelque vraisemblance aux paroles prononcées par Jésus; alors qu'au catéchisme, on nous l'enseigne, ce dogme de la Trinité, dès les premières leçons, comme une vérité élémentaire, toute simple, révélée par Jésus lui-même, et si claire, qu'elle n'a jamais été contredite par personne!

(D'autres pages.) Et ça! L'Immaculée conception... Une invention presque récente! Qui n'a pris naissance qu'au XII-siècle, dans le cerveau mystique de deux moines anglais! Qui n'a été discutée et formulée qu'au XIII t Dont l'unique point de départ est la faute grossière de je ne sais quel traducteur grec, lequel s'est servi à tort du mot grec-apOivoç *jeune fille,* pour traduire l'ancien mot hébreux, qui qualifiait naturellement Marie *de jeune femme...*

Vous souriez? Vous saviez tout ça? (Déçu.) Alors vous ne pouvez pas bien comprendre ce que j'ai pu éprouver à de pareilles lectures... Notez que je ne sais même pas encore si c'est exact. (Schertz fait signe que oui.) Mais que cela puisse être imprimé, tout au long, avec la signature d'un savant aussi sérieux, aussi circonspect que Brunois, c'est inouï! Le ton de l'article, surtout, est déroutant: ces objections sont rappelées là incidemment, pour appuyer la thèse, sans même être discutées, comme autant de vérités acquises aujourd'hui, comme autant de points d'histoire définitivement élucidés! Simplement, un renvoi, pour indiquer où les ignorants comme moi peuvent trouver la démonstration raisonnée de chacune de ces affirmations! Et je vous cite cet article parce que je viens de le lire. Mais de tous les côtés, dans tous les domaines, je me heurte à des réfutations!

Tout le savoir moderne est donc en contradiction absolue avec notre foi?

SCHERTZ (affectueusement). — Je vous croyais en relation avec un abbé de Buis, un prêtre instruit...

JEAN. — Bah... C'est un homme actif, un saint, qui n'a jamais eu un doute sérieux, et qui d'ailleurs, si cela lui arrivait, en triompherait tout de suite, par l'action. (Sourire rancunier.) Il m'a prêté des bouquins de théologie...

SCHERTZ. — Eh bien?

JEAN (levant les épaules).— J'y ai trouvé des arguments spécieux et verbeux, présentés comme s'ils étaient inattaquables, mais que la moindre réflexion crève comme des outres gonflées. Ça ne peut convaincre que des convaincus. Je vous scandalise?

SCHERTZ. — Mais non, aucunement. Je vous comprends très bien.

JEAN. — Vrai?

SCHERTZ. — Mieux que vous ne pouvez croire...

Jean ébauche un geste étonné que Schertz arrête de la main. SCHERTZ. — Continuez, voulez-vous?

JEAN. — Mais voilà... C'est tout... Chaque fois que je veux raisonner.. avec l'espoir de consoler ma foi, ou simplement chaque fois que je cherche à analyser mon inquiétude, je sens que je porte un nouveau coup à mes croyances. .. C'est en cherchant à prouver sa foi qu'on l'ébranle: j'en ai fait l'expérience. J'ai beau faire: ça croule...

SCHERTZ (vivement). — Non, non.

JEAN. — Ah, je vous assure que je ferai tout pour éviter ça! (Avec abandon et angoisse.) Il existe peut-être des gens qui peuvent se passer de religion? Moi pas. J'en ai besoin, besoin, comme de manger ou de dormir. Sans religion je serais, je ne sais pas, comme un arbre dont les racines n'auraient plus de sol, plus de nutrition possible! Tout s'en irait d'un seul coup... Ah, c'est terrible, mon cher; je me sens catholique jusqu'au fond des moelles! Je m'en aperçois mieux encore depuis que j'ai tant à lutter: tout ce que je pense, tout ce que je veux, tout ce que je fais, est déterminé en moi par un sens catholique qui fait partie de ma nature; et s'il m'arrivait de perdre ce sens-là, ma vie entière reposerait pour toujours sur une absurde contradiction!

SCHERTZ. — Mais enfin, cette crise morale a des intermittences? Il y a des jours encore où vous pouvez vous rapprocher de Dieu?

JEAN (perplexe). — Je ne sais pas comment vous dire.,, Au fond, je n'ai pas vraiment l'impression que je m'écarte de Dieu... même quand je doute de lui... (Souriant.) Je ne peux pas vous expliquer...

L'abbé fait signe qu'il comprend très bien.

JEAN (après avoir réfléchi). — En somme, le problème angoissant est celui-ci: Tout se tient dans la religion catholique: la foi, le dogme, la morale, l'émotion intérieure de la prière; tout se tient... (Schertz fait un geste de dénégation que Jean ne remarque pas...) Et si on en rejette une fraction, on perd l'ensemble!

L'abbé se lève, et fait quelques pas, les mains derrière le dos.

SCHERTZ. — Ach! mon ami, comme nous vivons une heure tragique de la vie religieuse des hommes!

Il s'arrête devant Jean et le considère, gravement.

SCHERTZ (d'une voix mesurée). — Voyons, pour résumer: d'une part, votre *raison,* qui se blesse à des points de dogme et qui refuse de les apeepter; et, d'autre part, votre *sensibilité religieuse,* vivace, très vjvace, qui a goûté Dieu, si je puis dire, et qui ne peut plus s'en passer?

JEAN. — Exactement. Sans compter une crainte instinctive, qui a ses racines dans mon enfance et dans mon atavisme, sans doute: la terreur de perdre la foi.

SCHERTZ. —Oui. Eh bien, mais c'est à peu près ce que j'ai éprouvé moi-même!

JEAN. — Ah? Quand?

SCHERZ. — Lorsque j'ai quitté le séminaire.

JEAN (impatiemment). — Et... maintenant?

SCHERTZ (montrant sa soutane et souriant). — Vous voyez...

Il repousse de la main l'interrogation de Jean.

SCHERTZ (posément). — Voulez-vous me laisser citer mon propre exemple?

Jean lui adresse un sourire reconnaissant. L'abbé se carre dans son fauteuil, le visage sur ses mains croisées, les paupières plissées, le regard lointain.

SCHERTZ. — Jusqu'à l'ordination, je n'avais pas beaucoup étudié les sciences, mais j'étais très attiré, depuis longtemps; et j ai commencé à étudier, aussitôt prêtre. Je me rends bien compte, à distance, de ce qui s'est passé; et cela arrive à beaucoup. (Avec respect.) C'est la *discipline scientifique* ! On la découvre tout à coup; on s'y soumet passionnément; elle prend possession de vous; elle vous forge un cerveau neuf. Et puis, plus tard, un jour, quand on se tourne vers le passé, tout est changé: les choses autrefois habituelles, on les regarde, et c'est comme si on les voyait pour la première fois: on les juge. .. Et, de ce jour-là, c'est fini, on *ne peut plus ne pas juger I* Pas vrai?... Voilà la *discipline scientifique!*

JEAN. — Oui: on ne peut plus s'empêcher de voir...

SCHERTZ (souriant). — Moi, je ne savais pas, j'ai cru que je pouvais retourner en arrière. J'ai fermé tous les livres, et je suis parti pour le monastère de Brligen. (Hésitant.) Une...

JEAN. — Une retraite?

SCHERTZ. — Une retraite. Cinq mois, pendant le plein hiver... D'abord j'ai tenté une consultation des Pères; beaucoup étaient instruits. Mais ils affirmaient, et moi je raisonnais; c'était toujours le même malentendu... Ils riaient à la fin, et disaient toujours: « Rien d'impossible pour Dieu. » Alors, quoi répondre?

L'un m'a dit, un jour: « Ce qui m'étonne, c'est qu'avec de pareilles pensées, vous n'ayez pas perdu la foi... » Ah, j'ai beaucoup réfléchi là-dessus. C'était vrai: ma foi n'était pas diminuée. Comme vous le disiez tout à l'heure pour vous. J'avais la conviction intérieure, — pour ainsi dire une certitude — que rien n'était modifié. Impossible d'éprouver un remords. Je me sentais soumis à quelque chose qui était plus fort que ma volonté, et, en même

temps, très élevé, et si respectable...

Alors, que faire? J'ai cherché à transiger.

JEAN (secouant la tête). — Une voie dangereuse...
r''

SCHERTZ. — J'étais bien obligé de reconnaître, devant les arguments scientifiques si nets, que la lutte était inutile. Et ne pas faire, comme certains prêtres savants, des demi-concessions, insuffisantes. Non: reculer courageusement, fier d'être sincère, et avec l'assentiment de Dieu au fond de la conscience. (Un temps.)

Ainsi, j'ai quitté Bûrgen, et je suis rentré à Berne, et je me suis appliqué à approfondir avec les livres et la réflexion, toutes ces questions. (Gaiement.) Ach! mon ami, quand on regarde, quelle inégalité vraiment des deux camps en présence! D'un côté, les adversaires de l'Église, — je parle seulement des vrais savants, ayant fait œuvre. — Et de l'autre, nos apologistes du catholicisme, qui se lamentent et brandissent de vieux arguments tout gâtés, et finalement menacent d'anathème! A qui, malgré soi, va la confiance? L'attitude de Rome est véritablement incompréhensible; il faut l'étudier de près pour s'en convaincre! Elle attaque la science moderne en ignorant tout des faits actuels. Elle ignore jusqu'à la plus élémentaire méthode: impossible de discuter. Pour cela même, voulant soutenir trop, elle rend sa thèse entière insoutenable. J'ai eu besoin de deux années pour acquérir cette conviction, mais je ne regrette pas: grâce à ces années de travail, j'ai reconquis pour toujours la paix intérieure.

JEAN. — La paix intérieure...

L'abbé se penche en avant, comme pour demander à Jean toute son attention.

SCHERTZ. — Mon ami, je suis parvenu à cette distinction capitale: s Il y a dans le sentiment religieux deux éléments tout à fait séparés par leur nature. Premièrement: le *sentiment religieux* dans sa pureté, qui est, si je puis dire, l'alliance conclue avec le divin, et, en même temps les rapports *intimes* et privés qui s'établissent entre Dieu et les

âmes religieuses. Bien, — Secondement: *l'élément,* je dirai *dogmatique,* les affirmations théoriques sur Dieu, et les rapports, — non plus intimes, mais *cultuels* — entre l'homme et Dieu. Comprenez-vous cela?

JEAN. — Oui.

SCHERTZ. — Eh bien, pour la sensibilité religieuse d'aujourd'hui, un seul de ces éléments est fondamental: c'est le premier, l'alliance personnelle avec Dieu.

JEAN. — Comment pouvez-vous dire: la sensibilité d'aujourd'hui? La religion n'est pas soumise à la mode!

SCHERTZ. — Ach, ceci est une parenthèse. La religion est soumise sinon à la mode, du moins au développement moral de l'humanité. Tenez: au moyen âge, est-ce qu'on ne puisait pas de grandes forces, simplement dans le sens littéral des dogmes? Aujourd'hui non; c'est un fait. Regardez les catholiques, ceux qui ont vraiment une vie intérieure: beaucoup d'entre eux ont de capitales ignorances, au sujet de la religion théorique; sans qu'ils s'en doutent, le dogme est chez eux au deuxième plan; et cela n'importe pas.

Reprenons. Je dis: pour vous, pour moi, pour un grand nombre de nos contemporains, le premier élément, la foi personnelle, est intacte. C'est la croyance dogmatique qui a perdu l'équilibre. Nous n'y pouvons rien: la religion romaine, telle qu'elle est fixée actuellement, est inacceptable pour beaucoup d'esprits ayant de la culture, et pour tous les esprits ayant des connaissances approfondies. Le Dieu qu'ils nous offrent est trop petitement humain: aujourd'hui, la croyance en un Dieu personnel, en un Dieu monarque, en un Dieu fabriquant l'univers, la croyance au péché et à l'enfer... Ach, non! Cette religion-là n'est plus à notre mesure! Elle ne contente plus, comment dire, notre soif de perfection.

Les croyances humaines sont obéissantes à l'évolution, comme toutes choses; elles marchent, allant du moins bien vers le mieux. Eh bien, la religion doit, de toute nécessité, être adaptée à l'intelligence actuelle. Rome est fautive de résister à cette adaptation.

JEAN (vivement). — Mais en condamnant, comme vous le faites, l'Église contemporaine, est-ce que c'est réellement vous qui avez raison?... N'est-ce pas, simplement, que vous êtes...

SCHERTZ (l'interrompant).— Comprenez bien ceci: dans les croyances des hommes, même en supposant que l'origine en soit divine, il y a forcément un élément humain. On commence seulement à en tenir compte. Ainsi, les orthodoxes avouent seulement depuis peu, que certains récits de la Bible et des Evangiles sont des histoires *figuré-es*. Je donnerai des exerhples: *I* Jésus descendant vers les régions inférieures de la terre... Ou bien Jésus emporté par Satan sur la montagne... Aucun théologien sérieux n'ose plus affirmer: « Oui, cette descente a eu lieu, matériellement... Oui, cette montagne a existé, matériellement. » Us avouent aujourd'hui: « C'est *figurativement.* »

Eh bien, cette manière d'appeler honnêtement *symbole* ce qui est manifestement symbolique, voilà ce qui est bon pour des gens comme vous ou moi. Mais il faut l'appliquer, non pas comme les orthodoxes, qui le font de mauvais gré et seulement pour les légendes vraiment grossières; il faut l'appliquer à tous les faits affirmés par la religion, *dès que ces faits sont inacceptables à la raison moderne.* Ainsi vous avez la solution de toutes les difficultés.

Long silence.

Jean réfléchit, sans détacher les yeux du visage énergique de l'abbé.

SCHERTZ. — D'ailleurs, il faut être bien persuadé, mon cher ami, qu'avant peu d'années, tous les théologiens instruits en arriveront là; et ils seront surpris que les catholiques du XIX siècle aient pu si longtemps accepter le sens littéral de tous ces récits poétiques. Ils diront: « Ce sont des visions, des histoires pleines de signification, mais *idéales;* les évangéhstes les ont accueillies sans critique, ainsi que pouvaient faire des gens anciens, dénués d'instruction, et crédules. »

JEAN. — Mais un fait est un fait. Les dogmes sont vrais, ou bien ils ne sont rien.

SCHERTZ.— Ach! Le *vrai* et le *réel,* c'est deux!.;. L'bbjectidn què vous faites est fréquente. Mais vous dites: *vé-rité;* et vous pensez: *authenticité.* Ce n'est pas la même chose. Il faut s'attacher à voir la vérité; notl pas dans le fait lui-même, mais dans la signification morale de te fait..: On peut accepter le sens fondamental que renferme le mystère de l'Incarnation, ou celui de la Résurrection, sans, pour cela, admettre que ce soient des événements authentiques, historiquement exacts, comme la capitulation de Sedan ou la proclamation de la République!

L'abbé se lève, tourne autour de la table et vient se camper devant le siège où Jean reste songeur.

L'abbé est ému. La gravité formaliste de son visage a disparu, laissant paraître l'intensité d'une flamme intérieure que Jean ne soupçonnait pas.

SCHERTZ (montrant, d'un grand geste, son crucifix).— Quand je suis agenouillé là, devant cette croix, et que je sens monter, du plus profond de moi, comme une vague, cet amour pour Jésus, et que ma bouche prononce: « Mon Sauveur! » Ach, ce n'est pas je vous assure, parce que je pense au dogme mystique de la Rédemption, à la façon d'un enfant du catéchisme!... Non... Mais je considère immensément, ce que Jésus a fait pour l'humanité: tout ce qui est vraiment bon dans l'homme d'aujourd'hui, tout ce qui promet de s'épanouir dans l'homme de demain, vient de lui! Et alors, je me penche, en toute raison satisfaite, devant *notre sauveur,* devant celui qui est le symbole du sacrifice et du désintéressement; devant la Douleur acceptée, qui rend l'homme pur!

Et quand je fais le matin, sur l'autel, ma communion de chaque jour, qui renouvelle ma force et m'élève le cœur pour la journée entière, mon sentiment est si intense que c'est bien exactement pour moi comme la Présence réelle de Dieu! Pourtant l'Eucharistie, ce n'est qu'un symbole, le symbole de l'action sensible et continue de Dieu sur mon âme; mais mon âme l'appelle, cette action, et la recherche, presqu'avidement!

Jean réfléchit. L'exaltation de l'abbé augmente, par opposition, son calme et son besoin de contradiction.

JEAN. — Je veux bien. Cependant un simple catholique, qui croit fermement aux faits matériels de l'Incarnation ou de l'Eucharistie, met dans ses prières et dans ses communions bien plus que vous ne pourrez jamais y mettre, avec vos restrictions!

SCHERTZ (vivement). — Non! L'essentiel, c'est de dégager la vérité *dans la mesure où elle peut être bonne* à chacun de nous.

Mettons-nous sur le terrain pratique: notre raison ne peut pas accepter le dogme, c'est un fait; au contraire, le symbole que nous en dégageons est clair, satisfait notre raison, et contribue à notre amélioration. Alors, comment hésiter?

JEAN. — Est-ce que ce n'est pas amoindrir la doctrine que de la dépouiller de ses formes traditionnelles? Le christianisme a toujours été, et reste une *doctrine.* « Allez et enseignez toutes les nations... » C'est l'acceptation intégrale de cette doctrine qui fait le chrétien.

SCHERTZ. — Mais c'est justement pour maintenir intégralement la doctrine, qu'il faut aujourd'hui en modifier la forme! L'histoire enseigne que les dogmes, pendant des siècles, ont pu se transformer, s'accroître, être soumis à l'évolution générale: vivre, en somme. Pourquoi maintenant les laisser immobiles dans la tradition, comme des momies? Puisque nous constatons que la religion actuelle n'est plus conforme aux besoins des consciences contemporaines, pourquoi n'aurions-nous pas le droit, à notre tour, d'ajouter quelque chose au travail des théologiens devanciers?

Quatre heures sonnent à Saint-Sulpice.

L'abbé se lève et touche l'épaule de Jean, qui regarde dans le vague.

SCHERTZ. — Nous recauserons de tout ça.

JEAN (comme au sortir d'un rêve). — Ah, je ne sais plus, moi... J'ai été si longtemps habitué à donner une valeur absolue aux formes traditionnelles... Il y a, dans la religion ainsi comprise, un manque d'unité qui me choque!

SCHERTZ (agrafant sa cape). — L'inégalité est partout. Pourquoi les hommes, tous si différents les uns des autres, n'auraient-ils pas des formules variables pour adorer le même Dieu? (Souriant.) Il faut partir

Laissez déposer, mon ami... Et rappelez-vous l'aveu deSaintPaul: « Nous ne voyons maintenant qu'au travers d'un miroir, en énigme... » « Videmus nunc per speculum, in œnigmate... »

Ils descendent dans la rue.

Plusieurs minutes de silence, côte à côte.

JEAN (brusquement). — Il faut être logique: pourquoi continuez-vous à pratiquer, s'il est avéré que ces pratiques n'ont qu'une importance figurative?

Schertz s'arrête net, sort le menton hors de son collet, et regarde Jean comme pour savoir s'il plaisante ou non. Son visage prend aussitôt une expression de souffrance.

SCHERTZ. — Ach, vous ne m'avez donc pas compris?

Il se recueille pendant quelques secondes.

SCHERTZ (pesant ses termes). — Parce qu'il serait insensé de renoncer à cette fontaine d'eau vive qu'est une religion *pratiquée* !... Il faut se comporter avec la religion comme si elle était vraie dans tous ses détails, parce qu'elle est vraie... en profondeur. Voyez, par exemple, notre prière catholique: où trouver semblable élan?

JEAN. — Vous n'avez plus besoin de formules!'

SCHERTZ. — Ne le croyez pas! C'est par les formules que le divin pénètre dans notre vie. Il faut qûe nous acceptions tous, indistinctement, fesr'formes du culte; mais que chacun, *selon l'état de sa conscience,* en fasse l'interprétation appropriée, et s'en serve selon ses besoins.

JEAN. — Alors, autant passer au protestantisme...

SCHERTZ. — Que non!Voyez cette religion individualiste et finalement anarchiste qu'est le protestantisme: là n'est pas réellement notre nature. Tandis que la forme du catholicisme, organisée, sociale... — que dire? — *communautaire...* Voilà la nature humaine!

JEAN. — Alors la libre-pensée toute pure!

SCHERTZ. — Non, mon ami. Nous, catholiques, nous n'aurons jamais le droit de faire cette rupture.

JEAN. — Le droit?

SCHERTZ (gravement). — Nous n'avons pas le droit de nous isoler des autres. Comment la religion a-t-elle acquis peu à peu ses indiscutables vertus sociales?Par les efforts de tous. Eh bien, rester à l'écart, c'est agir comme un individualiste.

JEAN. — Mais votre attitude est bien celle d'un individualiste!

SCHERTZ (sursautant). — Pas du tout! Choisir ses symboles, selon son développement personnel: oui; mais en se rappelant toujours que ce qui est symbole pour nous, a son équivalent dans les formules plus populaires. C'est ainsi qu'on reste lié à toutes les autres. Voilà le bon individualisme..;

Jean ne répond pas.

SCHERTZ. — Mon ami, songez donc à ce qu'elle est, cette religion! Songez que pour tant d'êtres humains, elle est la seule fenêtre ouverte sur la vie spirituelle! Combien sont-ils, ceux qui jamais ne pourront aller plus loin que l'image? Et vous voudriez commettre la mauvaise action de vous séparer d'eux? Mais dans chaque sentiment religieux, il y a un germe qui est le même: comme un gémissement, comme un élan plus ou moins vigoureux de l'âme vers l'infini... Nous sommes tous semblables devant Dieu!

...Faites comme moi. Je n'ignore pas quels inconvénients il y a dans la religion actuelle: mais je n y regarde pas. « Ora patrem tuum in abscondito...» Je pense que toutes les organisations des hommes ont des imperfections. Je pense que le catholicisme est, pour la majorité, très supérieur aux autres confessions, parce qu'il est vraiment, dans toute la valeur du terme, une *association.* Et j'accepte les pratiques, d'abord parce que j'y puise moimême des forces que je ne trouverais nulle part, et puis parce que, sans elles, le catholicisme cesserait d'être cette solidarité religieuse, dont tant d'âmes ont le besoin...

L'abbé se tait.

Ils viennent de pénétrer dans les galeries de la Sorbonne, encombrées d'étudiants.

Jean cherche à mettre un peu d'ordre dans ses idées: — « Ce qu'il y a de certain, oui, c'est qu'il faut chercher... Jusqu'ici j'ai fait tout ce que j'ai pu pour me refuser à penser; je croyais qu'il n'y avait rien à gagner par la réflexion... C'est une erreur: on ne peut pas retourner en arrière, revenir aux sentiments religieux de son enfance... C'est impossible, voilà un fait acquis... Tâchons au contraire d'aller de l'avant: il y a un moyen de reconstruire, puisque Schertz. ..

« Mais je me suis aperçu que je ne connais pas le premier mot de tout ça... C'est le grand point, *savoir...* Il faut que je traj vaille ça... Les dogmes... Je n'en ai retenu que le côté extérieur, cultuel. L'abbé parle toujours du fond, du fond qui est sous la forme... La forme, jusqu'ici m'a caché le fond... Approfondir, d'abord... Approfondir jusqu'au point où le sens du dogme et les exigences de la raison sont conciliables: voilà... « C'est la seule chance d'équilibre qui rne reste,., »

« A Monsieur l'abbé Schertz, Professeur de Chimie Biologique, « Institut Catholique, Berne (Suisse).

« Paris, lundi de Pâques.

« Mon cher ami,

« Je vous remercie de l'affectueux intérêt que vous prenez à la santé de mon père. Il va mieux. Il a dû renoncer à ses jours de consultation et à son cours; il n'a gardé que ses matinées à l'hôpital. C'est encore beaucoup pour son état. Néanmoins ses confrères estiment qu'avec une surveillance attentive, une rebmin'est pas à craindre avant plusieurs années.

« Je suis bien en retard avec vous; ne m'en gardez pas rigueur; je suis tellement occupé cet hiver! Vos lettres me font toujours le même plaisir; elles me rappellent nos bonnes soirées d'il y a deux ans, nos discussions, nos lectures à haute voix! Hélas, cher ami, tout cela me paraît si loin... Non que j'aie perdu le bienfait de votre influence: rassurez-vous, je crois que vous m'avez pour toujours apaisé, et que je vous dois, pour la vie entière, une foi compréhensive et calme, robuste en son fond, conciliante en sa forme, le vrai soutien de tous les jours. Mais l'engrenage de ces études médicales est impitoyable: il m'est impossible d'ouvrir un livre qui ne soit pas technique!

« J'en ai d'autant moins le temps, que j'ai tenu à ne pas interrompre mes sciences naturelles; ces études m'ont toujours passionné, infiniment plus que celles de médecine, et je ne veux pas me contenter de ce brevet élémentaire qu'est la licence. Mon patron me pousse beaucoup à concourir pour l'internat dès l'an prochain. Je préférerais consacrer tout mon effort à l'agrégation. La médecine est un chemin tout tracé pour moi; le professorat de sciences naturelles, qui répond plus complètement à mes goûts, est une carrière assez aléatoire. Je ne sais que résoudre. Je ne suis pas seul en cause, vous le savez, et ma décision engage une autre vie que la mienne... Ces perplexités, que je ne puis confier à personne, assombrissent souvent mon horizon.

« J'ai été bien heureux de vous savoir définitivement occupé selon vos désirs. Je regrette seulement que vos congés soient si rares: quand nous reverrons-nous, maintenant? En y pensant, je me défends mal d'un regret égoïste: je songe à tout ce que votre amitié représentait pour moi, et que je n'ai pas remplacé.

« Au revoir, cher grand ami. Envoyez-moi une bonne et longue réponse, et ne doutez pas de mon fidèle attachement.

Jean Barois. »

L'ANNEAU

I

Une fin d'après-midi, en mai.

Jean rentre chez lui, dans le petit appartement qu'il habite depuis que son père a quitté Paris. Sous la porte, une lettre de Mme Pasquelin:

« Buis-la-Dame, dimanche, 15 mai.

« Mon cher Jean,

« Je ne sais pas quelles nouvelles ton père te donne de sa santé, mais j'en suis assez préoccupée, je ne trouve pas qu'il aille bien..,

Jean courbe les épaules. Cette lettre, il voudrait maintenant ne pas l'avoir ou-

verte.

(' « Depuis le printemps, surtout depuis la petite crise du mois dernier, nous le trouvons bien changé. Il a encore maigri. L'entrain qu'il avait montré tout l'hiver est tombé. Il ne suit plus sérieusement son régime; il dit qu'il est fini, qu'il ne guérira pas. C'est navrant de voir un homme qui a été si actif, inoccupé tout le jour, et seul avec son domestique, dans cette grande maison pleine de souvenirs. Nous voulions l'installer ici, il aurait profité du jardin; mais il veut rester chez lui.. « Mon cher enfant, tout cela est bien triste. Je veux te parler franchement... »

Ses mains se mettent à trembler, ses yeux se brouillent.

«... Je crois bien qu'il faut dès maintenant prévoir le cas où ton père ne se relèverait pas, et c'est pourquoi je t'écris.

« Je sais combien vous avez tous souffert, dans la famille, de la froideur de ses sentiments religieux; et j'estime que c'est un devoir pour nous, ses plus vieux amis, ses plus proches voisins, de nous préoccuper de ce lamentable état de choses. Aussi depuis que ton père est auprès de nous, je m'efforce à chaque occasion d'amener la conversation sur ce grand sujet. Mais il faudrait que tu joignes tes efforts aux nôtres, en abordant avec précaution la question religieuse dans tes lettres... »

Son bras retombe avec lassitude. Une sourde animosité.

Il passe une page. Ses yeux tombent sur: « Cécile va bien... »

— « Cécile... »

Un regard vers la cheminée, où il avait mis sa photographie. Elle n'y est plus...

— « C'est vrai, je l'ai cachée depuis qu'Huguette vient ici... Huguette!... Six heures, elle ne va pas tarder à venir... »

Un malaise poignant: Cécile et Huguette confondues dans sa pensée; les deux noms ensemble sur ses lèvres... Il passe nerveusement la main sur son front:

— « Ça ne peut pas durer... » Et, tout à coup, le sentiment très net que c'est déjà fini: ça ne pouvait durer que parce qu'il n'y réfléchissait pas vraiment...

«... Cécile va bien, elle a un peu grandi ces derniers temps, ce qui l'a fatiguée. Elle va plusieurs fois par semaine avec son ouvrage passer l'après-midi auprès de ton père. Elle s'emploie de son mieux pendant ces longs tête-à-tête. ... »

Son regard mécontent se fixe.

Il aperçoit le docteur, étendu près de la cheminée; le jour baisse; Cécile est assise devant la fenêtre; son petit front bombé penche obstinément sur son ouvrage; elle insinue des mots préparés d'avance...

Cette vision lui est odieuse.

— « Pourquoi employer Cécile à cette besogne? » Il se lève, fait quelques pas à travers la chambre; puis il se dirige vers son bureau et ouvre un tiroir fermé à clef.

La photographie de Cécile...

Il s'approche de la lampe.

C'est une ancienne épreuve: Cécile accoudée à un dossier gothique, les mains croisées, la tête un peu de biais, les yeux souriants; elle est coiffée comme autrefois: un gros nœud sur la nuque.

Long, long regard. Exaltation croissante... Non, rien n'est changé; elle seule existe; rien autre ne compte!

Huguette! Pauvre Guette... Il sourit en pensant à la petite peine qu'elle aura, lorsqu'il lui dira: — « C'est fini, laisse-moi; reprends ta vie, je reprends la mienne... Je retourne vers celle que je n'ai cessé de porter en moi. »

Une demi-heure plus tard.

La pointe d'une ombrelle gratte à la porte.

Huguette, en toilette claire, un grand chapeau chargé de fleurs.

HUGUETTE. — Bonjour mon loup, ça va? C'est comme ça que tu me dis bonjour? Prends garde à mon chapeau...

Il la voit avec un recul inouï... Presque sans émotion.

Elle a jeté son ombrelle en travers du lit et se dégante posément.

HUGUETTE. — Ce n'est pas tout ça, mon petit... Je ne peux pas dîner avec toi. J'ai laissé Simone au Vachette, avec son nouvel ami, tu sais... Il a trois fauteuils pour ce soir à Cluny, et on dîne ensemble avant...

T'es pas fâché?...

JEAN. — Mais non...

Elle s'avance vers lui. La lampe, basse, éclaire les courbes lisses de sa robe. En haut, dans l'ombre, ses mains nues et sa bouche entr'ouverte. fraîche...

Ah, ce brusque désir d'elle! Souvenir brutal de telle place de chair plus pâle, plus satinée...

...Il la saisit, il enfonce son visage dans ses cheveux...

Il pense: « Non c'est impossible que ça finisse comme ça... Encore une nuit, et demain, demain... »

Elle s'échappe de ses bras, en riant.

HUGUETTE. — Laisse, que je me lave les mains...

Il la regarde aller vers le coin obscur de la toilette, relever soigneusement ses manches, et poser sans hésitation ses bagues dans un cendrier qui est là.

Une animosité soudaine... Il pense: « Comme elle est chez elle!... Ah, rompre, s'évader!... Tout de suite!... Ce soir!... »

Résolution définitive, qui l'apaise et l'éloigne d'elle.

Il soupire doucement. Il la regarde, attentive à ses ongles, le visage froncé, enlaidie.

C'est fini, irrémédiablement: — quelque chose de cassé, de tout à fait cassé...

HUGUETTE. — Accompagne-moi jusqu'au tramway?...

Ils sortent.

La rue de Rennes. Sept heures. Une cohue tumultueuse: la ruée des banlieusards vers la gare Montparnasse.

Jean marche devant, pour fendre le flot.

HUGUETTE. — Voilà mon tram'... Alors c'est convenu? Si tu ne viens pas me chercher à la sortie de Cluny, je rentre directement... A tout à l'heure, mon loup... Zut, le voilà qui file!

Elle bondit, bouscule des gens...

Il suit des yeux sa silhouette noire, qui saute sur la plateforme éclairée, cueillie par le geste arrondi du conducteur. Il est pris d'un tremblement de tout le corps.

Le tramway s'éloigne dans la nuit piquée de lumières.

Il reste là, debout, devant la terrasse d'un café. L'odeur acidulée des ab-sinthes. Des gens passent. On glapit les feuilles du soir.

II

A Buis.

Cécile est seule dans la maison du docteur. Immobile, au guet, l'épaule appuyée à la fenêtre entre-bâillée...

Jean et Mme Pasquelin ont surgi dans la trouée du portail.

— « Les voilà... »

D'instinct elle s'est rejetée en arrière, oppressée, le regard tendu, un sourire attendri aux lèvres...

Il marche vite... Il n'a pas changé... Il enveloppe la maison d'un regard vif, qui se heurte aux volets clos de la chambre du docteur.

Cécile court au devant de lui.

Adossée au départ de la rampe, les bras tombants, glacée, elle entend, derrière la porte, son pas fiévreux qui gravit le perron.

Il ouvre et s'arrête, tout pâle. Ses yeux n'expriment aucune joie; ils interrogent anxieusement.

CÉCILE. — Il est là-haut... il dort...

JEAN (la gorge moins serrée). — Il est là-haut? Il dort?

Son œil s'adoucit, s'émeut d'amour. Il tend sa main brûlante. Un long regard, enfin, extrêmement doux, plein de choses, où vient se fondre le regard souriant de Cécile.

Madame PASQUELIN (ouvrant la porte du salon). — Entre là, puisqu'il dort...

Jean pense: « Ils disent: il... » Et c'est comme s'il pensait: « Mon père va mourir »...

MADAME PASQUELIN. — Assieds-toi donc. J'ai fait ouvrir le salon; nous nous tenons là, pour qu'il n'entende pas de bruit... Ces dernières nuits, j ai couché dans la chambre de ta pauvre grand'mère, pour être plus près... (Elle ne s'assied pas. Coup d'œil tendre.) Restez là, mes enfants, je monte. Dès que ton père sera réveillé, je viendrai te le dire.

(De la porte, avec une sorte de pudeur.) Cécile est bien contente de te voir!

Seuls.

Une seconde de silence gêné.

Cécile est debout, tête basse, une main appuyée à un guéridon, l'autre au corsage, piquant et repiquant une aiguille oubliée là.

Jean approche et prend sa main.

Jean. — Nous payons cher le bonheur de nous revoir!

Elle relève son visage en larmes et porte à ses lèvres un doigt qui tremble.

Qu'il ne parle pas! Aucune parole ne peut dire...

L'embarras domine leur tendresse; ils se demandent s'ils ne s'attendaient pas à plus de joie...

Jean la guide vers le canapé. Elle s'assied, et reste droite, haletante... Il a pris sa main. Ils ne bougent plus.

Silence. Heure douloureuse et douce. ..

Jean pense: — ' On a marché là-haut... Comment est-i/? Très changé?... »

Il évoque le masque du docteur: son regard dur et fin; sa bouche, autoritaire jusque dans le baiser; son sourire décidé et courageux; mais tant de bonté secrète!

Il regarde les meubles du salon. Et, un à un, les souvenirs...

— « Ce fauteuil bas... Grand'mère un soir... Grand'mère qui est morte! — Et bientôt je dirai: Mon père *habitait* cette chambre, *habitait* cette maison, *vivait*... Et après, plus tard, ils diront: Jean *habitait, vivait*... »

Il frissonne

Il oubliait cette présence tiède, toute proche... La confiance qu'elle a mise en lui, le pénètre tout à coup comme un cordial. Cette main qu'il tient abandonnée et moite, il la porte sans défense à ses lèvres. Plusieurs fois... pieusement d'abord, avec recueillement; puis avec une émotion grandissante, un bouleversement, une violence irrésistible, accélérée, qui lui délie le cœur.

Cécile renverse la tête. Le front enivré vacille et glisse sur l'épaule de Jean.

Alors dévotement, les lèvres sur les paupières closes... Longuement, longuement...

Des pas, des bruits de porte.

Cécile ouvre les yeux, s'écarte.

MADAME Pasquelin (d'une voix naturelle). — Jean... ton père est éveillé.

La chambre du docteur.

Mme Pasquelin, ouvrant la porte avec

précaution, s'efface.

Jean hésite au seuil: une seconde d'atroce angoisse.

Il entre, seul.

Tout de suite, un allègement: le sourire de son père.

Le malade est soulevé sur des oreillers, les bras étendus. Pas très changé. La respiration est courte. Il regarde Jean s'approcher et lui sourit encore.

LE DOCTEUR (très bas, voix rauque). — Bien fatigué, vois-tu... bien, bien fatigué...

Il tend la main. Jean, qui se penchait pour l'embrasser, avance, la sienne. Le malade s'en empare, et soudain, les traits mortellement graves, il attire passionnément cette main, ce bras, tout son fils contre lui.

LE DOCTEUR (sanglot déchirant). — Mon petit!

Il tient ce visage d'homme entre ses paumes, et il n'y voit rien qu'un visage d'autrefois, un visage d'enfant. Il le palpe fiévreusement, il le serre fort, il l'appuie contre ses lèvres gercées, il le presse à droite, à gauche, contre le poil rude de ses joues.

LE DOCTEUR (retombant épuisé, avec un bref soupir). — Ah...

Il fait signe à Jean de ne pas bouger, de ne pas appeler; ce n'est rien... Et il s'immobilise, la tête en arrière, les paupières 5 doucement closes, la bouche entr'ouverte, les poings comprimant les battements du cœur.

Jean, raide, le long du lit, regarde fixement son père. Une stupeur curieuse anime son chagrin:

— « Qu'est-ce qui le change à ce point? La maigreur? Non, autre chose... Quoi?... »

Les pommettes du malade rosissent; il ouvre les yeux. Il aperçoit Jean: le front se plisse, la bouche se contracte. Puis les traits se détendent en un sanglotement paisible.

LE DOCTEUR. — Mon petit... mon petit-

Ces larmes, ce balbutiement de tendresse-.. Un inexplicable malaise envahit Jean: est-ce qu'il ne reste plus rien de son père?

Quelques minutes passent.

Elles suffisent pour mettre le chagrin de Jean en déroute: la vie, plus forte que la mort. Malgré lui, devant ce lit, c'est à Cécile qu'il pense tout à coup; son arrivée, le choc de leurs yeux... Un désir le saisit, impérieux, mais encore immatériel: aspiration vers il ne sait quelle étreinte des âmes, quelle pénétration intégrale et réciproque de toute pensés... Pourtant sur les lèvres il garde la tiédeur satinée de ses paupières 1 Un brusque goût de; vivre le soulève et le heurte impatiemment contre ce lit, qui barre son élan... Puis un subit retour sur lui-même, et le rouge au visage I

Le docteur essuie ses joues mouillées; son regard naïf et tendre ne quitte pas le visage de Jean.

LE DOCTEUR. — Dis-moi... On t'a fait venir n'est-ce pas?... Mais si, je sais... Qui? le docteur?... non?... ta marraine?

Jean secoue la tête évasivement.

LE DOCTEUR (gravité soudaine et implacable). — Ils ont bien fait. Ça n'ira plus bien longtemps... Je t'attendais.

Jean, par émotion, ou par contenance, se penche vers la main abandonnée sur le lit, _t l'embrasse.

Le docteur, l'air soucieux, dégage sa main pour se dresser sur les coudes: quelque chose d'important qu'il ne veut pas remettre..

LE DOCTEUR. — Je t'attendais. Ecoute-moi mon petit... Je ne te laisse pas grand'chose...

Jean ne comprend pas tout de suite. Puis il ébauche un mouvement de recul.

Le malade fait signe qu'il se fatigue, qu'il ne faut pas l'interroger.

LE Docteur (avec de courtes pauses, les yeux fermés, comme s'il récitait). — J'aurais pu te laisser davantage. Je n'ai pas su. De quoi vivre tout de même. Et un nom honorable, c'est quelque chose...

Maintenant, écoute: Cécile et toi, n'est-ce pas?

Jean tressaille. Le docteur le regarde avec un sourire très tendre.

LE DOCTEUR. — Elle m'a tout raconté, cette petite. Elle te rendra heureux, je suis content. Toi, tâche qu'elle soit heureuse aussi, un peu... C'est plus difficile. Tu verras... Les femmeo, on cherche à les comprendre, et c'est impossible. Il faut seulement consentir à ceci: qu'elles sont *autres*.. C'est déjà bien difficile!— Je me fais des reproches, moi, pour ta mère... (Long silence.)

Maintenant, ta santé. Tu as été... oui.. . Et tu n'as pas fait ton volontariat. Mais c'est par excès de prudence. Tu es guéri, complètement, tu m'entends? — J'en ai parlé à ta marraine, en toute sincérité.. . Pourtant, mon petit, il faudra y penser quelquefois, ne pas te surmener, surtout plus tard, vers la quarantaine... Ça sera toujours ton point faible. Tu me promets?...

Une pause. Sourire paisible.

Rappelle-toi tout ça. C'est tout.

Il se laisse glisser au milieu des oreillers et allonge les bras avec un soupir de satisfaction. Mais bientôt, quelque chose le préoccupe à nouveau.

LE DOCTEUR (rouvrant les yeux). — Elle a été bien bonne pour moi, ta marraine, tu sais... Elle a fait beaucoup, beaucoup... Elle te dna.

Cependant il ne résiste pas au plaisir de l'annoncer lui-même.

Un sourire, d'abord esquissé comme avec souffrance, s'épanouit graduellement jusqu'à illuminer les yeux, le front, toute la face, d'un rayonnement ingénu.

Il fait signe qu'il veut parler de plus près. Jean se penche sur le lit. Le docteur lui prend le visage et 1 approche de sa bouche i LE DOCTEUR. — Jean... Ta marraine ne t'a rien dit? (Solennel.) Je me suis confessé, hier.

Il recule un peu la figure de Jean pour savourer sur ses traits l'émotion que cet aveu lui cause. Puis il l'attire à nouveau:

Le Docteur. — Je devais communier aujourd'hui... Mais quand ils m'ont dit que tu venais, je t'ai attendu... Demain, avec toi... avec vous tous-..

Jean se redresse; il fait l'effort de sourire joyeusement, et détourne les yeux. Une déception confuse, irraisonnée, poignante...

LE DOCTEUR (avec un regard lointain, un peu craintif). — Tu sais mon petit, on a beau dire... (Secouant la tête. ) C'est un x terrible...

Le lendemain.;

La chambre du docteur. Aspect nu et grave.

L'office est terminé.

Mme Pasquelin, raidie contre toute émotion, remet en ordre la commode qui a servi d'autel.

Le malade est assis, soulevé sur ses oreillers. Le jour des fenêtres tombe à plein, écrase la figure, fait luire le blanc de l'œil. Le front se penche, les cheveux sont en désordre; la barbe est longue, les joues creuses. Le regard, sans lorgnon, clignotant et décentré, est pensif, exalté et puéril.

Cécile et Jean se sont approchés du lit.

Ce matin leur amour ne les tourmente plus; il fait partie d'euxmêmes; il est absolu, définitif. Une certitude les possède, d'aimer l'un et l'autre pour la première et pour la dernière fois.

Depuis hier, dans l'état du malade, un inexplicable et indiscutable changement: un calme surprenant, une détente. Indice de mieux qui les épouvante 1

Le regard lointain qu'ils examinent en silence, passe sur eux et s'arrête; mais ils ne se sentent pas atteints par lui; il les traverse, les dépasse, tendu au-delà, au-delà...

Puis un sourire affectueux, mais forcé, empreint d'un irrésistible éloignement.

LE DOCTEUR (d'une voix sans timbre et pourtant nette). — Vous voilà tous les deux là... C'est bien... C'est bien... Donnez-moi vos mains.

Son sourire se fige, conventionnel. Il semble tenir un rôle et s'en rendre compte, et se hâter pour en avoir fini.

Il joue avec les deux mains qu'il a rassemblées entre les siennes.

Mme Pasquelin s'est arrêtée au pied du lit, les traits altérés.

LE DOCTEUR (à Mme Pasquelin). — N'est-ce pas? C'est très bien... Les deux petits...

Cécile en larmes, s'abat sur l'épaule de sa mère, qui attire Jean contre elle. Ils forment un groupe enlacé.

Les yeux du mourant, qui vaguaient, effleurent lentement Cécile, puis Mme Pasquelin, et soudain se fixent sur Jean avec une hostilité catégorique, une lueur aigue de rancune... puis une supplica-

tion déchirante, aussitôt dissipée.

Jean a compris cet éclair: — « Tu vis, toi!... »

Une pitié sans bornes...

Il voudrait donner cette vie... Il se dégage, et passionnément s'incline vers le front blême.

Mais le docteur ne bouge pas. Son masque a repris sa sérénité, son indifférence. Tardivement, il semble s'apercevoir du baiser de Jean, et ses lèvres, avec effort, essayent un bref sourire, sans que ses yeux expriment une émotion humaine.

Jean se retourne vers Cécile et ouvre les bras.

III

' A M. Jean Barois.

« Buis-la-Dame (Oise) ''Berne, le 25 juin.

« Très cher ami!

« La part que j'ai prise, si naturelle, à votre deuil, ne méritait certes pas une lettre aussi reconnaissante et si affectueuse. Je vous en remercie du profond du cœur-Je suis particulièrement touché de la confiance que vous me témoignez, sur le grave sujet dont vous me faites confident, et heureux de pouvoir exprimer mon avis très net.

« Non vraiment, je considère qu'il n'y a pas obstacle de conviction entre cette jeune fille et vous. Vous êtes rendu hésitant par la nature un peu rudimentaire de sa croyance et par la place trop importante qu'elle donne aux pratiques.

« Je ne vous comprends pas. Le sentiment religieux est un. Il ne sert pas d'analyser les variations qu'il peut avoir, Il y a une hauteur où tous les élans se rencontrent et se confondent, malgré que différents soient les, points de départ.

« Vous opposez que si elle connaissait votre conception actuelle de la religion elle retirerait sa parole. Je le crois peut être. Mais ce serait par une erreur de jugement, et rien d'autre.

« Il serait donc, selon moi, très nuisible de l'avertir. Elle ne serait pas susceptible de comprendre quelle sorte de distinction vous faites entre la croyance légendaire et la base morale et humaine du sentiment religieux. Elle croirait au sacrilège, par naïveté. Ce serait provo-

quer une catastrophe par une sincérité imprudente, qui, dans l'actualité, n'est pas nécessaire. Vous seul, élevé par I instruction et le raisonnement au-dessus du mouvement instinctif de la croyance, vous devez prendre, avec toute conscience, la décision et la responsabilité de votre bonheur.

« Que vous avez tort de craindre! Vous oubliez qu'il y a entre vous deux des ressemblances profondes! Même hérédité. Même éducation. Au surplus, vous avez une nature tellement religieuse par votre tempérament propre, que vous pourrez toujours, sans effort, suivre et approuver avec sympathie l'état d'âme de votre future femme. Et elle aussi fera évolution: non seulement l'écartement enre vous n'ira pas s'agrandissant, mais au contraire se diminuant.

« Cette idée m'est venut avec certitude du récit de la communion que vous avez accomplie l'un près de l'autre devant le lit de votre auguste père mourant. En vous mettant à genoux, vous à côté d'elle, chacun croyait au fond de lui-même à une chose différente: elle, la chair ressuscitée du Christ; vous, le symbole d'amour surhumain des hommes. — Et tout d'un coup, si élevés sont vos sentiments, qu'une même intensité d'émotion les soulève, les emporte mélangés, et il n y a plus de séparation entre vos deux âmes! Ainsi, exactement, sera votre vie dans l'avenir.

« Excusez, très cher ami, le manque de suite de cette lettre. Je. n'écris pas souvent en français.

« Je suis depuis des années le confident de votre espoir qui a fait ses preuves de fidélité et de bien fondé; il ne faut pas que des scrupules exagérés anéantissent ce bonheur, que vous méritez tous les deux.

« Votre très fidèlement attaché et dévoué,

Hermann Schertz! »

LA CHAINE

« *Le mariage n'est dangereux que pour l'homme qui a des idées.* » Herzog.

I

« A Monsieur l'Abbé Schertt « Professeur de Chimie Biologique à l'Institut Catholique

« Berne (Suisse)

« Cher «mi,

« Vous avez mille fois raison de me reprocher ce long silence. Votre rappel me prouve que votre affection n'en est pas altérée, et c'est, avant tout, ce qui m'importe.

« Je vous remercie tout d'abord de l'intérêt que vous portez à la santé de ma femme. Depuis deux ans, elle n'a cessé d'être pour moi un sujet d'inquiétude. Son accident a eu des conséquences plus graves que je ne pouvais l'imaginer, lorsque je vous en ai fait part. Des troubles de tous ordres en ont dérivé. Après dix-huit mois de soins, elle en reste encore ébranlée, au point que nous devons peut-être renoncer à l'espoir de jamais avoir d'enfant.

« C'est pour elle une bien cruelle épreuve et qui a sur son moral un pénible retentissement.

« Ce n'est pas que je veuille chercher dans ces préoccupations privées une excuse à la rareté de mes lettres. Bien des fois j'ai voulu vous écrire je ne l'ai pas fait, parce que je me sentais si éloigné des convictions religieuses que nous partagions autrefois, que je ne savais pas comment vous l'apprendre. H faut se décider pourtant; nous sommes l'un et l'autre capables, n'est-il pas vrai? de mettre notre amitié à l'abri d'une divergence d'opinions. « J'ai eu, dans ma viv religieuse, trois grandes étapes: « A dix-sept ans, quand, pour la première fois, j'ai eu la noion que tout n'était pas clair dans cette religion « révélée » j quand j'ai compris que le doute n'était pas une imagination coupable, que l'on chasse en secouant la tête, mais une hantise tenace, impérieuse comme la vérité; une pointe fichée au plus profond de la croyance, et qui l'épuise, goutte à goutte.

« Puis, à vingt ans, quand je vous ai connu, quand je me suis accroché désespérément à votre interprétation conciliante du catholicisme. Vous vous souvenez, cher ami, avec quel frémissement j'ai saisi cette perche que vous me tendiez? Je vous dois quelques années vraiment sereines. Mon mariage, au début, n'a fait que consolider votre œuvre; au contact de la foi absolue de ma femme, je me suis trouvé tout naturellement enclin au respect des choses religieuses; votre conception symboliste m'offrait l'heureux compromis dont j'avais besoin, pour accepter le voisinage d'une orthodoxie, dont ma raison ne cessait de repousser les affirmations dogmatiques.

« Mais ce calme n'était qu'apparent. Une réaction inconsciente travaillait en moi.

« Comment ai-je été amené à tout remettre en question? Je ne le vois pas clairement.

« L'attitude que nous avions prise ne pouvait être définitive. Ce terrain symboliste est trop glissant: on ne peut y faire qu'un arrêt provisoire. A force d'enlever à la tradition catholique tout ce qui ne peut plus satisfaire les exigences de la conscience moderne, il ne reste bientôt plus rien du tout. Du jour où l'on admet que l'on puisse abandonner le sens littéral des dogmes — et comment ne pas admettre cet abandon, si l'on consent à réfléchir? — on légitime du même coup toutes les indépendances d'interprétation, le libre-examen, la libre-pensée toute entière.

Sans doute l'avez-vous senti comme moi? Je ne puis imaginer que vous trouviez encore la paix de conscience dans ce parti-pris équivoque. C'est jouer sur le sens traditionnel des mots; c'est une échappatoire... Il était trop fragile, votre lien entre le présent et le passé! Comment s'attarder à mi-chemin de l'affranchissement? Vouloir conserver la religion catholique pour sa valeur sentimentale, ou pour le groupement social qu'elle représente encore, ce n'est plus faire œuvre de croyant, mais de folkloriste! Je ne nie pas l'importance historique du christianisme: mais il faut loyalement avouer aujourd'hui, qu'il n'y a plus rien de vivant à tirer de ces formules, — pour ceux du moins, dont le jugement garde une activité propre.

« Aussi n'ai-je pas tardé à m'apercevoir que cette foi d'enfance et de i race dont j'avais cru si longtemps l'armature nécessaire, m'était insensiblement devenue étrangère. Et c'est le dernier bienfait de votre action sur mon développement moral, de m'avoir permis d'atteindre sans déchirement la négation définitive. Je vous dois-de pouvoir enfin regarder froidement ces dogmes morts, auxquels j'avais tant prêté de ma propre vie!

« Il faut aussi tenir compte de l'influence que mon entrée à Venceslas a pu apporter, indirectement, à la revision de mes croyances. Cela peut paraître paradoxal, puisque c'est un collège dirigé par des ecclésiastiques; mais les professeurs sont choisis dans l'Université, l'enseignement y est relativement très libre, et le cours que je fais ne subit aucun contrôle.

« J'avais brigué cette chaire, sans exactement me représenter les difficultés que j'affrontais. Je n'avais guère l'habitude de parler en public. Mais, dès les premières leçons, j'ai senti passer sur mes élèves ce frémissement d'attention qui ne trompe pas...

« Voici la seconde année que leur curiosité ne s'est pas démentie. Je leur consacre tout mon temps, et, je puis le dire, le meilleur de moi. Tout ce que m'apportent chaque jour, mes études, mes réflexions privées, passe dans mes leçons. Je veux que ceux qui suivent mon cours emportent de leur bref contact avec moi, autre chose que quelques connaissances exactes; je fais le rêve d'élever leur niveau moral, d'exalter leurs personnalités, de marquer à jamais ces âmes qui s'offrent à l'empreinte: et vraiment je crois obtenir un résultat qui n'est pas indigne de tout mon effort.

« Ce cours n'est donc pas ce que vous semblez croire, lorsque vous me demandez s'il me laisse le loisir de travailler pour moi. Il n'a rien d'une besogne professionnelle: c'est la grande joie de ma vie, c'est mon œuvre, c'est la consolation de tous mes ennuis. (Et, quoique je ne veuille pas insister sur la plaie secrète que mon affranchissement a creusée dans ma vie conjugale, vous devinez aisément que les chagrins de. cet ordre ne me sont pas épargnés.)

« Voici, mon cher ami, ce qu'est mon existence. Où en êtes-vous, vous-même? J'espère ne pas vous Avoir peiné en vous ouvrant toute ma pensée actuelle?

« Je n'ai d'ailleurs fait que mettre en pratique un passage de Saint Luc, que vous connaissez bien:

« *Personne ne met du vin nouveau dans des outres vieilles; autrement le vin nouveau rompra les vieilles outres...*

« *Mais il faut mettre le vin nouveau dans des outres neuves; et l'un et l'autre seront conservés.* »

« Je vous serre très affectueusement les mains.

Jean Barois. »

« A Monsieur Jean Barois « Professeur de Sciences Naturelles au Collège Venceslas

« Paris

« Très cher ami!

« Quelle indicible surprise et quelle douloureuse émotion a provoqué votre lettre, je ne saurais l'écrire! Il me semble que vous avez dû souffrir beaucoup pour devenir ainsi!

« Mais je garde encore confiance en votre jugement, et je pense que vous reviendrez un jour ou l'autre à des conceptions moins absolues. En effet, celui qui, comme vous et moi, n'est plus possédé par la foi intégrale, n'a devant lui que deux routes: ou bien l'anarchie morale, l'absence complète de toute règle et mesure; ou bien l'interprétation symboliste, qui concilie la tradition et l'intelligence contemporaine, et qui permet de conserver la haute et estimable organisation catholique. Notre religion constitue le seul ensemble auquel nous puissions relier nos élans individuels, le seul aussi qui donne à l'obligation morale une raison objective: en dehors du catholicisme, il n'y a pas de science, il n'y a pas de groupement philosophique, qui donne une raison satisfaisante au devoir.

« Pourquoi secouer les épaules, et vouloir échapper à toute autorité?

« Je refuse, comme vous, d'être un croyant automatique; mais est-ce qu'il faut pour cela refuser tout le catholicisme? Votre noble Renan l'a exprimé: « Garder du christianisme tout ce qui peut se pratiquer sans la foi au surnaturel. »

« J'ai regretté, pendant la lecture de votre lettre, l'enrôlement de votre ami Monsieur l'abbé Joziers dans les Missions. Il vous a bien manqué. Je sais que son orthodoxie est rigoureuse; mais il aurait aperçu la crise que vous avez traversée, et son cœur lui aurait inspiré le moyen de vous tendre la main avec efficacité.

« Je vous tends aussi la mienne, très cher ami, comme une fois déjà, avec tout mon encouragement. J'espère que vous ne la repousserez pas, et dans ce souhait je termine cette lettre, en vous adressant mes sentiments de dévouement et de fidèle amitié.

« Hermann Schertz.

« P. S. — Vous avez incomplètement lu l'Évangile, car ceci est le verset suivant, qui est capital:

— « *Et personne, ayant bu du vin vieux, n'en demande aussitôt du nouveau, parce qu'il dit: Le vieux est meilleur.* »

« A Monsieur l'Abbé Schertz « Professeur de Chimie Biologique à l'Institut Catholique

« Berne (Suisse)

« Cher ami,

« Vous comparez mon affranchissement au geste d'un gamin révolté contre une férule gênante... S'il est vrai que, depuis mon mariage, j'ai souvent eu à souffrir d'un contact plus direct et plus fréquent avec les exigences orthodoxes, croyez bien que je n'ai pas obéi à un sentiment aussi personnel, lorsque j'ai été conduit à rejeter définitivement ce qui me restait de catholicisme.

« Vous vous leurrez, en voulant interpréter au mieux de vos convenances individuelles, une religion, qui s'est nettement formulée elle-même, et qui, sans aucune ambiguïté possible, rejette et condamne d'avance toute interprétation comme la vôtre. Car l'Eglise, avec une intransigeance préventive dont il faut bien reconnaître la logique, a pris soin d'expulser de cette communauté où vous revendiquez une place, les demi-croyants que nous étions — et que vous êtes encore...

« L'assurance de votre lettre m'autorise à vous rappeler certains paragraphes de la constitution « Dei filius » du Concile du Vatican de 1870, qui me paraissent particulièrement significatifs et que je viens de recopier à votre intention:

« Si quelqu'un ne reçoit pas *dans leur intégrité, avec toutes leurs parties,* comme sacrées et canoniques, les Livres de l'Écriture, comme le Saint Concile de Trente les a énumérées, ou nie qu'ils soient divinement inspirés: qu'il soit anathème!

« Si quelqu'un dit qu'il ne peut y avoir de miracles, et par conséquent, que *tous les récits de miracles,* même ceux que contient l'Écriture sacrée, *doivent être relégués parmi les fables ou les mythes;* ou que les miracles ne peuvent jamais être connus avec certitude, et que l'origine de la religion chrétienne n'est pas valablement prouvée par eux: qu'il soit anathème!

Si quelqu'un dit qu'il peut se faire qu'on doive quelquefois, selon le progrès de la science, attribuer aux dogmes proposés par l'Eglise *un autre sens que celui* qu'a entendu et qu'entend l'Église: qu'il soit anathème!

« Enfin ceci, d'une limpidité cristalline:

« Car la doctrine de la foi que Dieu a révélée n'a pas été livrée comme *une invention philosophique aux perfectionnements de l'esprit humain,* mais a été transmise *comme un dépôt divin* à l'Epouse du Christ pour *être fidèlement gardée* et infailliblement enseignée. Aussi doit-on toujours retenir *le sens des dogmes sacrés* que la Sainte Mère Église a déterminés *une fois pour toutes,* et ne jamais s'en écarter *sous prétexte et au nom d'une intelligence supérieure à ces dogmes.*

« C'est donc, cher ami, l'Église qui nous ferme ses bras.

« Pourquoi se cramponner, par je ne sais quelle tendresse sentimentale qui n'est guère payée de retour, à cette vieille nourrice qui nous a repoussés, qui tient pour criminels les efforts que nous avons faits vers elle?

« Réfléchissez encore une fois à tout cela. Tôt ou tard, j'en ai la certitude, vous en viendrez à penser comme moi. Vous vous apercevrez que vous n'avez accompli que la moitié du trajet vers la lumière, et d'un bond, vous ferez le reste.

« Je vous attends dehors, à l'air libre.

« Croyez, cher ami, à toute ma fidèle affection.

Jean Barois. » e

II

La chambre à coucher, à l'aube.

Jean soulève les paupières, et cherche d'un œil clignotant l'interstice des rideaux.

JEAN (bâillant). — Quelle heure est-il donc?

CÉCILE (d'une voix nette). — Six heures et demie.

JEAN. — Pas tard... Tu as mal dormi?

CÉCILE. — Non, mon chéri.

Il répond par un sourire indifférent et se pelotonne au fond du lit.

CÉCILE. — Samedi... Tu n'as pas de cours ce matin?

JEAN. — Non.

CÉCILE (tendre). — Mon chéri... J'ai quelque chose à te demander...

JEAN. — Quoi donc?

Un silence. — Elle s'est couchée contre lui, comme autrefois, a posé son visage au creux de l'épaule, et reste blottie, sans bouger.

CÉCILE. — Ecoute.

JEAN. — Eh bien?

CÉCILE. — Tu ne vas te fâcher, dis?... Tu ne vas pas me faire de la peine...

Jean se soulève sur un coude et l'examine avec inquiétude. Il connaît ce regard obstiné, voilé de tendresse.

JEAN. — Qu'est-ce qu'il y a encore?

CÉCILE. — Ah, si tu commences comme ça...

JEAN. — Allons, voyons, parle... Qu'est-ce qu'il y a?

Elle n'aime pas être contrainte. Son sourire est aigre. Elle réfléchit une seconde, et se décide.

CÉCILE. — Tu ne peux pas me refuser ça...

JEAN. — Qu'est-ce que c'est?

CÉCILE. — Voilà... Tu sais qu'en ce moment je fais une neuvaine...

JEAN (le masque assombri). — Non.

CÉCILE (décontenancée). — Tu ne le savais pas?

JEAN. — Me l'as-tu dit?

CÉCILE. — Tu as bien dû t'en apercevoir...

Un silence.

JEAN (froidement). — Une neuvaine... Pourquoi?... Pour avoir un enfant?...

(Une pause.) Ainsi, tu en es là!

Cécile se jette contre sa poitrine, lui ferme la bouche d'un baiser bref, presqu'agressif.

CÉCILE (lui parlant au visage, avec une violence soudaine). — Mon chéri, mon chéri, ne me dis rien, laisse-moi... Vois-tu, je suis sûre que je serai exaucée... Mais il faut que toi aussi... Je ne te demande pas grand'chose: de venir avec moi ce soir, à Notre-Dame des Victoires... Simplement une fois, pour le neuvième jour.

Elle s'écarte et, sans le lâcher, contemple Jean, qui secoue la tête avec tristesse.

JEAN (doucement). — Tu sais bien.. .

CÉCILE (lui mettant sa main brûlante sur les lèvres). — Tais-toi... Tais-toi...

JEAN. —...que ce n'est pas possible.

CÉCILE (hors d'elle). — Mais tais-toi donc!Ne me dis rien... (Se coulant contre lui sans le regarder.) Tu ne peux pas me refuser ça... Un enfant, pense donc, mon chéri, entre nous, à nous... un enfant!... — M'accompagner seulement, sans rien faire, sans rien dire; ce n'est pas grand'chose!

Tais-toi, ne me dis rien: c'est promis.

JEAN (froidement). — Non. Je ne peux pas faire ça.

Un silence.

Brusquement Cécile éclate en sanglots.

JEAN (agacé). — Ah, ne pleure pas, ça n'avance à rien...

Elle fait un effort pour retenir ses laimes.

JEAN (lui prenant les poignets). — Tu ne comprends donc pas ce que tu veux me faire faire? Tu es donc aveuglée à ce point que tu ne vois pas la laideur du geste que tu me proposes?

CÉCILE (suffoquant). — Qu'est-ce que ça te fait?... Puisque je t'en supplie. ..

JEAN. — Voyons, Cécile, réfléchis seulement une seconde. Tu sais bien, n'est-ce pas, que je ne crois pas à l'efficacité de cette prière, de ces

cierges? Alors? Veux-tu me contraindre à jouer la comédie?

CÉCILE (dans ses larmes). — Qu'est-ce que ça te fait?... Puisque je t'en supplie...

JEAN. — Comment as-tu pu croire que j'accepterais?.. Tu ne comprends donc pas, qu'en me demandant des choses pareilles, après toutes les pénibles discussions que nous avons eues ensemble, tu nous avilis tous les deux?

CÉCILE (sanglotant toujours). — Puisque je t'en supplie...

JEAN (avec brusquerie). — Non.

Cécile lève sur lui des yeux hagards.

Un silence.

JE4N (sombre). — Je t'ai expliqué ça vingt fois... Ce qu'il y a de plus propre en moi, c'est justement cette loyauté dans le doute... C'est d'attacher une si grande importance à tout acte de foi, que je ne peux plus en faire le simulacre par complaisance... Tu ne comprends rien, rien, à ce que j'éprouve!

CÉCILE (vivement). — Mais, à cette heure-là, tu ne rencontreras personne.. Jean ne saisit pas tout de suite.

Long regard d'étonnement, puis de véritable détresse.

JEAN. — C'est toi qui me donnes des raisons pareilles!

Ils demeurent allongés l'un près de l'autre, mêlant leurs tiédeurs, mais l'un à l'autre fermés, rancuneux, hostiles.

Jean (cherchant à raisonner). — Voyons, réfléchis un instant... Cette neuvaine, je ne t'empêche pas de la faire. Je refuse-seulement d'y prendre part... C'est le moindre de mes droits...

CÉCILE (violente et têtue). — Tu parles toujours de tes droits, parle donc aussi de tes devoirs! D'ailleurs, je n'ai rien à t expliquer... Tu ne comprendrais pas. Mais il faut, il faut absolument que tu viennes avec moi ce soir; sans quoi tout est perdu!

JEAN. — Mais c'est stupide! En me menant là-bas, à mon corps défendant, qui penses-tu tromper?

CÉCILE (suppliante). — Jean, je t'en conjure, viens avec moi ce soir!

JEAN (sautant du lit). — Non, non, et non! Je ne m'oppose pas à tes croyances, mais laisse-moi libre d'agir selon les miennes 1

CÉCILE (un grand cri). — Ah, ce n'est pas la même chose!

Jean se retourne vers le lit où Cécile sanglote éperdûment.

Jean (avec une tristesse profonde). — *Ce n'est pas la même chose...* Voilà ce qui est cause de tout! Jamais tu rie consentiras à respecter ce que tu ne comprends pas...

(Levant la main.) Ah, ma pauvre enfant, tu peux me rendre justice, je n'ai jamais prononcé une parole qui puisse ébranler ta foi! Mais, bon Dieu, il y a des instants où je souhaite de toute ma rancune que tu apprennes un jour, à tes dépens, ce que c'est que le doute — juste assez pour perdre le goût de l'absolu, et ce besoin de dominer, du haut de ta certitude!

11 s'aperçoit dans une glace, ébouriffé, pieds nus, jetant l'anathème vers le lit défait... Exaspéré contre lui autant que contre elle, il s'enfuit en claquant la porte

Jean, seul à son bureau.

Il a des notes éparpillées devant lut.

Il écrit une page entière sans lever les yeux, puis repose sa

Elume avec humeur. Malgré tout son effort, il ne travaille pas: il esogne, machinalement; son application se perd dans le vide. Il pense:

— « C'est stupide... Je ne peux rien faire ce matin..i Et tout ça, pour cette histoire de neuvaine... »

Il repousse ses fiches, et reste un instant songeur.

— « Ce serait trop bête... Tout l'avenir dépend de moments comme ceux-ci. Il faut que j'aie ma liberté d'action, c'est bien le moins! Aujourd'hui ceci, demain autre chose ï non I »

Il se lève, par énervement fait quelques pas, les bras croisés, jusqu'à la fenêtre, où il stoppe net, les yeux vagues dans le ciel pluvieux.

— « Mais qu'est-ce qu'elle peut s'imaginer avec sa rieuvaine? Toujours cette action directe des prières sur la volonté de Dieu... C'est d'un enfantillage!... Vraiment elle a une façon de croire, qui ocrait dighe dc3 Clivages do l'abbé Joasiers I Cet abonnement de neuf jours... ce nombre neuf... Elle doit s'être procuré un formulaire spécial pour femmes stériles!... Prodigieux! »

Il hausse les épaules, se dirige vers la bibliothèque, et debout, appuyé au battant vitré, semble s'attarder à la recherche d'un livre.

— « Avoir une attitude loyale vis-à-vis de soi-même. Les femmes ne comprennent rien à ce sentiment-là! « *Qa est-ce que ça te fait, puisque je t'en supplie....* » La dignité pour soi... la dignité de la vie, pour soi-même... »

Il prend un volume, au hasard, et regagne son fauteuil.

L'heure du déjeuner.

Jean se met à table, seul

Il pense: — « Elle va rester dans sa chambre, à bouder. Elle espère que je serai sensible à cette comédie!... (Excédé.) Quand tout ça finira-t-il! »

Mais Cécile paraît.

Et Jean, levant les yeux au bruit de la porte, aperçoit un pauvre visage ravagé de douleur, plombé, maigri, labouré de larmes.

Tout ressentiment s'évanouit: une compassion soudaine, comme devant la faute d'un enfant entièrement irresponsable: une immense pitié, jaillie du plus profond de sa tendresse instinctive... presqu'une résurrection, mais si triste si décolorée, de l'amour d'autrefois, — qui est mort.

Sans aucun cabotinage, elle s'assied à sa place, livide.

Le repas.

Elle s efforce de toucher aux plats. Dè longs silences. Devant la femme de chambre, quelques mots rapides sur sa migraine.

Jean l'examine à la dérobée: la courbe nette et têtue du front baissé; les paupières bouffies, sèches et rotlges; les lèvres feriflées, la bouche béante, vraiment déformée par la douleur...

Il pense avec angoisse: — « Comme je la torture!... A tort ou à raison, peu importé!... Elle souffre par moi, ét c'est abominable 1 Ah, à quoi bon vouloir qu'elle comprenne? je n'arriverai jamais qu'à lui faire mal. Plutôt céder que de la martyriser odieusement, pour rien 1 Ert somme que derisnde-t-elle? guère plus que ce que j'ai fait souvent, cet été, en l'accompagnant le dimanche à la messe.., Tant pis pour elle, si elle ne voit pas la sottise, la laideur de cette démarche forcée...

« Allons, je ne m'obstine pas... »

Et tout de suite, par cette seule résolution intérieure, une détente, un allègement joyeux. Il goûte une jouissance volup tueuse à s'évader de son égoisme, à êtr le meilleur des deux, celui qui comprend, qui pardonne, qui cède.

Il la regarde avec douceur. Elle mange docilement, sans lever les yeux.

— « Jolie, dans ses larmes... C'est monstrueux de laisser pleurer une femme! Mon père disait: « Les femmes sont *autres,* on l'oublie trop souvent. » Il avait raison; voilà ce qu'on obtient à vouloir les traiter en égales: de la souffrance inutile... Oui, il avait raison. Il faudrait négliger ce qui nous sépare d'elles, et s'acharner à découvrir ce qui peut nous en rapprocher...

« Oui, oui: mais pour que ce soit possible, et facile, il faudrait encore s'aimer... »

Il se lève de table.

Elle attendait, indifférente, les yeux sur la nappe.

Il pense: — « Elle va fuir dans sa chambre... Je la suivrai, je lui dirai que je veux bien. »

Mais, comme d'habitude, Cécile se dirige vers le cabinet de Jean, où l'on a porté le café. Et elle reste debout devant le plateau, les bras tombés.

Jean va vers elle.

Il a fait un dur effort; il a piétiné un peu de sa conscience, un peu de son amour-propre, un peu de l'avenir. Il escompte cette joie qu'il lui apporte. Elle va s'abattre contre son épaule avec un sanglot attendri, et il sera payé par l'éclair reconnaissant de ses yeux.

Il se penche, il entoure sa taille. Elle se laisse manier sans résistance.

JEAN (avec un tremblement dans la voix). — Ecoute... C'est bien, j'irai ce soir avec toi, où tu voudras. Pourvu que tu ne pleures plus...

Mais elle se dégage et le repousse brutalement.

CÉCILE. — Ah, je sens que tu seras mon ennemi, toujours!

Il la considère, abasourdi.

CÉCILE (martelant les mots). — Je sais qu'il faudra que nous nous quittions, un jour, dans un an, dans deux ans, dans dix... je ne sais pas... mais, un jour, certainement, il le faudra! Et je te détesterai! (Éclatant en larmes.) Tu me fais déjà horreur...

Elle ébauche un geste vague des mains en avant, comme si elle allait tomber, et vient s'appuyer au bord de la table.

JEAN (amer). —C'est bien... Je pensais te faire plaisir.

Elle relève la tête, comme s'éveillant d'un cauchemar, et son visage s'adoucit. Elle s'agrippe au bras de Jean.

CÉCILE (balbutiant). — Ah oui, pour ce soir? C'est vrai, je te remercie.. (Elle se baisse, et furtivement lui embrasse la main.) Merci, mon chéri.

Et brisée, le mouchoir sur les lèvres, elle quitte la pièce lentement; de la porte, elle cherche à lui sourire.

Jean, hébété, fixe machinalement cette porte fermée.

Puis il secoue le front et les épaules, va vers la fenêtre, l'ouvre brusquement, malgré la pluie, et se penche dehors, comme quelqu'un qui s'évade d'un trou sans air.

Notre-Dame des Victoires. 8 heures du soir.

Un sépulcre. Les herses flamboyantes aveuglent, endorment, mais n'éclairent pas.

Là, le soir, de tous les coins de Paris, les détresses qu'aucun courage ne porte plus, et les espoirs tenaces que tout a déjoués, viennent s'ensevelir côte à côte, dans l'ombre qu'épaissit la fumée des cires.

Cécile, prosternée; Jean, debout: l'un et l'autre courbés sous le poids de l'irrémédiable.

Le même soir.

Jean, revenu à sa table de travail, s'y attarde, — pour être seul.

La porte s'ouvre.

Cécile entre sans bruit, lès pieds nus.

CÉCILE. — Tu ne viens pas te coucher? (Naïvement.) Tu me boudes?

Elle rit gentiment, d'un air puni.

Désarmé par tant d'inconscience, Jean ne peut s'empêcher de sourire.

Elle est en peignoir. Aucune trace de larmes. Sa coiffure de nuit la rajeunit: cheveux lâches, pinces à la nuque par un gros papillon noir. Elle a quinze ans, ce soir; elle est la frêle fiancée de Buis.

Comme une enfant, elle saute, et se perche sur les genoux de Jean.

CÉCILE. — Je ne veux pas m'endormir toute seule, après une journée pareille. Je veux que tu me dises que tout est oublié... que tout est fini...

Jean est las de paroles.

Sans répondre, il embrasse doucement ce front cahn, qu'elle tend. Plus que jamais, ce soir, il se sent un vieil homme.

CÉCILE. — Là-bas, il fait trop froid. Je vais t'attendre. Continue, mon chéri, il ne faut pas que je t'empêche de travailler. Je vais rester sur ton genou, je ne bougerai pas.

Elle se blottit, elle s'abandonne. Le bras de Jean qui l'encercle, sent fondre le pli de sa taille, mouvante et tiède.

Ses mules de paille ont glissé; il prend dans le creux chaud de sa main, les petits pieds frileux.

CÉCILE. — Tu vois, je suis gelée...

Elle rit: un rire saccadé, provocant. Puis elle se laisse emporter, la tête en arrière, riant toujours.

Maintenant, leurs yeux se croisent. Un choc bref: sous les paupières baissées de Cécile, Jean a heurté une petite lueur de joie triomphante.

Il pense brusquement:

— « Ah!... le neuvième soir... Il (allait aussi que... »

Pas même un sentiment de rancune; il la garde allongée contre lui.

Il vient de toucher du regard toutes les possibilités de la bêtise humaine, et il se sent si loin de Cécile, si loin!...

— « Les femmes sont *autres*,.. »

III

Quelques feuillets, d'une écriture cursive et nerveuse, au fond d'un tiroir du bureau de Jean: *Les femmes : êtres inférieurs, irrémédiablement. Leur sensiblerie est en elles, comme un ver dans un fruit. Qui attaque tout: qui rend impuissante leur intelligence, et infirme leur cœur. Un cerveau de petite fille, confit à l'ombre d'une ville de province: toutes les affirmations de la sottise ignorante. Ça ne se décrasse pas. Les femmes aiment le mijstère, par instinct.*

*Contre, rien ne peut. Encore l'aiment-elles bassement. Si, la nuit, elles ont peur des voleurs, une veilleuse leur rend la sécurité. Le geste de l'autruche: leur geste naturel. Il leur faut une foi pour être assurées, pour n'avoir pas à chercher au delà. — (N'imaginant même pas qu'on puisse avoir soif de « vérification... ») On ne doit se marier que lorsqu'on est bien fermement dirigé dans sa voie, et certain de n'en pas changer. Modifier sa direction après le mariage, c'est bouleverser deux vies pour une; c'est creuser entre deux êtres, que tout oblige à rester liés, un gou0re où tout le bonheur s'abîme, — sans le combler.*

L, *r* année suivante.

A Buis, le lundi de Pâques.

Le petit salon de Mme Pasquelin. Midi. Jean et Cécile viennent d'arriver pour passer quelques jours.

L'abbé Joziers, revenu de Madagascar depuis deux mois, est venu déjeuner avec eux.

MADAME PASQUELIN. — Allons.. . Approchez-vous... Venez vous chauffer... Il faisait si beau ce matin!

Le ciel s'est subitement assombri, une rafale de grêle tambourine sur les vitres.

L'abbÉ JOZIERS (de la fenêtre). — C'est une giboulée, ça ne durera pas... (A Jean.) Ce grand ami-là, comme il a changé depuis cinq ans!

JEAN. — C'est vous que je n'aurais pas reconnu!Maigri, jauni...

L'abbÉ (riant). — Merci!

MADAME PASQUELIN. — Et encore, depuis un mois, il a vraiment meilleure mine... Il serait mort au milieu de ses nègres, si je ne l'avais fait rappeler d'autorité par Monseigneur.

L'abbÉ (à Jean). — C'est vrai, mon cher, j'ai failli rester là-bas. Et puis le bon Dieu, prévenu par Mme Pasquelin, a dû se dire: « Mais ce gaillardlà, on peut encore en faire quelque chose... Bon pour le service! » Et me voilà...

JEAN (sérieux). — Il s'agit de réparer les avaries.

L'abbÉ. — Oh, ça y est... Radoubé, remis à flot... (Se frappant la poitrine.) La coque était bonne! Tenez avanthier, j'ai été jusqu'à SaintCyr, à pied;

les jambes sont solides. Aujourd'hui, je compte aller à Beaumont, pour M. le Curé. Vous voyez, il n'est même plus question de ménagements.

(Il regarde longuement Jean tout en parlant.) Comme il a changé! JEAN. — Tant que ça?

L'abbÉ. — Cette moustache, maintenant! Et puis, je ne sais pas, quelque chose de nouveau, de différent... Le regard... Non, toute la physionomie...

MADAME PASQUELIN (prenant Cécile à part). — Eh bien, toi? Comment vas-tu?

CÉCILE. — Pas mal.

MADAME PASQUELIN. — Enfin, toujours rien?

CÉCILE (les larmes aux yeux). — Non.

Une pause.

MADAME PASQUELIN (plus bas; coup d'œil vers Jean, qui bavarde avec abbé). — Et... lui?...

Cécile répond par un geste découragé. Profond soupir.

Après déjeuner.

L'abbÉ JOZIERS (s'approchant de la fenêtre). — Voilà le beau temps, il faut que je me sauve. Je vais jusqu'au presbytère de Beaumont. Jean, m'accompagnez-vous un bout de chemin?

JEAN. — Bien volontiers.

Les nuages sont passés. Une brise fraîche achève de sécher les grêlons fondus.

Un ciel lavé, immense et clair, d'un blanc à peine bleuté, s'étend sur la ville. Les rues sont propres, le soleil d'avril fait sourire les façades. Des volets blancs luisent, laqués par la pluie. Lundi de Pâques: jour férié. Des familles en promenade.

JEAN. — Nous prenons le raccourci du cimetière?

L'ABBÉ. — Oui... (Passant sa main sous le bras de Jean.) Ça m'a fait plaisir ce déjeuner. Je craignais, d'après une de vos lettres,.-et puis, d'après les réticences de votre belle-mère... (Insistant, à son habitude, sur certains mots.) Mais je vois que vous êtes *heureux,* l'un *et* l'autre, ainsi que vous le méritez *tous les deux...*

Jean le regarde presque gaiement; et l'abbé prend ce sourire pour un acquies-

cement. Quelques pas silencieux.

JEAN (avec un petit rire sec). — Le bonheur? Eh bien non, non: ce n'est pas précisément le bonheur!

L'abbé tressaille et s'arrête.

L'ABBÉ. — Vous plaisantez?

JEAN (sourire amer). — Vaut-il pas mieux en rire?

L'ABBÉ (stupéfait, un peu scandalisé). — Jean...

JEAN (haussant les épaules). — Elle est si bête, notre histoire!

L'ABBÉ. — Vous m'effrayez, Jean.

JEAN. — Que voulez-vous, c'est l'impasse...

L'abbé. — L'impasse?... Mais vous vous aimez pourtant?

JEAN (sombre). — Je n'en sais rien.

Le chemin de traverse se rétrécit. L'abbé passe devant, sans répondre. Devant le calvaire, il se signe.

Ils traversent le cimetière en biais, par des sentiers mangés d'herbe.

Une porte basse ouvre en pleine campagne. La grand'route; sur l'un des accotements, des poteaux télégraphiques à perte de vue, divisent en mesures les portées des fils. Un soleil splendide et jeune, baigne les prés, les chaumes, les labours assombris par la pluie. Des pâturages, coupés de raies d'argent, dévalent jusqu'à l'Oise, dont les rives sont encore inondées: l'eau, abritée du vent, reflète un ciel immobile, d'un gris fin; les saules immergés jusqu'au menton, lèvent leurs grosses têtes noires ébouriffées.

L'abbé s'approche de Jean, qui s'est arrêté devant le paysage. Leurs regards se croisent: celui de l'abbé est préoccupé et plein de reproche.

JEAN. — Je sais bien que je suis fautif. J'ai voulu réaliser, à vingt-deux ans, un rêve stupide, fait à seize... Ça ne pouvait rien apporter de bon.

L'abbÉ. — Au contraire, cette amitié d'enfance...

JEAN (l'interrompant avec amertume). — Permettez, permettez... Je connais bien la question, je vous assure: j'ai eu le loisir de l'approfondir!

L'abbé se tait et reprend silencieusement la marche. Cette assurance d'homme le déconcerte.

Jean devine sa surprise et y prend un

mauvais plaisir: l'air vif, le soleil, la promenade, le grisent un peu. Il devient loquace.

JEAN. — A seize ans, voyez-vous, on se fait de l'amour une idée follement mystique! On place son rêve si loin, tellement hors des possibilités de la vie, qu'on ne pourrait rien trouver dans la réalité qui le satisfasse; alors on se fabrique, de toutes pièces, un objet imaginaire! Ça se fait tout seul: on prend la première venue, la plus proche... On se garde bien de chercher quel est son véritable caractère! Non... On l'enferme comme une idole dans le cercle clos de son imagination, on la pare de toutes les qualités que l'on souhaite à l'Élue, — et puis on s'agenouille devant, avec un bandeau sur les yeux... (Il rit.)

L'abbÉ. — Mon pauvre Jean, que me racontez-vous donc?

JEAN. — L'intoxication est lente et sûre... Le temps passe, le bandeau ne tombe pas. Alors un beau jour, pour la remercier d'avoir plus ou moins longtemps personnifié vos aspirations amoureuses, sans hésiter, le sourire aux lèvres, on épouse une fillette qui vous est essentiellement étrangère...

(Une pause) Et puis, quand on a stupidement engagé sa vie entière... Il s'arrête et regarde le prêtre bien en face.

JEAN. — ...*en-ga-gé sa vie...* Sentez-vous ce que c'est?

L'abbé baisse la tête.

JEAN. —... Quand on se trouve enfin devant celle qu'on a choisie, et qu'on veut l'aimer, cette fois, pour de bon, dans la réalité de tous les jours, alors on s'aperçoit que l'on n'a rien de commun avec elle... Une inconnue! Peut-être une ennemie... Et c'est l'impasse 1

L'abbÉ. — Une inconnue, une inconnue... Voyons, ne me dites pas ça vous avez été élevés l'un *près* de l'autre!

JEAN (avec âpreté). — Oui, et nous nous connaissions moins que l'on ne se connaît dans la plupart des mariages de présentation; parce que, dans ces cas-là, on emploie fébrilement le temps des fiançailles, à s'expliquer, à tâcher de se comprendre. C'est toujours ça... Tandis que nous n'y avons même pas pensé: nous croyions que c'était fait depuis toujours

L'abbÉ. — Pourtant au début, vos premières lettres...

JEAN. — Au début? Je me suis aperçu très vite que nous étions très différents, mais sans la moindre inquiétude, je l'avoue...

L'abbÉ. —...?

JEAN. — Si vous saviez l'exaltation qui vous aveugle à ces moments-là! Ce bonheur, après lequel j'avais vu tout le monde courir en vain, je voulais si intensément qu'il fût pour moi, j'attendais avec tant de certitude cette exception de la vie en ma faveur! J'étais d'avance résolu à tout trouver parfait.

Et puis, dans les premiers temps du mariage, le rôle de l'homme est si facile! Il prend si aisément de l'influence sur sa femme! Mais qu'il se hâte! Les femmes les plus naïves ont un sens merveilleux qui les avertit vite de leur force, et les fait ressaisir bientôt tout 1 empire qu'elles ont laissé prendre... Les premiers mois, allez, sont bien trompeurs! La femme, avec une inconsciente habileté, sait retenir et répéter. Elle vous tend un miroir fidèle... Mon Dieu, on s'y regarde avec plaisir... Jusqu'au jour où l'on découvre que ce qu'elle vous présente n'est qu'une image, — votre propre image... Et si pâle, si fragile, si effacée déjà...

L'abbÉ. — Vous l'aimiez pourtant?

JEAN. — Je ne crois pas... C'est *l'amour* que j'aimais.

L'abbÉ. — Elle vous aimait, *elle,* sans réserve!

Jean ne répond pas.

L'abbÉ. — Elle vous aimait, et elle vous aime encore! J'en ai eu a preuve tout à l'heure, dans son sourire, dans son regard...

JEAN. — Ça, non. — Vous avez surpris, entre nous, un peu d'entrain factice... (Avec lassitude.) Un armistice, tacitement conclu pour notre retour ici, rien de plus.

L ABBÉ. — Elle vous a aimé, Jean, je le sais bien!

JEAN. — Oui, oui... (Haussant les épaules.) A sa façon... Petite flamme permise, qu'elle a patiemment attisée pendant des années, dans la solitude, avec la permission de sa mère et de son confesseur... Petit amour bien poétique,

bien « mois de Marie »...

L'abbÉ. — Jean!

JEAN. — Laissez, je vous parle franchement. Cet amour-là, je ne le nie pas; mais il n'était pas capable de faire un miracle: et il en faudrait un, je vous assure, pour que nos deux pensées s'accordent, pour que nos deux vies viennent à n'en faire qu'une seule!

L'abbÉ. — Mais elle était si jeune I

JEAN (avec un rire nerveux). —Ah c'est vrai: « Elle était si jeune! » (11 fait quelques pas et se retourne fébrilement.) Je le croyais! Je pensais: « Tout ce qui me déplaît en elle, est provisoire. .. » Quelle erreur!... Cécile avait, en effet, le cœur et le cerveau d'une gamine de seize ans, qui *veut.* juger la vie, et dont toute l'expérience, tous les points d'appui, sont ce peq de chose qu'elle a pu glaner, le dimanche, au catéchisme de persévérance...

L'abbÉ. «--Jean!

JEAN (avec une animation hostile). — Mais ce que je ne prévoyais pas,') c'est que cet état embryonnaire était pour elle le point terminus, et qu'elle avait atteint son point mort!

Voilà pourtant l'exacte vérité!

Jean s'est arrêté, dans une attitude de combat, les jambes écartées, le buste frémissant, la tête en arrière, l'œil dur, les mains soulevées à la hauteur de la poitrine, et les doigts ouverts comme s'il soupesait un bloc compact.

JEAN. — Elle était très fière de sa petite jugeotte! Parbleu! Elle l'avait formée à des sources inattaquables: au sermon, dans les entretiens de quelques bonnes gens de province, ou bien dans ces bouquins théoriques à l'usage des jeunes filles chrétiennes, dans lesquels il n'y a rien, rien, qui, de près ou de loin, corresponde aux réalités qu'elles devront vivre!

L'abbé fait un pas, et pose la main sur le bras de Jean. Il le regarde au visage.

L'abbe. — Jean, Jean... Vous ne parleriez pas ainsi si vous n'aviez vous-même terriblement évolué... (Baissant la voix.) Je suis sûr que vous ne pratiquez plus!

Un silence.

JEAN (sur un ton affectueux, mais ferme.) — Non.

L'abbe (avec douleur). — Ah, je comprends *tout,* maintenant!

Le chemin monte; on aperçoit le clocher de Beaumont.

L'abbé accélère l'allure, comme s'il cherchait à être seul.

L'un derrière l'autre, ils atteignent le haut du plateau. Un vent léger, venu de loin, les accueille. Sur le bord de la route, les fils télégraphiques tendus dans la brise, chantent.

Les maisons du hameau sont éparpillées à travers champs. L église est à cent mètres, gardée par les sapins pointus du presbytère.

Jean laisse l'abbé prendre de l'avance, et s'assied sur un tas de cailloux.

Son dos chauffe au soleil. Le vent lui souffle sa fraîcheur au visage. A ses pieds, de petites feuilles sèches roulent, avec un froissement de soie.

Devant lui, la plaine.

Les ombres s'allongent, obliques. A travers les houppes défeuillées des ormes, à travers les peupliers en rideaux, brillent des façades blanches, des toits bleus. Presque personne. Une charrette avance sur un chemin qu'il ne voit pas, et les roues grincent dans la boue des ornières. Au loin, un cheval gris et un cheval roux traînent la charrue sur les courbes molles d'un vallonnement, et soulèvent sans bruit des flocons d'ouate brune. Une flaque attardée luit entre des troncs. Les nids désertés font des nœuds dans l'écheveau des branches. Les laboureurs ont atteint le bout de leur champ: avec des gestes lents, ils virent et repartent; ils montent vers Jean, et le cheval gris, dissimulant tout l'attelage, semble venir seul.

Le vent s'est tu. Les cahots de la charrette ont cessé. Les feuilles mortes reposent.

Du silence.

L'abbé revient, le front incliné.

Jean se lève et va vers lui. Le prêtre lui tend les mains; ses yeux sont pleins de larmes.

Ils redescendent la côte, sans mot dire. L'abbé marche droit devant lui, la tête basse.

JEAN (avec douceur). — Mon cher abbé, je vous ai fait de la peine. Mais tôt

ou tard, il fallait bien vous l'apprendre..
.

L'abbé fait un geste évasif et triste.

JEAN. — Je connais le reproche habituel des croyants: « Vous vous êtes débarrassé d'une religion qui entravait votre bon plaisir. » Ce n'est pas mon cas. J'ai lutté pendant des années; vous en avez été témoin... Il le fallait. Maintenant c'est fini. J'ai repris mon équilibre.

L'abbé tourne la tête et regarde Jean avec une insistance involontaire, comme s'il cherchait à voir l'homme nouveau qu'il est devenu.

L ABBÉ (avec désespoir). — Vous, que j'ai quitté si *droit,* en si *bon* chemin!..

JEAN. — Vous ne devez pas me mépriser. Croire ou ne pas croire, au fond, ce n'est pas ça qui importe: l'essentiel, c'est la façon dont on croit ou la façon dont on ne croit pas...

L'abbÉ. — Mais comment, comment est-ce arrivé?...

JEAN. — Je ne peux pas expliquer. J'ai eu la foi, c'est certain; maintenant, je ne peux plus m'imaginer cet état-là. Des idées qui passent comme des courants, et qui vous poussent tout naturellement dans le même sens... Et puis, ça dépend aussi des natures... Certains hommes sont, plus que d'autres, susceptibles d'accepter une formule toute faite; comme le bernard-l'ermite, vous savez, qui s'installe dans la première coquille vide qu'il rencontre, et qui s'y moule. D'autres, au contraire, ont besoin de sécréter eux-mêmes leur carapace...

L'abbÉ (sombre). — Ce sont *vos études* qui vous ont perdu... Le poison de l'orgueil scientifique! Ah, et combien d autres...! A force de s'absorber dans l'examen du monde *matériel,* on s'aveugle jusqu'à perdre le sens *surnaturel,* et bientôt la foi!

JEAN. — C'est possible. Quand on se sert quotidiennement des méthodes scientifiques, et qu'on a éprouvé mille fois combien elles sont propres à la recherche de la vérité, comment ne serait-on pas amené à les appliquer aux problèmes religieux?
(Tristement.) Est-ce ma faute, si la foi résiste mal à un sérieux examen critique?

L'abbÉ (vivement). — Ah, il ne sait plus comprendre qu'avec son intelligence! L'examen critique, *la raison* ! Est-ce que ce n'est pas *à l'aide de la raison* que les théologiens établissent les preuves de l'existence de Dieu et de la Révélation?

JEAN (à mi-voix). — C'est par elle aussi qu'on les renverse...

L'abbÉ. — Mais lorsqu'il m'est prouvé, à *mot,* que ma raison ne peut à elle seule, embrasser dans son entier le mystère des dogmes, ni toutes les choses de l'âme, ni la solution chrétienne du problème de nos destinées, j'y vois *au contraire,* une preuve irréfutable de l'Autorité supra-humaine qui nous a *révélé* la lumière!

Jean se tait.

L'abbÉ (prenant avantage de ce silence). — Et d'ailleurs, pouvez-vous me citer *une seule* vérité scientifique *certaine,* qui soit en opposition *réelle* avec un de nos dogmes?

Est-ce votre science qui vous a démontré qu'il n'y avait pas de Dieu?

JEAN (se décidant à répondre). — Pas absolument.

L'abbÉ. — Ah!

JEAN. — La scierke se cbhtente de prouver que tout, dans l'univers, se passe cbmrhe si votre Dieu personnel n'existait pas.

L'abbé. — Mais la science; mon pauvre ami, *uniquement* assujettie à l'étude des lois naturelles est) quand on *sait* voir, le plus éclatant témoignage de l'existence d'un Dieu!

JEAN (avec tristesse et fermeté). — Oh, pardon, pardon... ne rious payons pas de mots; De çe que je crois reconnaître un Ordre, des Lois, n'allez pas conclure que. je crois en Dieu: c'est un tour de passe-passe qu'on a trop employé! Non, non, nous sommes 1 un et 1 autre persuadés que l'univers obéit à des lois, soit ', — mais mon opinion, toute experimentale, n'est nullement compatible avec les données de la religion catholique, où Dieu est considéré comme un Être suprême, ayant une action persbnnelle, et des qualités précises! Ne confondons Jjas. Saris quoi là religion siérait èhcorè la science, tomme èlle

l'était jadis, à l'éveil de l'ihtèlligèhce humaine. (Souriant à demi.) Et ce n'est pas le cas...

L'abbÉ (avec feu). — Alors quand, *de bonne foi,* vous mettez votre raison en face du christianisme...
t,

JEÀN (vivcrheht). — Mon cher abbé, ndiis discuteribns ainsi jusqu'à l'aube, sans nous cohvamcrè.
(Souriant.) Je suis bien revenu de ces controverses iriterminablès..: Il y a entre un croyant et un athée, un abîme tel, qu'ils se combattraient toute une vie sans s'être compris. J'ai été souvent mis aii pied du mur par" des théologiens avertis et bien armés. Le plus souvent, je ne trouvais, je l'avoue, pas grand'chose à leur répondre. Mais cela n'ébranlait en rien ma éortvictioh. Je savais, avec certitude; qu'i'/ *i) avait une réponse,* et qu'il aurait suffi d'un hasard, d'urie association d'idées heureuse, otl d'une soirée de réflexion pour la trouver. — Des arguments? Mais on en trouve toujours» et pour toutes les causes, en cherchant un peu...

L'abbé fait un geste d'impuissance définitive; Jean sourit affectueusement, et s'approche de lui, jusqu'à lui prendre lé bras.

JEAN. — Voyez-vous, on ne se convertit pas pour des ràisons logiques: voilà là certitude à laquelle je suis arrivé. On se contente d'étayer, par dés arguments logiques, une conviction que l'on porte en soi: et cette conviction n'est pas motivée, comme on le croit, par des syllogismes et des raisonnements, mais par une disposition naturelle, plus forte que toutes les dialectiques.

Je crois que l'on naît prédisposé à la foi ou au doute; et que tous les raisonnements ne peuvent pas grand'chose, ni pour, ni contre.,.

L'abbé ne répond pas.

L'air a fraîchi tout à fait. Le soir tombe vite. Le soleil n'est plus qu'une ligne orangée, parmi les brumes violettes, au ras de l'horizon.

Devant eux, s'étend un blé naissant, d'un vert uni, à peine duveté par le brouillard qui se lève; et ur cette nappe soyeuse, se mêlent le reflet rosé du jour qui meurt, et l'éclat laiteux de la lune.

Ils pressent le pas.

Dans un chaume, des corbeaux s'élèvent, en rafale, pour s'abattre plus loin, sur des pommiers noirs.

Un long silence.

L'abbÉ. — Et... pour votre femme... que va-t-il arriver?

JEAN (simplement). — Ma femme? Mais il y a trois ans, au moins, que e pense tout ce que je vous ai dit ce soir.. ..Alors? Il n'y a aucune raison pour que ça change...

L'abbé hoche la tête, incrédule.

LA RUPTURE

I

Au Côllêgè Venceslas,

Huit heures du matin: l'heure de la classe.

Jêan monte allègrerrient sur l'estrade et s'installe

UN ÉLÈVE (s'approchant). — Pardon, Monsieur..! M. le Directeur ne vous a pas remis un cahier pour moi?

JLAN. — Neri, pourquoi?

L'ÉLÈVE. — M. le Directeur m'avait demandé mes notes, hier soir... Il devait me les rendre ce matin.

JEAN. — Quelles notes? Celles que vous prenez à mon cours?

L'ÉLÈVE. — Oui, Monsieur.

JEAN (le congédiant). — On ne m'a rien apporté.

Sur les bancs, un bouillonnement de cuve qui fermente. Il faut quelques minutes pour que les individualités, éparses depuis la veille, s'agglomèrent à nouveau. Les têtes se dressent et s'abaissent. Puis l'ordre renaît. Quelques pensées parasités semblent bien encore voleter par-ci par-là, à la surface. Mais le silence s'établit: la rtiasse est étale.

Jean, levant les yeux, heurte cifiquàhte regards convergents vers lui. I! se sent cloué à sa chaire pâr ce faisceau d'attentes braquées. Muette injonction, qui accélère les battements de son cœur et déclanche son élan.

JEAN. — Je vous demande aujourd'hui, Messieurs» une attention plus soutenue que jamais.

Il respire largement, enveloppe sa classe d'un coup d'œil de conquête, et poursuit.

Nous avons terminé l'autre jour, l'ensemble des leçons que je désirais consacrer à *Vorigine des espèces*. Je sais que vous avez compris l'importance de ce problème capital. Mais je ne puis me résoudre à clore ce chapitre de notre cours, sans un regard en arrière, sans une courte récapitulation des points qui me paraissent...

La porte s'ouvre; toute la classe est debout. Le Directeur entre.

Jean s'est levé, surpris.

M. l'abbé Miriel, directeur du Collège Venceslas: Un prêtre de soixante ans passés. Grande aisance d'allure, malgré son âge et sa forte charpente.

Un masque fin, quelque peu empâté. Le front dégarni et taché de rousseurs. Entre des paupières qui se lèvent et qui s'abaissent très vite, un regard pâle, d'une lucidité avertie et sans indulgence. Sur les lèvres minces, un sourire d'enfant, factice peut-être, mais d'un grand charme.

LE DIRECTEUR (aux jeunes gens). — Asseyez-vous, mes enfants.

Je vous prie de m'excuser, Monsieur Barois: j'avais oublié de rendre ce cahier à l'un de vos élèves... (Sourire bonhomme.) Et, ma foi, puisque je suis entré, l'envie me prend de ne pas m'en retourner sans tirer quelque profit de ma visite... Voulez-vous me permettre d'entendre un peu de votre leçon du jour? —...Non, non, ne vous dérangez pas. (Il avise un banc vide, en retrait. ) Je serai très bien là... (S'asseyant.) Et je vous en prie, que ma présence ne change rien à vos habitudes...

Jean a rougi, puis pâli.

La suspicion du procédé ne lui échappe pas. Il lutte, une seconde, contre la tentation d'atténuer le sens de la leçon préparée. Mais, bravement, avec un léger tremblement de défi dans la voix, il reprend son cours.

JEAN (se tournant vers le Directeur). — Je m'apprêtais, Monsieur le Directeur, à résumer les quelques leçons que nous avons employées à l'étude de l'origine des espèces. (L'abbé incline la tête, en signe d'assentiment.) (A ses élèves.) Je vous ai expliqué la place essentielle que Lamarck, et après lui, Darwin, doivent occuper dans cette science

des origines, qui ne s'est constituée qu'après eux, et toute entière de leur héritage; Lamarck surtout; et je crois vous avoir prouvé que sa théorie de l'évolution, ou mieux, du transformisme, — découverte plus générale et moins sujette à controverses que celle de la sélection naturelle, — doit être considérée comme une vérité scientifique *définitivement acquise.*

Il jette un regard vers le Directeur.

L'abbé écoute, les paupières baissées, ses deux mains blanches posées devant lui, impénétrable.

JEAN. — Nous avons vu en effet, qu'avant Lamarck, la science n'expliquait aucun des phénomènes de la vie. On avait dû supposer que toutes les espèces, aujourd'hui connues, avaient été créées successivement, et chacune en possession de tous ses caractères actuels. Lamarck a véritablement trouvé le fil d'Ariane du labyrinthe universel.

J'ai longuement développé devant vous, les raisons qui doivent aujourd'hui nous faire accepter avec certitude l'existence de cette filière indéterminée d'êtres, qui nous relie à la matière universelle. Depuis la monère initiale, à peine distincte des molécules du milieu organique dont elle était formée, — ancêtre informe de nos cellules, auprès de laquelle les plus simples expressions actuellement connues de la vie, sont des produits infiniment complexes, — jusqu'aux mécanismes les plus compliqués de la physiologie et de la psychologie humaine, à travers des milliers de siècles, la pensée de Lamarck a retrouvé et fixé l'échelle des êtres et leur progression ininterrompue.

Puis, — et ceci a un intérêt d'actualité — je vous ai mis en garde contre la prétendue crise que le transformisme aurait subi, depuis la découverte des variations brusques. Vous vous souvenez, qu'à des intervalles d'immobilité de l'espèce, peuvent succéder de brusques mutations, qui s'expliquent par l'accumulation d'efforts orientés dans le même sens, pendant des séries de générations. Je vous ai démontré que si l'on veut, de bonne foi, atteindre le fond de la question, cette théorie est en tous points conciliable avec la doctrine de Lamarck.

Une pause.

Depuis l'arrivée du Directeur, Jean a senti sa classe lui échapper. Sa parole frappe une trame distendue; et lui-même, à s'appuyer sur ce vide, perd peu à peu l'équilibre.

Alors, renonçant à récapituler ses leçons précédentes, il change résolument de sujet.

JKAN. — J'ai cru utile de procéder rapidement à cette revision.

Mais le but de notre leçon d'aujourd'hui est autre.

Dès les premiers mots, sa volonté qui s'exprime dans sa voix, ressaisit les mailles dénouées. La trame brusquement retendue, offre à nouveau aux mots qu'il jette son élasticité de raquette.

JEAN. — Je veux surtout graver dans vos mémoires, et 4 telle façon qu'elles n'en puissent jamais perdre l'empreinte, l'importance essentielle du transformisme; son utilité indispensable pour la formation des intelligences modernes; pourquoi il est, en quelque sorte, le noyau de toute la science biologique; et comment l'on doit reconnaître, sans dépasser les limites d'une scrupuleuse exactitude scientifique, que cette nouvelle façon d'envisager la vie universelle a pu modifier entièrement les bases de la philosophie contemporaine, et renouveler dans leur fond et dans leur forme, la plupart des concepts de l'esprit humain.

Entre Jean et sa classe, s'est rétabli un incessant échange de courants. Il la sent onduler et frémir à son commandement.

Le Directeur lève les yeux. Jean croise son regard qui n'exprime rien.

JEAN. — Du jour où nous avons compris l'activité ininterrompue de « ce qui est », nous ne pouvons plus concevoir la vie comme un principe, créateur de mouvement, qui viendrait animer une inertie. Lourde erreur, dont nous portons encore le poids sur nos épaules, et qui, dès 1 origine de la pensée, a faussé toute l'observation des phénomènes vivants! — La vie n'est pas un phénomène dont on puisse concevoir le dé-

but, puisque c'est un phénomène qui se poursuit sans discontinuer. Ce qui revient à dire: le monde *est;* il a toujours été, et i! ne peut pas ne plus être; *il n'a pu être créé:* l'inerte n'existe pas.

Du jour où nous avons compris qu'un être, à deux instants de sa courbe, ne peut en aucune façon être identique à lui-même, nous perdons de ce fait tous les points d'appui, que l'illusion individualiste des hommes avait échafaudés, pour soutenir la gageure du libre arbitre; et nous ne pouvons plus concevoir un être qui jouirait d'une liberté absolue.

Du jour où nous avons compris que notre faculté raisonnante n'est que l'apport, à travers les âges, des expériences ancestrales, apport transmis en nous sans contrôle par les lois multiples et capricieuses de l'hérédité, nous ne pouvons plus accorder la même créance aux notions absolues de l'ancienne métaphysique et de l'ancienne morale.

Car le transformisme, dont la loi domine tout, domine aussi l'évolution de la conscience humaine.

Et c'est pourquoi Le Dantec, l'un des esprits les plus avertis et les plus indépendants de la science contemporaine, a pu déclarer: « Pour un transformiste convaincu, la plupart des questions qui se posent naturellement à l'esprit humain, changent de sens: quelques-unes même, n'ont plus de sens du tout »

Le Directeur se lève d'un mouvement sec, malgré sa carrure. Il tourne vers la chaire son masque sévère, où les yeux sont à demi-clos.

LE PJRECTEUR. — Très intéressant, Monsieur Barois... Vous mettez à votre enseignement une louable chaleur, qui le rend très vivant... (Aigre sourire.) Nous en recauserons d'ailleurs... (Aux élèves, avec une bonhomie paternelle.) Ce qu'il faut retenir de tout cela, mes enfants, — et j'anticipe sans doute sur a conclusion que Monsieur Barois allait tirer de sa leçon, — c'est l'impeccable ordonnance du plan suprême... Notre pauvre raison n'approche qu'en tâtonnant de ces grandes lois; mais elle en reste confondue... Et cet acte d'humilité devant les merveilles du Créateur est d'autant plus nécessaire, que nous vivons en un siècle

où les progrès des découvertes scientifiques tendent trop à nous faire perdre le sentiment de notre petitesse et de la relativité de notre savoir... (Il s'incline avec une extrême réserve.) Je vous laisse, Monsieur Barois... Au revoir..

La porte est à peine refermée, qu'un remous houleux fait osciller l'âme mobile de la classe.

Jean, debout, rassemble d'un vif coup d'œil le fajsceau des regards qui s'éparpillaient.

Communion silencieuse et passionnée, qu'aucun blâme administratif ne pourra atteindre.

JEAN (simpjpmerçt). — Je continue.
,.

II

A Buis, chez Mme Pasquelin, pendant les grandes vacances.

Cécile est dans sa chambre, debout, en chemise, devant la fenêtre ouverte.

D'un geste inconscient elle caresse la courbe déformée de son 'ventre. Les traits, autrefois vifs, sont voilés d'indifférence: le regard lointain des femmes alourdies.

Neuf heures du matin: un ciel lisse, d'où coule un soleil jaune et fluide comme du miel.

On frappe à la porte, qui s'ouvre aussitôt

CÉCILE (rougissant comme une enfant). — C'est toi, maman?...

MADAME PASQUELIN. — Oui, c'est moi!

Au ton de sa mère, Cécile lève les sourcils avec angoisse.

Madame PASQUELIN. — Tiens, regarde! (Elle brandit une brochure blanche, et saisissant son face-à-main, elle épèle): « Bulletin du Congrès de la Libre-Pensée!... Monsieur Barois, chez Madame Pasquelin!... Buisla-Dame, Oise »...

(Un temps.) Où est-il?

CÉCILE. — Jean? Je ne sais pas.

MADAME PASQUELIN. — Tu ne l'as pas vu encore î

CÉCILE. — Non.

MADAME PASQUELIN. — Il n'est plus dans sa chambre

CÉCILE. — Il aura été faire sa promenade.

MADAME PASQUELIN. — Alors,

non seulement, vous avez chacun votre chambre, mais il ne vient même plus te dire bonjour, avant d'aller se promener?

Cécile s'assied; geste résigné et las.

MADAME PASQUELIN (jetant la brochure sur les genoux de Cécile). — Eh bien, tu lui remettras *ça,* toi, si tu veux... Et tu lui diras, de ma part, qu'il se fasse adresser *ça* ailleurs que chez moi...

D'ailleurs, je ne sais pas ce qui se passe... (Soulevant une enveloppe décachetée.) Je reçois ce matin un mot de l'abbé Miriel...

CÉCILE. — Le directeur de Jean?

MADAME PASQUELIN. — Il prend ses vacances en ce moment à l'évêché de Beauvais, chez son frère, « et serait heureux, si j'avais ces jours-ci l'occasion de l'y rencontrer. » Il désire me « faire uns communication personnelle »...

CÉCILE (inquiète). — Que peut-il vouloir te dire?

MADAME PASQUELIN (sombre). — Hé, je n'en sais rien, ma pauvre enfant Mais je vais y aller cet après-midi, je veux en avoir le cœur net.

Elle se pencjy brusquement, saisit le front de sa fille et y colle ses lèvres sèches, avec une petite aspiration bruyante qui ressemble à un sanglot. Puis, relevant un visage clos et courroucé elle quitte la pièce à pas sonnants.

Deux heures plus tard.
Cécile achève sa toilette.

JEAN (entrant). — Bonjour.

CÉCILE. — Tu as vu maman?

JEAN. — Non, je suis sorti de bonne heure

CÉCILE (désignant le bulletin). — Maman a monté ça pour toi.

La physionomie de Jean s'éveille.

JEAN. — Ah oui, je sais... Je l'attendais... Merci.

Il rompt la bande, s'assied sur le lit et feuillete les pages avec intérêt.

Cécile le suit d'un regard curieux et hostile.
Il surprend l'interrogation et ne s'y dérobe pas.

JEAN. — C'est le programme d'un congrès qui se tient à Londres cette année, en décembre...

CÉCILE (sur la défensive). — Mais..

. en quoi cela te concerne-t-il?

JEAN (tranchant). — Ça m'intéresse. (Mouvement de Cécile.) Et puis on m'a demandé d'en faire un rapport, pour une revue

CÉCILE (nettement). — Qui, on?

JEAN (brusque). — Breil-Zoeger.

CÉCILE. — J'en étais sûre!

JEAN (glacial). — Oh, ie t'en prie, Cécile-

Un silence.
Jean s'est remis à feuilleter le bulletin.

CÉCILE (avec désespoir). — Je ne veux pas que tu t'occupes de ça!

Jean, sans cesser de lire, grimace un mauvais sourire. JEAN — Comment dis-tu? Tu ne *veux* pas?...

Il met la brochure dans sa poche et s'avance vers elle.

JEAN (sans acrimonie). — Écoute, ma petite, laisse-moi tranquille avec cette histoire...

Ce congrès ne se tient que tous les dix ans... (Il se promène de long en large, sans la regarder.) C'est un mouvement international, dont tu ne peux pas soupçonner le retentissement. — De plus, les matières inscrites cette année au programme, m'intéressent personnellement beaucoup. Zœger m'avait proposé d'y prendre une part active, comme correspondant spécial de la *Revue internationale des Idées,* qui est, en France, l'organe de ce mouvement. J'ai failli accepter... (Mouvement de Cécile)...et puis, j'ai refusé à cause de mon cours à Venceslas. Mais, le moins que je veuille faire, c'est d'assister aux dernières séances, qui auront justement lieu pendant les vacances du jour de l'an, et de publier sur les conclusions du congrès, un rapport pour la section française. C'est convenu, il n'y a plus à y revenir.

Elle ne répond rien.

Il fait quelques pas en silence, et se décide enfin à lever les yeux vers elle.

Elle est écroulée comme un animal qu'on vient d'abattre. Ses prunelles dilatées s'emplissent d'angoisse, comme si elle allait s'évanouir.

Il s'élance, il la relève, il l'étend sur son lit.

Une pitié subite, poignante, impérieuse...

JEAN (avec une résignation morne).

— C'est bien, c'est bien.. Remetstoi... Je n'irai pas, c'est entendu...

Elle reste un instant immobile, les yeux clos. Puis elle leregarde, sourit simplement, et prend sa main. Mais il s'ecarte. Il s'approche de la fenêtre. Ah, elle est la plus forte! Avec cette souffrance vraie qui la ronge, et qu'elle étale, elle est invincible!

Il entrevoit tout ce que son renoncement lui fait perdre: l'occasion unique d'entendre résumer, combattre, défendre, passer au crible de la contradiction publique, cet ensemble d'idées, dont, depuis cinq ans, il cherche dans les ténèbres à se faire une doctrine vitale... Un immense écœurementPitié pour elle, soit: mais pitié pour lui!

JEAN (sans se retourner, d'une voix sourde et violente). — Vois-tu... Voilà pourquoi je ne serai jamais qu'un raté! Et ce n'est même pas ta faute, *tu ne peux pas jaire autrement...* Toutes les réalités les plus pressantes de ma vie, tu ne les aperçois pas, tu ne les soupçonneras jamais! Pour toi, ce seront toujours des manies inutiles, ou, ce qui est pis, honteuses, criminelles.. C'est ta nature, c'est comme ça que tu es vraiment toi!

L'atmosphère que tu crées autour de moi, j'y étouffe!... Tout mon courage, toute mon activité s'y dissolvent... Le seul bonheur que tu peux m'offrir, la petite affection dont tu es capable, ne pourront jamais que me nuire, me rapetisser à ta mesure! Voilà la vérité, l'atroce vérité... Du fait que tu es là, dans ma vie, elle est gâchée, quoi que je fasse 1... Et, quoi que je fasse, tu resteras là, dans ma vie, toujours! Tu briseras mes lueur, pour comprendre ce que tu es!... Toute ta vie tu pleureras sur tes petits chagrins à toi...

(Explosion.) Et moi, par ta faute, je suis foutu, — irrémédiablement foutu!

Elle n'a pas fait un mouvement.

Rien autre dans son regard qu'une douloureuse surprise...

Alors, il hausse les épaules. Et, la bouche sèche, les épaules lourdes, il quitte la chambre.
même pas, tu n'auras jamais une

III

« A M. l'Abbé Miriel Directeur du Collège Venceslas « Paris.

« 17 Août,

« Monsieur le Directeur,

« Vous me permettrez tout d'abord d'être surpris que vous ayez cherché un tiers pour me faire connaître votre opinion sur mon enseignement Sans insister davantage sur un procédé qui manque de courtoisie, pour ne pas dire plus, je veux tout de suite aborder avec vous les critiques que vous formulez à mon endroit. Je ne risque pas de m'égarer, puisque vous avez pris soin de résumer vos griefs en une note, dont j'ai obtenu communication, et qui se termine, si j'ai bien compris, par un ultimatum formel.

« Voici la quatrième année que je suis chargé par vous d'enseigner les sciences naturelles à des jeunes gens de dix-sept et de dix-huit ans. Je n'ai pas voulu me contenter d'un cours uniquement pratique, car il y a, pour le maître, une obligation supérieure à celle de préparer strictement les matières d'un examen: c'est de porter à un degré plus élevé l'éducation générale de ses élèves, et de donner des motifs d'exaltation à leurs personnalités naissantes.

« Je ne désavoue nullement l'orientation que j'ai cherché à donner à mes leçons.

« Si je me suis, en maints endroits, évadé hors des barrières que l'on a dressées, dans les établissements catholiques, autour des sciences naturelles, ce n'est donc pas par mégarde. J'estime qu'il n'y a pas d'autre arrêt pour la pensée que les limites mêmes de son élan, et que, pour ce vol, on ne prendra jamais trop d'essor.

« Votre blâme m'a donné l'occasion d'apercevoir qu'en matière d'enseignement scientifique, un homme sincère ne peut s'engager à professer selon certaines règles convenues. Un jour ou l'autre, en effet, il est amené à conclure; et ce jour-là, toute sa vie intellectuelle tend à s'exprimer: s'il a quelque dignité, comment apporterait-il, à ceux qui l'écoutent, autre chose que le résultat de ses propres réflexions, de sa propre expérience? Qu'on le veuille ou non, l'analyse scientifique des phénomènes de la vie mène droit à la philosophie. — C'est même, selon moi, la seule philosophie qui compte

« Or il faut, pour traiter ces questions avec l'ampleur qu'elles réclament, une liberté de pensée et d'expression qui, j'en conviens, n'est guère conciliable avec l'esprit de votre maison. Je suis donc prêt à reconnaître qu'à ce point de vue, j'ai outrepassé le mandat qui m'était confié.

« Mais, comme je ne saurais modifier l'esprit de mon cours, et que je tiens essentiellement à me présenter devant mes élèves, tel que je suis, en homme libre qui s'adresse à des intelligences libres, je ne vois pas d'autre solution que de vous donner ma démission.

« Veuillez agréer, Monsieur le Directeur, l'assurance de mes sentiments distingués.

Jean Barois. »

Cinq heures.

Au jardin.

Mme Pasquelin et Cécile cousent à l'ombre d'un parasol de toile, près de l'espalier qui borde l'enclos.

Assises sur des chaises voisines, elles parlent bas, sans mouvoir les lèvres.

Jean paraît au perron, sa lettre dépliée à la main. Il franchit, en approchant, comme la résistance d'une zone hostile.

Un silence l'accueille.

JEAN. — Je veux vous tenir au courant de ma réponse à l'abbé Miriel. Je lui envoie ma démission.

L'assurance de sa voix fait frissonner les deux femmes. Mais Mme Pasquelin, d'instinct plus combattif, dissimule d'abord son anxiété.

Madame PASQUELIN. — Ta démission? Tu plaisantes?

Cécile a laissé tomber son ouvrage sur ses genoux. Elle présente le front, lisse et bombé comme une cuirasse.

Depuis hier elle vit dans une stupeur désespérée. Le jugement du Directeur de Venceslas lui a fait prendre conscience de toute la réalité: elle s'inquiète peu de la situation compromise; elle ne pense qu'au salut éternel: Jean est un *athée* !...

JEAN. — Vous semblez surprises. Je me demande pourtant ce que vous pouviez prévoir? L'ultimatum...

MADAME PASQUELIN (avec vivacité). — Oh, il n'a jamais été question d'ultimatum. Tu dramatises tout!

L'abbé Miriel a été très peiné de ce que tu osais dire à tes élèves; mais il n'a jamais pensé à te congédier. Il ne le voudrait pas... ne fût-ce que par égard pour moi. Il exige seulement que tu fasses ton cours autrement; (souriant) tu avoueras qu'il sait mieux que toi ce que tu dois faire, puisqu'il est ton Directeur...

Jean détourne les yeux sans répondre.

Mme Pasquelin veut prendre avantage de ce silence. Et avec une bonhomie factice, elle cherche à pallier le débat.

MADAME PASQUELIN. — Allons, voyons, ne fais pas de sottises. Tu t'es monté la tête. Le Directeur lui-même n'attache pas à ces incartades plus d'importance qu'il ne faut; il est prêt à les oublier. (Son sourire feint est douloureux à voir.) Allons, ne t'entête pas... Déchire cette lettre, et va lui en écrire une autre...

JEAN (avec lassitude). — Ne discutons pas. Ma décision est prise.

MADAME PASQUELIN (violemment). — Tu ne peux pas faire ça! N'est-ce pas, Cécile?

JEAN. — C'est fait.

MADAME PASQUELIN. — Non. Je te défends d'envoyer cette lettre.

JEAN (perdant patience). — Mais enfin, si l'on vous demandait à l'une ou à l'autre, de renier vos croyances religieuses pour conserver un emploi, qu'est-ce que vous répondriez?

Madame Pasquelin (furieuse). — Comme si c'était la même chose!

JEAN. — Oui, je sais: Ce n'est pas « la même chose ». Eh.bien, vous vous trompez: c'est tellement la même chose, que je n'ai pas hésité une seconde! J'aurais même dû comprendre plus tôt que je n'étais pas à ma place dans ce collège de prêtres, et m'en aller de moi-même. Je regrette de m'être laissé aveugler si longtemps.

Mme Pasquelin reste perplexe. Le masque de Jean, son regard froncé, sa bouche volontaire, l'effraient. Elle maîtrisa sa colère.

MADAME PASQUELIN. — Jean, je t'en supplie... Si tu perds ce poste, qu'est-ce que tu feras?

JEAN. — Oh, soyez sans crainte; je ne manque ni de projets, ni de moyens de dépenser mon activité.

Madame PASQUELIN. — De beaux projets! Tu ne pourras que t'ancrer plus profondément dans tes mauvaises idées!

JEAN (saisissant l'occasion). — Certes! Maintenant que je suis libre (il soulève sa lettre,) je ne me plierai plus à toutes les concessions, à tous les compromis auxquels j'ai consenti jusqu'ici, et dont j'ai honte vis-à-vis de moi-même... C'était une transition, soit: mais le temps en est révolu,

Cécile, atteinte au vif, s'est redressée.

CÉCILE. — « Maintenant que tu es libre », Jean? Et moi?

JEAN (interloqué). — Toi? Eh bien?

Ils se toisent, heurtant deux regards où ne subsiste aucune trace des tendresses passées.

CECILE. — J'ai été trompée par toi! J'ai été trompée par ton passé, par tes paroles, par ton attitude! Ne l'oublie pas!

MADAME PASQUELIN (se jetant à la traverse). — Crois-tu qu'elle puisse tolérer que son mari soit un athée, un ennemi de notre religion? Mais c'est abominable!Élevé comme tu l'as été!

JEAN (répondant à Cécile seule, sur un ton angoissé et sombre). — Ce qui est fait est fait. Tu souffres? Moi aussi..

.

Je ne peux pas empêcher mes idées d'évoluer, d'être vivantes... Ce n'est pas moi qui dois les diriger, mais elles qui doivent diriger mai vie!

CÉCILE (durement). — Non. Tant que je serai là, non!

MADAME PASQUELIN (affermie par la résistance inattendue de sa fille). — Non! Elle te quitterait plutôt! N'est-ce pas, Cécile?

Cécile, oppressée, hésite une demi-seconde, puis fait un brusque signe d'assentiment.

Jean guettait sa réponse: il hausse les épaules.

Court silence.

Mme Pasquelin regarde Cécile avec un sentiment nouveau. Au fond obscur de son âme maternelle, il y a eu un bref éclair, un espoir, qui oriente malgré elle ses paroles.

Madame PASQUELIN. — C'est trop bête à la fin! Tu viens empoisonner notre vie, avec tes idées... Tes idées! Tout le monde en a, des idées! Tu n'as qu'à avoir celles de tout le monde! (Jouant le dernier atout.) Si tu ne renonces pas à cette lettre, si tu n'es pas décidé à reprendre l'existence d'autrefois, comme autrefois, Cécile ne rentrera pas à Paris avec toi!

JEAN. — Tu entends, Cécile?

Cécile est liée par son acquiescement,

CÉCILE. — Maman a raison.

JEAN. — Si je donne ma démission, tu ne rentreras pas à Paris avec moi?

CÉCILE. — Non.

JEAN (froidement, à sa belle-mère). — Vous voyez la belle besogne que vous faites.

Il saisit une chaise, l'approche de Cécile, et s y plante à califourchon.

JEAN. — Écoute Cécile, et pas de bêtises... Je te jure que je ne plaisante pas; (Longue aspiration.) Je pourrais te promettre des concessions nouvelles, pour sauver notre vie commune. Mais non, je veux continuer à agir loyalement. J'ai accepté pour toi le maximum des sacrifices que je peux faire il est impossible que je persiste dans cette voie sans perdre toute dignité, toute propreté morale! Ce que tu me demandes, c'est de jouer pendant toute ma vie une lugubre comédie: c'est de paraître, par une attitude passive, par une simulation continuelle, approuver une religion que je ne peux plus pratiquer. Il faut que tu comprennes une fois pour toutes, qu'il y a là quelque chose qui dépasse les convenances personnelles. Un honnête homme ne peut pas s'engager à exprimer toute sa vie le contraire de sa pensée: fût-ce par affection... Tu ne peux pas me faire un grief de cette loyauté morale, même si elle te fait souffrir!

Pause.

Veux-tu rentrer avec moi à Paris, en octobre, comme c'était convenu? CÉCILE (désespérément raidie). — Non.

JEAN (écartant de la main Mme Pasquelin). — Cécile: écoute-moi bien! (Un temps.) Si tu refuses de m'accompagner à Paris, si tu romps sciemment les seuls liens que je veuille encore ménager, alors, *rien ne me retiendra plus*... Et j'irai passer l'hiver à Londres, au congrès dont je t'ai parlé.

MADAME PASQUELIN (éclatant). — Mais tu veux donc la tuer! Dans la situation où elle..

Cécile s'est dressée et s'est rapprochée de sa mère

CÉCILE (sanglotant). — C'est tout réfléchi. J'aime mieux te perdre tout à fait que de vivre avec un païen!

Jean se lève.

Il les contemple toutes deux, frappé soudain de leur ressemblance... Ce front busqué, cet œil rond et noir, et ce regard contrarié, dont l'émotion accuse l'asymétrie, ce regard incertain, qui dans la discussion se dérobe...

jEAN (tristement). — Tu l'auras voulu, Cécile, tu 1 auras voulu... Réfléchis jusqu'à ce soir. En me laissant partir seul, tu lèveras tous mes scrupules: tu me rendras toute ma liberté. Je vais mettre ma lettre à la poste.

« A M. Breil-Zoeger « Directeur de la *Revue Internationale des Idées* "78, boulevard Saint-Germain

« Paris 20 Août.

« Cher ami,

« De grands changements sont survenus, en quelques jours, dans ma vie. J'ai donné ma démission de professeur à Venceslas, et je me trouve, à tous égards, beaucoup plus libre que je ne pouvais le prévoir. Je puis disposer à ma guise de mon hiver, et faire un long séjour à Londres. J'accepterais donc très volontiers la place active que tu m'avais primitivement réservée au Congrès, si cette place est encore sans titulaire.

« Je ne resterai pas dans l'Oise jusqu'à la fin des vacances, comme je te l'avais annoncé. Je rentre à Paris ce soir.

« Peux-tu me consacrer une matinée de cette semaine?

' Bien à toi,

J, Barois. »

A Londres.

Une chambre d'hôtel.

Le soir. Un plafonnier électrique verse une lumière impitoyable. Les rideaux tirés feutrent les bruits de la rue.

Breil-Zoeger est étendu sur son lit. Soulevé sur un coude, il concentre son regard sur une femme d'une cinquantaine d'années, assise à une petite table, et qui relit le compte-rendu sténographié de la séance du jour.

Jean va et vient, les bras croisés, — sous pression.

LA STÉNOGRAPHE (lisant). —...ce qu'en 1879, un Suisse, Vinet, écrivait déjà: « C'est de révolte en révolte que les sociétés se perfectionnent, que la civilisation s'établit, que la justice règne... Liberté de la presse, liberté de l'industrie, liberté du commerce, liberté de l'enseignement, toutes ces libertés, comme les pluies fécondes de l'été, arrivent sur les ailes de la tempête! »

JEAN (interrompant). —...Ici, quelques applaudissements; surtout les Suédois, les Danois, les Russes. Alors le président a pris la parole, il a résumé les débats...

Zoeger, les sourcils froncés, ponctue d'un signe d'assentiment chaque membre de phrase.

JEAN. —...Il a expliqué que.tu venais d'être subitement immobilisé par une crise héphatique; puis il a donné lecture du mot où tu me désignais pour parler demain à ta place, et la proposition a passé, à l'unanimité.

ZOEGER. — Woldsmuth t'a communiqué les chiffres exacts?

JEAN. — Oui. Et j'ai prévenu Backerston que je ne siégerais pas à la commission des réformes.

Zoeger approuve de la tête.

Breil-Zoeger: la trentaine.

Né à Nancy, de parents alsaciens. Mais, dans la coupe du visage, quelque chose de japonais, qu'accentue sa maladie de foie: un teint jaune, un masque élargi aux pommettes, des sourcils bridés, une moustache maigre et tombante, un menton pointu.

L'arcade sourcillière est très saillante: au fond des orbites, les prunelles, toujours dilatées, d'un noir luisant et dur, ont une expression fiévreuse, aiguë, aride, qui contraste avec la douceur générale des traits.

La voix est monotone, sans timbre, agréable au premier abord, — mais d'une implacable sécheresse.

ZOEGER. — Madame David, cherchez donc les notes que vous avez sténographiées ces jours-ci... Un dossier vert: «Problème religieux en France.»

— Merci.

JEAN. — Tu préfères que je dicte devant toi, comme ce matin?

ZOEGER. — Oui, ça vaut mieux.

JEAN. — J'ai préparé la deuxième et la troisième partie, mais en intervertissant l'ordre de ton plan. Je t'expliquerai...

Breil-Zoeger s'allonge avec une grimace de souffrance,

JEAN. — Tu souffres?

ZOEGER. — Par intermittences... ,

Quelques instants de silence.

JEAN (tirant des papiers de sa poche). — Nous en étions à la seconde partie:

« Causes De L'Ébranlement GÉnÉral De La Foi ». Vous y êtes. Madame David?

(A Zoeger.) Première cause: l'extension qu'ont prise depuis cinquante ans *les études des sciences naturelles.* A mesure que l'effort humain restreint le nombre des ignorances, dont l'homme, depuis des siècles, avait constitué sa croyance en Dieu, cette part divine se réduit inévitablement...

ZOEGER. — Tu pourrais rappeler brièvement...

JEAN. — Notez, Madame...

ZOEGER. —...quelques données scientifiques qui permettent de démontrer, dès maintenant, l'impuissance de leur Dieu sur le cours inéluctable des phénomènes, et par suite l'impossibilité du miracle, l'inefficacité des prières, et cœtera...

JEAN. — Si tu veux...

Seconde cause: *Les travaux historiques.*

ZOEGER. — Passe rapidement..

JEAN. — Non, c'est un point très important. Je tiens à rappeler le grand pas qui s'est trouvé fait, le jour où l'on a pu, textes en mains, décomposer la formation des légendes, et montrer que, dans cette formation, il n'est entré que des éléments humains, groupés autour d'un fait très simple, mais que la naïveté populaire a enveloppé de merveilleux.

Pour placer ensuite cette idée: Comment peut-on « croire », quand on a suivi d'âge en âge l'histoire des religions, et aperçu les diverses crédulités, toutes intransigeantes, par lesquelles le pauvre

cerveau des hommes a déjà passé?

ZOEGER. — Bien,

JEAN. — Puis une transition: le progrès scientifique ne peut atteindre que les intelligences cultivées; il n'aurait pas suffi, pour ébranler une religion qui a tant de racines dans les cœurs français.

Et j'en arrive... (On frappe.)...aux facteurs économiques et sociaux...
(Allant ouvrir.) Qu'est-ce que c'est?

UNE VOIX. — Le *Times*... Demander des renseignements sur l'indisposition de M. Breil-Zoeger... Sur le discours de demain...

JEAN. — Adressez-vous au 29, le secrétaire-adjoint. Monsieur Woldsmuth. (Revenant vers le lit.) Où en étais-je? Ah, troisième cause: *Facteurs économiques et sociaux.* Le développement prodigieux des industries a fait sortir des campagnes des milliers de jeunes hommes, qui rompent ainsi, brutalement, les liens familiaux traditionnels...

ZOEGER. — Insiste; c'est capital, si l'on songe au nombre considérable d'usines qui fonctionnent dans un pays civilisé, — nombre qui doit fatalement s'accroître encore, et dans des proportions incalculables.

Il feuillète son dossier, en tire une fiche, et change de position, avec une contraction douloureuse.

ZOEGER (lisant). — « L'ouvrier industriel est, par fonction, rationaliste. Jeté dans un grand centre d'action, où les spéculations métaphysiques n'ont plus leur place; vivant au milieu de machines, dont les ronflements célèbrent le triomphe du travail, de l'intelligence, des mathématiques, sur la nature... » (Tendant la feuille.) Tiens, si ça peut te servir..

Continue.

JEAN. — C'est là que je veux placer le tableau, dont je t'ai parlé: La nation française, actuellement divisée en deux camps bien tranchés: d'un côté, les incrédules; de l'autre, les croyants.

Les *incrédules,* qui comprennent tout le prolétariat, déjà cité, et tous les intellectuels. Majorité numérique incontestable. Puis...

ZOEGER. — Ajoute donc, parmi les incrédules, les demi-instruits, les « Homais »; il y a là une réhabilitation à ébaucher... Il est vraiment trop facile de les ridiculiser, ces malheureux, parce qu'ils n'ont pas eu le loisir d'appuyer sur des études véritables leur crédulité instinctive, et que pourtant, par leur simple bon-sens, par le seul équilibre de leur santé morale, ils sont irrésistiblement poussés vers les solutions moins confuses de la science.

JEAN. — Oui, très juste.'

Quant aux *croyants,* ils sont naturellement recrutés parmi les deux classes conservatrices: paysans et bourgeois. Les paysans vivent loin des villes, dans un cadre immuable où les traditions se perpétuent toutes seules. Les bourgeois, eux, sont en réaction systématique contre toute évolution; ils sont intéressés à la conservation intégrale de l'ordre établi, et particulièrement attachés à l'Eglise catholique, qui musèle depuis des siècles les appétits des déshérités; de plus, ils ont l'habitude d'expliquer la vie par des formules toutes faites, et leur bien-être serait compromis s'ils y laissaient pénétrer le doute...

SflMais, entre ces deux camps distincts, oscille un nombre considérable *d'indécis,* écartelés entre les exigences de leur logique... (On frappe. Avec impatience.) Entrez!

UN DOMESTIQUE. — Here is the mail, Sir...

JEAN. — Mettez ça là, je vous prie.

Le domestique dépose le courrier et sort.

JEAN (reprenant ses allées et venues). —... Les indécis... écartelés entre les exigences de leur logique et certains besoins mystiques qu'ils ont hérité. C'est eux qui donnent à la crise religieuse de la France contemporaine son caractère trouble... et douloureux... trouble... douloureux...

Son regard, brusquement, est tombé sur la pile de journaux et de lettres écroulée sur la table: il a reconnu l'écriture de Mme Pasquelin.

JEAN. — Tu permets?...

Il décacheté: t.'. J

« Buis-la-Dame, 14 janvier.

« Mon cher Jean,

« Cécile est accouchée hier d'une fille... »

Il s'arrête. Ses yeux se brouillent; le passé lui saute au visage...

«...Elle me prie de t'en avertir. Elle me charge de te dire que si tu veux voir ta fille, tu peux venir. J'ajoute que ma maison t'est ouverte, comme par le passé, pour tout le temps que tu jugeras bon. Peut-être as-tu compris déjà que tu t'es engagé sur une fausse route, et songes-tu à réparer un peu le mal que tu nous fais, à Cécile et à moi? Tu nous trouveras dans l'état d'esprit où tu nous as laissées: prêtes à tout oublier, le jour où tu reconnaîtras ton égarement.

« M. Pasquelin »!

ZOEGER. — Un ennui?

JEAN. — Non, non...

Voyons, je continue, où en étais-je?... (Sa voix se troue. Il fait un violent appel à son énergie.) Voulez-vous relire, Madame?

MADAME DAVID. — «...un nombre considérable *d'indécis,* écartelés entre les exigences de leur logique et certains besoins mystiques, qu'ils ont hérités. C'est eux qui donnent à la crise religieuse de la France... »

Mais Jean, assis sur le coin d'une malle, n'entend qu'un bourdonnement confus.

La gare de Buis-la-Dame.

Jean descend du train. Personne n'est venu l'attendre.

Seul dans l'omnibus aux vitres branlantes, il fait lentement l'ascension de la ville. Il regarde, le cœur serré. Des rues. Des enseignes connues. Rien n'a changé. La ville émerge d'un nuage que trois mois d'absence ont épaissi: elle émerge comme un souvenir de sa petite enfance...

Il croise frileusement son gros pardessus de voyage, qui garde le goût salé de la traversée.

La maison est fermée.

Une bonne, qu'il ne connaît pas, entr'ouvre la porte. Il se glisse comme un voleur.

Dans l'escalier, il s'arrête, la main crispée sur la rampe, frappé au vif par les cris d'un nouveau-né.

Il se raidit, il atteint le palier.

Une porte s'ouvre.

Madame Pasquelin. — Ah, c'est toi...? Entre.

Cécile est couchée. L'enfant n'est pas dans la chambre. Il y a un grand feu bruyant dans la cheminée.

Mme Pasquelin referme la porte.

Jean s'avance vers le lit.

JEAN. — Bonjour, Cécile.

Elle répond par un sourire embarrassé. Il se penche, l'embrasse au front.

JEAN. — La petite... va bien?

CÉCILE. — Oui.

Mme Pasquelin est debout, Jean sent la dureté de ce regard posé sur lui.

3EAN. — Quand est-ce que...?

CÉCILE. — Lundi soir.

JEAN (comptant sur ses doigts). — Il y a six jours. (Un temps.) J'ai reçu la lettre jeudi. On avait besoin de moi...Je suis parti aussitôt que j'ai pu...

Un silence.

JEAN. — Tu as beaucoup souffert?

CÉCILE. — Ah, oui...

Autre silence.

MADAME PASQUELIN (brusque). — Est-ce que tu dînes ici ce soir?

JEAN. Mais... oui... je pensais...

MADAME PASQUELIN (imperceptible nuance de satisfaction).— Tu restes quelques jours?

JEAN. — Si vous voulez.

MADAME PASQUELIN. — Bien.

Elle sort donner des ordres.

Ils restent seuls. Une gêne angoissée.

Leurs yeux se croisent. Jean se courbe à nouveau, l'embrasse tendrement, tristement. Cécile fond en larmes.

JEAN (à mi-voix). — Je resterai ici le temps que tu voudras... Jusqu'à ce que tu sois relevée... Et puis...

Il s'arrête. Il ne sait pas lui-même ce qu'il doit proposer.

Un silence.

CÉCILE (très bas, avec désespoir). — Tu n'as même pas demandé à embrasser ta fille I

Mais Mme Pasquelin rentre, la petite dans les bras. MADAME PASQUELIN (à Cécile). — Nous oublions l'heure, avec tout ça!

Jean, qui s'avançait, reçoit le « tout ça » au visage.

Il sait qu'il doit se pencher, embrasser son enfant. Il ne le peut pas... Moitié par respect humain, devant sa belle-mère; moitié par une sorte de répugnance physique, invincible.

Avec une fausse désinvolture, il caresse, du doigt, la joue môTIe, le menton rouge enfoui dans la bavette mouillée.

JEAN. — Elle est très gentille... *(y í V'- W4*

Il s'est reculé.

Une question l'obsède: le prénom qu'ils vont donner à son enfant. Il ne songe pas que la déclaration légale est faite.

JEAN. — Comment s'appellera-t-elle?

MADAME PASQUELIN (d'un ton péremptoire). — Elle s'appelle Marie.

JEAN (comme s'il avait un effort à faire pour graver ce nom dans sa mémoire). — Marie...

Il regarde de loin ce sein gonflé qu'il ne connaît pas, où les doigts minuscules sont crispés en possesseurs. Il regarde ce petit être de chair, qui se hâte, avide de vivre. Il regarde Cécile, et ce visage nouveau, pâle, un peu engraissé, rajeuni: son visage d'autrefois...

Puis, à un geste qu'elle fait pour soutenir l'enfant, il aperçoit à sa main, la bague... Ils étaient fiancés; il arrivait de Paris, l'écrin dans la poche; il avait trouvé Cécile seule; et il s'était agenouillé de tout son être devant elle, pour lui mettre au doigt cette bague, l'anneau, la chaîne...

Tout un passé de jeunesse, de tendresse... Ah, ce désir sincère et fou qu'il avait, de donner et de prendre le bonheur!...

Il soulève un suaire: il viole l'ensevelissement des deux qu'ils ont été.

Il se sent autre. Elle aussi... Tous les deux, si différents!

Et que faire?

VI

Vingt jours plus tard.
La chambre de Cécile

CÉCILE. —... Je ne céderai pas.

JEAN. — Céci.e!

CÉcile. — Non!

JEAN. — Tu es sous l'influence de ta mère. Rentrons à Paris, seuls, le plus tôt possible, et je suis sûr...

CÉCILE. —Je ne partirai pas avant que le baptême ait eu lieu.

JEAN. — Soit.

CÉCILE. — Et que tu y aies assisté!

Un silence.

JEAN. — Je t'ai dit: non.

CÉCILE. — Alors, tu peux partir seul.

Autre silence.

Cécile s'approche de la fenêtre, soulève le rideau, et reste immobile, le dos tourné, le front à la vitre.

JEAN (avec lassitude). — Ecoute... Des discussions, nous en avons tous les jours... Scènes muettes, allusions blessantes, crises de larmes... Je suis à bout. .. Une de plus, pourquoi faire?.;. '.. -i-

Cécile ne bouge pas.

JEAN (d'une voix qu'il contraint au calme). — Il faut éviter l'irréparable... Je te répète que je suis prêt à reprendre la vie commune, notre vie d'autrefois. Je suis prêt à faire beaucoup de concessions.

CÉCILE (se retournant). — Tu mens. Tu les refuses toutes.

JEAN (tristement). — Comme tu es montée, Cécile...

Nouvelle pause.

JEAN. — Tu sais très bien, au contraire, que je suis prêt à faire des concessions pour sortir de la situation rjpus sommes. Et en voici la preuve: si j'étais seul et libre, je soirs"irirais'entièrement cette petite à l'Influence de la religion; je l'élèverai de telle façon qu'elle 'rie se trouve pas, un jour, acculée aux atroces débats de conscience par lesquels j'ai passé...

CÉCILE (frémissante). — Tais-toi, tu me fais horreur!

JEAN — Je te dis: voilà ce que je ferais, — si j'étais seul.

Mais nous sommes deux, c'est notre enfant; tu as sur elle les mêmes droits que moi, je ne l'oublie pas. Je te laisserai donc libre de lui donner la. foi que tu possèdes toi-même. Seulement je me refuse à t'y aider, par une attitude hypocrite. Cela me parait plus que légitime...

CÉCILE (farouche). — Non, non, non! C'est *ma* fille, toi tu n'as aucun, aucun droit sur elle! Je ne t'en reconnais aucun! Tu les as tous perdus maintenant; c'est comme si elle avait un père infirme, ou dans un asile...

JEAN (découragé). — Cécile... Sommes-nous vraiment si loin, si définitivement loin l'un de l'autre?

CÉCILE. — Ah, oui, nous sommes loin!Et je suis lasse de lutter... Toute notre vie, ce sera la même chose... Aujourd'hui le baptême, demain le catéchisme, après-demain la première communion... J'aurai à la défendre contre toi, chaque jour, chaque minute... La défendre contre ton exemple, contre le scandale de ta vie... Non, non, je n'ai plus qu'un devoir, moi, c'est de sauver ma fille, de la sauver de toi!

JEAN — Mais que voudrais-tu donc?

Cécile s'avance vers lui, les traits égarés.

CÉC LE. — Ce que je veux? Ah, je veux que tout ça finisse, que tout ça finisse, mon Dieu! Je ne te demande pas de redevenir ce que tu étais, je ne sais pas si tu en serais encore capable, je ne le crois pas... Mais je veux au moins que tu n'affiches pas publiquement ces épouvantables idées qui te sont venues! Je veux que tu assistes au baptême de ton enfant! Je veux que tu me promettes...

Elle éclate en larmes, fait quelques pas en chancelant et s'abat sur son priedieu, le visage enfoui dans ses bras.

CÉCILE (sanglotant). —...Que j'aie un mari, enfin, dont je n'aie pas honte. .. Que j'aie un mari, comme toutes les femmes... Que nous soyons un ménage comme les autres, enfin!...

JEAN. — Je réclame seulement pour moi la liberté que je te laisse,

CÉCILE (se relevant, hors d'elle). — Ça, jamais, jamais!

JEAN (après un silence). — Alors?

Elle ne répond pas.

JEAN. — Tu as voulu, en m'épousant, prendre de la vie plus que tu ne:; pouvais porter!

CÉCILE. — C'est toi qui m'as trompée! Tu m'as menti! A moi, tu n'as rien à reprocher: je suis telle que tu m'as choisie...

JEAN (haussant les épaules; d'une voix presque basse). — Est-ce que l'on peut être jamais assez certain de l'avenir de sa pensée, pour prendre, en ces matières, des engagements éternels...?

CÉCILE (qui a écouté avec épouvante). — Apostat!

Jean la considère sans rien dire. Il mesure l'abîme.

Quelques pas à travers la chambre.

Puis il s'arrête devant elle.

JEAN (décidé à %n finir). — Alors?

Cécile se tait, les mains crispées sur le front.

JEAN (glacial). — Alors?

CÉCILE (éclatant). — Va-t-en!Va-t-en! Un silence.

JEAN (d'une voix morne). — Ah, Cécile, ne me tente pas..

CKCILE (sanglotant). — Va-t-en!

JEAN. — Quoi, va-t-en?... Le divorce?

Cécile cesse de pleurer, écarte les doigts de son visage, et le considère avec effroi.

JIAN (les mains aux poches, avec un mauvais sourire). — Tu crois donc qu'il suffit de crier: « Va-t-en!... » Tu n'as pas l'air de te douter que, pour permettre à une femme de vivre à sa guise, et de garder son enfant, il faut un procès... il faut des jugements...

Il parle... Mais il a brusquement senti croître en lui, malgré lui, malgré les mots qu'il dit, une ivresse nouvelle, le goût démesuré d une liberté toute proche, un furieux appétit de vivre encore!

Il parle... Mais, au loin, devant lui, il aperçoit, et son regard ne s'en détache plus, il aperçoit au loin... la trouée lumineuse!

VII ″Etude de M″ Mougin, Notaire, « à Buis-la-Dame (Oise)

« 12 février.

« Monsieur, Je suis heureux de pouvoir vous apprendre, qu'après un dernier entretien avec Mad ame Barois et Madame Pasquelin, et devant la menace d'un procès en divorce que ces dames désirent éviter à tous prix, il a été accédé à toutes les exigences que vous m'aviez chargé de défendre, et convenu ce qui suit:

« 1 Vous reprenez toute votre indépendance. Madame Barois n'a pas l'intention d'habiter Paris, et se fixera à Buis auprès de sa Mère.

« 2 Madame Bai ois s'occupera en toute liberté de l'éducation de sa fille; à cette seule condition, exigée par vous, que vous serez autorisé à reprendre votre fille chez vous, pendant une année complète, lorsque celleci aura atteint sa dix-huitième année.

« 3 Madame Barois s'engagea ne pas refuser la rente de 12.000 francs que vous la contraigniez à accepter annuellement. Elle est bien résolue d'ailleurs à ne rien distraire de cette somme, ni pour elle-même ni pour l'entretien de sa fille, mais à la totaliser sur la tête de l'enfant.

« Cette dernière clause a donné lieu à un long débat. Madame Barois n'y a souscrit que pour éviter le procès, et sur mon affirmation formelle que c'était pour vous une condition dirimante. Ces dames désiraient tout au moins réserver leur acceptation, afin que je puisse vous avertir de la diminution exacte causée par cet abandon à vos propres revenus (réduits à environ 5.000 francs). J'ai dû, pour éviter une nouvelle perte de temps que je savais inutile, leur avouer que j'avais cru devoir attirer votre attention sur ce point, et que vous n'aviez pas consenti à modifier vos dispositions.

« Sur la demande de Madame Barois je lui ai remis une note écrite, relative à ces divers engagements.

« Je pense m'être ainsi acquitté, selon vos desiderata, de la mission que vous m'aviez confiée. Je reste tout dévoué à vos ordres, et vous prie de recevoir mes salutations empressées.

MOUGIN. »

DEUXIÈME PARTIE LE SEMEUR

I

« A M L. Breil-Zoeger,

« Hôtel des Pins, Arcachon.

« Paris, 20 mai 189S.

« Cher Ami,

« Je te remercie tardivement de ta sympathie, au cours des récents événements. Je n'ai guère eu de loisirs: il faut avoir rompu les mille liens qui amarrent une vie au monde extérieur et à son passé, — si simple que semble cette vie, — pour imaginer la ténacité de ces fils, leur multiplicité mouvante et insaisissable. J'ai employé à cette dernière lutte deux grands mois, j'y ai mis un acharnement désespéré, j'ai brisé toutes les chaînes: me voici libre!

« Tu ne peux savoir ce que j'éprouve à pousser ce cri de triomphe, toi dont la vie rétive n'a jamais supporté d'entrave. ″Iaca-« Libre!

« J'atteins cet affranchissement en pleine jeunesse encore, en plein courage, après un long apprentissage de la servitude, après deux années pendant lesquelles j'ai obscurément et patiemment désiré cette liberté. Elle se donne à moi, enfin, sans restrictions, je l'étreins, je la possède, je m'initie passionnément à elle, je me rive à elle pour toujours!

« Je me suis terré, seul, sans laisser d'adresse. Depuis des semaines je n'ai pas vu une figure d'autrefois, ni entendu le son d'une voix qui m'ait rappelé le passé!

« Et tout me pénètre à la fois... Un printemps merveilleux emplit ma chambre, m'entoure de soleil, d'effluves de sève, de beauté! Jamais je n'ai ressenti rien de pareil...

« Ne, jn'ecris pas, cher ami, laisse-moi m'enivrer de solitude jusqu'à l'automne. Mais ne doute pas de ma fidèle amitié.

Jean Barois. »

Novembre.

Rue Jacob: vieille maison, porte étroite.

— M. Barois?

— Au quatrième. Vous verrez sa carte.

Un escalier branlant, parcimonieusement éclairé. Au quatrième, trois portes pareilles; un seul paillasson.

Harbaroux furète dans l'ombre des chambranles; ses yeux perçants déchiffrent:

JEAN BAROIS
DOCTEUR EN MÉDECINE ET AGREGE ES-SCIENCES
PROFESSEUR AU COLLÈGE VENCESLAS
80, BOULEVARD MALESHERBES.
(Les deux dernières lignes barrées au crayon.)

Il sonne.

Barois. — Tu es le premier!Entre...

Jean Barois: trente-deux ans.

La plénitude robuste de la jeunesse.

En moins d'un an, la physionomie s'est modifiée: un souci l'habitait; elle resplendit maintenant comme un ciel éclairci. De l'énergie en rayonne librement, et de la joie: affranchissement, certitude, confiance passionnée en l'avenir.

Une pièce claire et froide. Aux murs, des planches de sapin, portant des livres. L'éclat cru d'une lampe à gaz, dans un globe. Des fauteuils de rotin.

Sur la cheminée, un moulage, seul: l'« Esclave enchaîné», de Michel-Ange, étirant hors de la matière son corps douloureux, aux épaules rebelles.

Au fond, une porte basse, ouverte sur une chambrette où pendent des vêtements.

HARBAROUX. — Je n'étais pas encore venu chez toi.

BAROIS. —wPendant six mois, j'ai vécu comme un ours...

Harbaroux considère les sièges disposés en rond, et grimace un sourire.

Harbaroux: un gnome malingre.

La figure, sans âge, est d'une laideur, mais d'une intelligence sataniques. Un visage étroit, s'élargissant aux tempes, puis s'effilant en lame jusqu'à la pointe d'une barbiche rouss5tre. Des oreilles dressées de faune. La fente des paupières, la bouche, sont comme des trous, brutalement creusés avec une spatule dans de la cire à modeler. Regard aigu, tenace, sans douceur.

Bibliothécaire à l'Arsenal. Travailleur acharné. S'est d'abord spécialisé dans le droit du Moyen Age. Puis s'est consacré à l'histoire de la Révolution.

HARBAROUX. — Je voulais te voir seul... Ne penses-tu pas qu'il y aurait intérêt à préciser d'avance, ensemble, les sujets que nous aurons à aborder ce soir avec les autres?

Barois (après réflexion). —. Non, au contraire.

HARBAROUX (dont le masque se contracte et se détend comme un ressort)— Ah!Pourtant..

BAROIS. — Une réunion comme celle de ce soir est, par nature, préparatoire. Ce n'est pas son efficacité pratique qui importe

Harbaroux. — Alors?

BAROIS. — Ce qui importe, selon moi, c'est que dès aujourd'hui il s'établisse, entre ces diverses énergies que nous venons grouper ici, un courant spontané... Comment dire? Que nous sentions, du seul fait de notre réunion, se dégager un élan commun.

HARBAROUX. — Ça ne dépend pas de notre volonté.

BAROIS (vivement). — Non: mais nous avons plus de chances de créer cette atmosphère, en laissant nos rapports s'établir librement, en nous abandonnant à nos impulsions, sans orientation préconçue. (Sourire confiant.) Laisse faire...

Barois parle posément, en achevant ses phrases, comme un homme habitué à prendre la parole en public. Sans qu'il élève la voix, la fermeté du ton maîtrise l'attention.

HARBAROUX (haussant les épaules). — Des bavardages exaltés... Chacun suivant son idée... Chacun, à tour de rôle, infligeant aux autres sa conférence... Et tout à coup, il sera deux heures du matin!

Une soirée perdue...

Barois fait un geste: « Et quand ce serait »?...

Puis, sans répondre, il allume une cigarette, d'un geste rapide qui lui est devenu coutumier. Son regard dur, mais rêveur, suit un instant l'onde bleuâtre de la première bouffée dans l'air vierge de la pièce.

HARBAROUX. — Tu fumes donc maintenant?

BAROIS. — Oui.

Un temps.

HARBAROUX. — Soit, soit... Moi, j'aurais préféré prévoir, diviser In besogne... Je crois que la fondation d'une revue demande plus de...

:.i..) Un coup de sonnette.

BAROIS (se levant). — Dis-le donc.. .: de méthode?

Il va ouvrir.

Harbaroux, resté seul, soliloque en grimaçant.

UNE vOIx ÉRAILLÉE (dans le corridor). — Mon cher... Saisissant! Dans Lamennais, par hasard... Ne trouverez rien de mieux!...

Cresteil d'AHize paraît de dos, volubile et gesticulant. Pour entrer, il tourne sur lui-même, et clignote en recevant au visage la lumière crue du gaz.

François Cresteil d'AHize: vingt-huit ans.

Une taille élancée, prolongée par un cou maigre qui porte fièrement une tête petite, au crâne bombé par derrière.

Un visage court, triangulaire. Des traits tourmentés: le front large, coupé de rides; l'œil ardent et tendre; le nez provoquant; la moustache tombante, châtain foncé, cachant une bouche dédaigneuse, un sourire nerveux, désabusé.

Le parler haut, l'élégance désinvolte d'un officier de cavalerie; le geste enthousiaste, excessif.

U a quitté l'armée, assailli de doutes, écartelé entre son éducation et l'irrésistible besoin d'affranchir sa pensée; il s'est séparé des siens, rompant net la tradition catholique et royaliste des Àllize.

L'âpre rancune d'un récent évadé.

Il s'avance vers Harbaroux, prompt et souple, courbant sa haute taille, les mains chaleureusement offertes.

CRESTEIL. — Vous avez entendu, Harbaroux? J'ai trouvé ça, tout à l'heure, dans les « Paroles d'un croyant ».

Sans s'inquiéter de Barois, qui s'éclipse, appelé par un nouveau coup de sonnette, il plonge la main dans ses basques, et en extrait un volume débroché.

CRESTEIL (debout, déclamant de mémoire). — « Prêtez l'oreille! Et dites-moi d'où vient ce bruit confus, vague, étrange, que l'on entend de tous côtés! »

Breil-Zoeger, Woldsmuth, Roll et Barois, qui viennent d'entrer, s'arrêtent, collés au mur, surpris et amusés.

CRESTEiL (continuant, sans les voir).

« Posez la main sur la terre, et dites-moi pourquoi elle a tressailli?

« Quelque chose que nous ne savons pas se remue dans le monde.

« Est-ce que chacun n'est pas dans l'attente? Est-ce qu'il y a un cœur qui ne batte pas?

(Pathétique, le bras levé.) « Fils de l'homme! monte sur les hauteurs, et annonce ce que tu vois!»

Il aperçoit les nouveaux arrivants, et les enveloppe d'un regard illuminé qui les électrise.

CRESTEIL. — Je propose de graver ces lignes sous le titre de notre revue! Ce sera le plus beau et le plus concis des manifestes!

BAROIS (du fond de la pièce, frémissant). — Entendu!

Ils se regardent en souriant. L'ironie n'a pas de place ici, ce soir.

Quelques minutes d'expansion. Du premier coup, les cloisons étanches ont cédé: venus pour fusionner, le premier tressaillement de l'un d'eux les unit.

Zoeger s'avance au centre du groupe: son visage oriental est plus jaune que jamais. Une apparence de timidité: sourire indécis, geste gêné et court; — mais, au creux des orbites, dans l'ombre mordorée des paupières qu'il plisse comme on bande un arc, ses prunelles noires, mouvantes, fiévreuses, implacables.

ZOEGER. — Voyons, asseyons-nous. Procédons avec un peu d'ordre. Il manque?

BAROIS. — Portal.

Sourires sympathiques.

ZOEGER (sans indulgence). — Nous ne l'attendrons pas.

Il se trouve installé au bureau de Barois, comme s'il présidait.

Harbaroux s'est assis près de lui: il veut prendre des notes.

Cresteil, pour gesticuler plus à l'aise, demeure adossé à la bibliothèque, le front haut, les bras croisés, drapé dans sa redingote comme un demi-solde.

Roll, le typographe, s'est carré dans un fauteuil de jonc: il regarde, il écoute. Ses doigts, par contenance, tortillent sa moustache de jeune ouvrier parisien.

Woldsmuth, silencieux, les épaules basses, se tient à 1 écart dans l'encoignure de la cheminée, si menu qu'il semble assis.

Barois lui tend un siège. Lui-même se campe au milieu de la pièce, à califourchon sur un escabeau.

BAROIS (ouvrant une boîte sur le bureau). — Voilà des cigarettes... Nous y sommes? (Sourires.) Quand vous êtes arrivés, nous discutions, Harbaroux et moi, sur ceci: faut-il que notre première réunion soit simplement une prise de contact, libre et fraternelle... (Donnant la parole à Harbaroux.) Ou bien...

HARBAROUX. — Ou bien une première séance de travail utile, d'après un plan prémédité?

BAROIS. — Je crois que la bonne direction vient de nous être donnée par Cresteil.

CRESTEIL. — Par Lamennais...

BAROIS. — Nous ne voulons pas seulement fonder un groupement de travail; ce serait trop peu. Nous voulons, avant tout, n'est-ce pas? associer nos tempéraments. Il y faut de la spontanéité. (Cordial.) Nous voici entre nous, animés des mêmes désirs, guidés par la même conscience: que chacun apporte au foyer commun sa flamme personnelle...

Il hésite un instant, puis reprend:

Je continue, puisque j'ai commencé un véritable discours... D'où est venue l'idée première de ce groupement? (Il se tourne vers Breil-Zoeger.)

ZOEGER (vivement). — De toi.

BAROIS (souriant). — Non, nous en avons pris l'initiative ensemble...

Mais je voulais dire ceci: l'idée était dans l'air. Elle répond à une série de besoins particuliers, qui sont les mêmes pour nous tous. Les uns comme les autres, nous sentons que nous avons quelque chose à dire, que nous avons un rôle à tenir.

CRESTEIL (sombre). — Oui, le moment est venu de donner à notre vie intellectuelle un retentissement social!

Pas un sourire.

BAROIS. — Et pourtant, dès que nous cherchons à nous exprimer, à rendre le public témoin de notre effort, nous nous heurtons, comme de simples débutants, à des coteries établies, à des agglomérations de fonctionnaires littéraires, qui se sont fait un monopole de penser et d'écrire, qui ont accaparé jusqu'aux moindres porte-voix, et ne se les laissent plus arracher des lèvres! N'est-ce pas vrai?

ZOEGER.— Le seul remède: créer nous-mêmes notre organe d expansion.

HARBAROUX. — C'est un problème d'ordre économique: pouvoir écouler sa production, sans user son temps à des démarches...

BAROIS. —...qui échouent...

CRESTEIL. —... et à de fausses camaraderies, qui avilissent!

BAROIS (posément). — Nous n'avons plus vingt ans, nous venons de passer la trentaine. C'est très important.

L'ardeur qu'aujourd'hui nous mettons, d'abord à consolider, ensuite à imposer et à défendre nos idées, ce n'est plus un trop plein de jeunesse qui mousse et qui déborde: c est la flamme même, l'essence de nos sensibilités; c'est l'attitude résolue et définitive que nous avons prise dans la vie.

Tous approuvent gravement.

CRESTEIL (avec un grand geste du bras étendu). — Et quel merveilleux coup de fouet ce doit être, que de se sentir périodiquement lu, suivi, discuté!

ZOEGER (qui, d'instinct, résume). — Agir!

HARBAROUX (sourire machiavélique). — Seulement, en pratique, tout ça, c'est assez difficile...

BAROIS (acceptant le défi). — Non. En pratique, notre projet est réalisable. (Un silence. Fermement.) Nous disposons d'un capital...

ZOEGER (de sa voix douce et nette). — Tu disposes...

BAROIS. — Nous disposons d'un capital, assez mince il est vrai, mais que j'estime pourtant suffisant, grâce au désintéressement de notre camarade Roll... (Mouvement deRoll)... ou, s'il préfère, grâce au désintéressement de la « Société collectiviste d impression » qu'il dirige. De plus, notre collaboration est gratuite. Nous n'aurons en somme que des frais réduits: matière première et main-d'œuvre. Nous pouvons donc nous en tirer, et vivre le temps qu'il faut pour nous faire une place au soleil. Après il faudra la défendre; mais nous serons mieux outillés pour la lutte.

ZOEGER. — C'est donc cette année, au début, qu'il importe de donnei notre maximum.

BAROIS. — Parfaitement. Les différences de nos natures, malgré des tendances générales qui sont les mêmes... (Coup de sonnette. Il se lève.)...nous assurent cette variété qui est indispensable à la composition d une revue.

Il sort.

ZOEGER (sèchement, comme un verdict). — Nous devons réussir.

CRESTEIL (enthousiaste). — Le succès dépend de notre élan, de notre foi!...

HARBAROUX. — Dis plutôt: de la

persévérance de nos efforts.

ZOEGER (avec une raide inclinaison de tête). — La foi n'a jamais accompli de miracles, qu'en apparence. Mais la volonté, oui, chaque fois qu'elle s'affirme puissamment.

Portal, poussé par Barois, fait enfin son entrée, un cigare à la bouche, souriant avec bonhomie.

PORTAL. — Voilà, voilà... (Il serre des mains.) Déjà commencé? Pas possible, vous dînez à six heures, au Quartier, comme dans Balzac...

Pierre Portal: un gars d'Alsace, blond, poupard; des yeux bleu faïence, des yeux de « bonne nature ». La moustache en frange, soyeuse et couleur d'argent dédoré, virilise à peine un sourire de gosse.

Ami de toutes les femmes: teint clair, un peu fripé; regard chaud, insistant, et, par flambées, sourdement sensuel.

Quelque lourdeur: dans la démarche, dans le geste, dans la voix; dans la plaisanterie.

Des convictions ardenteb, mais sans violence, fondées sur le bon sens, sur une vue juste des droits et des devoirs.

Au Palais, secrétaire de Fauquet-Talon, avocat politique intègre et énergique, deux fois ministre.

BAROIS (présentant). — Portal... Notre ami Roll...

Roll salue d'un mouvement gauche.

Depuis qu'il s'est atsis, il n'a pas dit un mot. Il fixe alternativement celui qui parle. L'attitude, la physionomie, trahissent *b* l'effort d'une intelligence moyenne, tendue à la limite de ce qu'elle peut, et s'y cramponnant.

BAROIS (affectueusement). — Eh bien, Roll, que pensez-vous de nos projets?

*-A*

Il pâlit d'un coup, comme s'il avait été outragé. Puis il rougit, décroise les jambes, et se penche en avant, pour parler. Mais il ne dit rien... Et, brusquement, il se décide.

ROLL. — A l'atelier, on en voit des revues! Tous les ans, des nouvelles! Mais pas encore comme la vôtre.

CRESTEIL. — Tant mieux.

ROLL (hésitant). — Des revues pour des amateurs, des revues qui ne

s'occupent d'aucun problème...(Sur un ton indéfinissable:) Des *dilettantes...* Il manque une revue qui soit au courant du grand mouvement social... (Une pause, puis un geste mass '.) Enfin, quoi, des hommes qui comprennent c qui s' prépare...

Cresteil, déclamatoire et farouche, fait un pas en avant.

Cresteil. — « Quelque chose que nous ne savons pas, se remue dans le monde! »

Barois. — « Fils de l'homme, monte sur les hauteurs! »...

Cresteil, Barois, Roll (ensemble). — .« et annonce ce que tu vois! »

Ils se regardent: à peine un sourire de respect humain, qui voile une sincérité touchante.

ZOEGER (posément, sur un ton qui rappelle à l'ordre). — Il faut qu'avant six mois notre revue soit devenue l'alliée de tous les groupes isolés, s'occupant de philosophie positive ou de sociologie...

HARBAROUX (qui fume en grimaçant, la tête de biais, les yeux clignotants). —... de sociologie *pratique.*

BAROIS. — Naturellement.

PORTAL. —. Il y a plus d'efforts individuels qu'on ne croit...

ZOEGER. — Il s'agit de les centraliser.

PORTAL. —...Tous les organisateurs de ligues sociales, d'unions morales, d'universités populaires...

CRESTEIL. —...tous les croyants sans église...

WOLDSMUTH (timidement). —... les pacifistes...

BAROIS. — En un mot, tous les généreux. Voilà notre clientèle. (S'enflammant.) Il y a vraiment un grand rôle à jouer. Coordonner ces forces qui souvent se perdent, les canaliser dans la même direction. Un beau programme!

ZOEGER. — Nous devons le réaliser, simplement, par la diffusion de notre pensée.

BAROIS. — Et par l'exemple d'une sincérité absolue.

PORTAL (souriant). — Ça, c'est quelquefois dangereux...

BAROIS. — Oh que non! Je crois à la contagion de la franchise...

Examiner tous les problèmes, ouvertement.

Ainsi, pour ma part, je pense, avec les réactionnaires, que nous traversons une crise morale. Eh bien, je suis résolu à l'avouer tout de suite. Je suis prêt à reconnaître que la morale a chancelé. C'est un fait. Je l'ateribue, pour la masse, à l'anémie générale des croyances religieuses, — tt pour nous, à la défaveur, au discrédit des principes abstraits que jadis. nos professeurs de métaphysique nous offraient arbitrairement comme autant d'axiomes.

(A Zoeger.) Tu sais, ce que nous disions l'autre jour...

PORTAL. — Mais cet aveu n'a d'intérêt que si vous proposez un remède.

BAROIS. — Ça, c'est autre chose... Cependant on peut déjà proposer certains palliatifs.

ZOEGER. — Mieux que ça. On peut montrer que, dès maintenant, il n'est pas impossible de concevoir une direction morale positive.

PORTAL. — Basée sur?

ZOEGER. — Mais, d'une part, sur l'état actuel de la science, et, d'autre part, sur l'évidence, déjà bien établie, de certaines lois de la vie...

PORTAL. — Lois bien vagues encore, et d'une application éthique difficile!

ZOEGER (qui n'aime pas à être contredit). — Pardon, mon cher, pas si vagues. Nous les préciserons, en les classant: d'abord, conservation et développement de l'individu; ensuite, adaptation de l'individu à l'existence collective, qui lui est essentielle.

HARBAROUX (approuvant). — Double devoir, auquel il faut consentir...

ZOEGER. —...L'homme oscillant entre ces deux pôles, et trouvant dans ce va-et-vient, son équilibre moral.

BAROIS. — Oui, c'est là certainement qu'est le ralliement, l'unité morale de l'avenir...

Cresteil s'avance, le front hautain, les bras soulevés: un mouvement d'expansion, naturelle et charmante.

CRESTEIL. — Ah, mes amis, quand je vous entends parler comme ce soir, je me dis que si nous arrivons à faire comprendre, non seulement ce que nous *voulons,* mais surtout ce que nous *valons...*

Portal sourit.

...Oui, parfaitement: si nous faisons bien connaître la *qualité morale* de notre élan, nous attirerons infailliblement à nous, en auefaues mois, tous les chercheurs solitaires... tous ceux qui ont quelque chose là! (Il frappe son thorax osseux).

BAROIS (dont la flamme intérieure se traduit trop volontiers par un transport oratoire). — Et nous y arriverons, en exaltant la dignité de chacun! En contribuant à restituer leur sens plein à quelques mots français, comme *droiture* et *probité,* que nous avons laissé se décolorer dans le magasin des accessoires romantiques! En affirmant, dans tous les domaines, les droits de la pensée libre! *y*

Regards et sourires qui s'étreignent. Effusion générale.
Puis détente.

Barois emplit les verres de bière fraîche; l'aigreur fermentée se mêle à la fumée des cigarettes.

PORTAL (reposant son verre. Avec bonne humeur). — Et le titre?

BAROIS. — Mais il est décidé. Nous nous sommes rangés à la proposition de Cresteil: Le Semeur. (Souriant vers Cresteil.) L'image n'est peut-être pas très neuve...

Cresteil. — Merci.

Barois. — Mais elle est simple, et répond bien à notre attitude.

ZOEGER. — Est-ce que Barois vous a communiqué la pensée qu'il a eue pour le premier numéro?

BAROIS. — Non, pas encore. Un projet, qui, je l'avoue, me tient fort au cœur... J'espère que vous y souscrirez tous, comme Breil-Zoeger.

Voici: Je voudrais consacrer nos premières pages à la glorification de l'un de nos aînés...

Plusieurs VOIX. — Qui? Luce?

Barois. — Luce.

CRESTEIL. — Ah, parfait!

BAROIS. — Attendez. J'y verrais plusieurs avantages. D'abord, ce serait manifester, par un choix significatif, quel est notre point de vue, et auquel de

nos contemporains nous tendons délibérément la main. Puis, du même coup, nous affirmerions que nous ne sommes pas des démolisseurs systématiques ni des utopistes impuissants, puisque notre idéal a trouvé dans la réalité une sorte d'incarnation, puisqu'il en existe, à côté de nous, un vivant exemple.

PORTAL. — Je vous comprends. Mais n'aurons-nous pas l'air d'acheter pour nos débuts un patronage illustre?

CRESTEIL (vivement). — La personnalité de Luce est à l'abri de...

BAROIS. — Ecoutez, Portal, vraiment, si les mots désuets que j'employais tout à l'heure, droiture, propreté morale, dignité personnelle, ont jamus été applicables à quelqu'un, c'est bien à Luce! Et puis, il n'est pas question de lui demander un mot d'introduction auprès du public ni une signature à mettre en vedette. Il s'agit de lui rendre un hommage spontané et collectif. Je propose même qu'il ne soit averti de rien.

PORTAL. — C'est tout différent.

BAROIS. — Aucun de nous ne le connaît directement. Nous ne savons de lui que ses livres, ses actes, sa vie publique. De plus, c'est un isolé: en philosophie, il ne se rattache à aucun système; en politique, au Sénat, il n'a adopté aucun groupement. L'honneur que nous voulons lui faire, n'atteindra donc que lui seul, l'homme qu'il est.

N'oublions pas que nous lui devons tous une part importante de notre formation morale. J'ai pensé qu'au moment de nous jeter à notre tour dans la lutte, nous lui devions ce geste de gratitude. — Vous m'approuvez, Cresteil?

CRESTEIL (souriant à un souvenir). — Entièrement... Et j'ai bien envie de rappeler un détail personnel... C'est Luce, qui, à l'improviste, a présidé la distribution des prix, à la fin de ma rhétorique. Il y a une douzaine d années; il venait d'être nommé... je ne sais plus quoi...

BAROIS. — Suppléant au Collège de France, sans doute.

CRESTEIL. — Je le vois encore, sur l'estrade, au milieu des vieux professeurs, lui très jeune, à peine de quinze ans notre aîné... Un visage d'une ardeur,

et en même temps d'une gravité inoubliables. Il s'est mis à parler, très familièrement, sans élever la voix, i îîis avec une autorité extraordinaire. En quelques minutes, il a su prés nter en raccourci une vision si claire de l'homme, de la vie, de l'univers; et le sujet coïncidait si heureusement avec mes préoccupations du moment, que j'y ai trouvé, je crois bien, l'orientation de mon existence.

Deux mois après, j'entrais en philosophie, mis d'avance en garde contre le spiritualisme universitaire.

ZOEGER (ricanant). — Celui que Coulangheon appelait: « une espèce de folie des grandeurs... »

CRESTEIL. — J'étais sauvé...

Un silence.

BAROIS.:— Donc, c'est convenu. Notre premier fascicule débutera par jan « Hommage à Marc-Elie Luce », qui sera signé: *Le Semeur.*

HARBAROUX (à Roll). — Aurons-nous le premier numéro pour janvier?

ROLL. — Cinq semaines? Hum... Il faudra que j'aie vos articles avant le 10.

BAROIS. — Ce n'est pas impossible. .. Nous avons certainement tous quelque chose de prêt. (Se tournant vers Zoeger.) N'est-ce pas?

ZOEGER. — Moi, je n'ai pas rédigé, mais j'ai tous mes matériaux.

PORTAI.. — Sur?

Zoeger dévisage Portal; il hésite à répondre. Son œil froid passe la revue des physionomies, curieusement attentives. Alors il desserre les lèvres.

ZOEGER. — Voici.

Sa voix lente, privée d'accent, paraîtrait molle, sans une résonnance finale qui déconcerte, une sécheresse tranchante comme un couperet qui tombe.

ZOEGER. — Je crois qu'il est utile, pour un premier numéro, que nos études soient délibérément tendancieuses, qu'elles affirment nettement notre tour d'esprit..

Regard circulaire qui s'assure l'approbation de tous.

ZOEGER. — Pour moi, j'ai donc l'intention de donner un article qui prépare en quelque sorte les suivants. Je me contenterai de développer cette idée générale: que, — notre seul point de départ logique pour étudier l'homme étant le milieu vital où il évolue, — la philosophie moderne, la seule qui puisse renouveler le domaine philosophique, doit être biologique, doit être une philosophie à notre niveau, au plan que l'homme occupe dans la nature; qu'en outre, cette philosophie a l'avantage d'être à cycle ouvert, puisqu'elle émane spontanément de l'état actuel des sciences; et que, nourrissant ses raisonnements des seuls faits contrôlables, elle est nécessairement alimentée par le progrès scientifique, et amenée à se transformer avec lui.

PORTAL. — Voilà qui écartera tout de suite de notre revue les neuf dixièmes des métaphysiciens...

ZOEGER (incisif). — C'est ce qu'il faut.

HARBAROUX (saisissant l'occasion). — Ce serait une bonne chose que chacun de nous puisse ainsi donner, dès aujourd'hui, un aperçu de ses projets... Notre premier fascicule se trouverait à peu près constitué dès ce soir. Est-ce ton avis, Barois?

BAROIS (depuis un instant soucieux). — Mais oui.

HARBAROUX (spontanément). — Moi, j'ai une trentaine de pages sur le mouvement des Communes au XII siècle, et son analogie avec les troubles sociaux de ces cinquante dernières années.

Et vous, Cresteil?

Cresteil vient s'adosser à la cheminée, dans une pose un peu prétentieuse; mais dès qu'il parle, sa voix passionnée, son regard lumineux, ses gestes violents, forcent l'attention.

CRESTEIL. — Je voudrais reprendre la question de « l'art pour l'art »... Vous savez, à propos du récent manifeste de Tolstoï. Montrer qu'elle est généralement mal posée; revendiquer avant tout, pour l'artiste, le droit — le devoir — de ne se préoccuper de rien autre, lorsqu'il secrète, que de faire beau: car c'est l'émotion désintéressée qui crée. Mais je me hâterais de concilier les uns et les autres, en prouvant que l'utile est infailliblement la conséquence du mobile esthétique. L'artiste n'a pas à prévoir, en travaillant, ce qui pourra résulter *socialement* de son œuvre.

ZOEGER (très attentif). — Pas plus que le savant.

CRESTEIL, — Pas plus que le savant. Ils ont à atteindre, l'un la beauté, l'autre la vérité: deux faces d'un même but. Aux masses às'en accommoder ensuite... (De haut.)... à y conformer leurs petites combinaisons sociales...

ZOEGER. — C'est très juste.

BAROIS (à Cresteil). — Je pensais que vous vous réserviez la paraphrase de votre citation de Lamennais?

CRESTEIL (souriant). — Non, je vous la laisse.

BAROIS (gaîment). — Je l'accepte.

J'y pensais, tout en vous écoutant. Je crois qu'il y a quelque chose à en tirer: exposer pourquoi nous l'inscrivons ainsi en exergue, et en quoi elle exprime si bien le caractère essentiel de notre tentative.

CRESTEIL. — Ce serait bien en place dans un premier numéro.

BAROIS (dont le regard s'avive). — N'est-ce pas?

PORTAL. — Quelle citation?

Harbaroux (grincheux). — Vous n'étiez pas arrivé

PORTAL. — Expliquez-nous votre idée, Barois.

ZOEGER. — Oui, explique-toi.

BAROIS (souriant à sa propre pensée, à mesure qu'il l'exprime). — Je reprendrais mot à mot le texte: ynOVt

« Quelque chose que nous ne savons pas se remue dans le monde... »

Quel est ce frisson?JL'éternel mouvement de la pensée humaine, le progrès... — Vous voyez le développement...— La gestation d'une œuvre Infinie, à laquelle s'agglomèrent chacun de nos efforts, chacune de nos émotions réalisées... Et ce mouvement porte obscurément en lui toutes les solutions_ue nous cherchons, toutes ces vérités de demain, qui se Térobent encore à nos explorations, mais qui, à leur jour, comme Tombent les fruits mûrs, se dévoileront l'une après l'autre, devant l'interrogation humaine!

CRESTEIL.;— Oui, un hymne au progrès!

BAROIS (encouragé, se laissant définitivement aller à son improvisation). — Et je dirais encore ceci: Il en est,

parmi nous qui sont doués d'une sorte de prescience, qui distinguent déjà ce que d'autres n'aperçoivent pas encore. C'est à ceux-là que Lamennais crie:

« Fils de l'homme, monte sur les hauteurs et annonce ce que tu vois! »

Et je ferais un rapide tableau de notre vision de l'avenir... « Annonce ce que tu vois... »

Je vois: l'extension monstrueuse des puissances de l'argent; toutes les revendications les plus légitimes, écrasées et maintenues sous sa tyrannie...

Je vois: l'ébranlement de la masse laborieuse, dont le tumulte grandissant n'est que mal couvert par cette parade bruyante des partis politiques, qui, jusqu'ici, réussit seule à capter l'attention...

Je vois: la poussée régulière d'une majorité humaine, brutale, inculte, enivrée d'illu ions, affamée de sécurité et de bonheur matériel, contre une minorité aveugle, encore puissante par la force des choses établies, mais dont la stabilité relative ne repose, en fait, que sur le régime capitaliste. Donc: poussée générale contre l'état capitaliste, c'est-à-dire contre l'organisation sociale de tout le monde actuel, — car aujourd'hui il y a, en somme, unité de régime dans tous les pays civilisés; — poussée formidable, dont l'histoire n'enregistre pas de précédent, et qui ne peut pas ne pas être victorieuse, parce qu'elle est la force nouvelle, le jet même de la sève humaine, *l'élan actuel* contre un monde fatigué, étiolé par l'affinement!

ROLL (brusquement, la gorge serrée). — Bravo!

Sourires.

Barois s'est levé, grisé par le son et la cadence de ses paroles, surexcité par les regards qui le tiennent en vedette: les jambes écartées, le buste offert, le menton haut, son visage mâle frémissant d'activité, un joyeux défi dans les yeux, — il vibre...

Ivresse d'orateur, qui lui manquait depuis des mois.

BAROIS. — Enfin, après cette vue d'ensemble, il faudrait terminer par un coup d'œil sur les individus.

Que trouve-t-on en chacun de nous? Le désordre, l'incertitude.

L'amélioration matérielle a démesurément développé nos faiblesses, et jamais encore elles ne se sont épanouies avec un pouvoir si dissolvant. Une épouvante inavouée de l'inconnu, plane sur la plupart des êtres cultivés: un combat se livre en chacun d'eux: toutes les forces vives des âmes, se sont soulevées, consciemment ou non, contre la survivance des impératifs mythologiques... Combat multiple, plus ou moins obscur, mais universel, et qui rend intelligibles les excès du déséquilibre social... Combat onéreux surtout, parce qu'il aboutit, dans tous les domaines, à un sensible abaisse ment de la conscience individuelle et, finalement, à une déperdition inquiétante d'énergie!...

(Il s'arrête, passe rapidement en revue les visages rayonnants, et sourit.) Voilà.

Une seconde de vie intense... Et brusquement, sans raison apparente, comme un fil trop tendu, son enthousiasme casse net.

Il s'assied, souriant, gêné, très las.

Quelques instants silencieux.

Il débouche une cannette, emplit les verres, et vide le sien d'un trait.

Puis il se tourne vers Portal.

BAROIS (avec un entrain forcé)..— Et vous, Portal, avez-vous pensé à nous?

PORTAL (riant). — Ma foi, non! Faites votre premier numéro sans moi Je collaborerai au second.

Cresteil. — Lâcheur...

PORTAL. — Parole! Mon sujet n'est pas mûr, mais j'en ai un... (Sourires.) Vous ne me croyez pas?Tenez, voilà mon idée... Ce n'est pas exactement un article que je veux écrire... Des croquis, des notes,sur les types que je vois tous les jours, sur ceux que je connais bien, le Palais, les députés, les gens du monde... La moyenne, enfin...

CRESTEIL. — La sainte et irréductible moyenne!

PORTAL.— Oui; ceux qui sont « bien pensants », parce qu'ils ne peuvent pas être « pensants » tout court... Ces légions d'êtres, relativement instruits, policés par les usages comme des galets roulés... Ces êtres qui, pour la plupart, occupent une place dans la société, souvent même une fonction importante, et qui, cependant, vivent leur vie, à la li. çon des bêtes de somme... (S'amusant, progressivement, du portrait qu'il trace)... Qui s en vont, devant eux, les yeux mi-clos entre leurs œillères, n'ayant jamais réfléchi par eux-mêmes, n'ayant jamais eu la hardiesse de réviser les vagues croyances qu'on leur a fait enfiler avec leur première culotte... Et qui mourront, dociles et incertains, n'ayant même pas eu conscience de leur incertitude, n'ayant rien aperçu de ce qui domine la vie: l'instinct, l'amour, la mort...

ZOEGER (implacable). — Hâtez-vous de les caricaturer, Portal! Ils encombrent, ceux-là, ils empoisonnent! Nous les charrierons vite hors du chemin...

ROLL (sombre). — Ils se croyent à l'abri, comme des vers dans une carcasse pourrie.

L'âpreté de leur ton contraste avec l'ironique bonhomie de Portal. Il reste un peu inquiet d'avoir attisé cette haine.

HARBAROUX. — Ils sont condamnés. Regardez-les: de père en fils, on les voit se débiliter, devenir de plus en plus amorphes, inexistants, incapables de participer à quelqu'effort neuf!

Barois se jette brusquement dans la discussion.

BAROIS. — Oui, Harbaroux, quand vous les regardez de loin, quand vous les croisez sur la route! Mais quand on a vécu au milieu d'eux, mes amis, ah!comme leur existence confite est encore vivace! (Levant le poing.) Et nuisible!

ZOEGER (avec un mauvais sourire). — Non. Ils ne sont pas si dangereux que ça. Nous les avons exclus de tout, isolés, circonscrits. Dans les incendies de forêts, on fait la part du feu: la fraction sacrifiée continue à flamber; mais elle se consume sur elle-même, sans atteindre le reste. C'est exactement la même chose.

BAROIS (lourdement). — Ah, il faut *en avoir été* pour comprendre cette masse immuable, cette puissance inerte qu'ils sont encore!

CRESTEIL — C'est rudement vrai, ce que Barois dit là!

BAROIS. — Leurs nécropoles lézardées abriteront encore des générations et des générations, avant que leur race ne disparaisse! Heureux, s'ils n'arrivent pas à en sortir, pour ressaisir et aveugler une fois de plus 1 opinion... Sait-on jamais?

Un silence

HARBAROUX (méthodique). — Ne pensez-vous pas qu'il faudrait noter nos projets par écrit?

Pas de réponse; on ne semble pas avoir entendu.

Il est tard.

Aux généreux bouillonnements a succédé une vague somnolence; il plane une impalpable tristesse, un relent aigre d'enthousiasme refroidi.

CRESTEIL. — Notre premier numéro va éclater comme une fanfare!

Sa voix, de plus en plus enrouée, a perdu son timbre triomphal; elle sombre dans le silence, qui se referme sur elle, comme une eau morte.

ROLL (les yeux gonflés de fatigue). — Permettez-moi de me retirer... L'atelier, demain, à sept heures...

HARBAROUX. — Vous savez, il va être deux heures... (A CresteiL) Au revoir.

CRESTEIL. — Mais nous partons tous...

Triste départ.

Barois, resté seul, ouvre la fenêtre, et s'accoude au bord de la nuit glacée.

Dans l'escalier.

Descente silencieuse: Portal marche en tête, tenant un bougeoir. Tout à coup, il se retourne, avec une gaîté de noctambule

PORTAL. — Et Woldsmuth? on l'a oublié... Qu'est-ce qu'il va nous donner d'intéressant, Woldsmuth?

Le monôme s'arrête, amusé. Les têtes se lèvent vers Woldsmuth, qui ferme le cortège. Le flambeau remonte de main à main, jusqu'à lui.

Sa face d'épagneul frisé apparaît, posée sur la rampe, dans la pénombre des étages supérieurs: au milieu des cheveux, des sourcils et de la barbe en broussaille, ses yeux, vivants et doux, clignotent derrière le lorgnon.

Il se tait.

Puis soudain, comme les autres

semblent bien décidés à attendre, son visage change; une brusque roseur paraît sur les pommettes, les paupières se baissent, palpitent, et se relèvent sur un regard ardent et pitoyable.

WOLDSMUTH (avec une fermeté inattendue). — Je recopierai simple-, ment une bien triste lettre que j'ai reçue de Russie... On a chassé six cents familles juives qui habitaient un faubourg de Kiev. Pourquoi? Parce qu'un enfant chrétien a été trouvé mort, et qu'on a accusé les Juifs de lavoir tué pour fabriquer des azimes... Oui, là-bas, c'est ainsi... Alors les Juifs ont été chassés, après un massacre... Et il y a cent-vingt: six nouveaux-nés qui sont morts, parce que ceux qui avaient des enfants i jeunes à porter, allaient moins vite, et ils ont dû camper deux nuits dans la neige...

Oui, là-bas, c'est ainsi... On ne le sait pas, en France..

III A Auteuil.

Huit heures du matin.

Une vaste bâtisse, au fond d'un jardin blanc de givre, où s'ébrouent une demi-douzaine d'enfants.

LUCE (apparaissant sur le perron) — Allons, mes petits... Il est l'heure... Au travail!

Une galopade joyeuse. Les deux aînés, — une fillette de treize ans, un gamin de douze, — arrivent les premiers. Leur essoufflement, dans l'air froid, les enveloppe de buée. Les autres rejoignent, un à un, jusqu'à la dernière de la bande, une petite fille de six ans.

Le poêle de la salle à manger ronfle. Sur la grande table cirée s'alignent les encriers, les sous-mains, des livres de classe.

Debout à la porte de son cabinet, le père regarde.

Ils s'entr'aident gentiment, sans tapage, en liberté.

Puis le silence s'établit tout seul.

Luce, traversant la pièce, monte au premier étage.

Une chambre d'enfant. Les rideaux tirés.

Au chevet du lit, une femme, encore jeune, assise.

Luce l'interroge du regard. Elle fait signe que la petite vient de s'endormir.

Quelques secondes passent.

La mère tressaille: un coup de timbre.

, Le docteur?

Luce est allé jusqu'à la porte.

LA FEMME DE CHAMBRE. — Un jeune homme à qui Monsieur a donné rendez-vous... Monsieur Barois...

Barois est seul, dans le cabinet de Luce.

Une pièce sans draperies; un bureau encombré de revues étrangères, de volumes neufs, de lettres. Aux murs, des reproductions, des plans, des cartes; deux panneaux couverts de livres.

Chaque bruit du monde a son écho là.

Entrée de Luce.

Marc-Élie Luce: de petite taille. Une tête forte, mal proportionnée au corps.

Deux yeux clairs, étrangement enfoncés entre un front immense et une barbe en éventail: les yeux sont d'un gris fin, caressants et limpides; le front, dégarni, très large, bombé, surplombe le masque, accapare le crâne; la barbe est épaisse, d'un blond qui commence à blanchir.

Quarante-sept ans.

Fils d'un pasteur sans église. A commencé ses études de théologie, mais les a interrompues, faute de vocation, et jparce_ au'il ne pouvait accepter aucun credo confessionnel. En a seu I lernent gardé le goût fervent des questions morales.

A publié, très jeune, cinq gros volumes: « Le passé et l'avenir de la croyance », œuvre considérable, qui lui a fait attribuer une chaire d'histoire religieuse au Collège de France.

S'est fait connaître à Auteuil par son dévouement à l'Université populaire qu'il y avait créée, et aux œuvres sociales de l'arrondissement. S'est laissé porter au Conseil Général, puis au Sénat, où il est parmi les plus jeunes: ne sVst affilié à aucun parti; revendiqué à tour de rôle, par tous ceux qui veulent assurer le triomphe de quelque noble pensée.

A fait paraître, successivement: « Les régions supérieures du socialisme ». « Le sens de la vie » et « Le sens de la mort ».

Il s'avance vers Barois et lui tend la main, avec une cordialité simple et imposante.

BAROIS. — Votre lettre nous a infiniment touchés, Monsieur, et je suis le porte-parole de tous...

LUCE (interrompant sans façon). — Asseyez-vous; je suis très content de faire votre connaissance.

Un parler gras, pesant, où perce l'origine franc-comtoise.

LUCE. — J'ai lu votre *Semeur*. (Il sourit en regardant Barois bien en face, sans fausse modestie). C'est très dangereux de recevoir les éloges de plus jeunes que soi: on y est trop sensible...

Un temps.

Il a pris sur son bureau le premier numéro, et le feuillète en parlant.

LUCE. — Un bien beau sous-titre: « Pour la culture des qualités humaines ". ..!

Il est assis, les jambes entr'ouvertes, les coudes sur les genoux, le *Semeur* entre les mains.

Barois contemple ce front, dur et comme gonflé, familièrement penché sur leur œuvre naissante... Orgueil.

Luce parcourt encore une fois la brochure, et s'arrête aux notes qu'il a crayonnées en marge. Il semble réfléchir, soupeser les feuillets... Il se redresse enfin, regarde Barois et remet le *Semeur* sur la table.

LUCE (simplement). — Disposez de moi, je suis avec vous.

L'accent alourdit encore la gravité de ce pacte. Barois se tait, pris au dépourvu, très troublé. Il répugne à formuler un remercîment banal.

Ils se dévisagent: long regard ému...

BAROIS (après un court silence). — Ah! si mes camarades avaient pu entendre ces mots-là, et le timbre de votre voix!

LUCE (souriant). — Quel âge avez-vous?

BAROIS. — Trente-deux ans.

Luce l'examine avec ce sourire intéressé et sans ironie qu'il promène à travers le monde: une sorte d'étonnement enfantin, une curiosité amoureuse des choses, et pour laquelle tout est inédit et admirable. I.i

Un temps.

LUCE, — Oui, vous avez raison. Il manquait un organe comme votre *Semeur*. Mais vous assumez un rôle énorme...

BAROIS. — Pourquoi?

LUCE. — Justement parce que vous serez les seuls à aborder les véritables problèmes contemporains. Vous serez très lus: lourde tâche... Songez que chacune de vos paroles aura une répercussion et que cette répercussion ne vous appartiendra pas, que vous ne pourrez pas la diriger... Bien plus, que vous l'ignorerez le plus souvent!

(Comme à lui-même.) Ah, on écrit toujours trop vite. Semer, semer... Il faut trier, analyser minutieusement ses graines, pour être à peu près sûr de ne lancer que les bonnes...

BAROIS (fièrement). — Cette responsabilité-là, nous l'avons pesée et acceptée.

LUCE (sans répondre). — Vos amis ont le même âge que vous?

BAROIS. — A peu près.

LUCE (maniant la revue). — Quel est ce Breil-Zoeger? Est-ce un parent du sculpteur?

BAROIS. — Son fils.

LUCE. — Ah! Mon père connaissait le sien; c'était un des familiers de Renan... Votre ami ne fait pas de sculpture?

BAROIS. — Non. Il est agrégé de philosophie. Nous avons travaillé l'agrégation de sciences, ensemble.

LUCE. — Son « Introduction à une philosophie positive » iêvèle un tempé ament très personnel.

(Avec sévérité.) Mais c'est d'un sectaire.

Mouvement de Barois.

Luce relève le front, et considère Barois, presque affectueusement,

LUCE. — Vous permettez que je vous dise toute ma pensée?

Barois. — Je vous en prie.

LUCE. — Je voudrais étendre le reproche à tout votre groupe.. (Avec douceur.) A vous, en particulier.

Barois. — Comment cela?

LUCE. — Vous avez pris, dès le premier numéro, une attitude très franche, très courageuse, — mais un peu jacobine...

Barois. — Une attitude combattive.

LUCE. — Elle me plairait sans réserves si elle n'était que combattive. Mais_elje_est... agressive, N'est-ce pas vrai?

BAROIS. — Nous sommes tous ardents, convaincus, prêts à lutter pour nos idées. Il ne me déplaît pas de montrer quelque intransigeance... (Luce se taisant, il continue.) Je crois qu'une doctrine puissante et jeune, est, par nature, intolérante: une conviction qui commence par admettre la légitimité d'une conviction adverse, se condamne à n'être pas agissante elle est sans force, sans efficacité.

LUCE (fermement). — Pourtant c'est l'esprit de tolérance qu'il faut essayer d'établir entre les hommes: nous avons tous le droit d'être ce que nous sommes, sans que notre voisin puisse nous l'interdire, au nom de ses principes personnels!

BAROIS (involontairement brusque). — Oui, la tolérance, la liberté poui tous, c'est parfait, — en principe... Mais voyez où conduit le scepticisme souriant des dilettantes? Est-ce que l'Église serait encore ce qu'elle est dans notre société moderne, si...

LUCE (vivement). —-Vous savez si je suis hostile à l'esprit clérical! Je suis né en 48, au milieu de décembre; et j'ai toujours eu plaisir à penser que j'avais été conçu en pleine effervescence libérale. J'abhorre toutes les soutanes et toutes les fausses enseignes, quelles qu'elles soient. Eh bien, pourtant, ce qui m'écarte des églises, bien plus que leurs erreurs, "c'est Tour uitûléjcance. (Un temps. Posément.) Non, je ne serai jamais partisan d'opposer le mal au mal. Il suffit de réclamer pour tous la liberté de la pensée, et d'en donner l'exemple.

Voyez l'église catholique: elle a eu des siècles de domination; et cependant, pour ébranler ce pouvoir colossal, il a suffi que ses adversaires eussei.t à leur tour acquis le droit de proclamer ce qu'ils pensaient!

Barois écoute; mais, visiblement, ce silence attentif lui pès

LUCE (conciliant). — Que l'erreur reste libre, mais que la vérité soit libre aussi; voilà tout. Et ne nous préoccupons pas trop des suites. La vérité sera toujours victorieuse, à son heure...

(Après un temps.) Ne le croyez-vous pas?

BAROIS. — Ah, parbleu, je sais bien que, dans l'absolu, vous avez raison! Mais nous ne sommes pas maîtres de certains sentiments qui nous trahissent...

Un instant de silence.

Luce semble attendre une explication.

BAROIS (presque violemment). — Je le sais bien, que je ne suis pas tolérant! J_e ne le suis plus!

(Baissant la voix.) Il faut savoir ce que j'ai souffert, pour me comprendre...

Un esprit affranchi, qui se trouve obligé de vivre dans l'intimité de personnes pieuses, — qui se voit, chaque jour, plus étroitement enserré dans ce tissu élastique et si résistant de la foi catholique, — qui sent, à propos de tout, la religion *s'infiltrer* dans sa vie, pénétrer ceux qui l'entourent, *modeler le cœur et l'âme des siens,* laisser partout son empreinte et sa direction! Celui-là, oui, il a le droit de parler de tolérance! Non pas celui qui a quelques concessions à faire, par affection; mais *celui dont la vie quotidienne n'est qu'une seule concession ininterrompue!*

Celui-là, — il a le droit de parler de tolérance!...

(Il se contient, lève les yeux vers Luce, et sourit péniblement.) Et alors, il en parle, Monsieur, comme on parle de la Vertu parfaite, comme on parle d'un idéal qui n'est pas humainement réalisable!

LUCE (après un instant de silence, avec douceur). — Vous ne vivez pas seul?

Le visage énergique de Barois, crispé par les souvenirs, s'illumine d'un coup; son regard s'attendrit.

BAROIS. — Si, maintenant, je suis libre! (Souriant.) Mais depuis trop peu de temps encore, pour être redevenu tolérant...

(Pause.) Excusez-moi d'avoir pris cette discussion trop à cœur...

LUCE. — C'est moi qui, sans le savoir, ai ranimé de tristes émotions...

Échange de regards affectueux.

BAKOIS (spontanément). — Ça me fait du bien. J'ai besoin de conseils... Il y a beaucoup plus de quinze années entre nous, Monsieur... Vous *vivez,* vous, depuis vingt-cinq ans. Moi, je viens seulement de rompre, après des sursauts douloureux, toutes mes chaînes... Toutes! (Son geste cassant scinde sa vie en deux: là, le passé; ici, l'avenir. Il étend la main.) Alors, vous comprenez, j'ai devant moi une vie toute neuve, qui me paraît immense à donner le vertige... Ma première pensée, en fondant cette revue, a été de me rapprocher de vous, comme du seul point de repère que j'aperçoive à l'horizon.

LUCE (hésitant). — Je ne pourrai vous donner que ma propre expérience... (Il sourit, et montre du doigt les cartes de géographie pendues aux murailles.) J'ai toujours pensé que la vie était comme une de ces cartes des pays que je ne connais pas: pour se diriger, il suffit de s'appliquer à la lire... L'attention, l'ordre dans les pensées, la mesure, la persévérance... Voilà tout, c'est très simple.

(Reprenant sur son bureau le numéro du *Semeur*.) Vous êtes très bien parti, vous avez beaucoup d'atouts en main. Vous êtes entouré d'intelligences aigues et originales. Tout cela est très bien... (Réfléchissant.) Si,, /""javais un conseil à vous donner, pourtant, ce serait celui-ci: ne vous Jâissez pas trop influencer par les autres... Oui, c'est quelquefois le danger de ces groupements. II y faut une conscience commune, c'est évident; vous l'avez: un même élan vous a rassemblés et lancés en avant. Mais ne jetez pas votre personnalité dans le creuset commun. Conservez-vous à vousmême, obstinément; ne cultivez en vous que ce qui vous est propre.'

Nous avons tous une faculté particulière, un don si vous voulez, par lequel nous resterons toujours absolument distincts des autres êtres. C'est ce don-là qu'il faut arriver à trouver en soi et à exalter, à l'exclusion du reste.

BAROIS. — Mais n'est-ce pas se restreindre? Ne faut-il pas, au contraire, essayer de sortir de soi, le plus possible?

LUCE. — Je ne crois pas...

LA FEMME De CHAMBRE (entr'ouvrant la porte). — Madame fait prévenir monsieur que le docteur est là.

LUCE. ——Bien.

(A Barois.) J'estime qu'il faut resfer *le*

*même,* avec acharnement, — mais *grandir* !Tendre à devenir l'exemplaire le plus parfait du type spécial d'humanité que l'on représente.

Barois (se levant). — Mais ne faut-il pas agir, parler, écrire, manifester sa force?

LUCE. — Oh, une personnalité vigoureuse s'exprime toujours... Ne vous illusionnez pas sur l'utilité de la production quand même. Est-ce qu'une belle vie ne vaut pas une belle œuvre? J'ai cru aussi qu'il fallait besogner. Peu à peu j'ai changé d'avis...

Il accompagne Barois vers la porte. En passant près de la fenêtre, il écarte le rideau de percale blanche.

LUCE. — Tenez, dans mon jardin, c'est la même chose: il faut soigner la sève, l'enrichir d'année en année: et alors, si l'arbre doit porter des fruits, vous les voyez se multiplier d'euxmêmes...

Ils traversent la salle à manger.

Les petites têtes, penchées sur les devoirs, se redressent, curieuses.

LUCE (enveloppant la table d'un vaste regard). — Mes enfants...

Barois s'incline en souriant.

LUCE (devinant sa pensée). — Oui, c'est beaucoup... Et j'en ai deux autres encore.jJl.Vfa des/ours où j'aperçois tous ces yeux-là fixés sur moi, et j'en suis épouVanté?5(oecouant la tête.) Il faut s'en remettre à la logique de la vie, qui doit être juste.

(Il s'est approché de la table.) Celle-là, c'est mon aînée, une grande fille déjà... Celui-là, Monsieur Barois, c'est un mathématicien... (Il passe amoureusement sa main sur ces têtes de cheveux fins, et se retourne tout-à-coup vers Barois.) — C'est si beau, la vie... ./'/'......, 1

En juin 1896.

Cinq heures du soir.

Une brasserie du boulevard Saint-Michel.

Rez-de-chaussée, vaste et sombre, style Heidelberg: tables massives, escabeaux, vitraux armoriés. Un peuple bruyant d'étudiants et de femmes.

A l'entresol, une pièce basse, réservée une fois par semaine au groupe du *Semeur.*

Cresteil, Harbaroux et Breil-Zoeger

sont attablés près d'une large baie en demi-cercle, ouverte, au ras du parquet, sur le vaet-vient du boulevard.

Entrée de Barois, une lourde serviette sous le bras.

Poignées de mains.

Barois s'assied, et tire des papiers de sa serviette.

Barois. — Portal n'est pas arrivé?

ZOEGER. — Pas vu

BAROIS. — Ni Woldsmuth?

HARBAROUX. — Voilà plusieurs jours que je vais à la Bibliothèque Nationale sans le rencontrer.

BAROIS. — Il m'a envoyé une dizaine de pages tout à fait curieuses, à propos des « Lois sur l'Instruction ». (Il tend un paquet à Cresteil.) Voici vos épreuves. C'est un peu "serré, mais nous avons tant de copie cette fois-ci... (A Harbaroux.) Tiens...

HARBAROUX. — Merci. Quand les veux-tu?

BAROIS. — Roll les demande pour la fin de la semaine. (A Breil-Zoeger.) Voici les tiennes. A ce propos, je voudrais te dire un mot. (Aux autres.) Vous permettez?

Il se lève et emmène Breil-Zoeger au fond de la pièce.

Barois (baissant la voix; affectueusement). — C'est au sujet de ton étude sur le « Déterminisme vital »... Excellent d'ailleurs; je crois que tu n'as rien écrit de plus plein et de plus sobre. J'ai commis l'indiscrétion d'en lire une partie à Luce, hier soir; j'avais tes épreuves dans ma poche... Il a trouvé ça très fort.

ZOEGER (satisfait). —. Tu lui as lu le passage sur Pasteur?

BAROIS. — Non. Et justement je voulais t'en parler avant que tu ne fasses tes corrections...

Zoeger fronce les sourcils.

BAROIS (un peu gêné). — Franchement, je trouve cette page-là trop dure...

ZOEGER (avec un geste sec). — Je ne touche pas au savant; je m'occupe de Pasteur métaphysicien.

Barois. — J'entends bien. Mais tu juges Pasteur comme tu jugerais l'un de nos contemporains, un de ses élèves.

Je ne dis pas que sa conception philosophique de l'univers.. Mais tu oublies trop que notre matérialisme scientifique, c'est à ce spiritualiste impénitent que nous le devons!

ZOEGER (geste qui déblaye). — Je sais comme toi ce que nous lui *devons,* — quoique cette façon de parler ne corresponde pour moi à aucune reconnaissance sentimentale... (Un rire bref, qui dans cette face jaune, montre des dents luisantes.)

Pasteur a cru devoir prendre publiquement une attitude métaphysique bien accusée: nous avons le droit de la juger. Merci bien! On nous a trop souvent opposé son discours de réception à l'Académie, pour que nous ayons, à cet égard, le moindre scrupule!

Barois. — Pasteur avait une hérédité et une éducation qui 1 ont empêché d'aller, — comme nous avons pu le faire depuis, et grâce à lui — jusqu'aux conclusions philosophiques de ses découvertes. Il n y a pas-à lui tenir rigueur de n'avoir plus été assez jeune pour se transformer luimême.

Il le regarde et attend quelques secondes. Zoeger se détourne sans répondre.

BAROIS. — Tes premières pages sont injustes, Zoeger

ZOEGER. — Tu subis l'influence de Luce.

BAROIS. — Je ne m'en défends pas.

ZOEGER. — Tant pis. Luce manque souvent de fermeté, et quelquefois de pénétration, par manie de tolérance, *j*

BAROIS.— Soit. (Un temps.) N'y pensons plus, tu es libre. (Souriant.) Libre et responsable...

Il rejoint sa table et s'assied.

Le garçon apporte les consommations.

BAROIS. — Etes-vous sûrs que Portal viendra ce soir?

CRESTEIL. — Il me l'a dit.

ZOEGER. — Ne l'attendons pas.

BAROIS. —-C'est que j'ai de bonnes nouvelles à vous annoncer, et j aurais voulu que le groupe fût au complet.. . Oui, mes amis, au point de vue matériel, notre *Semeur* continue à être en excellente voie. Je viens d'achever nos comptes semestriels. (Soulevant un registre.) Ils sont à votre disposition.

Nous avons débuté, il y a six mois, avec 38 abonnements. Nous en avons 562 ce mois-ci. De plus, il s'est vendu, le mois dernier, 800 livraisons, tant à Paris, qu'en province. Et nos 1.500 numéros de juin sont déjà épuisés.

CRESTEIL. — La collaboration de Luce nous a certainement été d'un solide appui.

Barois. — C'est évident. JDepuis le premier article qu'il nous a donné jl y a quatre mois, les abonnements ont exactement doublé. Le Semeur de juillet se tirera à 2.000. Je vous propose même de donner à ce numéro 220 pages au lieu de 180.

ZOEGER. — Pourquoi?

Barois. — Voici. Les lettres reçues à propos de la revue augmentent dans une proportion considérable. J'en ai eu près de 300 à lire ce mois-ci! Je les ai classées, avec l'aide d'Harbaroux, selon les articles qui les avaient inspirées, et je transmettrai à chacun de vous celles qui le concernent. Vous verrez qu'il y en a beaucoup d'intéressantes. Je crois qu'il conviendrait de leur faire une place dans la constitution de nos numéros. Nous sommes sérieusement lus et discutés; ces lettres en sont la preuve; il faut en être fiers et ne pas enfouir dans nos tiroirs cette participation du public à notre effort. Je vous offre donc de publier chaque mois la partie la plus significative de notre correspondance, accompagnée, lorsqu'il y aura lieu... (Entrée de Portal.) Bonjour... accompagnée d'une note rédigée par l'auteur de l'article.

Portal, distrait et la figure sérieuse contre son habitude, serre la main de Cresteil, de Barois, puis s'assied.

HARBAROUX. — Et moi, vous ne me dites pas bonjour?

PORTAL (se relevant). — Je vous demande pardon. (Il sourit à peine, et se rassied.)

ZOEGER. — Nous ne vous espérions plus.

PORTAL (nerveux). — Oui, j'ai beaucoup à faire en ce moment. Je sors seulement de la bibliothèque du Palais. (Il lève les yeux et surprend des interrogations muettes.) Il y a peut-être du nouveau...

BAROIS. — Du nouveau?

PORTAL. — Oui. J'ai entrevu ces jours-ci des choses... pénibles. Je vous raconterai. Une erreur judiciaire? On ne sait pas.. Ce serait assez grave...

Ils se taisent, intrigués.

PORTAL (baissant la voix). — Il s'agirait de Dreyfus...

CRESTEIL. — Dreyfus, innocent?

BAROIS. — C'est fou!

HARBAROUX. — Une plaisanterie, voyons!

PORTAL. — Je n'affirme rien. Je vous dis le peu que je sais; et d'ailleurs, jusqu'ici, personne ne semble en savoir plus long que moi. Mais on s'inquiète, on cherche... Il paraîtrait même que l'État-Major fait une enquête. Fauquet-Talon s'en occupe activement: il m'a demandé un rapport détaillé sur le procès d'il y a dix-huit mois.

Un silence.

ZOEGER (posément, à Portal). — Il peut se glisser une erreur dans les jugements des tribunaux civils, qui fonctionnent tous les jours, pour qui la justice est une espèce de besogne. Mais un conseil de guerre, une réunion d'hommes choisis, qui ne sont pas des professionnels de la justice, qui, par conséquent sont sur leur garde, qui nécessairement y mettent une extrême circonspection...

BAROIS.— Et surtout pour une affaire de trahison, si importante... C'est un canard.

CRESTEIL. — Ça? Je vais vous le dire: c'est un coup machiné par...

WOLDSMUTH (d'une voix émue, mais sans hésitation). —...par les Juifs?

CRESTEIL (froidement). —...par la famille de Dreyfus.

BAROIS. — Tiens, vous êtes donc là, Woldsmuth? Je ne vous avais pas vu entrer.

HARBAROUX. — Ni moi.

Zoeger. — Ni moi.

Poignées de mains.

PORTAL (à Woldsmuth). — Est-ce que vous avez aussi entendu parler de cette histoire?

Woldsmuth lève vers Portal son masque poilu, qu'assombrit une vague souffrance. Il fait oui, en baissant ses paupières ourlées de rose.

BAROIS (vivement). — Mais vous êtes bien d'avis qu'une erreur.est invraisemblable?

Woldsmuth fait un geste résigné et dubitatif, comme s'il disait: « Que sait-on? Tout est possible... »

Léger malaise, accentué par un instant de silence.

BAROIS. — Tenez, Woldsmuth, je vous ai apporté vos épreuves.

PORTAL (à Woldsmuth). — Est-ce que vous connaissiez un peu ce Dreyfus?

WOLDSMUTH (avec un regard plus clignotant que jamais). — Non. (Un temps.) Mais j'étais à la dégradation... Et *j'ai vu.*

BAROIS (agacé). — Vu quoi?

Les yeux de Woldsmuth s'emplissent de petites larmes. Il ne répond pas. Il regarde Earois, Harbaroux, Cresteil, Zoeger, l'un après l'autre, lentement, timidement.

Il se sent seul: un sourire résigné de vaincu.

II

« A Monsieur J. BAROIS, 99 *bis,* rue Jacob, Paris.

« 20 Octobre 1896

« Mon cher ami,

« Je suis dans l'impossibilité de me rendre chez vous; (un petit accident, sans gravité, mais qui m'immobilise pour quelques jours). J'aurais cependant bien besoin de vous voir. Aunez-vous la bonté de monter mes six étages, demain, ou après demain au plus tard?

« Excusez mon sans-gêne. C'est urgent. « Votre très dévoué,

Ulric Woldsmuth. »

Le lendemain.

Une vieille maison, presqu'une cité, rue de la Perle, en plein Marais. Au sixième étage de l'escalier F, sous les toits, au fond d'un corridor, un petit logement, n" 14.

Barois sonne.

Une jeune femme vient lui ouvrir.

Trois chambres en enfilade. Dans la première, une vieille à cheveux gris, étale une lessive sur des ficelles. Dans la seconde, deux lits, deux matelats par terre; une machine à écrire devant la fenêtre. La troisième porte est fermée.

Au moment de l'ouvrir, la jeune femme se tourne vers Barois.

JULIA. — Il dort, Monsieur... Si vous n'étisz pas trop pressé?...

BAROIS (vivement). — Ne le réveillez pas, je serais désolé... Je vais attendre.

IULIA. — Ça lui fait tant de bien!

Barois la considère curieusement. Il ignorait que Woldsmuth fut marié.

Julia Woldsmuth: Vingt-cinq ans. Un type étrange.

Au premier abord, elle paraît très grande et très maigre-Pour tant le torse, sans corset dans une étoffe noire, est chàTrnreT7 court. Mais les jambes, et surtout les bras, sont d'une longueur anormaTeT..

Le visage s'effile en avant comme une lame. Ses cheveux annelés, rudes et noirs, qu'elle masse sur la nuque, allongent encore la forme de la tête. La ligne accusée du nez prolonge celle un peu fuyante du front. Les yeux très fendus mais à peine ouverts, glissent en montant vers les tempes. La lèvre supérieure, d'un dessin énigmatique, comme immobilisée dans un perpétuel début de sourire, surplombe la lèvre inférieure, sans la joindre.

D'un geste décidé, elle indique à Barois l'unique chaise de la chambre, et, sans gêne aucune, s'accroupit sur l'un des lits défaits.

Barois (prudemment). — Comment cet... accident est-il arrivé, Madame?

JULIA. — Mademoiselle.

BAROIS (souriant). — Je vous demande pardon.

JULIA (sans se troubler). — Nous n'avons pas su. (Montrant les lits.) Il était minuit passé, nous étions couchées, mère et moi... (Montrant la chambre de Woldsmuth.) Nous avons entendu une petite explosion. Mais nous ne nous sommes pas inquiétées. Au contraire, j'étais contente de penser que mon oncle s'était remis à travailler, qu'il oubliait un peu cette affaire... Et puis, le matin, il nous a appelées: il avait la figure toute coupée par les éclats du verre, et brûlée...

BAROIS (intrigué). — Une explosion de quoi?

JULIA (sèchement). — Une cornue qui a éclaté au feu.

Barois se souvient tout à coup que Woldsmuth a été préparateur de chimie.

Léger silence.

BAROIS. — Je ne voudrais pas interrompre vos occupations. Mademoiselle. ..

Elle est accoudée au milieu des draps, les jambes croisées, et elle le dévisage librement, d'un regard sympathique et sans équivoque.

JULIA. — Nullement... Je suis heureuse de cette occasion. J'entends depuis longtemps parler de vous. J'ai lu vos études et vos chroniques dans le *Semeur...* (Un temps. Sans le regarder, elle conclut, avec une franchise un peu distante.) Vous avez une belle vie.

Sa voix est gutturale, comme celle de Woldsmuth, avec, en plus, une désinvolture un peu rude.

Il ne répond rien. Etrange créature...,

BAROIS (après un silence). — Woldsmuth ne m'avait pas dit qu'il s'occupait encore de chimie.

Julia tourne précipitamment la tête: un peu de fièvre dans ses prunelles fluides...

JULIA. — Il ne raconte rien, parce qu'il travaille, il cherche... Il se dit: « Quand j'aurai trouvé, je parlerai... »

Barois ne questionne pas, mais son attitude interroge.

JULIA. — Il n'a pourtant aucun mystère à faire avec vous, Monsieur Barois. Vous êtes un biologiste. (D'une voix plus chaude.) Oncle pense qu'un jour l'homme arrivera, en réunissant certaines conditions dans un milieu parfaitement approprié, a créer de la vie. .. (Un sourire très simple.)

BAROIS. — A créer de la vie?

JULIA. — Ne le croyez-vous pas?

BAROIS (surpris). — Je sais que cette hypothèse n'est pas invraisemblable, mais...

JULIA (vivement). — Oncle en est sûr.

BAROIS. — C'est un beau rêve, Mademoiselle. Et, en somme, il n'y a aucune raison pour qu'il soit irréalisable. .. (Réfléchissant tout haut.) On sai taujourd'hui que jadis la température de la terre a été trop élevée pour que la synthèse vivante y ait été possible. Il y a donc eu un moment où la vie n'existait pas, puis un moment où la vie a existé.

JULIA. — Voilà. Et c'est cet instant précis où la vie est apparue, qu'il s'agit de reproduire...

BAROIS (rectifiant). — Permettez. Je ne dis pas tout à fait: l'instant où la vie est apparue... Je dirai: l'instant où, sous l'influence de certaines conditions, *qui restent à trouver,* la synthèse vivante s'est faite, entre des éléments qui existaient déjà de toute éternité.

JULIA (attentive). — Pourquoi cette distinction?

BAROIS (un peu gêné du tour technique de la conversation). — Mon dieu, Mademoiselle, parce que je crois que la locution courante: « la vie est apparue », est dangereuse.. Elle correspond trop à cette manie que l'on a de toujours poser le problème d'un « commencement »...

Elle a croisé les jambes, posé le coude sur un genou, et tient son menton dans sa main.

JULIA. — Miis il est nécessaire, pour concevoir que la substance vivante existe, de supposer qu'elle a « commencé » d'être.

BAROIS (vivement). — Au contraire. Pour moi, c'est l'idée d'un début qui me semble impossible à concevoir! Tandis que j'accepte sans effort l'idée d'une substance qui « est », qui se transforme, qui évoluera éternellement.

JULIA. —...Tout l'univers se tenant..

.

BAROIS. —...ne formant qu'une seule substance cosmique, qui transmettrait la vie à tout ce qui émane d'elle... (Un temps.) Vous travaillez sans doute avec votre oncle, Mademoiselle? JULIA. — Un peu.

BAROIS. — Vous expérimentez les rayons du radium?

JULIA. — Oui.

BAROIS (rêveur). — Il est certain que les découvertes de la chimie n'ont pas laissé subsister grand'chose de l'abîme qui séparait autrefois la vie de la mort...

Un silence.

JULIA (montrant la machine à écrire). — Vous permettez que je continue mon travail? J'espère que vous n'attendrez plus longtemps...

Elle s'installe. Le cliquetis de la dactylographie emplit la pièce.

Sa silhouette se profile en sombre sur le vitrage blême. Une lumière frisante éclaire ses mains: des mains étrangères, plus claires au-dedans, d'une agilité simiesque; des doigts s'effilant en ongles jaunes, plats et longs.

Cinq minutes s'écoulent.

LA VOIX DE WOLDSMUTH. — Julia!

Julia ouvre la porte.

JULIA. — Oncle, voici Monsieur Barois, justement...

Elle s'efface pour qu'il passe.

L'embrasure est étroite. Elle ne semble pas s'en apercevoir: aucun mouvement féminin de retrait. Au contraire, elle avance la tête, si près qu'il sent son souffle sur sa joue.

fuLlA (bas). — Ne dites pas que je vous ai demandé d'attendre.

Il acquiesce des yeux.

La chambre de Woldsmuth est agrandie par un avant-corps vitré, ancien atelier de photographie transformé en laboratoire.

Barois s'avance vers le fond de la chambre, qui forme alcôve.

Un corps d'enfant soulève à peine les draps; si menu que la grosse tête en linge, posée sur l'oreiller, ne semble pas lui appartenir.

BAROIS. — Mon pauvre ami... Vous souffrez?

WOLDSMUTH. — Non. (Gardant sa main.) Julia va vous donner un siège... Barois la devance et tire une chaise près du lit.

Julia sort.

WOLDSMUTH (fierté tendre, qui s'efforce de paraître paternelle). — Ma nièce.

C'est bien son timbre; mais, lui, il est méconnaissable. Un pansement d'ouate recouvre les cheveux, le nez, la barbe, ne laissant vivre qu'un sourire à demi-couvert, et les yeux marrons, sous les sourcils en broussaille.

WOLDSMUTH. — Je vous remercie d'être venu, Barois...

BAROIS. — C'est tout naturel, mon cher. Qu'y a-t-il donc?

WOLDSMUTH (la voix changée). — Ah Barois! Il faut que tous les honnêtes gens sachent enfin ce qui se passe. .. Il est là-bas, il va mourir de, privation. .. Et il est innocent!

BAROIS (souriant à cette hantise de malade). — Encore ce Dreyfus?

WOLDSMUTH (dressé sur les coudes, fébrile). — Je vous en prie, Barois, je vous en supplie, au nom de tout ce qui est noble et juste, abandonnez tout parti-pris, oubliez tout ce que vous avez appris par les journaux il y a deux ans, et tout ce qu'on raconte... Je vous en supplie, Barois, écoutezmoi! (Se laissant retomber sur l'oreiller.) Ah, on dit toujours: le bien de l'humanité. .. Oui, c'est facile de s'intéresser à l'humanité en général, à la masse anonyme, à ceux dont on ne verra jamais la souffrance! (Rire nerveux.) Mais ce n'est rien, ça, non. Aimer son vrai prochain, aimer ceux dont la souffrance se trouve, un beau jour, là, tout près de nous... Ça, c'est aimer, c'est être bon! (Se redressant.) Barois, je vous en supplie, oubliez tout ce que vous savez, et écoutez-moi!

Toute la vie de cet homme, bloc informe de bandelettes, s est réfugiée dans le regard, seul libre: regard mouvant et ardent, qui implore et qui scrute.

Barois ému, tend affectueusement la main.

BAROIS. — Je vous écoute. Ne vous exaltez pas...

Woldsmuth se recueille un instant.

Puis il tire de sous ses draps une liasse de pages dactylographiées qu'il essaye de feuilleter. Mais l'ombre, maintenant, s est. épaissie au fond de la pièce.

Woldsmuth (appelant). — Julia! Un peu de lumière, je te prie...

La machine à écrire stoppe.

Julia paraît, portant un petit fumeron à essence, qu'elle pose vivement sur la table de nuit.

WOLDSMUTH. — Merci.

Elle lui jette un sourire froid. Il la suit tendrement des yeux à travers ses linges, jusqu'à ce qu'elle ait disparu. Puis il tourne la tête vers Barois

WOLDSMUTH. — Il faut que je reprenne tout, comme si vous n'aviez jamais rien su... (Changeant de ton.) Remontons au début de l'année 1894. D'abord les faits, n'est-ce pas?

Donc, au Ministère de la Guerre, on constate des fuites de pièces Puis, un jour, le chef de la section de statistique remet au ministre une lettre qui aurait été trouvée parmi les papiers de l'ambassade d'Allemagne. Une lettre autographe, une sorte de bordereau, une liste des documents que l'auteur de la lettre propose de livrer à son correspondant.

Voilà le point de départ. Bien.'

On cherche un coupable. Sur cinq documents cités dans le bordereau, trois ont trait à l'artillerie: on cherche donc parmi les artilleurs de l'Etat Major. D'après une analogie d'écriture, les soupçons se portent sur I Dreyfus. Il est juif et peu aimé. Première enquête qui n'aboutit à rien.

BAROIS. — Vous le dites.

WOLDSMUTH. — La preuve, c'est que l'acte d'accusation n'a rien trouvé de suspect, ni dans la vie privée de Dreyfus, ni dans ses relations. Rien que des présomptions...

BAROIS. — Vous avez lu l'acte d'accusation?

WOLDSMUTH (montrant un feuillet). — J'en ai la copie. Je vous la remettrai.

Un silence.

WOLDSMUTH. — On procède alors à deux expertises des écritures. L'un des experts ne pense pas que le bordereau soit de Dreyfus. L'autre croit qu'il peut être de sa main: mais son rapport débute par une restriction capitale. (Il cherche dans les papiers.) Voici le texte: «...si l'on écarte l'hypo:hèse d'un document forgé avec le plus grand soin. .. »

Ce qui veut dire, n'est-ce pas? L'écriture ressemble beaucoup à celle de Dreyfus, mais je ne peux pas dire si elle est de lui ou d'un imitateur.

Vous me suivez, Barois?

BAROIS (très froid). — Je vous suis.

WOLDSMUTH. — Sur ces deux expertises contradictoires, on décide l'arrestation. Oui. Sans attendre un supplément d'enquête, sans même surveiller les allées et venues de celui qu'on soupçonne... On est moralement convaincu que c'est lui. Ça suffit. On l'arrête.

Là, un incident dramatique, que je veux vous raconter.

Dreyfus est convoqué, un matin, au ministère, pour une inspection générale. On lui a recommandé, contre toutes les règles, de se présenter en civil. Premier étonnement. Remarquez que s'il avait été coupable, sa méfiance se serait éveillée et il aurait eu le temps de fuir. Mais non. Il arrive, tranquillement, à l'heure dite, et ne trouve aucun des camarades habituellement convoqués avec lui. Nouvelle surprise.

On l'introduit hâtivement dans le cabinet du chef d'État-Major général. Le général n'y est pas; mais des inconnus, en civils, sont là, massés dans un coin, et le dévisagent. Un commandant, sans lui parler de l'inspection, lui dit: « J'ai mal au doigt, voulez-vous écrire une lettre à ma place? »

Étrange moment pour demander à un subordonné ce service d'ami...

Il plane une sorte de mystère. Les paroles, les attitudes, tout est insolite.

Dreyfus s'assied, interloqué.

Aussitôt le commandant commence une dictée: des phrases choisies parmi celles du bordereau incriminé. Naturellement Dreyfus ne les reconnaît pas; mais la voix hostile de l'officier supérieur et cette atmosphère de drame qui l'enserre depuis son arrivée, le troublent: son écriture s'en ressent. Le commandant se penche vers lui, et crie: « Vous tremblez! » Dreyfus, ne comprenant pas ce mouvement d'humeur, s'excuse: « J'ai froid aux doigts... »

La dictée continue. Dreyfus s'applique à écrire mieux. Le commandant, déçu, l'interrompt: « Faites attention, c'est grave! » Et brusquement: « Au nom de la loi, je vous arrête!»

BAROIS (impressionné). — Mais ce récit, d'où le tenez-vous? UEcIair l'a raconté les faits tout autrement.

(Il se lève et fait quelques pas dans la chambre obscure.) Qui vous dit que votre histoire est la vraie?

WOLDSMUTH. — Je sais d'où viennent les renseignements de VEclair. La scène a été dénaturée.

(Baissant la voix.) Barois, j'ai eu entre les mains la photographie de la dictée.. . Oui! Eh bien, l'émotion qu'elle révèle est presque insignifiante et très explicable. — En tous cas, je vous'affirme qu'un traître qui se sent découvert, et à qui l'on veut faire écrire les mots mêmes dont il s'est servi pour trahir, ne se maîtrise pas à ce point, ce n'est pas possible!

Barois ne répond pas.

WOLDSMUTH. — Et puis, je sais encore autre chose. Le mandat d'arresrion, a. été signé un jour *avant* l'épreuve de la dictée; et l'arrestation etait si bien décidée, quoi qu'il pût arriver ce matin-là, que la cellule de la prison était prête depuis la veille!

Barois ne répond toujours rien.

Il est assis au chevet du ht, les bras croisés, le buste droit, la tête un peu en arrière, les sourcils dressés, son menton volontaire, levé, provoquant.

Un instant de silence.

Woldsmuth parcourt ses notes. Puis il relève la tête, et se penche vers Barois.

WOLDSMUTH. — Donc, Dreyfus est incarcéré. Pendant quinze jours, au risque d'un transport cérébral, on refuse de lui expliquer son arrestation, on ne lui dit pas ce dont il est accusé.

Pendant ces quinze jours on enquête, on cherche partout. On le questionne, on le cuisine, sans résultat. On perquisitionne chez lui. On interroge sa femme avec une cruauté impitoyable, en lui laissant ignorer où est son mari, en lui persuadant même qu'elle signerait l'arrêt de sa mort si elle informait qui que ce soit de sa disparition.

Enfin, le quinzième jour, on montre à Dreyfus le bordereau. Il nie avec violence, avec désespoir: peu importe; l'instruction préparatoire est terminée.

Le parquet du Conseil de guerre est saisi. Une nouvelle instruction commence. Dreyfus est de nouveau questionné, pressé, retourné en tous sens; des témoins sont entendus; on cherche des complices, sans succès. L'enquête n'aboutit à rien de sérieux.

Alors, Barois, le ministre de la Guerre jette une première fois sa parole dans la balance. Au cours d'une interview de presse,il déclare,lui, ministre, que la culpabilité de Dreyfus est «absolument certaine», mais qu'il ne peut s'expliquer davantage.

Quelques semaines plus tard, Dreyfus est jugé à huis-clos, condamné, dégradé, déporté.

BAROIS. — Eh bien, voyons, mon cher, vous n'êtes pas ébranlé par cette condamnation? Si vraiment aucune charge sérieuse ne s'élevait contre Dreyfus, pensez-vous que des officiers...

WOLDSMUTH (avec angoisse). — Oui, je dis, j'affirme, qu'aprèsjquatre_ jours de débats, il a été indubitablement établi que Dreyfus n avait eu aucune relation suspecte, que ses voyages à l'étranger, ses besoins d'argent, ses habitudes de jeu, ses liaisons amoureuses, tout ce que l'on avait lancé dans la presse antisémite, pour influencer défavorablement l'opinion, étaient des racontars sans fondement.

BAROIS (haussant les épaules). — Et, malgré ça, il se serait trouvé deux colonels, deux commandants, deux capitaines, pour... Voyons, mon cher, voyons!...

Dans le regard enflammé du malade passe comme une satisfaction de n'avoir pas convaincu Barois: plus la résistance sera vive, plus la certitude et la révolte finales, seront fortes.

WOLDSMUTH (soulevant les feuillets dactylographiés). — Toute la vérité est là.

BAROIS. — Qu'est-ce que c'est?

WOLDSMUTH. — Un mémoire, Barois, un simple mémoire... Rédigé par un inconnu, un admirable cœur, un esprit d'une clarté, d'une logique invincibles.

BASOIS. — Comment l'appelez-vous?

WOLDSMUTH (respectueusement). — Bernard Lazare.

Barois fait un geste qui signifie: « Je ne connais pas. »

WOLDSMUTH. — Il faut que vous m'écoutiez jusqu'au bout. Je n'ai pas fini; je commence... Je vous ai appelé, pour que vous sachiez, vous, ce qui se passe: mais pour autre chose aussi. (Avec une autorité inattendue, imposante.) Barois, il faut vaincre cette conspiration de mensonges, de sous-entendus et de silences, qui bâillonne la vérité. Il faut qu'une parole accréditée se fasse entendre... Qu'un homme, dont la droiture est reconnue de tous, soit averti, soit convaincu, et que sa conscience crie tout haut, pour nous tous!

Il s'est soulevé sur les mains, et à travers ses linges, il fixe Barois, pour voir s'il a compris son désir.

Le masque de Barois, éclairé à plein par la petite flamme, reste dur et impassible.

WOLDSMUTH (précisant, avec une supplication de la voix). — Il faut, en un mot, que Luce reçoive la visite de Bernard Lazare. (Mouvement de Barois.) Il faut qu'il consente à l'entendre, sans parti-pris, avec sa seule bonne foi et sa probité.

(Brandissant les feuillets.) Il faut que cet appel soit imprimé à cent mille exemplaires! 11 y a là une mission de justice, à laquelle ni moi, ni vous, ni lui, ne pouvons plus nous dérober!

Barois fait mine de se lever.

WOLOSMUiH. — Attendez, Barois, ne vous prononcez pas. Non, non, ne me dites rien... Patientez, écoutez... (Suppliant.) Ne vous raidissez pas, Barois... Vous allez être juge: soyez seulement impartial... Je veux vous lire des fragments, je veux que vous soyez pénétré par cette longue cla meur vers la justice...

(Fébrilement.) Voyons... Ceci, d'abord:
' Le capitaine Dreyfus a été arrêté à la suite de *deux expertises contradictoires.*

« L'instruction a été conduite de la façon la plus arbitraire. Elle n'a abouti qu'à *montrer l'inanité absolue des racontars faits sur le capitaine Dreyfus, et le mensonge des rapports policiers que des témoins ont démenti et que l accusation n'a pas osé retenir.*

« La base de l'accusation reste donc une *feuille de papier pelure* — sorte de bordereau d'envoi, de style et d'orthographe bizarres, — *déchirée en quatre morceaux et soigneusement recollée.*

« D'où venait cette pièce? D'après le rapport de M. Besson d'Ormescheville, le général Joux, en la remettant à l'officier de police judiciaire, déclara qu'elle ayait été adressée à une puissance étrangère, qu'elle lui était parvenue, mais que, d'après les ordres formels du ministère de la Guerre, il ne pouvait indiquer par quels moyens ce document était tombé en sa possession.

i *L'accusation ne sait donc pas comment ce document non daté, non signé, est parti des mains de l'inculpé. La défense ignore par quelles voies il est revenu de l'ambassade qui le possédait. A qui la lettre était-elle adressée? Qui l'a volée ou livrée ? A toutes ces questions pas de réponse.* » (i). (S'interrompant.) Ailleurs, déjà, il avait démontré l'invraisemblance de cette pièce. (Reprenant sa lecture.) Tenez:
« Ce document lui-même est-il vraisemblable? *Non.*

« Examinons son origine, ou plutôt l'origine qu'on lui attribue. D après M. Montville *(Journal du 16 Septembre 18%)* il aurait été trouvé, à l'ambassade d'Allemagne, par un garçon de bureau qui avait l'habitude de livrer à des agents français, le contenu des corbeilles à papier. Y a-t-il jamais eu à l'ambassade d'Allemagne quelqu'un qui se soit livré à ce trafic? Oui. Cela était-il resté ignoré de l'ambassade? Non. Quand cette ambassade en eut-elle connaissance? *Un an environ avant l'affaire Dreyfus.* Dans quelles circonstances? Je vais le dire (2). » (S'interrompant.) Je vous passe le récit du procès de Mme Millescamps en police correctionnelle. Vous le lirez...
(Reprenant:)
« Donc, un an avant l'affaire Dreyfus, on savait à l'ambassade d'Allemagne que les détritus de papier étaient communiqués à des agents français. Mais on ignorait, un an après, si celui qui se livrait à ce commerce n'était pas toujours à l'ambassade. On avait, par conséquent, la plu? extrême méfiance, et on prenait les plus grandes précautions.
(1) Bernard Lazare, *La vérité sur l'affaire Dreyfus.* Stock, réédition de iSgS (p. 80 et suiv.). (2) Op. cit. p. 72.
« Est-il donc admissible qu'on ait déchiré en quatre morceaux et jeté au panier un papier aussi compromettant pour un auxiliaire précieux et qu'on devait tenir essentiellement à conserver, alors qu'on savait que, selon toute probabilité, ces fragments seraient livrés au bureau de renseignements du ministère de la Guerre?
» L'origine qu'on attribue à ce borde-

reau n'est donc pas plausible, *à moins qu'on admette sa confection par un faussaire en relations avec un personnage, depuis longtemps acquis, du bas personnel de l'ambassade d'Allemagne, et ayant pu par cette entremise introduire ce bordereau fabriqué, énamérant des pièces qui jamais n'ont été livrées, et le faire sortir ensuite par des procédés habituels.*

« Etudions maintenant la vraisemblance du document. Voit-on la nécessité, pour celui qui aurait trahi, de faire accompagner son envoi d'un bordereau inutile et compromettant? Généralement la préoccupation d'un espion ou d'un traître est de ne laisser aucune trace de ses actes. S'il livre des documents, il les mettra entre les mains d'une série d'intermédiaires chargés de les faire parvenir à destination, *mais jamais il n'écrira.* Il faut remarquer d'ailleurs que l'acte d'accusation est fort embarrassé pour expliquer la façon dont un tel bordereau aurait pu être transmis. Est-ce par la poste? Quelle folie! Est-ce par l'intermédiaire de quelqu'un? Alors, quel besoin de remettre un bordereau? Quelle nécessité d'écrire, au lieu de donner les pièces de la main à la main?

L'absurdité de ces deux hypothèses est telle, que l'acte d'accusation a mieux aimé s'en abstenir. » (i). (S'interrompant.) Vous me suivez, Barois?

Barois, sans répondre, l'invite à poursuivre d'un geste rude.

Il ne cherche plus à prendre une attitude. Les coudes sur les genoux, le dos ployé, le menton enfoncé dans les mains, son regard dur impitoyablement rivé à cette tête inexpressive en tarlatane dont pas un détail ne lui échappe, les narines palpitantes, les lèvres entr'ouvertes et crispées sous la moustache, il écoute, il attend la suite, le cœur battant d'anxiété, espérant encore que tout cela n'est pas vrai.

WOLDSMUTH (après l'avoir examiné silencieusement). — Je continue...

« A-t-on trouvé, pendant les deux mois d'enquête, que le capitaine Dreyfus ait eu des relations suspectes? *Non.* Cependant l'étrange missive dit: « Sans

nouvelles m'indiquant que vous désirez me voir. » Il (i) Oi. cit. t. ?4. s voyait donc le correspondant mystérieux? On a scruté sa vie, suivi tous ses pas, examiné toutes ses actions, *on n'a pu citer aucune fréquentation compromettante...*

« *Jamais l'accusation n'a pu produire un fait, alléguer une charge pouvant faire supposer que le capitaine Dreyfus ait eu des relations quelconques avec un agent étranger,* MÊME POUR LE SERVICE DE L'État-major!

«...*Quelles raisons ont pu pousser le capitaine Dreyfus à commettre la trahison dont on l'accuse? Etait-il besogneux? Non. Il était riche. Avait-il des passions et des vices à satisfaire? Aucun. Etait-il avare? Non, il vivait largement et n'a pas augmenté sa fortune. Est-ce un malade, un impulsif susceptible d'agir sans raison? Non, c'est un calme, un pondéré, un être de courage et d'énergie. Quels puissants motifs cet heureux avait-il pour risquer tout ce bonheur? Aucun.*

« *A cet homme que rien ne pousse au mal, que rien n'accuse, que l'enquête établit probe, travailleur, de vie régulière et honnête;* à cet homme, on montre un p ipier mystérieux, louche, de provenance obscure: On lui dit: « C'est toi qui as écrit ceci. Trois experts l'attestent, et deux le nient. » Cet homme, s'appuyant sur sa vie passée, affirme qu'il n'a pas commis pareil acte, il proteste de son innocence; *on reconnaît l'honorabilité de son existence,* et, sur le témoignage contradictoire de ces experts en écriture, on le condamne à la déportation perpétuelle! » (i). t,

Un silence.

Woldsmuth. — Et voici maintenant ce que Lazare écrit sur la communication secrète:

« Cela n'eût pas suffi, en effet.

« Aussi, mis' en présence de ces seules charges, *le Conseil de guerre penchait vers l'acquittement.*

« C'est alors que le général Mercier, *malgré les promesses formelles faites au ministre des Affaires étrangères,* se décida à communiquer en secret — *hors la présence même de l'avocat,* — aux juges du Conseil de guerre, dans la chambre des délibérations, la pièce, su-

prême accusation, qu'il avait gardée jusqu'à ce moment. Quelle était cette pièce?

« *Elle était,* dit l'Eclair, *relative au service d'espionnage à Paris, et contenait celte phrase* '. « DÉCIDÉMENT CET ANIMAL DE DREYFUS DEVIENT TROP EXIGEANT. »

« Cette lettre existe-t-elle? Oui. A-t-elle été communiquée secrètement aux juges? Oui.

« La phrase citée par *l'Eclair* est-elle contenue dans cette missive? « *J'affirme que non.*

« *J'assure que celui qui a livré au journal ''Eclair* cette pièce dont on redoutait à tel point — en raison de complications diplomatiques possibles — la divulgation, que l'on dut, à cause de son existence même, exiger le huisclos, — j'assure que celui-là n'a pas craint, ajoutant une infamie à celles déjà commises, de falsifier ce document capital, dont la publication devait achever de convaincre chacun de la culpabilité du malheureux, qui, depuis deux ans, subit un martyre sans nom.*

« La lettre apportée aux. juges *ne contenait pas le nom de Dreyfus,* MAIS SEULEMENT L'INIALE D.

« L'*Eclair,* dans son numéro du 10 Novembre 1896 ne conteste pas mon affirmation, mais il faut cependant que je la précise:

« La lettre *révélée pour la première fois, malgré le double huis-clos, si je puis dire, par l'Eclair* est arrivée au ministère de la Guerre par l'intermédiaire du ministre des Affaires étrangères, *huit mois environ avant l'affaire Dreyfus.*

« Il est si vrai qu'elle ne contenait pas le nom de Dreyfus, qu'on s'appliqua pendant quelque temps à filer et à surveiller un malheureux garçon de bureau du ministère de la Guerre, dont le nom commençait par un D. Cette filature fut rapidement abandonnée, ainsi qu'une ou deux autres, posterieurement entreprises, puis la lettre fut oubliée. *Aucun soupçon ne se portait sur Dreyfus* (nouvelle preuve qu'on ne se méfiait pas de lui dès l'origine) *et on ne songea à cette missive qu'après la saisie du bordereau et son attribution au capitaine Dreyfus.*

« Le récit de *l'Eclair* du 15 Septembre 1896 n'est donc pas exact.

« Faut-il maintenant examiner la vraisemblance de cette lettre?

« Supposons qu'une puissance étrangère soit assez heureuse pour s'attacher un officier d'Etat-Major, et que cet officier lui livre les pièces les plus confidentielles. Il sera pour cette puissance d'un prix inestimable, elle fera tout pour se l'attacher, et prendra, de concert avec lui, toutes les précautions nécessaires pour qu'il ne puisse être soupçonné... D'autre part, cette puissance étrangère se fera un devoir, commandé par la plus élémentaire prudence, de ne pas compromettre elle-même, par d'inutiles confidences un homme si précieux, et elle se gardera bien plus encore de confier à une lettre qui peut s'égarer ou être saisie, le nom de l'officier susceptible de lui rendre de si grands services.

« Il reste donc acquis, jusqu'à ce que le gouvernement l'ait nié, que la condamnation du capitaine Dreyfus, que nulle preuve suffisante ne provoquait, a été obtenue en mettant sous les yeux des juges une lettre *systématiquement soustraite à l'accusé, systématiquement soustraite au défenseur.*

« *Au cours du procès, ils l'ont ignorée : ils n'ont donc pu la discuter contester soit son origine, soit l'attribution qu'on faisait d'une initiale à un homme que rien d'autre ne désignait.*

« Est-il admissible qu'on puisse condamner quelqu'un en lui refusant les éléments nécessaires à sa défense? N est-il pas monstrueux qu'on puisse, hors la salle d'audience, peser sur l'esprit, sur la décision, sur la sentence des juges? Est-il permis à qui que ce soit d'entrer dans la chambre des délibérés et de dire au magistrat : « Oublie ce que tu viens d'entendre en faveur de l'homme que tu as à juger. Nous avons, nous, en main, des pièces que, *par raison d'Etat ou de haute politique, nous lui avons cachées, et sur lesquelles nous te demandons le secret. Ces pièces nous en affirmons l'authenticité, la réalité. »* Et un tribunal, là-dessus, a prononcé la sentence! Nul de ses membres ne s'est levé et n'a dit : « On nous demande là une chose contraire à toute équité, nous

ne devons pas y consentir!»

« Et l'on avait à tel point égaré l'opinion, on lui avait tellement présenté l'homme qu'on avait condamné comme le dernier des misérables, indigne de toute pitié, que l'opinion ne songea pas à s'émouvoir de la façon dont celui qu'on lui présentait comme le plus odieux des traîtres, avait été condamné. Ceux-mêmes dont le patriotisme s'inquiète lorsqu'on touche à un officier, oublièrent les procédés employés dans cette circonstance, parce qu'on les avait convaincus, au nom de la patrie offensée, de la nécessité du châtiment, par tous les moyens.

« S'il n'en eût pas été ainsi, des milliers de voix se seraient élevées, — et elles s'élèveront peut-être demain, après que les préventions auront été dissipées, — pour protester au nom de la justice. Elles auraient dit : « Si l'on admet de semblables abus de pouvoir, des mesures aussi arbitraires, la liberté de chacun est compromise, elle est à la merci du ministère public, et on enlève à tout citoyen accusé les garanties les plus élémentaires de la défense. » i).

Barois a laissé glisser son front dans ses mains. Immobile, le visage altéré de pitié et de chagrin, il fixe désespérément, à ses pieds, un carreau du carrelage, fendu en deux et soudé par la poussière.

WOLDSMUTH. — (Sa voix grave, cassée par la fatigue et l'exaltation, reprend, avec une sombre tristesse) :

« Il est encore temps de se ressaisir. Qu'il ne soit pas dit que, ayant devant soi un juif, on a oublié la justice. C'est au nom de cette justice que je proteste, au nom de cette justice qu'on a méconnue.

(i) Op. cit. pp. 83 à 89. *Le capitaine Dreyfus est un innocent et on a obtenu sa condamnation par des moyens illégaux : il faut que son procès soit révisé.* «...Et ce n'est plus à huis clos qu'il devra être jugé, mais devant la France entière.

« J'en appelle donc de la sentence du Conseil de Guerre...

« Des faits nouveaux viennent d'être apportés au débat : ils suffisent juridiquement pour faire casser le jugement : mais

au-dessus des subtilités juridiques, il y a des choses plus hautes : ce sont les droits de l'homme à sauvegarder sa liberté, et à défendre son innocence, si on l'accuse injustement!» (i).

Woldsmuth, à la limite de l'effort, retombe au creux de l'oreiller. Il a baissé les paupières; et, tout à coup, dans ce bonhomme en chiffons, il n'y a plus rien de vivant, que le tremblement des petites mains, immobiles sur le drap.. Barois se lève et, lourdement, fait quelques pas.

Puis il s'approche du lit et s'arrête, les jambes écartées, le buste frémissant, les mains entr'ouvertes à hauteur de la poitrine.

Il respire fortement, avant de pouvoir parler.

BAROIS. — En tous cas, il faut chercher, il faut savoir! Le doute est horrible...'

Je vous promets que Luce recevra votre ami.dès demain.

22 octobre 1896.

« Mon cher Barois,

« Monsieur Bernard Lazare vient de passer l'après-midi dans mon cabinet. Vous savez dans quelles dispositions d'esprit j'étais hier soir : je ne puis en changer si brusquement. Mais je confesse que cet entretien m'a profondément remué.

« Tout cela m'apparaît si î,rave, si plein de périls, qu'il me semblerait criminel d'improviser une attitude, ou de prendre une décision e. la légère. J'ai donc refusé, pour le moment, de prêter mon nom à quoi que ce soit, tout en assurant M. Lazare de ma sympathie, qui est complète. On devine en lui un de ces hommes, pour qui tout l'appareil des puissances, la raison d'Etat, les puissances temporelles, les puissances politiques, les autorités de tout ordre, intellectuelles, mentales mêmes, ne pèsent pas une once devant un mouvement de la conscience propre (i). C'est, de plus, un esprit lucide, dont l'argumentation est troublante.

« Il n'est pas possible de penser sans anxiété qu'une aussi effroyable injustice pourrait avoir été commise sous nos yeux. Je ne pourrais pas vivre plus longtemps en compagnie d'une semblable inquiétude.

Je veux savoir.

« Je veux être rassuré. Je reste persuadé que la vérité est autre, qu'il y a quelque chose que nous ignorons et qui nous délivrera de cette angoisse. Aussi vais-je me consacrer à une sérieuse enquête personnelle, dont je vous communique-rai les résultats.

« D'ici là, mon cher ami, ne me par-lez plus de cette pénible affaire; laissez-*moï* toute la lucidité et le calme que je veux mettre à cette recherche. Je vous le demande instamment. Et si vous me permettez un conseil, n'en (i) Cette der-nière phrase, depuis: « pour qui » est empruntée à Péguy. *Not e jeunesse,* p. 96.

parlez pas davantage autour de vous: l'opinion n'a été que trop agitée déjà au sujet de cette histoire, et il ne peut rien sortir de bon de ces basfonds soulevés.

« Mon fils aîné va tout à fait bien. Mais voici que la santé de notre chère petite Antoinette nous tourmente à nou-veau; je crois que nous serons obligés de tenter l'opération. C'est un gros sou-ci pour moi, mon cher Barois, et pour ma pauvre Lucie. Le calme bonheur est à peu près impossible dans une famille nombreuse...

« De cœur avec vous, mon cher Ba-rois,— et plus un mot de tout cela, je vous en conjure.

Marc-elie Luce. »

A Auteuil, un matin de juillet, 1897.

Le cabinet de Luce.

La chaleur matinale d'un beau jour; l'air tremble dans les fenêtres ouvertes: entre les rideaux de percale blanche, l'éblouissement de la verdure enso-leillée, où piaillent les moineaux et les enfants.

Barois assis, attentif et silencieux.

Luce à son bureau.les mains sur le bord de la table, le buste en arrière, mais la tête légèrement penchée, comme si le poids du crâne l'entraînait en avant; dans l'ombre du front, ses yeux de vi-sionnaire levés vers Barois.

LUCE (d'une voix contenue). — Vous comprenez, Barois, que je ne pro-nonce pas des mots si graves sans que ma conviction soit absolue.

Quand vous êtes venu, il y a huit

mois, et que vous m'avez envoyé Ber-nard Lazare, je sentais déjà combien l'affaire était dangereuse. Je connais-sais, depuis l'article de *l'Eclair,* l'hypothèse d'un dossier secret... (Apre-ment.) Mais je me refusais à y croire! Les avertissements précis de Lazare m'ont fait peur. J'ai voulu savoir. (Douloureusement.) Je sais.

Un temps.

(Elevant la voix.) II y a huit mois, je *n'osais* pas supposer que des juges mi-litaires, conscients de leur responsabili-té, eussent pu accepter dans leurs débats l'intervention de leur propre ministre; encore moins la production par lui de pièces secrètes, à l'insu de l'accusé et de son défenseur.

Depuis, mon pauvre Barois, j'en ai ap-pris bien davantage... J'ai appris, non seulement qu'il y avait eu un dossier se-cret, volontairement caché à la défense par les juges du conseil de guerre; mais de plus, que ce dossier ne contenait même pas cette révélation indubitable, qui, sans pouvoir servir d'excuse à la faute judiciaire, eût du moins soulagé nos consciences! Qu'il ne contenait au-cun document grave contre l'accusé, rien d'autre que des présomptions, faci-les à interpréter, soit pour, soit contre lui!

Ses mains ponctuent l'affirmation, d'un battement sec des doigts sur le bois de la table.

(Gravement.) Je vous jure que ceci est la vérité.

Barois n'a pas tressailli. Les jambes écartées, les mains sur les genoux, il écoute. Sur son visage énergique, dans son regard ardent, une curiosité passion-née, mais aucune surprise.

LUCE (posant la main sur une liasse sanglée). — Je ne peux pas vous ra-conter par le menu l'enquête que j'ai faite. Voilà huit mois que je ne me suis pas occupé d'autre chose. (Bref sourire. ) Vous le savez, puisque je n'ai même pas pu régulièrement donner au *Semeur* cet article hebdomadaire que je vous avais promis...

Mon mandat de sénateur, et d'anciennes camaraderies, m'ont per-mis de pénétrer partout, de contrôler moi-même toutes mes informations. La-

zare m'a procuré une photographie des pièces les plus importantes. J'ai pu les examiner, seul, au calme, sur ce bureau. J'ai fait faire, par surcroît, des exper-tises d'écritures par les meilleurs spé-cialistes d'Europe. (Palpant un dossier. ) Tout ca est là. Je connais maintenant l'affaire à fond: (pesant ses mots) et il ne me reste plus de doute... plus un seul!

BAROIS (se levant). — Il faut qu'on le sache! Il faut le dire! Au ministère, d'abord.

Luce reste un instant silencieux. Puis il fixe Barois: un bon sourire, doux et triste, qui se perd dans sa barbe. Il se penche, expansif.

LUCE. — Lundi dernier, — à cette heure-ci, tenez — j'étais au Ministère de la Guerre, face à face,avec un vieux camarade, un officier qui est au-jourd'hui tout-puissant à l'Etat-Major. I

Je ne l'avais pas revu depuis environ deux ans. Il m'avait accueilli par une explosion d'amitié. Au seul nom de Dreyfus, il s'est dressé, aigre et violent, me coupant la parole, refusant la dis-cussion, »e démenant comme si j'étais venu lui chercher une querelle person-nelle, j'ai été péniblement impression-né; mais je venais pour parler, et j'ai dit tout ce que je voulais dire, tout ce que j'avais patiemment recueilli, véri-fié, tout ce dont j'étais sûr. Il marchait à travers son cabinet, les bras croisés, fai-sant craquer le vernis de ses bottes, mais silencieux, désarmé par la précision de mes renseignements. Enfin il est revenu s'asseoir, et, le plus calmement qu'il a pu, il m'a posé des questions sur l'état de l'opinion au Sénat, dans le monde des savants, des professeurs, autour de moi. Il avait l'air d'hésiter encore, de vouloir dénombrer ses adversaires avant de prendre un parti. Je lui ai saisi la main, je l'ai supplié, au nom de notre amitié, au nom de la justice: « Il est temps encore... Le scandale est immi-nent, mais il n'a pas éclaté. Vous pou-vez le conjurer en prenant les devants: que l'initiative de la revision vienne de l'armée, et tout est sauvé. On a le droit de se tromper, mais il faut savoir recon-naître librement son erreur, et la réparer. .. » Je me heurtais à un silence vague-ment inquiet, mais têtu, glacial.

Brusquement il s'est levé, il a mis un tiers entre nous; et il m'a congédié poliment, sans un mot d'éclaircissement, ni d'espoir...

Son visage se crispe. Un temps.

LUCE. — Alors, Barois, je suis revenu, tout doucement, à pied, en suivant la Seine. (Avec angoisse.) Et pendant un long moment, mon cher, je me suis demandé... si ce n'était pas lui qui avait raison...

Barois ébauche un geste de surprise.

LUCE (levant la main, et la laissant retomber avec découragement). — J'ai si nettement entrevu ce que sera cette affaire, du jour où notre doute sur la culpabilité de Dreyfus sera public!

BAROIS (vivement). — Ce sera sa réhabilitation!

LUCE. — Soit. Mais ne nous leurrons pas. Ce sera autre chose encore autre chose surtout.

(Avec lourdeur.) Ce sera, mon ami, *la lutte du bon droit contre la société française...* Une lutte acharnée, et psut-être, en un sens, criminelle?...

BAROIS (violemment). — Oh, comment pouvez-vous...

LUCE (interrompant). — Ecoutez-moi... Si Dreyfus est innocent, ce qui est certain... (Scrupuleux.) — ou à peu près certain... — sur qui retombe faute?

Qui vient prendre sa place d'accusé? C'est l'Etat-Major de l'armée française.

BAROIS. — Eh bien?

LUCE. — Et derrière l'Etat-Major, c'est le gouvernement actuel de la République, c'est-à-dire l'ordre établi, auquel nous devons notre vie nationale depuis vingt-cinq ans...

Barois se tait. Un temps.

LUCE. — Je n'oublierai jamais, Barois, ce retour le long des quais... Devant moi, ce dilemme terrible: connaître la vérité et fermer les yeux; se résigner au respect d'un jugement inique, parce qu'il a été rendu, solennellement, par l'armée et par le gouvernement, avec — il faut bien le dire — l'approbation passionnée de l'opinion. Ou bien attaquer, preuves en mains, l'erreur judiciaire, déchaîner le scandale, et, délibérément, comme un révolutionnaire, assaillir de front cet ensemble sacré: l'ordre constitué de la nation!

Barois médite quelques secondes; puis un brusque sursaut des épaules.

BAROIS. — Il n'y a pas à hésiter!

LUCE (avec simplicité). — J'ai hésité cependant. Je n'ai pas pu faire si vite bon marché de cette paix relative dans laquelle nous vivons depuis tant d'années.

(Regardant Barois avec attention.) Je comprends votre révolte, qui ne prend rien autre en considération, que la justice. Pourtant, laissez-moi vous le dire, Barois, nos attitudes ne peuvent pas être tout à fait les mêmes: dans votre ardeur à prendre parti, il y a... comme un sentiment privé... Je ne crois pas me tromper. .. Il y a comme une satisfaction personnelle, comme une revanche, enfin...

BAROIS (souriant). — C'est vrai, vous avez raison... Oui, j'ai eu plaisir à me placer ouvertement de l'autre côté de la barricade... (Sérieux.) Car il n'y a pas de doute, notre adversaire d'aujourd'hui, c'est bien mon adversaire d'autrefois: la routine, l'autocratisme, l'indifférence pour tout ce qui est élevé et sincère! Ah, vraie ou illusoire, que notre conviction est plus belle!

LUCE. — Je vous comprends bien. Mais ne me reprochez pas d'hésiter, au moment où il va falloir exposer tant de laideurs aux yeux de tous, aux yeux des étrangers...

Barois ne répond pas; son regard et son sourire semblent dire: « Je vous admire de toute mon âme; que parlez-vous de reproche?... »

LUCE (sans lever la tête). — Cette semaine, Barois, j'ai passé par une crise de conscience terrible... J'ai été balloté entre mille sentiments contraires... (Douloureusement.) Jusqu'à me laisser émouvoir par mon intérêt propre...Oui, mon cher, j'ai fait le compte de ce que je risque,comme individu, si je parle, si j'attache ce monstrueux grelot... et j'ai eu un vilain frisson...

EAROIS. — Vous exagérez.

LUCE. — Non. Il y a beaucoup de chances, vu l'état de l'opinion, pour qu'en quelques mois je sois irrémédiablement coulé J'ai neuf enfants mon ami...

Barois ne proteste plus.

LUCE. — Vous voyez, vous êtes de mon avis...

(D'une voix chaude.) Et pourtant, les circonstances sont telles que je ne peux pas me dérober, sans faillir à la direction même de ma vie. J'ai aimé la vérité par-dessus tout, et avec elle la justice, qui en est la réalisation pratique. J'ai toujours eu cette conviction, cent fois contrôlée par les faits, que le devoir indiscutable et le seul bonheur qui ne déçoive pas, c'est de tendre vers la vérité de toutes ses forces, et d'y conformer aveuglément sa conduite: tôt ou tard, malgré les apparences, on s'aperçoit que c'était la bonne voie. (Lentement.) Il faut que chacun de nous consente à sa vie: et la mienne m'interdit de me taire. Ah, jamais je n'ai si clairement compris que, si le travail de tous permet à quelques-uns de vivre dans le recueillement, et si ces efforts solitaires sont nécessaires, puisque, bout à bout, ils forment le progrès, — en revanche, ce privilège ne va pas sans créer des obligations intransgressibles! Il faut les reconnaître, lorsqu'elles se présentent: en voici une!

Barois approuve d'une simple inclinaison de tête.

Luce se lève.

LUCE. — Je ne veux pas me poser en redresseur de torts. Je veux seulement que mon cri d'alarme avertisse le gouvernement, et provoque dans l'opinion un revirement de conscience qui s'impose. Après quoi, je suis résolu à livrer mon enquête telle quelle, comme un outil de travail, — et à m'effacer. Vous me comprenez? (Avec une expression de souffrance réelle.) Simplement rejeter ce doute qui m'étouffe!

Si Dreyfus est coupable, — et je le souhaite encore de toutes mes forces — qu'on le prouve, en débats publics: nous nous inclinerons. Mais avant tout, que l'on dissipe cet air irrespirable!

Il s'avance pesamment jusqu'à la fenêtre ouverte, et baigne son regard dans les fraîcheurs vertes du jardin.

Quelques instants passent.

Il se retourne vers Barois, comme s'il se souvenait tout à coup du but de sa convocation; et, familièrement, il lui met ses deux mains sur les épaules.

LUCE. — Barois, j'ai besoin d'un organe où lancer cet appel à la loyauté... (Hésitant.) Consentiriez-vous à jeter votre *Semeur* dans la mêlée?

Une telle fierté relève le visage de Barois, que Luce se hâte de parler.

LUCE. — Non, non, écoutez-moi, mon ami. Il faut réfléchir.

Voilà deux ans que, pour créer cette revue, vous vous êtes donné, sans restriction. Votre *Semeur* est en plein élan. Eh bien, s'il devient mon porte-voix, tout est compromis; c'est la faillite probable de tous vos efforts...

BaroiVs'est dressé, trop bouleversé pour répondre. Une joie soudaine, un orgueil immense... V

Ils se regardent. Luce,a compris! Autour d'eux l'atmosphère s'alourdit. Dans le silence où bat leur double cœur, ils ouvrent les bras et s'étreignent.

C'est le commencement des exaltations surhumaines...

'

Huit jours plus tard.

Dans la cour de la maison qu'habite Barois, rue Jacob.

Au fond d'une remise ouverte, Woldsmuth et quelques acolytes, sont assis à une table. Breil-Zoeger, Harbaroux, Cresteil, Portal, vont et viennent. 4çJ

Derrière eux. en piles blanches, 80. 000 numéros du *Semeur* sont entassés. Odeur humide de l'impression fraîche.

D'autres ballots, cordés, sont prêts pour la province.

Le long des murs, une centaine de tnmardeurs attendent en file indienne, comme à l'entrée d'une soupe populaire.

Trois heures.

La distribution commence.

Barois griffonne des chiffres sur un registre.

Les placards disparaissent, par blocs de 300, sous l'aisselle des coureurs, qui s'enfuient aussitôt vers la rue, sur leurs savates molles.

Déjà les premiers sont hors de la zone où ils doivent se taire, et, boulevard Saint-Germain, rue des Saints-Pères, sur les quais, les cris éclatent: une clameur rauque, dispersée par cent bouches haletantes:

— Numéro spécial!... « LE SEMEUR »!... Révélation sur l'affaire Dreyfus!.. . « CONSCIENCE », lettre au peuple français, de MAP.C-EL1E LUCE, sénateur, membre de l'Institut, professeur au Collège de France...

Les passants se retournent, s'arrêtent. Les boutiques béent. Des enfants courent. Des mains se tendent.

Un vent d'orage semble éparpiller les feuilles.

En deux heures, le vol des papillons blancs s'est abattu jusque dans les quartiers extrêmes, sur la chaussée, sur les tables, au fond des poches.

Les aboyeurs reviennent, assoiffés, les bras vides.

La cour s'emplit à nouveau. Le vin coule.

Les dernières piles sont entamées, épuisées, emportées.

L'essaim bourdonnant s'échappe une seconde fois, secouant,

dans le soir d'été, la torpeur de la ville chaude.

La foule s'exalte. Les boulevards grouillent.

Veillée de guerre...

Déjà, en mille endroits, des pensées françaises, soulevées par cette vague d'héroïsme, s'entrechoquent.

Jne irrésistible explosion de passions a ébranlé le cœur nocI turne de Paris.

## LA TOURMENTE

### I

Les nouveaux bureaux du *Semeur* rue de l'Université.

Quatre fenêtres, à l'entresol, portant, fixés aux appuis, de larges plaques de tôle, où se lit, en majuscules noires sur fond blanc: « LE SEMEUR ».

Petit appartement de cinq pièces.

Dans les deux premières, des scribes, des employés, un vaet-vient commercial. La troisième, plus vaste, sert de salle de rédaction. Sur la cour, le cabinet de Barois et une chambre où travaille la sténographe.

Le 17 janvier 1898. Cinq heures du soir

La salle de rédaction: une grande table, semée d'encriers et de buvards; au mur, un exemplaire déployé de Y *Aurore* du 13: « *J'accuse...* », et deux affiches, imprimées par Roll, reproduisant en caractères gras, la péroraison de la lettre de Zola.

Conversation bruyante: Barois, Harbaroux, Cresteil, BreilZoeger, Portal, et d'autres collaborateurs.

— Cavaignac a affirmé que Dreyfus avait fait des aveux, le matin de la dégradation.

— C'est faux!

— Pourtant je suis sûr qu'il est de bonne foi...

— On lui a persuadé qu'il y a un témoignage contemporain

— D'ailleurs, il ne dit pas qu'il a vu le document!

BAROIS. — Comment! Il existerait, depuis 1894, un témoignage aussi accablant, dont la publication suffirait à annuler, d'un coup, tout le branlebas, — et depuis quatre ans personne n'aurait pensé à le produire?

Cresteil. — Ça saute aux yeux!

BAROIS. — Voici les faits, tels qu'ils se sont passés...

Le silence s'établit aussitôt.

BAROIS. — Je les tiens de Luce dont l'enquête est sérieuse. Vous allez voir comme tout cela est simple.

Dreyfus s'est trouvé, le matin de la dégradation, une heure de suite avec Lebrun-Renault, capitaine de la garde républicaine. Il a protesté de son innocence avec la dernière énergie. Il a même annoncé qu'il allait la crier publiquement, si bien que le capitaine, inquiet d'un scandale possible, a cru devoir prévenir le colonel.

Ensuite Dreyfus a raconté une nouvelle épreuve, analogue à celle de la dictée, qu'il avait eu à subir quelques jours auparavant: le ministre, espérant toujours obtenir une certitude qui allégerait sa responsabilité personnelle, lui avait envoyé dans sa cellule le commandant du Paty de Clam, pour lui demander « *si ce n'était pas par patriotisme qu'il aurait proposé des documents à l'Allemagne* » dans le but de s'en procurer d'autres plus importants, — ce qui eût atténué sa faute et motivé un adoucissement de peine. Lebrun-Renault ne connaissait naturellement pas cette démarche. Dreyfus, qui attendait de minute en minute le commencement du supplice, était dans un état de surexcitation facile à imaginer, et parlait fébrilement sans beaucoup de suite. On comprend très bien comment ses paroles ont pu être mal comprises, mal rapportées, dénaturées en passant de bouche en bouche, et comment a pu naître l'histoire d'un échange de documents avec l'étranger.

Quant à Lebrun-Renault il n'a jamais parlé d'aveux, à cette époque. Le général Darras a fait demander, le matin même, après la dégradation, s'il n'y avait pas eu d'incident particulier; on lui a répondu que non, et il en a aussitôt rendu compte au ministre. De même, le rapport que Lebrun-Renault a fait, sa mission accomplie, au Gouverneur de Paris, — rapport que Luce a vu, — porte la mention: « Rien à *signaler.* »

Pensez-vous que s'il avait recueilli un aveu, sous quelque forme que ce fût, il ne se serait pas hâté de le dire? Et quand le ministre de la guerre a appris, le lendemain, les bruits vagues qui couraient dans la presse, est-ce que, s'ils avaient été le moins du monde fondés, il ne s'en serait pas préoccupé? Est-ce qu'il n'aurait pas tout de suite ordonné une enquête, afin d'avoir ce témoignage décisif? Est-ce qu'il n'aurait pas cherché à presser de nouveau Dreyfus, afin d'avoir des détails complémentaires, et afin de savoir, — question essentielle pour la sécurité nationale, — quels étaient exactement les documents livrés à la puissance étrangère?

Non, vraiment, plus on y réfléchit et plus apparaît l'irréalité de cette histoire des aveux!

CRESTEIL. — "Vous devriez publier une interview de Luce sur ce sujet.

Barois. — Il trouve que ce n'est pas encore le moment. Il attend la déposition de Casimir-Périer, au procès Zola.

JULIA Woldsmuth (paraissant à la porte). — On demande M. Barois à l'appareil.

Il se lève et sort.

ZOEGER. — Quoi qu'il en soit, j'estime que l'attitude de Cavaignac est très heureuse pour nous.

PORTAL. — Heureuse pour nous?

ZOEGER. — Evidemment. Voilà un ancien ministre de la Guerre, qui, devant la Chambre, en pleine tribune, est venu affirmer solennellement qu'il

existe une pièce décisive, d'après laquelle la culpabilité de Dreyfus ne peut pas être mise en doute. Eh bien, le jour où il sera publiquement démontré que c'est faux, que la pièce en question n'existe pas, ou que, si elle existe, c'est un document refait après coup pour les besoins de la cause et antidaté, — ce jour-là, l'opinion du pays sera fortement ébranlée! J'en fais mon affaire. Ou alors c'est qu'on nous aura changé la France!

CRESTEIL (tristement). — Vous n'avez jamais rien dit de si vrai...

PORTAL. — Tout ça va être discuté au procès Zola.

"-Rentrée de Barois.

BAROIS (assez troublé). — C'est Woldsmuth qui me téléphonait... Il vient d'apprendre qu'il est question de limiter la plainte contre Zola, en ne relevant que ses imputations relatives au conseil de guerre de 1894, et en négligeant les autres. Je me demande dans quel but...

PORTAL (se levant). — C'est très important!

CRESTEIL. — Mais ils n'en ont pas le droit!

PORTAL. — Je vous demande pardon.

CRESTEIL. — En quoi cela modifierait-il...?

BAROIS. — Laissez Portal s'expliquer.

PORTAL. — Ce serait très grave. Le gouvernement cherche par tous les moyens possibles, à entraver le développement de cette affaire. Or il y a un article de loi, formel, d'après lequel l'accusé ne peut fournir d'autres preuves que celles des faits articulés et qualifiés *dans la citation.* Autrement dit, en restreignant les termes de l'assignation, on circonscrit à volonté l'extension des débats.

CRESTEIL. — Avec ce procédé, on pourrait arriver à réduire la défense de Zola à presque rien!

PORTAL. — Mais parfaitement!

BAROIS. — C'est monstrueux... C'est un étranglement du procès

CRESTEIL (indigné) — Ce sont des finasseries de procureur!

PORTAL. — C'est la loi.

Consternation générale.

Zoeger (posément). — Pour ma part

je n'y crois pas. Les accusations sont trop outrageantes pour être escamotées. Impossible de ne pas poursuivre celui qui a écrit et publié ça!

Il s'approche du tableau où s'étale, en gros caractères, la lettre de Zola. (Lisant.) « J'accuse le lieutenant-colonel du Paty de Clam d'avoir été l'ouvrier diabolique de l'erreur judiciaire... 1 » ... « J'accuse le général Mercier de s'être rendu complice...!»,... « J'accuse le général Billot d'avoir eu entre les mains les preuves certaines de l'innocence de Dreyfus et de les avoir étouffées...! » ... « J'accuse le général de Boîsdeffre...! » ... « J'accuse le général de Pellieux...! » ... « Enquête scélérate! » ... « Enquête de la plus monstrueuse partialité...! »... « J'accuse les bureaux de la Guerre d'avoir mené dans la presse... une campagne abominable, pour égarer l'opinion et couvrir leur faute... » CRESTEIL. — Et le défi de la fin: ... « En portant ces accusations, je n'ignore pas que je me mets sous le coup des articles 30 et 31 de la loi, etc..

« Je n'ai qu'une passion, celle de la lumière, au nom de l'humanité qui a tant souffert et qui a droit au bonheur. Ma protestation enflammée n'est que le cri de mon âme. Qu'on ose donc me traduire en Cour d'Assises, et que l'enquête ait lieu au grand jour! ».

« J'attends! (l) »

BAROIS. — Et vous croyez qu'un gouvernement peut avaler ça, sans broncher?

PORTAL. — En tout cas, Barois, il y aurait intérêt, avant que la citation ne soit rédigée, à dénoncer publiquement la supercherie

ZOEGER. — Il faudrait que ton article éclate comme un pétard, demain à la première heure.

BAROIS. — Je vais m'y mettre. — Portal, voulez-vous me rechercher le texte exact de cette loi dont vous parlez?

PORTAL. '— Puis-je téléphoner à la bibliothèque du Palais?

BAROIS (ouvrant la porte). — Mademoiselle Julia?

PORTAL. — C'est pour moi, Mademoiselle. Voudriez-vous me demander le 889-21?

BAROIS (se dirigeant vers son bureau). — Je Vous laisse... Serez-vous ce soir boulevard Saint-Michel?

DIVERSES VOIX. — Oui...

BAROIS. — Je vous apporterai mon travail avant de le porter à Roll. Nous le reverrons ensemble. A ce soir... *i* (i) L'Aurore (13 janvier 1898). *Lettre ouverte d'Emile Zola au Président de la République* : « *J'accuse...* 1

Une heure plus tard.

La salle de rédaction est vide. Les employés sont partis. Le garçon de bureau balaye, en attendant l'heure de la fermeture.

Barois travaille dans son cabinet.

Brusquement, la porte s'ouvre: Julia blême, le visage angoissé; et, en même temps qu'elle, par la porte ouverte, une rumeur étrange.

IULIA. — Monsieur Barois... une émeute... Vous entendez...

Barois, surpris, gagne les pièces qui donnent sur la rue. Il ouvre une fenêtre et se penche dans la nuit. Un murmure confus.

La flamme jaune d'un réverbère, toute proche, l'aveugle. Ses yeux s'habituent peu à peu à l'obscurité: devant lui, la chaussée est encore déserte; mais, là-bas, entre les façades d'ombre, coule une masse noire qui bourdonne.

Il s'apprête à descendre, par curiosité. Le brouhaha se rapproche; des chants; quelques cris:

« Dreyfus!... »

Le groupe isolé qui dirige la colonne n'est plus qu'à cinquante mètres de la maison. Barois aperçoit des visages et des bras levés vers lui.

— Conspuez le *Semeur* ! Conspuez Barois! Conspuez!

Il recule précipitamment. BAROIS. — Les volets! Vite!

Il aide le garçon, affolé.

Au moment où il va barricader la dernière croisée, une canne, lancée dans les carreaux, le couvre de débris de verre.

La foule est sous les fenêtres, à quatre ou cinq mètres de lui. Il distingue le timbre différent des voix.

— *Le Semeur* ! Vendu! Traître! A mort!

Des pierres, des bâtons, font sauter les vitres en éclat, et frappent le bois des volets.

Il reste planté au milieu de la pièce, l'oreille tendue:

— Mort à Zola! Mort à Dreyfus!

Dans la pénombre, il devine Julia, debout, immobile. Il la pousse vers son cabinet.

BAROIS. — Demandez le numéro du commissariat...

Les projectiles doivent être épuisés. Les vociférations redoublent de violence, rythmées par les piétinements:

— Mort à Luce! Mort aux traîtres!

— Mort à Barois! Vendus!

BAROIS (très pâle, au garçon). — Verrouillez la porte, et gardez le vestibule!

Il se dirige vers son cabinet, ouvre un tiroir et prend un revolver.

Puis il rejoint le garçon

BAROIS (rage froide). — Le premier qui ose entrei, je le tue comme un chien.

Sonnerie du téléphone

BAROIS (à l'appareil). — Allo!le commissaire? Bien... Je suis le Directeur du *Semeur*. Il y a une émeute, rue de l'Université, sous mes fenêtres.. Ah, déjà? Bon, merci...

Je ne sais pas; mille, quinze cents peut-être...

Le tapage continue: martèlement cadencé des semelles sur le pavé, dominé par une sorte de rugissement, d'où se détachenl. en notes plus aigues, des cris:

— Mort à Dreyfus! Mort à Zola! Mort aux vendus!

Subitement la clameur hésite, et cesse. Quelques instants de tumulte confus: on-devine l'intervention des agents.

Puis des cris éclatent, isolés, interrompus, de moins en moins distincts.

Le piétinement s'éloigne.

L'émeute est dispersée

Barois tourne un commutateur et aperçoit Julia, tout contre lui, debout, appuyée à une table.

Elle est tellement enlaidie par l'émotion, qu'il la fixe une seconde, pour la reconnaître: les traits crispés, le teint de plomb, le visage vieilli, durci, farouche, avec une expression bestiale et passionnée... L'instinct à nu... Quelque chose de sensuel, d'effroyablement sensuel...

Il pense: « Voilà son masque, dans l'amour... »

Le regard qu'il lui jette est brutal et pénétrant comme un viol: et elle le reçoit, comme une femelle consentante.

Puis, détente nerveuse, elle s'abat sur un siège en sanglotant.

Il quitte la pièce, sans prononcer un mot. Ses mains tremblent d'énervement. Il ouvre les volets.

La rue est calme, à peine plus animée qu'à l'ordinaire, si ce n'est, aux fenêtres et aux balcons, par des groupes de curieux.

Sous les réverbères brisés, dont le vent couche et tord les flammes, les agents font les cent pas.

LE GARÇON. — Monsieur, c'est le concierge avec le Commissaire, pour les constatations...

Il 17 février 1898.

Au Palais de Justice: la Cour d'Assises, 10 journée du procès Zola.

L'audience est suspendue.

Salle comble. Une foule tassée, grouillante, bavarde, gesticulant sur place. Un semis d'uniformes, d'aiguillettes dorées, parmi des toilettes de femmes. On se montre des têtes connues: généraux de l'État-Major, actrices en vedette, journalistes comédiens, députés. Le barrage noir des avocats sépare cette houle chatoyante du prétoire vide, que domine le Christ mélodramatique de Bonnat.

Une atmosphère acre, étouffante, que traverse et secoue par instants une onde brusque de sympathie ou de haine, violente comme un courant électrique.

Dans les premiers rangs de l'auditoire, un groupe attentif, parlant bas: Hàrbaroux, Barois, Breil-Zoeger, Cresteil d'Allize, Woldsmuth; et parmi ces hommes, la silhouette sibylline de Julia.

Trois heures.

Un remous profond, venu des portes, soulève la foule. Un flot neuf d'arrivants s'insinue dans les moindres interstices du fmblic massé; des étudiants à bérets, des avocats en robe, escaadant les hautes cloisons de l'enceinte réservée, se juchent en grappes, sur la crête des portants, sur l'entablement des fenêtres.

Luce, patiemment, s'enfonce à son

tour dans la cohue, qui murmure avec hostilité son nom, et parvient à gagner la place que Barois lui a réservée près de lui.

£tluce (bas, à Barois). — Je viens de là-bas... ça va être rude. La majorité du jury penche pour l'acquittement. A l'État-Major, ils s'en rendent compte, ils sont très alarmés... Ils vont essayer de frapper un grand coup, aujourd'hui ou demain...

Un brusque silence, qui ne se prolonge pas: l'entrée de la Cour.

L'hémicycle se peuple: les magistrats, en robe rouge; les jurés, deux par deux, d'une gravité endimanchée de cortège municipal.

Emile Zola s'assied au banc des accusés, près du gérant de l'Aurore; derrière eux, les avocats: M Labori, Albert et Georges Clémenceau, entourés de leurs secrétaires.

Un sourd grondement ébranle la salle.

Zola et Labori se penchent vers la droite, où vient de retentir un coup de sifflet. Zola a les deux mains jointes sur le pommeau de sa canne, et les jambes croisées; sa face de hérisson, plissée de rides, est soucieuse; à chaque mouvement de sa physionomie, le lorgnon brille, aiguisant la vivacité des prunelles. Il parcourt lentement des yeux cette multitude qui le hait, et son regard s'attarde, se repose un instant sur le groupe du *Semeur*.

Dans l'allée centrale, un uniforme s'avance. Des voix murmurent: — « Pellieux... Pellieux... »

A pas décidés, le général se dirige vers la barre des témoins et s'arrête militairement.

BAROIS (à Luce). — Voilà... C'est Pellieux qu'ils lancent à l'assaut!

L'émotion de la salle est si bruyante, que le général se retourne, d'un geste impatient, et la toise, imposant tout à coup, par son visage martial, par sa prestance de grand seigneur, par l'indiscutable autorité de toute sa personne, un silence, qui, d'ailleurs, est de courte durée.

Le Président, gros homme à figure ronde, dont les lèvres rasées, entre les favoris, sont minces et closes, fait un mouvement de colère; mais il est impuissant à rétablir le calme.

Dans le brouhaha, qui peu à peu s'éteint, on distingue la voix nette du général articulant certains mots:

« —... Les termes stricts de la légalité... l'affaire Dreyfus... Je demande à parler... (i) ».

(i) La suite des débats reproduit scrupuleusement le compte-rendu sténographique de la 10 audience. (Le Procès Zola. *Compte-rendu stérwg. in-extenso. Paris, Stock.* 1898. *Tome II, pages* 118 *à* 125.)

DES VOIX. — Chut! chut!

M. LE GÉNÉRAL DE PELLIEUX. —... « Je répéterai le mot si typique du colonel Henry: « On veut de la lumière? Allons-y! »

Son timbre métallique, provoquant, sonne dans la vaste enceinte, devenue enfin silencieuse et immobile.

M. LE GÉNÉRAL DE PELLIEUX. — « Au moment de l'interpellation Castelin, il s'est produit un fait que je tiens à signaler. On a eu, au ministère de la Guerre, — et remarquez que je ne parle pas de l'affaire Dreyfus, — la preuve absolue de la culpabilité de Dreyfus, absolue! et cette preuve, je l'ai vue! »

Il s'est tourné vers les jurés, puis vers la défense, puis vers le public. Un sourire de défi anime son masque dur d'escrimeur.

M. LE GÉNÉRAL DE PELLIEUX. — « Au moment de cette interpellation, il est arrivé au Ministère de la Guerre un papier dont l'origine ne peut être contestée, et qui dit — je vous dirai ce qu'il y a dedans: — « Il va se produire une interpellation sur l'affaire, Dreyfus. Ne dites jamais les relations que nous avons eues avec ce juif. »

« Et, Messieurs, la note est signée! Elle n'est pas signée d'un nom connu, mais elle est appuyée d'une carte de visite, et, au dos de cette carte de visite, il y a un rendez-vous insignifiant, signé d'un nom de convention, qui est le même que celui qui est porté sur la pièce, et la carte de visite porte le nom de la personne... »

Une légère pause.

L'auditoire a eu un bref frémissement, et il demeure haletant, considé-

rant tour à tour le tribunal, le témoin, Zola qui n'a pu réprimer un mouvement d'indignation, et les jurés, sur la figure banale desquels il y a comme un bien-être, une impression de soulagement.

M. LE GÉNÉRAL DE PELLIEUX (d'une voix triomphante qui claironne). — « Eh bien! Messieurs, on a cherché la revision du procès par une voie détournée; je viens vous donner ce fait. Je l'affirme sur mon honneur! Et j'en appelle à M. le général de Boisdeffre pour appuyer ma déposition.

« Voilà ce que je voulais dire 1 »

V

Un trépignement général, prolongé, au-dessus duquel crépite un tonnerre d'applaudissements.

Luce reste les bras croisés, très pâle, son large front penché en avant, les yeux tristement levés vers le prétoire. Ses amis échan gent des regards violents, chargés de révolte; mais ils demeurent abattus, immobilisés par ce coup de massue que rien ne faisait prévoir.

BREIL-ZOËGER (à mi-voix). — C'est un faux!

Barois (avec un haut-le-corps). — Parbleu! (Il montre du doigt un groupe d'officiers, sanglés dans leurs dolmens, levant leurs mains gantées de blanc pour applaudir frénétiquement.) Mais essaye donc de leur faire admettre ça!

Labori s'est dressé, de toute sa stature d'athlète, offrant aux coups son poitrail de lutteur. On n'entend pas ce qu'il dit. Il semble donner de son front bas contre un mur. Sa bouche est ouverte, toute ronde. Avec des gestes véhéments il s'adresse au Président qui paraît vouloir lui couper la parole.

Enfin, dans une accalmie, on distingue une interruption du Président, lancée d'une voix tranchante i

M. LE PRÉsident, — « Mais, maître Labori...»

M LABORI (exaspéré). — « Oh, Monsieur le Président...»

M. LE PRÉSIDENT (avec hauteur). — Le témoin vient de parler. Avezvous une question à poser? »

M LABORI. — « Permettez, Monsieur le Président, ici...»

Le timbre cuivré du général de Pellieux domine le colloque, — cinglant comme Un coup de cravache.

M. LE GÉNÉRAL De PELLIEUX. — « Je demande que l'on appelle M. le général de Boisdeffre! »

M LABORI (d'une voix tonnante, qui impose enfin le silence). — « Je demande, Monsieur le Président, et aujourd'hui l'incident sê présente avec une gravité telle que la défense ne peut pas ne pas insister, — que la parole me soit donnée un moment, non pas seulement pour répondre à M. le général de Pellieux — encore qu'on ne réponde pas à une affirmation, — mais pour tirer immédiatement, au point de vue de l'affaire, la cotiséquence nécessaire qui se dégage des paroles de M. le général de Pellieux.

« Je vous demande la permission, Monsieur le Président, de dire deux mots. »

M. LE PRESIDENT (acerbe). — « Deux mots seulement-..

M LABORI. — « Deux mots seulement. »

M. LE PRÉSIDENT. — « A moins que vous n'ayez une question à poser? »

M LABORI (éclatant). — « Comment aurais-je des questions à poser, en réponse à un fait absolument nouveau qui est jeté dans le débat? J'en ai une cependant, et c'est à cette question que je vais arriver. »

M. LE GÉNÉRAL DE PELLIEUX. — « Vous avez jeté dans le débat un fait nouveau, en lisant un acte d'accusation de M. le commandant d'Ormescheville, qui était du huis-clos. »

M LABORI (triomphant). — « Nous avançons, nous avançons! »

M. LE GÉNÉRAL GONSE. — « Je demande la parole. »

M. LE PRÉSIDENT. — « Tout à l'heure, général. »

M LABORI. — « Je dis simplement ceci: Il vient de se produire à la barre un fait d'une gravité exceptionnelle; c'est un point sur lequel nous sommes tous d'accord. M. le général de Pellieux n'a pas parlé de l'affaire Dreyfus, il a parlé d'un fait postérieur à l'affaire Dreyfus; il n'est pas possible que ce fait ne soit pas discuté ici, ou ailleurs, dans une autre enceinte. Après une pareille chose, il ne s'agit plus de restreindre ni de rétrécir un débat d'assises. Que M. le général de Pellieux me permette, très respectueusement, de lui faire observer, qu'il n'est pas une pièce, quelle qu'elle soit, qui ait une valeur quelconque, et qui, scientifiquement, constitue une preuve, avant qu'elle ait été contradictoirement discutée. Qu'il me permette d'ajouter que nous sommes maintenant dans cette affaire, — qui, quoi qu'on veuille et quoi qu'on fasse, prend des proportions d'une affaire d'État, — en présence de deux pièces ou de deux dossiers également graves l'un et l'autre, parce qu'ils sont secrets: un dossier secret, qui a été l'instrument de la condamnation de Dreyfus en 1894, sans contradiction, sans discussion, sans défense; un second dossier secret, cpii sert depuis des semaines à empêcher qu'on apporte ici autre chose que des affirmations. » Une pause.

« Quelque respect que j'aie pour la parole de soldat de M. le général de Pellieux, je ne puis accorder la moindre importance à cette pièce. »

Un tollé furieux éclate dans la salle; des ricanements soufflètent l'avocat.

M LABORI (faisant face à la tourmente, et, d'une voix violente, implacable, articulant tous les mots). — « Tant que nous ne la connaîtrons pas, tant que nous ne l'aurons pas discutée, tant qu'elle n'aura pas été publiquement connue, elle ne comptera pas! Et c'est au nom du droit éternel, au nom des principes que tout le monde a vénérés depuis les temps les plus reculés et depuis que la civilisation existe, que je prononce ces paroles! »

Une légère oscillation du public. L'opinion hésite. Plusieurs « Très bien! » se font entendre.

M LABORI (plus calme). — « Par conséquent, j'arrive à un point qui, maintenant, est d'une précision telle, que ma tranquillité à tous les points de vue augmente. Je n'ai, en ce qui me concerne, qu'une préoccupation dans cette affaire: c'est celle de l'obscurité constante, c'est celle de l'angoisse publique augmentant tous les jours, grâce à des ténèbres qui s'épaississent quotidiennement, je ne dis pas par des mensonges, mais je dis par des équivoques.

« Que Dreyfus soit coupable ou innocent. qu'Esterhazy soit coupable ou innocent, ce sont là sans doute des questions de la plus haute gravité. Nous pouvons, les uns et les autres, M. le général de Pellieux, M. le Ministre de la Guerre, M. le général Gonse, moi-même, avoir là-dessus des convictions, et nous pourrons y persévérer éternellement, si l'éclaircissement complet, si la lumière absolue n'est pas faite.

« Mais ce qu'il est indispensable d'éviter, c'est que l'émotion du pays augmente et se perpétue.

« Eh bien! maintenant, sans que le huis-clos puisse être invoqué, sans que les arrêts de la Cour puissent être mis en avant, nous avons un moyen d'arriver à la lumière, à la lumière partielle.:. (Avec un grand éclat.) « Car, quoiqu'il advienne, la revision du procès Dreyfus s'imposera! »

Violentes manifestations. Des cris éclatent: « Non! non! —. La patrie avant tout! »

Labori se redresse, d'un bond, face au public. Son regard est méprisant et brutal. Son poing de reître s'abat sur les dossiers ouverts devant lui.

M LABORI. — « Les protestations de la foule marquent bien qu'elle ne comprend pas la gravité de ce débat, au point de vue éternel de la civilisation et de l'humanité! »

Tumulte.

Quelques applaudissements, restreints et nourris. Labori se détourne et attend, les bras croisés, que le calme soit rétabli.

M LABORI (continuant). — « Si Dreyfus est coupable, et si la parole de ces généraux, que je crois de bonne foi — et c'est ce qui m'émeut, — si la parole de ces généraux est fondée, si elle se justifie en fait et en droit, ils en feront la preuve dans un jugement contradictoire. S'ils se trompent, au contraire, eh bien!ce sont les autres qui feront leur preuve. Et, voyez-vous, quand la lumière sera absolue, quand toutes les ténèbres seront dissipées, il y aura peut-être dans la France un ou deux hommes qui sont les coupables, qui seront responsables de tout le mal. Qu'ils soient d'un côté ou de l'autre, on les connaîtra, on les flétrira! Et puis, nous nous remettrons tranquillement à nos travaux de paix ou de guerre, Monsieur le général; car la guerre, n'est-il pas vrai, ce n'est pas quand on a des généraux à la barre, des généraux qui sont dignes de parler au nom de l'armée qu'ils commandent, ce n'est point à ce moment-là que personne la redoute; et ce n'est pas par la menace d'une guerre, qui n'est pas prochaine, quoi qu'on en dise, qu'on intimidera Messieurs les jurés!

« Je termine par une question. Vous voyez. Monsieur le Président, que e tendais à quelque chose de précis, et ici je vous remercie de m'avoir laissé la parole; je rends hommage à votre bienveillance, à votre courtoisie, à votre sentiment de la gravité de la situation.

« La question. Monsieur le Président, la voici: que M. le général de Pellieux s'explique sans réserve; et, la pièce, qu'on l'apporte ici!»

Un silence anxieux.

Mouvements d'émotion au banc des jurés, dont les yeux se dirigent vers le général de Pellieux.

Court silence.

M. LE PRÉSIDENT. — « M. le général Gonse, qu'est-ce que vous avez à dire?»

Le général Gonse se lève et s'approche du général de Pellieux, qui lui cède sa place à la barre.

Une physionomie soucieuse; un regard terne, mais agressif; une voix qui paraît étrangement molle après celle du général de Pellieux et celle de Labori.

M. LE GÉNÉRAL GONSE. — « Monsieur le Président, je confirme complètement la déposition que vient de faire le général de Pellieux.

« Le général de Pellieux a pris l'initiative, il a bien fait; je l'aurais prise à sa place pour éviter toute équivoque. L'armée ne craint pas du tout la lumière, elle ne craint pas du tout, pour sauver son honneur, de dire où est la vérité. »

Labori fait un geste d'assentiment et de confiance.

Des applaudissements.

M. LE GÉNÉRAL GONSE (avec lourdeur). — « Mais il faut de la prudence, et je ne crois pas qu'on puisse apporter publiquement ici des preuves de cette nature, qui existent, qui sont réelles, et qui sont absolues. »

Ces restrictions inattendues provoquent une houleuse inquiétude. Quelques murmures désapprobateurs. La majorité hésite, cherchant le vent.

M Clémenceau se lève posément.

M CLÉMENCEAU. — « Monsieur le Président, je vous demande la parole. »

Mais le général de Pellieux bondit à la barre, qu'il saisit fébrilement à deux mains, et son ton cassant domine tout.

M. LE GÉNÉRAL DE PELLIEUX. — « Messieurs, je demande à ajouter un mot! »

Le Président, d'un geste, donne la parole au général.

M Clémenceau se rassied.

M. LE GÉNÉRAL DE PELLIEUX. — « M Labori a parlé tout à l'heure de la revision, toujours à propos de la communication de cette pièce secrète au conseil de Guerre. On n'a pas apporté la preuve de cette communication... »

Cette fois l'assertion est si mal défendable, — après l'émouvante comparution de M Salle, à qui le Président a dû défendre de dire ce qu'il savait, et après la déposition formelle de M Demange,

— que la salle n'ose plus manifester, favorisant par un silence irrésolu les tonitruantes protestations des amis de Dreyfus.

Le général de Pellieux, surpris de cet accueil, hésite.

M. LE GÉNÉRAL DE PELLIEUX. — « Je ne sais pas...-»

Des ricanements l'interrompent.

Il fait un brusque demi-tour, offrant au public l'honnêteté de son visage rude, et, au fond des yeux caves, la franchise d'un regard hautain, habitué à d'autres horizons.

D'une voix sans réplique, d'une voix d'officier qui sait arrêter net une mutinerie de troupes, il cingle toutes les faces souriantes

M. LE GÉNÉRAL DE PELLIEUX. — « Je demande à ne pas être interrompu par des ricanements! »

Il reste quelques secondes impassible, immobilisant la foule sous son regard.

Puis, froidement, il se retourne vers le tribunal.

M. LE GÉNÉRAL DE PELLIEUX. — « Je ne sais pas si l'on a écouté avec suffisamment d'attention la déposition qu'a faite l'autre jour le colonel Henry. Le colonel Henry a fait remarquer que le colonel Sandherr lui avait remis un dossier secret; que ce dossier secret avait été scellé avant la séance du conseil de guerre, et qu'il n'avait jamais été ouvert. J'appelle l'attention de MM. les jlirés là-dessus.

« Maintenant, quant à la revision du procès Dreyfus sur cette pièce, qu'est-ce qu'il faut? la preuve... »

M. LE PRÉSIDENT. — « Nous n'avons pas à nous occuper de la revision. Cela ne peut pas se faire ici. »

M. LE GÉNÉRAL DE PELLIEUX. — « On ne parle que de cela... »

M. LE PRÉSIDENT. — « Je sais bien, mais elle ne peut pas se faire à l'audience d'une côUf d'assises, vous le savez. »

M. LE GÉNÉRAL DE PELLIEUX. —« Je m'incline. Je m'incline et j'ai dit.

M. LE PRÉSIDENT (s'adressant à M. le général GoHse). — « Vous n'avez plus rien à dire, général? »

M. LE GÉNÉRAL GONSE. — « Non, Monsieur le Président.

M. LE GÉNÉRAL DE PELLIEUX. — « Je demande qu'on appelle le général de Boisdeffre pour confirmer mes paroles. »

M. LE PRÉSIDENT. — « Voulez-vous lui faire dire de venir demain? »

Sans répondre, le général tourne à demi la tête vers la salle, et, par dessus l'épaule, à la cantonade, en chef qui a le droit de se faire servir à tout instant, il interpelle son officier d'ordonnance.

M. LE GÉNÉRAL DE PELLIEUX. — « Commandant Ducassé! Voulez-vous aller chercher le général de Boisdeffre, en voiture, — tout de suite! »

Il est l'Armée elle-même.

Son attitude implacable en impose à tous, à ses adversaires, à ses juges; la foule, subjuguée, hurle de joie, comme un chien qui vient d'être battu.

M CLÉMENCEAU (se levant). — « Monsieur le Président, j'aurais à répondre quelques mots aux observations de M. le général de Pellieux. »

Il s'arrête, interrompu une fois encore par le général.

Et, debout, d'aplomb sur les jambes, il suit, de cet œil vif et à peine ironique qui anime son visage plat de levantin, une courte joute entre Labori et le général de Pellieux, relative à la publication de l'acte d'accusation de 1894.

Labori, drapé dans les plis de sa robe, les bras dressés laissant voir la chemise jusqu'au coude, semble jtter l'anathème.

M LABORI. — « M. le général de Pellieux fait appeler ici M. le général de Boisdeffre: il a raison!

« Mais ce qu'il faut bien qu'on sache, et vous verrez qu'avant quarantehuit heures mes paroles se révéleront prophétiques, c'est qu'il ne sera pas possible d'arrêter le débat avec les paroles de M. le général de Pellieux, ni avec celles de M. le général de Boisdeffre. Ce ne sont pas des paroles d'hommes, quels qu'ils soient, qui donneront de la valeui à ces pièces secrètes. Ces pièces, il faudra, ou que l'on n'en parle pas, ou qu'on les montre; c'est pourquoi je dis à M. le général de Pellieux: « Apportez les pièces, ou n'en parlez plus!»

M Clémenceau lève tranquillement la main vers le Président

M CLÉMENCEAU. — « M. le Président, j'ai l'honneur de demander la parole...»

Sa sobre assurance impose, par contraste avec la superbe impétuosité de son confrère.

M CLÉMENCEAU. — «...Le général de Pellieux nous a dit qu'au moment de l'interpellation Castelin on avait eu des preuves *absolues*... Est-ce donc que, jusqu'alors, on n'avait eu que des preuves *relatives* ? »

Courte pause.

Il reste impassible, mais une ombre malicieuse plisse ses paupières bridées.

Zola, toujours appuyé sur sa canne, tourne légèrement la tête, et lui lance un bref sourire d'approbation.

LUCE (à Barois, bas). — Il sait sûrement que la pièce est fausse...

M CLÉMENCEAU (de sa voix paisible). — « Je demande à M. de Pellieux: Comment se fait-il, — car c'est

une question qu'on commence à se poser partout — comment se fait-il que ce soit dans un procès d'assises qu'une parole aussi sérieuse soit prononcée? Comment se fait-il que M. le général Billot, au cours de l'interpellation Castelin, n'ait pas parlé de ces pièces secrètes à la Chambre, et n'ait pas menacé la Chambre de la guerre, et que ce soit à une audience de la Cour d'Assises qu'on vienne prononcer 'es graves paroles que vous avez entendues hier, et que l'on vienne révéler les documents secrets? »

M. LE GÉNÉRAL DE PELLIEUX (agacé). — « Je n'ai pas menacé le pays de la guerre; tout cela, c'est jouer sur les mots. Que M. le général Billot n'ait pas parlé, lors de l'interpellation Castelin, de cette pièce ou d'autres, — car il y en a d'autres, le général de Boisderfre vous le dira, — cela ne me regarde pas; le général Billot fait ce qu'il veut. (S'adressant aux jurés.) « Ce qui est sûr, c'est que M. le général Bllot, à plusieurs reprises, l'a dit à la Chambre: « Dreyfus a été justement et légalement condamné! »

M LABORI (se dressant, prêt à bondir). — Ici, j'interviens pour dire qu'il y a au moins une de ces deux paroles qui est fausse, c'est: « légalement »!

M. LE GÉNÉRAL DE PELLIEUX (provoquant). — « Prouvez-le! »

M LABORI (brutal). — « C'est prouvé. »

M CLÉMENCEAU (plus ccintiliant). — « Nous avons voulu toujours prouver; on nous en a empêchés; et si M. le général de Pellieux veut que je m'explique sur ce point, je suis prêt à le faire. »

M. LE PRÉSIDENT (se hâtant, d'un geste sec). — « C'est inutilè. »

M LABORI (incàpable dé se contenir). — « C'est prouvé par lVI Salle, c'est prouvé par M Demange! C'est prouvé Sar les publications des journaux qu'on n'a pas démentis! C'èst prouvé par M. lë général Mercier, qui n'a pas osé dire en face de moi, le contraire! Je lui avais envoyé par les journaux, la veille, une provocation à laquellè 11 *a* répondu par le silence, à laquelle il a répondu par une distiriction,

qui, à elle toute seule, est une preuve décisive. Car, lorsque j'ai dit: « Le général Mercier a livré Une pièce au Conseil de Guèrrè, et publiquement le général Mercier s'en est vanté partout », M. le général Mercier, jetarit ericore dans le débat (je ne dis pas volontairement, mais peut-être inconsciemment) une équivoque, a répondu: « Ce n'est pas vrai ». Et je lui ai dit: « Qu'est-ce qui n'est pas vrai? Est-ce que c'est: *que vous ne l'avez pas dit partout, ou* est-ce que c'est au contraire: *que vous n'avez pas livré de pièces ?* » Et il a répondu: « *C'est seulement que je ne m'en suis pas vanté partout.* »

« Je dis que pour tout esprit de bonne foi, la preuve est faite. La preuve, c'est que personne, malgré toute l'émotion que l'affaire a jetée dans le pays, personne ne s'est levé pour dire ce que M. de Pellieux ici n'osé pas dire: je l'en défie f »

Une pause, (Souriant.) « Eh bien! moi, je dis que la preuve est faite. »

M. LE GÉNÉRAL DE PELLIEUX (hautain). — « Comment voulez-vous que je vous dise ce qui s'est passé au procès Dreyfus: je n'y étais pas!»

Labori regarde les jurés, puis le tribunal, enfin l'auditoire, comme pour prendre tout le monde à témoin de cette réponse évasive.

Puis il s'incline courtoisement devant le général, avec un sourire triomphant.

M LABORI. — « C'est bien, je vous remercie, mon général. »

M CLÉMENCEAU (intervenant). — « M. le Président, nous avons amené ici un témoin qui tenait de la' bouche d'un des membres du Conseil de Guerre qu'il y avait eu une pièce secrète communiquée aux juges On ne nous a pas permis de l'interrog'ér. »

M LABORI. — « J'ai dans mon dossier deux lettres qui disent la même chose. Et j'ai une lettre, qui est d'un ami du Président de la République*;* ce témoin a déclaré qu'il ne viendrait pas déposer, parce qu'on l'a prévenu, que, s'il racontait le fait, on viendrait dire qu'il est inexact. »

M CLÉMENCEAU. — « Et pourquoi le général Billot ne l'a-t-il pas dit à M. Scheurer-Kestner, quand il est allé le lui demander? Tout cela serait terminé aujourd'hui! »

M. LE PRÉSIDENT (nerveux).— «Vous direz tout cela dans votre plaidoirie.»

M. LE GÉNÉRAL GONSE (s'avançant à nouveau). — « J'ai un mot à dire au sujet de la déposition qui a été faite tout à l'heure, quand n parlé des notes. .« J'ai dit que les notes de l'Etat-Major étaient secrètes: elles sont toujours secrètes; nous ne correspondons dans les bureaux de l'État-Major que par des notes, qui ont toujours le caractère secret. Et, quand on dit: note sur cecj, note sur cela, cela veut cjire: note secrète.

« Maintenant, quand on vient dire que Dreyfus ne connaissait pas ce qui se passait dans les bureaux de l'Etat-Major en septembre 1893, c'est encore une erreur. Dreyfus a passé d'abord six mois.. . »

M. LE PRÉSIDENT (l'interrompant, sans courtoisie). —: « Nous n'avons pas à parler de l'affaire Dreyfus...

(Aux généraux de Pellieux et Gonse.) Vous pouvez vous asseoir, tous 1 es deux. »

Il y a un moment *de* stupeur.
Le Président en profite.

M. LE PRÉSIDENT (à rhuissier-audiencier, sur un ton sans réplique). — Faites venir le témoin suivant 1 »

L'huissier hésite.

Labori s'est dressé ej: se penche, les bras en croix, comme s'il ypulait, de sa personne, faire obstacle à ja suite des débats.

M LABORI. — « M. le Président, il est absolument impossible, après un événement... »

M. LE PRÉSIDENT (sèchement) — Continuons...

M LABORI (indigné). — « Oh, Monsieur le Président, ce n'est pas possible! Vous sentez très bien qu'un pareil incident termine le débat, s'il n'est pas vidé. Nous sommes par conséquent obligés d entendre M. le général de Boisdeffre. »

M LE PRÉSIDENT. — « Nous l'entendrons tout à l'heure.

(A l'huissier-audiencier.) « Faites venir le témoin suivant. »

M LABORI (tenace). — « Permettez, Monsieur le Président... »

M. LE PRÉSIDENT (furieux, à l'huissier-audiencier). — « Appelez le témoin suivant! »

L'huissier sort.

M LABORI. 'rf « M. le Président, je vous demande pardon, je pose dts conclusions tendant au sursis! »

Le commandant Esterhazy paraît, introduit par l'huissier.

M. LE PRÉSIDENT (à Labori). — « Il y sera statué quand Tes témoins auront été entendus!»

Esterhazy s'avance vers la barre. La salle éclate en applaudissements.

Il est voûté, d'une maigreur de tuberculeux, le teint jaunâtre, les pommettes fiévreuses, le regard mobile et brûlant.

Déjà le Président se tourne vers lui, lorsque Labori intervient une dernière fois, avec une énergie exaspérée.

M LABORI. — « Mais je demande à ce qu'il soit sursis à l'audition d'autres témoins, jusqu'à ce que M. le général de Boisdeffre ait été entendu! La Cour ne peut remettre à statuer jusqu'après qu'elle aura entendu d'autres témoins! »

Le Président, indécis, roule des yeux courroucés. Esterhazy, les bras croisés par contenance, attend, inquiet, ne comprenant pas ce qui se passe.

Labon s'est assis, et griffonne ses conclusions.

M. LE PRÉSIDENT (d'un ton dur et insolent). — « Y en a-t-il pour longtemps, à rédiger vos conclusions? »

M LABORI (sans lever la tête, rogue). — « Dix minutes. »
L'audience est suspendue.

Le Président fait signe à l'huissier de reconduire Esterhazy dans la salle des témoins.

L'auditoire énervé, tumultueux, l'acclame jusqu'à ce qu'il ait disparu.

Sans paraître s'apercevoir du tapage, les magistrats se lèvent et quittent gravement le prétoire, suivis des jurés, des accusés, et de la défense.

L'exaspération qui fermentait, à demi retenue par la présence de la Cour, se donne libre carrière.

Dans l'air surchauffé, devenu toxique, se croisent des appels, des commentaires passionnés, des vociférations: un vacarme assourdissant.

Les rédacteurs du *Semeur* se groupent autour de Luce.

Portal, en robe, vient les rejoindre; un pli désabusé attriste son visage honnête, plus blond, plus poupard que jamais sous la toque.

PORTAL (s'asseyant avec lassitude). — Encore une note secrète!

BAROIS. — Qu'est-ce que c'est que cette pièce?

ZOEGER (de sa voix grêle, aux finales blessantes). — Personne, que je sache, n'en a encore entendu parler.

LUCE. — Si, je connaissais son existence. Mais je ne pensais pas qu'on osât jamais s'en servir.

ZOEGER. — De qui est-elle?

LUCE. — Elle est soi-disant écrite par l'attaché militaire italien, et elle a soi-disant été saisie dans le courrier de l'attaché allemand...

BAROIS (vivement). — Elle pue le faux!

LUCE. — Oh, ça, elle est fausse, ce n'est pas douteux. Elle est arrivée au Ministère, je ne sais pas comment, mais avec un à-propos bien étrange... Juste la veille du jour où le ministre devait répondre à la Chambre à la première interpellation relative à l'affaire, et au moment où l'État-Major commençait à se préoccuper de l'incident!

ZOEGER. — Et puis, sa teneur...

JULIA. — Nous ne savons pas ce qu'il y a dedans. Le général a cité de mémoire.

LUCE. — Mais il a affirmé que le nom de Dreyfus était mentionné en toutes lettres. Or, c'est absolument invraisemblable: cela seul suffirait à éveiller les doutes! A l'heure où la presse s'occupait déjà activement de l'affaire, il est inadmissible de supposer que ces deux attachés aient librement parlé de Dreyfus dans leur correspondance privée. En admettant qu'ils aient eu réellement des relations avec Dreyfus, jamais ils n'auraienl commis cette imprudence inutile! surtout après les démentjs officiels donnés à plusieurs reprises, par leurs deux gouvernements!

BAROIS. — Ça saute aux yeux!

PORTAL. — Mais qui donc peut fabriquer de pareilles pièces?

ZOEGER (avec un ricanement impitoyable). — L'Etat-Majpr, parbleu!

HARBAROUX. — C'est une officine nationale de falsifications!

LUCE (posément). — Non, mes amis, non... Là,, je ne vous suis plu:!

Son expression simple et résolue en impose. Seul Zoeger secoue les épaules.

Zqeger. — Pourtant, permettez, les faits...

LUCE (très ferme, s'adressant à tous). — Non, mes amis, non... Mettonsnous en garde... L'Etat-Major n'est pas plus une bande de « faussaires », que nous ne sommes, nous, une bande de « vendus »... Jamais vous ne me ferez admettre que des hommes comme les généraux de Boisdeffre, Gonse, Billot, et les autres, puissent s'entendre pour fabriquer des pièces fausses I

Cresteil d'Allize, l'œil ardent, le sourire amer, le visage tourmenté, suit la querelle en lissant impatiemment sa longue moustache.

CRESTEIL. — A la bonne heure! Moi, j'ai connu le général de Pellieux, autrefois: c'est l'intégrité même.

LUCE. — D'ailleurs, il suffit de l'avoir vu et entendu, pour être certain que ce qu'il affirme, il le croit: son éloquence est indubitablement celle de la sincérité. Et, jusqu'à preuve du contraire, j'estime que les autres généraux sont tous dans le même cas.

CRESTEIL. — On les trompe. Ils sont les premières dupes de ce qu'ils avancent.

ZDEGER (sourire glacial). — Vous leur supposez un aveuglement qui n'est pas vraisemblable.

CRESTEIL (vivement). — Très vraisemblable au contraire! Ah, mon cher, si vous aviez fréquenté de près les officiers...

Tenez, le groupe, là, derrière nous... Regardez-les sans parti-pris.

Une expression d'assurance bornée, soit; ça, c'est l'habitude d'avoir' toujours, de droit, raison devant les hommes... Mais ces visages-là sont honnêtes, foncièrement!

LUCE. — Oui, regardez un peu la salle, Zoeger; c'est très instructif;

Que voulez-vous, ces gens-là ne sont pas accoutumés à des raisonnements subtils... Et, tout à coup, on leur présente un dilemme terrible: il y a un coupable, où est-il? Est-ce le Gouvernement, l'Armée, tous ces chefs qui viennent affirmer, solennellement, en donnant leur parole de soldats, que la condamnation de Dreyfus est juste? Ou bien est-ce ce petit juif inconnu, condamné par sept officiers, et dont on a dit tant de mal depuis trois ans qu'il en reste malgré tout quelque chose dans toutes les mémqires?

ZOEGER (hautain). — Il n est pas difficile de remarquer que l'Etat-Major a reculé, chaque fois qu'il a été mis en demeure d'avancer des preuves précises.

Tput le monde, même un officier, est capable de réfléchir jusque-là.

JULIA. — Et puis, qu'est-ce que peuvent ces paroles d'honneur, lancées à tout propos, contre une argumentation serrée comme celle des mémoires de Lazare, ou des brochures de Duclaux, ou de votre lettre à vous, Monsieur Luce!

ZOEGER. — Ou même, malgré son lyrisme, la lettre de Zola!

BAROIS. — Patience! Nous approchons du but.
(A Luce.) Aujourd'hui, nous avons fait un grand pas en avant!

Luce ne répond pas.

PORTAL. — Vous n'êtes pas exigeant, Barois...

BAROIS. — C'est pourtant très clair. Suivez-moi: le général de Boisdeffre va venir, puisqu'on est allé expressément le chercher. Dès les premiers mots, Labori va l'acculer à une impasse. Il ne pourra pas refuser de verser la pièce aux débats.

Ceci fait, on la discutera, et elle ne résistera pas longtemps à un examen approfondi. Alors l'Etat-Major, convaincu d'avoir apporté un faux à la barre, c'est le revirement immédiat de l'opinion! C'est la revision avant trois mois!

Il parle avec des gestes rapides, d'un ton incisif. Son œil rayonne d'insolence orgueilleuse. Tout son être palpite d'espoir.

LUCE (gagné par cet entrain). — Peut-être.

BAROIS (avec un grand rire clair). — Non, non, ne dites pas: peut-être. Cette fois, je suis certain que nous la tenons!

ZOEGER (cynique, à Barois). — Et si le général de Boisdeffre trouve un biais? Ce ne serait pas la première fois...

BAROIS. — Après ce qui s'est passé? Ce n'est plus possible... Vous avez bien vu que le général Gonse a couvert le général de Pelheux.!

WOLDSMUTH (qui s'était échappé à la suspension d'audience, et qui se glisse de nouveau à sa place). — Voilà des nouvelles... L'audience va reprendre. Le général de Boisdeffre vient d'arriver en voiture!

BAROIS. — Vous l'avez vu?

WOLDSMUTH. — Comme je vous vois. Il est en civil. Un huissier l'attendait sur les marches. Il est entré directement dans la salle des témoins.

JULIA (battant des mains, à Barois). — Vous voyez!

BAROIS (triomphant). — Cette fois, mes amis, pas de reculade possible! C'est la lutte ouverte, et, pour nous, la victoire!

Retour tumultueux des auditeurs et des avocats qui avaient quitté la salle.

La Cour, au milieu du brouhaha, fait sa rentrée; les magistrats, les jurés, s'installent. Les accusés sont introduits.

Labori gagne allègrement son banc, et reste un instant debout, un poing sur la hanche, penché vers Zola qui lui parle en souriant.

Le silence se fait de lui-même.

Les nerfs sont tendus jusqu'à l'exaspération. On sent que cette fois c'est vraiment la bataille décisive

Le Président se lève.

M. LE PRÉSIDENT. — « L'audience est reprise. » (Puis, rapidement, sans se rasseoir.)-« En l'absence de M. le général de Boisdeffre, la Cour remet la suite de l'affaire à demain. » (Un temps.) « L'audience est levée. »

D'abord une incompréhension totale: un instant de stupeur dont la Cour profite pour s'éclipser dignement.

Les jurés n'ont pas bougé. Zola s'est retourné, surpris, vers Labori qui reste adossé à son siège, figé dans une attitude vainement menaçante.

Enfin, tout le monde comprend: la bataille est ajournée, la bataille n'aura pas lieu...

Un hurlement de déception, signal d'un indescriptible désordre. Le public, debout, tape des pieds, hue, siffle, vocifère.

Puis, lorsque le prétoire est vide, il se rue frénétiquement vers les portes.

En quelques minutes la sortie est bouchée; des femmes, pressées dans la cohue, s'évanouissent; les visages sont en sueur; les yeux hagards: une véritable scène de panique.

Le *Semeur* est resté à sa place, consterné.

JULIA. — Les lâches!

ZOEGER. — Parbleu! Ils veulent attendre les ordres!

LUCE (tristement, à Barois). — Vous voyez? Ils sont les plus forts..

BAROIS (au comble de la rage). — Oh, mais cette fois,-ça ne se passera pas sans scandale! Je tiens mon article dp demain. C'est trop de cynisme, a la fin! Qui berne-t-on? Quand la Chambre s'émeut, quand elle force les IVJinjstres responsables à s'expljquer ouvertement, pour de bon, on lui repond: « Pas ici. Allez au Palais de Justice, vous saurez tout. » — Et puis, au Palais, toutes les fois qu'on veut remuer le fppd de ces débats obscurs, toutes les fois que la vérité monte péniblement jusqu'à la surface et sernble vpujoir sortir enfin, on la repousse du pies), on Ja renfonce dans son marécage: « La question ne sera pas posée!»

Ah, non! il faut que ça finisse! il faut que le pays comprenne à quel point on se fout de lui!

Sourde rumeur venue du vestibule.

WOLDSMUTH. — Il va y avoir du grabuge. Cpurons-y

CRESTEIL. — Par où passef?

BAROIS. — Par Jà! (A Julja.) Suivez-moi...

ZOEGER (enjambant les gradins). — Non, par là...

Barois (criant). — Rendez-vous autour de Zola, comme hier!

Ils s'éphappent comme ils peuvent de la salje des assises.

Un tumulte révolutionnaire ébranle les voûtes du Palais et se prolonge dans les galeries sonores, mal éclairées, grouillantes de monde.

Des gardes municipaux, en file, l'œil effaré, s'efforcent en vain de maintenir leur ligne de barrage. Des bandes se poussent, je heurtent, s'entremêlent dans la pénombre.

i Mille cris sè croisent:

— Misérables! Brigands! Traîtres!

— Vive Pellieux!

— Vive l'Armée!

— A bas les juifs!

Au moment où Baroi's et Luce rejoignent le groupe de Zola et de ses défenseurs, un remous, venu de loin, rompant le cordon de police, les écrase contre le mur.

Ba'rois essaye de protéger Julia.

Portal, qui connaît les aîtres, ouvre précipitamment la porte d'un vestiaire. Zola et ses fidèles s'y engouffrent.

Zola est adossé à un pilastre, nu-tête, très pâle, sans lorgnon, les paupières à demi plissées sur ses yeux fureteurs de myope, les lèvres serréès. Ses regards vont et viennent. Il aperçoit Luce, puis Barois, ét leur tend la main, brusquement, sans un mot.

Enfin les agents ont fait une trouée.

Le Préfet de police apparaît, dirigeant en personne le service d'ordre,

La petite phalange repart. Zoeger, Harbaroux, Woldsmuth, Cresteil, viennent se joindre à eux.

Par un détour, sous la conduite du Préfet, ils atteignent le grand escalier du boulevard du Palais.

Une foule compacte a envahi la Cour et les rues: tout le quartier, jusqu'aux murs.de l'Hôtel-Dieu, appartient aux manifestants: mouvante masse grise dans cette fin de journée d'hiver, que les réverbères pointillent déjà de halos jaunes.

Des cris, des hu'èès, des injures inintelligibles, coupées de sifflets stridents. Une clameur ininterrompue, que martèle comme un refrain: « A mort!... A mort!,.. »

Au seuil des marches, Zola, les traits crispés, se penche vers les siens.

— Les cannibales..

Puis, le cœur défaillant, mais d'un pied ferme, il descend les degrés, appuyé sur le bras d'un ami.

Un espace libre a pu être ménagé au bas du perron: sa voiture attend, enca-

drée de gardes à cheval.

Il veut se retourner, serrer quelques mains. Mais les hurlements redoublent...

— A l'eau!... A mort le traître!... A la Seine!...

— Mort à Zola!

Le Préfet de police, très nerveux, hâte le départ.

L'attelage démarre, au petit trot.

Des projectiles s'abattent, pulvérisant les vitres des portières. Des cris âpres, sanguinaires, poursuivent, comme une meute qu'on lance à la curée, le landeau qui disparaît dans le crépuscule.

Luce (la gorge serrée, à Barois). — Un peu de sang frais, et ce serait le massacre...

Le commandant Esterhazy paraît, suivi d'un général; on les acclame jusqu'à leur voiture.

Bientôt le cordon des agents est rompu. Barois essaye d'entraîner Julia et Luce; mais la foule est dense.

Les amis de Zola sont reconnus et conspués.

— Reinach!... Luce!.. Bruneau!... Mort aux traîtres!... Vive l'Armée!...

Des bandes sillonnent comme des courants, le flot des curieux" monômes d'étudiants, files de malandrins, conduits par des jeunes gens du Faubourg.

Sur tous les chapeaux, en exergue, comme un numéro de conscrit, s'étale une feuille qu'on distribue par milliers dans les rues:

RÉPONSE DE TOUS LES FRANÇAIS

A EMILE ZOLA

MERDE!..

Des officiers, en uniformes, se frayent un chemin au milieu des applaudissements.

Des isolés, qui ont le nez juif, sont pris, entourés et mal- menés par des gamins frénétiques, qui dansent autour d'eux des rondes de sauvages, en brandissant des torches en flammes, faites avec des *Aurores* roulées; l'effet est lugubre dans la nuit commençante.

Au coin du quai, Julia, Barois et Luce s'arrêtent pour attendre les autres.

Tout à coup, une jeune femme, élégamment mise, se précipite vers eux. Ils s'effacent, la croyant poursuivie, prêts à la protéger. Mais, en un clin d'œil, elle a foncé sur Luce, s'est accrochée à son vêtement, et lui a arraché sa rosette.

LA FEMME (s'enfuyant). — Vieille fripouille!

Luce la suit des yeux, avec un sourire navré.

Une heure plus tard

Luce, Barois, Julia, Breil-Zoeger et Cresteil, longent à petits pas, la grille du jardin de l'Infante.

La nuit est tout à fait venue. Un brouillard pluvieux mouille les épaules.

Barois passe familièrement son bras sous celui de Luce, qui marche, silencieux.

BAROIS. — Qu'est-ce qu'il y a, voyons? Du courage... Rien n'est perdu.

Il rit.

Luce le dévisage, à la lueur d'un bec de gaz: les traits de Barois reflètent une joie de vivre, une confiance, une activité sans bornes: c'est un accumulateur vivant.

LUCE (à Zoeger et à Julia). — Regardez-le: il dégage des étincelles... (Avec lassitude.) Ah, je vous envie, Barois. Moi, je ne peux plus, j'en ai assez. La France est comme une femme saoûie': elle ne voit plus clair, elle ne sait plus ce qui est vrai, elle ne sait plus où est la justice. Non, elle est tombée trop bas, c'est décourageant....

BAROIS (d'une voix timbrée, qui fouette les énergies). — Mais non! Avez-vous entendu ces cris, avez-vous vu cette foule en délire? Une nation qui est encore capable d'une telle effervescence pour des idée?, n'a pas déchu.

CRESTEIL. — Il a raison, le bougre!

ZOEGER. — Mais oui, parbleu! Il y a du tirage, c'est entendu: mais qui s'en étonnerait? C'est peut-être la première fois que la morale intervient dans la politique. Ça ne peut pas aller tout seul.'

BAROIS. — C'est une espèce de coup d'État...

LUCE (grave). — Oui, j'en ai l'impression depuis ie premier jour: nous assistons à une révolution.

ZOEGER (rectifiant). — Nous la *faisons*!

BAROIS (glorieusement). — Et comme toutes les révolutions, c'est une

minorité qui en prend l'initiative, et qui l'accomplit toute seule, à coup de - passion, à coup de volonté, à coup de persévérance!

Ah, c'est une belle vie, sacredié, qu'une lutte pareille!

Luce secoue la tête, évasivement.

Julia, spontanément, se rapproche de Barois et se pend à son bras; il ne semble pas s'en apercevoir.

BAROIS (avec un grand éclat de rire, jeune et crâne). — Oui, je l'accorde, la réalité, en ce moment surtout, est laide, féroce, injuste, inconerentê.: mais quoi! c'est d'elle pourtant que la beauté finale jaillira un jour!

(A Luce.) Vous me l'avez répété cent fois: le mensonge, tôt ou tard, trouve son châtiment dans la vie elle-même. Eh bien, je crois à la force inéluctable de la vérité!Et si, ce soir, la partie est perdue encore une fois, courage!

J_Nous la gagnerons peut-être au prochain tour!

III 31 Août 1898.

Paris: léthargique et dépeuplé.

Le café du boulevard Saint-Michel. Neuf heures du soir.

Le groupe du *Semeur* est réuni à l'entresol.

Devant les fenêtres, qui béent sur la nuit chaude, le store de la terrasse, fait, au premier plan une surface inclinée, transparente de lumière. Au delà, le quartier latin, nocturne et désert.

Des tramways, illuminés et vides, gravissent la pente du boulevard en grinçant sur leurs rails.

Barois a déballé devant lui sa serviette bourrée de paperasses. Les autres, en cercle autour de lui, piquent au tas, feuilletant brochures et journaux.

PORTAL (à Cresteil). — Vous avez des nouvelles de Luce?

Portal revient de sa Lorraine, où il a fait son séjour annuel.

CRESTEIL. — Oui, je l'ai vu dimanche, il m'a fait pitié: il a beaucoup vieilli depuis trois mois.

BAROIS. — Vous savez qu'on l'a prié — oh, très courtoisement — de renoncer à son cour du Collège de France, pour la rentrée? Il y a eu, à la fin de juin, trop de tapage autour de ses leçons. D'ailleurs tout le monde lui tourne le

dos: aux dernières séances du Sénat, ils n'étaient guère qu'une dizaine à lui serrer la main.

PORTAL. — Quelle incroyable incompréhension générale I

HARBARQUX (grimaçant la haine). — C'est la presse nationaliste qui est cause de tout. Ces gens-là ne laissent pas un instant l'opinion reprendre haleine, se ressaisir!

BAROIS. — Au contraire: ils refoulent systématiquement toute la générosité inhérente à notre race, tout ce qui avait jusqu'à présent placé la Fiance, à ses risques et gloire, en tête de la civilisation, sous prétexte de condamner l'anarchie et l'antimilitarisme, qu'ils ont la mauvaise foi de confondre avec les instincts les plus élémentaires de justice et de bonté!

Et tout le monde s'y est laissé prendre!

WOLDSMUTH (secouant sa tête de caniche, aux yeux tendres). — On obtient toujours ce qu'on veut d'un peuple, quand on sait l'exciter contre les juifs...

CRESTEIL. — Ce qui m'étonne, dans cette approbation commune, c'est que leur thèse est stupide; il suffit d'un minimum de bon sens pour l'anéantir: « L'Affaire Dreyfus est une immense machination montée par les Juifs... »

BAROIS. — Comme si une aussi prodigieuse aventure pouvait avoir été prévue, organisée de pied en cap...

CRESTEIL. — On leur objecte: « Mais, si Esterhazy était l'auteur du bordereau? » Ils ne se troublent pas pour si peu: « Eh bien, c'est que les Juifs l'auraient acheté d'avance et lui auraient fait adopter, à s'y méprendre, l'écriture de Dreyfus... »

C'est d'une insoutenable puérilité...

ZOEGER. — Le mal vient aussi de ce qu'on a compliqué l'Affaire à l'infini. Cette folie d'enquêtes et de contr'enquêtes, a complètement dénaturé sa véritable origine et son sens réel. On s'est lancé passionnément sur cent pistes adjacentes, contradictoires... Ce qu'il faudrait, maintenant, c'est un coup de théâtre, qui chavire net l'opinion, et la ramène à une vue d'ensemble.

CRESTEIL. — Oui: un coup de

théâtre...

BAROIS. — Nous en approchons peut-être avec cette histoire de Haute-Cour... (Tirant un papier de sa poche.) Tenez, j'ai encore reçu ça, ce matin... (Souriant.) Un anonyme plein d'attention...

HARBAROUX (qui a pris la feuille, lisant).

— « Je tiens de source sûre que le Ministre de la Guerre a proposé ce matin aux membres du Gouvernement de tiaduire les chefs du parti revisionniste devant la Haute-Cour.

« Votre nom est sur la liste, à côté de celui de M. Luce... »

BAEOIS. — C'est très flatteur.
HARBAROUX (lisant).

— « L'arrestation générale est fixée au 2 septembre, à la première heure.

« Vous avez le temps d'être loin. » Signé : « Un ami. »

BAROIS (riant à pleines dents). — Hein? Ça fouette le sang, au réveil, des petits billets de ce calibre!

ZOECER. — C'est ton article de samedi qui te vaut ça.

PORTAL. — Je ne l'ai pas lu... (A Cresteil.) De quoi s'agissait-il?

CRESTEIL. — De la fameuse séance de la Chambre, où, naïvement, le Ministre de la Guerre a cru sortir de son portefeuille cinq documents révélateurs, et n'a produit, en réalité, que cinq pièces fausse! Barois a magistralement établi pourquoi ces documents ne peuvent pas être authentiques...

Le gérant entr'ouvre la porte.

LE GÉRANT. — Monsieur Barois, il y a là un monsieur qui voudrait vous parler.

Barois le suit.

Au bas de l'escalier il aperçoit Luce.
BAROIS. — Vous, à cette heure? Qu'est-ce qu'il y a?

LUCE. — Du nouveau.
BAROIS. — La Haute-Cour?
1UCE. — Non... Qui avez-vous là-haut?

BAROIS. — Rien que le *Semeur.*
LUCE. — Alors, montons
En voyant entrer Luce, ils se dressent tous, d'un seul mouvement anxieux.

Luce, silencieusement, serre les mains tendues et s'assied avec une involontaire lassitude; le visage maigri, tiré, fait saillir plus volumineuse encore, la masse du front.

LUCE. — Je viens de recevoir des nouvelles... qui sont graves.

Ils se groupent autour de lui.

LUCE. — Hier ou avant-hier, il s'est passé, un drame imprévu au Ministère de la Guerre: le lieutenant-colonel Henry a été soupçonné par ses propres chefs, d'avoir falsifié les pièces du procès!

Une stupeur profonde.

LUjCE. — U y a eu aussitôt un interrogatoire d'Henry par le Ministre. Art-il avoué? Je n'en *suis* rien. — En tous cas, il est depuis hier soir.,, écrpué ai» Mont Valérien,

BAROIS. — Écroué? Henry?

Une sourde explosion de joie; quelques secondes d'exaltation enivrante.

ZOEGER (d'une voix étouffée). — Nouvelle enquête! Nouveaux débats!
BAROIS. — C'est la révision!

HARBAROUX (précis). — Mais... quelles pièces aurait-il falsifiées?

LUCE. — La lettre de l'attaché militaire italien, qui contenait, en toutes lettres, le nom de Dreyfus,

Barois. — Quoi? La fameuse preuve du général de Pellieux î

ZOEGER. — Celle que le Ministre a lue, il y a six semaines, en pleine tribune!

LUCE. — Fabriquée entièrement, — sauf l'en-tête et la signature, qui auraient été prises à une lettre insignifiante,

BAROIS (exultant). — Ah, ce serait trop beau (

WOLDSMUTH (en écho). — Oui... trop beau!... Je n'ai pas confiance.

LUCE. — Ce n'est pas tout. Si l'affaire s'engage sur cette voie, il y aura bien d'autres points à éclaircir 1

Qui a inventé l'histoire des aveux de Dreyfus? Pourquoi n'en a-t-il jamais été question avant 96, c'est-à-dire deux ans après la dégradation?

Qui a gratté et récrit l'adresse d'Esterhazy sur le petit bleu dénonciateur, pour pouvoir affirmer que Picquart cherchait à innocenter Dreyfus et accusait Esterhazy, à l'aide d'une pièce re-

touchée par lui?

WOLDSMUTH 0 yeux pleins de larmes). — Ce serait trop beau.., Je n'ai pas confiance...

LUCE. — En tous cas, l'arrestation a déjà des suites très importantes: Boisdeffre, Pellieux, Zurlinden démissionnent. Et il paraît que le Ministre lui-même va rendre son porte feuille.

Je le comprends, d'ailleurs: après avoir lu le faux, à la tribune, en toute bonne foi...

BAROIS (riant). — Mais c'est eux qu'il faut faire comparaître en Haute-Cour, à notre place!

LUCE. — D'autre part, Brisson est complètement retourné.

PORTAL. — Ah! enfin!

BAROIS. — Je l'ai toujours dit: le jour où un républicain de vieille race, comme Brisson, aura les yeux ouverts, il fera la revision, à lui seul 1

WOLDSMUTH. — Ce qui doit le ronger, c'est d'avoir fait tirer à un million d'exemplaires le faux Henry, pour l'afficher sur tous les murs de France...

HARBAROUX (ricanant). — Ah, ah, ah!... C'est vrai! Elle est sur toutes nos mairies! Elle est dans toutes les mémoires! Elle est citée avec attendrissement, ehaque jour, par toute là presse nationaliste! Ah, ah, ah!...

Et tout s'écroule d'un coup: là pièce est fausse!

PORTAL. — Sauve qui peut!

WOLDSMUTH (soudain taciturne). —Prenez garde. Je n'ai pas confiance...
BAROIS (riant). — Ah non, cette fois, Woldsmuth vous allez trop loio dans le pessimisme! Le Gouvernement n'a évidemment pas décidé l'arrestation d'Henry à la légère. Pour qu'on n'ait pas pu étouffer l'affaire, il faut que vraiment la vérité éclate avec une force irrésistible.

WOLDSMUTH (doucement). — Mais Henry n'est même pas en prison.4

BAROIS. — Comment?

LUCE. — Je vous dis qu'il est au Mont-Valérien!

CRESTEIL (les traits bouleversés, tout à coup). — Mais sacredié, Woldsmuth a raison! Il n'est qu'aux arrêts: sans quoi c'est au Cherche-Midi qu'il serait!

Ils se regardent, atterrés.

Les nerfs sont tellement tendus qu'un brusque abattement succède à leur triomphe.

LUCE (navré). — Ils ont peut-être voulu se réserver le temps de chercher un biais...

CRESTEIL. —...de façon à pouvoir traiter la falsification comme un simple manquement à la discipline..

PORTAL. — Ils vont nous échapper encore une fois, vous verrez!..:

WOLDSMUTH (secouant la tête). — Oui, oui... je n'ai pas confiance...

BAROIS (nerveux). — Taisez-vous donc, Woldsmuth! (Energique.) C'est à nous, maintenant, à faire assez de bruit autour de l'incident, pour qu'on ne puisse pas l'escamoter...

LUCE — Ah, si seulement Henry avait avoué, devant des témoins!

Une rumeur confuse rampe le long du boulevard Sont-ce des crieurs qui glapissent la dernière heure?

Malgré le silence désert, leurs abois se mêlent, lointains et inintelligibles.

PORTAL. — Chut! On dirait:... « Le colonel Henry... »

LUCE — Est-ce que la nouvelle s'ébruiterait déjà?

Ils se sont portés, d'un mouvement unanime, vers les fenêtres ouvertes, et, le corps penché, l'oreille tendue, ils écoutent, avec une soudaine angoisse.

ZOEGER (à la porte). — Garçon! Les journaux... vite!

Mais déjà Woldsmuth "s'est élancé dehors.

Les cris s'éloignent, par une rue transversale.

Quelques minutes s'écoulent.

Enfin Woldsmuth, hors d'haleine, échevelé, l'œil brillant, surgit au haut de l'escalier, brandissant une feuille d'où jaillit, en manchette énorme: SUICIDE. DU COLONEL HENRY
AU MONT-VALÉRIEN

BAROIS (rugissant). — Le voilà, l'aveu!

Il se tourne vers Luce, et tous deux, le cœur bondissant, s'étreignent, sans un mot.

PORTAL, ZOEGER, CRESTEIL (allongeant le bras vers Woldsmuth). — Donnez!

Mais tous se taisent.

Woldsmuth a tendu le journal à Luce, qui, très pâle, assujettissant son lorgnon d'un geste saccadé, s'avance sous le lustre. L'émotion alourdit sa voix.

LUCE (lisant). — « Hier soir, dans le cabinet du Ministre de la Guerre... le lieutenant-colonel Henry a été reconnu l'auteur de la lettre, datée d'octobre 1896... où le nom de Dreyfus est cité en toutes lettres.

« Le Ministre... a ordonné immédiatement l'arrestation du lieutenantcolonel Henry... qui, dès hier soir, a été conduit... à la forteresse du Mont-Valérien...

24ê j E À!N fc À R 0 I S

« Aujourd'hui.. lé planton chargé dè faire le service du lieutenantcolorie!., ayant pénétré dans sa cellule... à six heures du soir... l'a trouvé... étendu sur son lit... dans une mare de sang... Son rasoir à la main... et la gorge ouverte... en deux endroits... La mort... remontait à plusieurs heures...

« Le faussaire s'était fait justice... »

Le journal lui tombe des doigts.

Ils se l'arrachent; il passe de main en main: tous veulent avoir vu. /On cri sauvage de triomphe, un long hurlement, un véritable délire.rj LUCfc (la gorge serrée). — Henry mort, c'est fini: il y a des choses de l'affaire que personne ne saura jamais...

Ses paroles se perdent dans l'ivresse générale. Seul, Zoeger, qui a entendu, approuve d'un triste signe de tête.

Woldsmuth, à l'écart, incliné sur l'appui de la fenêtre, pleure silencieusement de joie, dans la nuit tiède.

Un an plus tard: le 6 août. 1899, veille de l'ouverture des débats de Rennes.

Dimanche après midi.
Aux bureaux du Semeur-.

Barois, seul, en manches de chemise, les mains aux poches, arpente son cabinet, préparant un article.
il est soUs-bressioh: Soft visage exalté-, zébré de tics, ses regards mobile, la joie de soft defni-SoUrire, toute sa personne enfin, rayonne dê sécurité triomphante.

Les mauvais jours sont passés.

Barois. Entre!
Ah.iWoldsmuth?.. Entrez, entrez...

Woldsmuth s'avance, tout menu dans son cache-poussière, la sacoche en bandoulière, une volumineuse serviette sous lê? bras»

BAROIS. — Qu'est-ce que vous êtes donc devenu depuis l'autre jour?

WOLDSMUTH (s'asseyant sur le premier siège rencontré). — J'arrive d'Allemagne.

BAROIS (sans surprise). — Vraiment?

(Un temps. Je comptais bien d'ailleurs vous voir ce soir, pour vous remettre là direction, comme c est convenu

WOLDSMUTH. — Vous prenez tous le rapide de nuit?

BAROIS, — Non, moi seul. Les autres sont déjà à Rennes depuis ce matin... Lucè avait à faire, ils l'ont accompagné.

WOLDSMUTH. — Quand dépose-t-il?

BAROIS. — Pas avant la 5 ou 6 audience...

Je suis resté pour vous passer la main et puis pour faire un dernier article, qui paraîtra demain.

WOLDSMUTH (vivement). — Ah, il y aura encore un numéro demain?

Barois, prenant cet intérêt pour de la curiosité, ramasse sur le bureau quelques feuilles volantes.

BAROIS. — Oh, presque rien, quelques lignes pour saluer l'ouverture des débats... Tenez, voilà ce que j'étais en train d'écrire:

« Nous touchons au but. Le cauchemar s'achève. Le dénouement, le verdict, n'intéresse plus; il est prévu, fatal comme le triomphe de l'équité.

« Il ne nous reste plus, aujourd'hui, que le souvenir d'avoir vécu un drame historique, à nul autre comparable; un drame à milliers de personnages, joué sur la scène du monde, et d'un intérêt si pathétique et si universel, que toute la nation, puis autour d'elle toute la civilisation, est venue y prend e part. Pour la dernière fois sans doute, l'humanité, divisée en deux masses inégales, s'est heurtée de front: — d'un côté, l'autorité, qui n'accepte le contrôle d'aucun raisonnement; — de l'autre, l'esprit d'examen, superbement dédaigneux de toutes précautions sociales.

« D'un côté, le passé, — de l'autre, l'avenir!

« Les générations futures diront « l'Affaire », de même que nous disions: « la Révolution »; et elles salueront, comme une coïncidence merveilleuse ce hasard qui donne à l'Ere nouvelle un millésime nouveau.

« Quel siècle, celui qu'inauguie une pareille victoire! »

Un simple coup de clairon, vous voyez...

Woldsmuth le considère avec stupeur.

Quelques secondes passent. Il approche timidement sa chaise.

WOLDSMUTH. — Dites-moi, Barois... Vous êtes donc pleinement rassuré?

BAROIS (soumnt). — Oh, pleinement!

WOLDSMUTH (affermissant sa voix). — Moi pas! Je n'ai pas confiance.

Barois, qui va et vient d'un air avantageux, s'arrête, surpris.

BAROIS (haussant les épaules). — Vous nous avez toujours répété ça.

WOLDSMUTH (vivement). — Jusqu'ici, je crois que...

BARoIS. — Mais tout est changé! Nous voici avec un gouvernement neuf, bien convaincu de l'innocence, et qui s'est donné pour mission de faire la lumière. Les débats, cette fois, seront publics, sans escamotage possible. Voyons!... Douter du verdict, dans de telles conditions, ce serait supposer la culpabilité de Dreyfus!

Il rit: un rire énergique et sans arrière-pensée; le rire du bon sens et de la certitude.

Woldsmuth le regarde silencieusement. Dans son masque poilu, poussiéreux, les yeux brillent, patients, tenaces.

WOLDSMUTH (affectueusement). — Asseyez-vous donc, Barois... Je vous parle sérieusement. Je vois beaucoup de monde, moi, vous savez... (Les yeux mi-clos, sur un ton voilé, traînant, indéfinissable)... je me renseigne...

BAROIS (brusque). — Moi aussi.

WOLDSMUTH (conciliant). — Eh bien, alors, vous avez remarqué... Hein? Leur presse!Tous les faux ont été démasqués, toutes les illégalités étalées au grand jour... N'importe, elle ne désarme pas! Il faut bien qu'elle renonce à ses affirmations, mais elle se venge: elle salit indistinctement tous ses adversaires. .. Le rapport de Ballot-Beaupré, qui résume si loyalement toute l'Affaire, croyez-vous seulement que leurs journaux l'aient publié? C'est l'enquête d'un « vendu », qui a touché les millions juifs, comme Duclaux, comme Anatole France, comme Zola...

BAROIS. — Et puis après? Quels sont les lecteurs qui s'y laissent prendre?

Pour toute réponse, Woldsmuth sort de sa poche un paquet de journaux nationalistes, et les jette sur la table.

BAROIS (agacé). — Ça ne prouve rien. Je vous répliquerai que, depuis deux mois, le *Semeur* a encaissé près de 3.000 abonnements nouveaux; vous le savez comme moi.

Un grand souffle de justice et de bonté passe, enfin, sur la France.

WOLDSMUTH (remuant tristement la tête). — Ce soufflera n'a pas effleuré les conseils de guerre...

BAROIS (après réflexion). — Soit. J'admets que les juges, parce qu'ils sont de braves militaires, aient d'avance une forte présomptiôh Contre les revisionnistes. Mais réfléchissez à ceci: l'Europe entière a les yeux fixés sur Rehneâ. Toute la civilisation juge avec eux. (Se levant.) Eh bien, il y a des situations qui obligent; ces messieurs Seront bien forcés de reconnaître que toutes les anciennes charges qui pesaient contre Dreyfus s'évanoUissent à l'examen, (Riant.) — et qu'il n'y en â pas de nouvelles!

WOLDSMUTH. — Ça dépend.

Barois enfonce les mains dans ses poches et reprend ses allées et Venues en haussant les épaules. Mais le ton résolu de Wolds muth l'intrigue: il vient se camper devant lui.

BAROIS. — Ça dépend de quoi?

Woldsmuth sourit péniblement.

WOLDSMUTH. — Asseyez-vous, Barois; vous avez l'air d'un' fauve en cage...

Barois, les sourcils froncés, regagne son bureau.

WOLDSMUTH. — Vous Vous rappelez l'histoire des pièces ultra-secrètes? (Geste de Barois.) Laissez-moi m'expliquer...

L'hypothèse est la suivante: On aurait volé à Berlin des lettres du Kaiser à Dreyfus et des lettres de Dreyfus au Kaiser... (Souriant.) Je n'insiste pas sur 1 enormité de cette supposition...

D'après cette légende, le véritable bordereau aurait été Une de ces lettres, écrite par Dreyfus sur papier ordinaire, et que l'Empereur aurait annoté de sa main dans les marges. Guillaume II s'apercevant du vol, aurait exigé la restitution immédiate des pièces saisies, en posant 1 alternative d'une déclaration de guerre. Alors, avant de rendre le dossier, pour garder Une preuve matérielle de la culpabilité manifeste de Dreyfus, on se serait hâté, au Ministère, de calquer le bordereau sur une feuille de papier pelure, sans reproduire, bien entendu, les annotations impériales... Et toute l'affaire serait, de ce fait, échafaudée sur une piecè câlquée, fausse si l'on veut, mais reproduisant le document *authentiqué* de la tfàhisOU.

BAROIS.

— L'hypothèse est tellement fragile que jamais, à mà connaissance, elle n'a été formulée eq termes explicites, ni officiellement, ni officieusement.

WOLDSMUTH. —r Je sais. Mais ça circule, colporté dans les salons par des officiers, des magistrats, des avocats, des gens du monde... Aucun d'eux n'avance rien de précis, mais « un ami très au courant leur a laissé entendre. ,. » C'est un colossal secret de Polichinelle, qui chemine, avec des silences renseignés, des sous-entendus, de petits rires énigmatiques,.. Tout ça prépare le terrain, peu à peu. Et demain, aux débats de Rennes, quand la défense voudra pousser ces messieurs de l'Etat-Major à s'expliquer enfin à fond, ils esquiveront le coup... Il suffit de quelques hésitations involontaires, de quelques sourires douloureux, et tout le monde traduira: « Supposez ce que vous voudrez. Plutôt passer pour un faussaire, que de déchaîner la guerre européenne... »

BAROIS. — La guerre! Mais aujourd'hui, il n'est plus question de sécurité nationale!... Après tout ce qui a été dit et écrit, depuis trois ans, sur les attachés militaires étrangers, sur l'espionnage et le contr'espionnage allemand, qui donc serait assez naïf pour croire qu'il reste encore une seule pièce diplomatique vraiment dangereuse à divulguer? Personne! Donc, si une pièce accusatrice décisive existait réellement, il est évident que l'Etat-major l'aurait mise en avant, depuis longtemps, pour en finir!

WOLDSMUTH (sombre). — Croyez-moi, vous voyez trop simple. De tous temps cette question diplomatique m'a préoccupé; c'est le fil secret de l'Affaire: un fil qui n'est à aucun endroit visible, mais auquel tous les événements viennent se rattacher. Il y a là un danger terrible!

Barois, ébranlé, hésite; puis se tait.

WOLDSMUTH. — Eh bien, mon cher, il est encore temps de prévenir le coup. J'ai peu à peu constitué un dossier: rien que des faits exacts, j'en réponds: ceux sur lesquels j'avais une hésitation, je viens d'aller les contrôler là-bas, en Allemagne...

BAROIS. — Ah, c'est pour ça, que...

Woldsmuth. — Qui, (Ouvrant sa serviette.) J'ai donc là, de quqianéantir d'avance le coup du « secret d'Etat ». Mais il est grand temps d'agir. Je vous apporte mon dossier. Publiez-le demain!

BAROIS (sérieux, après un instant de recueillement). — Je vous remercie, Woldsmuth... Mais je crois qu'aujourd'hui une pareille publication serait une faute capitale.

Woldsmuth fait un geste de découragement.

BAROIS. — Elle attirerait l'attention sur un point qui est, quoi que vous en pensiez, relégué dans l'ombre... Par esprit de riposte, on croirait peutêtre devoir y revenir; tout ça remuerait l'opinion: ce serait maladroit...

L'acquittement est inévitable. Eh bien, triomphons en beauté, sans ressusciter de mesquines polémiques...

Woldsmuth, les épaules basses, replie silencieusement sa serviette.

BAROIS. — Non, laissez-moi vos notes.

WOLDSMUTH. — A quoi bon?C'est préventivement qu'il faudrait s'en servir.

BAROIS. — Je les emporterai à Rennes pour les communiquer à Luce. Et, s'il est de votre avis, je vous promets...

WOLDSMUTH (une lueur d'espoir). — Oui, montrez-les à Luce, et répétez-lui bien exactement tout ce que je vous ai dit...

(Réfléchissant.) Mais il est impossible que vous les emportiez ce soir, telles quelles... Je n'ai pas eu le temps de les mettre au net... C'est un vrai fouillis.. . Je pensais faire le travail avec vous, pour le numéro de demain...

BAROIS. — Votre nièce est là, voulez-vous les lui dicter? Ce sera fait tout de suite...

WOLDSMUTH (dont le visage s'est éclairé subitement). — Ah? Julia est ici?

Barois se lève et ouvre la porte. BAROIS. — Julia?

JULIA (de la pièce voisine, sans se déranger). — Quoi?

.La familiarité du ton est si explicite, que Barois rougit et se tourne vivement vers Woldsmuth, qui, penché sur ses notes, n'a pas bronché.

BAROIS (maître de lui). — Voulez-vous venir un instant, je vous prie, pour sténographier...

Julia paraît. Elle aperçoit Woldsmuth. Un simple battement des paupières. Son visage insurgé signifie: « Je suis libre, n'est-ce pas? »

JULIA (durement). — Bonjour, oncle Ulric. Vous avez fait bon voyage?

Woldsmuth redresse la tête, mais sans la regarder. Elle surprend alors ce sourire affairé, oblique, dans un visage où tous les 'traits sont disjoints par la souffrance. Et elle comprend ce que jamais elle n'avait soupçonné...

CTest elle qui baisse les yeux, au moment où Woldsmuth lève les siens, pour répondre enfin.

WOLDSMUTH. — Hé, bonjour Julia... Tu vas bien?La maman va bien?...

JULIA (péniblement). — Très bien.

WOLDSMUTH. — Alors, veux-tu... Ce sont des fiches... Pour Barois...

BAROIS (qui n'a rien vu). — Allez donc dans son bureau, Woldsmuth, vous serez misux qu'ici... Moi, je vais finir cet article...

A Monsieur Ulric Woldsmuth, Rédacteur au *Semeur*
Rue de l'Université. Paris.

«Rennes, le 13 août 1899

« Mon cher Woldsmuth,

« Vous avez lu la sténo d'hier et d'avant-hier? Vous aviez donc raison, cher ami, mille fois raison! Mais qui pouvait se douter?

« Tous ces jours-ci nos adversaires ont attendu, passionnément, cet argument décisif contre Dreyfus, qui leur est promis depuis si longtemps Les généraux ont parlé: déception sur toute la ligne!Alors, comme l'opinion publique se refuse obstinément à admettre que cet argument n'existe pas, elle interprète certaines réticences de l'Etat-Major dans le sens que vous aviez prévu: et le tour est joué. Aujourd'hui on a été jusqu'à faire courir le bruit que l'Allemagne, au dernier moment, aurait imposé ce mutisme héroïque à nos officiers!

« Je vous expédie, en hâte, les feuillets que vous avez dictés à Julia avant mon départ. Ils sont, hélas, d'une urgente actualité. Breil-Zoeger qui rentre à Paris pour prendre votre place, vous les remettra ce soir, avec ce mot.

« Concertez-vous aussitôt avec Roll pour qu'ils paraissent, si possible, demain, et assurez-leur une large diffusion avant de quitter Paris. « Apportez-en deux mille numéros à Rennes, ce sera suffisant. « Bien tristement à vous,

Barots. »

Le lendemain, en première page du *Semeur*

GUILLAUME II ET LAFFAIRE DREYFUS.

Nous avons eu la surprise, ces dernières semaines, de voir sournoisement reparaître une hypothèse ingénieuse, qui expliquerait, pour certains cerveaux simplistes, toutes les obscurités de l'Affaire: c'est celle du bordereau sur papier fort, annoté par Guillaume II, saisi par un agent français sur le bureau impérial, qu'il a fallu rendre précipitamment devant la menace d'une guerre, et dont le bordereau sur papier pelure serait un calque, fait au Ministère de la Guerre, en vue du procès de 1894.

Nous ne prendrons pas la peine de relever les puériles invraisemblances de cette romanesque aventure.

Nous nous bornerons à poser trois questions: i Si le bordereau est un calque de l'écriture authentique de Dreyfus, pourquoi ressemble-t-il mal à l'écriture de Dreyfus, tandis qu'il reproduit identiquement l'écriture d'Estherhazy?
2 S'il est vrai que les faux d'Henry s'expliquent par la nécessité de substituer des pièces inoffensives aux autographes impériaux dont l'usage était impossible, comment se fait-il que, questionné' par le Ministre de la Guerre avant son arrestation, Henry n'ait pas dévoilé la légitimité de ses faux, afin de s'innocenter? Des généraux assistaient à l'interrogatoire; le général Roget en a pris la sténographie: Henry n'a donné aucun motif de ce genre à ses falsifications de pièces. 3 Si l'histoire du bordereau annoté est exacte, quand Brisson, bouleversé par le suicide d'Henry, a manifesté l'intention de reconnaître publiquement son erreur et de prendre en main la cause de la revision, pourquoi le Ministre de la Guerre, qui a fait à ce moment auprès de Brisson les plus inquiètes démarches pour empêcher ce geste, ne l'a-t-il pas simplement averti de l'intervention impériale, afin d'arrêter net ce revirement d'opinion si dangereux pour les anti-revisionnistes?

Ceci posé, nous nous contenterons d'aligner succinctement quelques faits chronologiques, dont la signification nous semble assez évidente pour se passer de commentaires:

I. — Le i novembre 1894, le nom de Dreyfus, espion de l'Italie ou bien de l'Allemagne, paraît pour la première fois dans les journaux. Les attachés militaires allemands et italiens s'étonnent: c'est un nom qu'ils ne connaissent même pas. Et en voici la preuve: l'ambassadeur d'Italie a remis, le 5 juin 1899, au Ministère des Affaires Etrangères, pour être transmise à la Cour de Cassation, la dépêche chiffrée, datée de 1894, de l'attaché italien qui travaillait en complète entente avec l'attaché allemand, et qui affirme secrètement à son Gouvernement *qu'aucun d'eux* n'a eu de relations avec ce nommé Dreyfus.

A la même époque, les Etats-Majors d'Allemagne, d'Italie et d'Autriche, ont fait une enquête dans tous les centres d'espionnage, sans pouvoir se procurer aucun renseignement sur ce Dreyfus.

II. — Le 9 novembre 1894, l'attaché allemand est mis en cause et nommé dans un journal français. L'ambassade d'Allemagne, après une nouvelle information, donne un premier démenti par une note à la presse. Remarquons que ce démenti n'a pu être donné à la légère: car l'Allemagne ne se serait pas exposée à avancer une dénégation, qui, ensuite et publiquement, eût pu être reconnue mensongère au cours des débats du Conseil de Guerre.

En outre, aux mêmes dates, le Chancelier de l'Empire a chargé son ambassadeur à Paris, de faire une déclaration officielle et spontanée » au Ministre des Affaires Etrangères.

III. — Le 28 novembre parait au *Figaro* l'interview du général Mercier. Le Ministre, cinq jours avant la fin de l'instruction qui devait conclure à la traduction de Dreyfus devant un conseil de guerre, y affirme la culpabilité de l'accusé: il a « des preuves certaines ; Dreyfus n'aurait offert ses documents, ni à l'Italie, ni à l'Autriche »...

L'Allemagne, nettement visée cette fois, proteste à nouveau et très énergiquement par voie diplomatique.

La presse française n'en ayant pas tenu compte, l'Empereur, l'Etat-Major allemand, la presse allemande, s'irritent de voir contestée la parole qu'ils ont solennellement donnée. Le 4 décembre, il y a, sur l'ordre de l'Empereur, une nouvelle entrevue entre l'ambassadeur et notre Ministre des Affaires Etrangères: une note officielle « proteste formellement contre les allégations qui mêlent l'ambassade d'Allemagne à l'affaire Dreyfus ».

IV. — Le procès a lieu.

Lorsqu'un dossier secret a été communiqué aux juges à l'insu de l'accusé et de la défense, nous affirmons qu'il n'y avait rien dans ce dossier qui pût accréditer l'histoire du bordereau annoté par l'Empereur.

Il est facile de s'en assurer en interrogeant sur ce point précis les membres du Conseil de Guerre de 1894, actuellement à Rennes.

V. — A la fin de décembre 1894, après le verdict, toute la presse accuse ouvertement l'Allemagne d'avoir exigé le huis-clos, parce que la culpabilité de Dreyfus l'intéresse directement: c'est un nouveau démenti à la parole de l'ambassadeur. Celui-ci, le 25 décembre, au lendemain de la condamnation, fait une nouvelle déclaration officielle à la presse.

Mais les journaux continuent leur campagne, parlant de pièce rendue pour éviter la guerre, etc...

VI. — Le 5 janvier 1895, jour de la dégradation, l'ambassadeur d'Allemagne reçoit une dépêche particulièrement solennelle du chancelier de l'Empire. En l'absence de notre Ministre des Affaires Etrangères, il la porte directement à notre Président du Conseil.

En voici le texte, inédit jusqu'à ce jour: S. M. l'Empereur, ayant toute confiance dans la loyauté du Président « et du gouvernement de la République, prie votre Excellence de dire à « M. Casimir Périer que, s'il est prouvé que l'Ambassade d'Allemagne n'a jamais été impliquée dans l'affaire Dreyfus, Sa Majesté espère que le Gou vemement de la République n'hésitera pas à le déclarer.

» Sans une déclaration formelle, les légendes que la presse continue à « semer sur le compte de l'Ambassade d'Allemagne, subsisteraient et com promettraient la situation du représentant de l'Empereur.

De Hohenlohe.

Ainsi donc, l'Empereur, à bout de patience, en appelait au Président de la République, lui-même.

L'Ambassadeur a été reçu à l'Élysée le lendemain, 6 janvier. Nous savons et certifions que M. Casimir-Perier voulut considérer l'incident comme étant personnel et non diplomatique, puisque son intervention directe était demandée par l'Empereur. Il a dit lui-même depuis, qu' « il était fait appel à sa loyauté d'homme privé... (Cassation. I. 329.)

Rappelons, à ce sujet, la déposition de M. Casimir-Perier devant la Cour de Cassation. Il a d'abord affirmé, formellement, qu'il n'avait rien à dissimuler de secret:

« J'ai pu constater que mon silence (au procès Zola) a accrédité cette « pensée, que j'ai, seul peut-être, connaissance *d'incidents,* de *faits* ou de t *documents,* qui pourraient déterminer la Justice.

« Dans l'état de division et de trouble où je vois mon pays, j'estime que t mon devoir est de me mettre sans *réserves* à la disposition de la juridiction « suprême... »

Ceci ne laisse pas subsister le soupçon que M. Casimir-Perier, comme on l'a prétendu, fût lié par une parole donnée; et cette déclaration, dans sa bouche d'honnête homme, est d'une singulière netteté. Il raconte ensuite la conversation diplomatique qui eut lieu, et qui motIva une note officielle de l'Agence Havas, mettant une fois pour toutes hors de cause les ambassades étrangères à Paris. Et, le surlendemain, le Kaiser se déclara satisfait.

Rappelons aussi la déposition, à la Cour de Cassation, de M. Hanotaux, qui était Ministre des Affaires Etrangères pendant le procès de 1894. Interrogé comme suit: "Avez-vous connaissance de certaines lettres d'un souverain étranger, écrites à l'époque du procès Dreyfus, et desquelles ressortirait la culpabilité de cet accusé?» — il répondit formellement: Je n'en ai eu aucune connaissance. Je n'ai jamais rien vu de pareil. On ne m'a jamais rien offert de tel. Je n'ai jamais été consulté sur l'existence ou la valeur de tels documents. En un mot, toute cette histoire est une fable; « elle a d'ailleurs été démentie à diverses reprises par des notes communi quées aux journaux. »

Rappelons enfin pour terminer, la déposition à la Cour de Cassation de M. Paléologue, qui a été l'intermédiaire quotidien, pendant le procès Dreyfus, entre les Affaires Etrangères et la Guerre: *tf* Ni avant, ni après le procès Dreyfus, je n'ai été informé de l'existence « d'une lettre de l'Empereur d'Allemagne, ni de lettres de Dreyfus adressées « à ce souverain. Les allégations auxquelles M. le Président fait allusion me « paraissent complètement erronées. La nature de mes fonctions me permet 1 d'affirmer que, s'il avait existé des documents de ce genre, je ne l'eusse « pas ignoré, sans doute.

VII. — Le 17 novembre 1897, l'ambassadeur d'Allemagne déclare à notre Ministre des Affaires Etrangères que l'attaché militaire allemand, colonel de Schwartzkoppen, *attestait sur l'honneur n'avoir jamais eu, ni directement, ni indirectement,* aucune relation avec Dreyfus. »

VIII. — En 1898, avant le procès Zola, l'Empereur, impatienté, voulut faire une manifestation décisive, *personnelle.*

Son entourage l'en empêcha, connaissant l'état des esprits en France, et craignant qu'une insulte grave ne fût faite à la personne même du souverain,et n'entraînât à des complications inquiétantes. Il exigea néanmoins qu'une parole officielle (ut donnée publiquement, en plein Reichstag.

Voici la déclaration du Secrétaire d'Etat aux Affaires Etrangères de l'Empire, à la séance du 24 janvier 1898:

« Vous comprendrez que je n'aborde ce sujet qu'avec de grandes précau« tions. Agir autrement pourrait être interprêté comme une immixtion de « notre part dans les affaires de la France Je crois d'autant plus devoir « observer une réserve complète à ce sujet qu'on peut s'attendre à ce que les « procès ouverts en France jettent la lumière sur toute l'affaire. Je me bornerai donc à déclarer *de la façon la plus formelle et la plus coté gorique,* qu'entre l'ex-capitaine Dreyfus, actuellement détenu à l'Ile du Diable, et n'importe quels agents allemands, il n'a *jamais* existé de rela« tions, ni de liaisons, *de quelque nature qu'elles soient.* »

IX. — Cinq jours plus tard, l'Empereur vint lui-même chez notre ambassadeur à Berlin, *pour lui apporter sa déclaration personnelle, et le prier de la communiquer officiellement à notre Gouvernement.*

X. — Enfin, à l'heure actuelle, l'état d'esprit autour du Souverain est le même. L'Empereur éprouve le plus impatient désir de faire un geste personnel; mais on l'en empêche, et on l'en empêchera jusqu'au bout, pour ne pas risquer que la France, par une seconde condamnation, ne donne au Kaiser un nouveau démenti qu'il ne pourrait pas supporter sans une rupture diplomatique. Cependant on est prêt à renouveler, par notes officielles, toutes les déclarations déjà faites.

Si l'on consent à supposer un instant que l'Empereur ait été réellement compromis dans une affaire d'espionnage, on peut admettre, à la rigueur, qu'il ait été, pour certaines nécessités politiques, contraint de nier la vérité par un démenti officiel.

Mais, ce mensonge diplomatique une fois commis et enregistré, aurait-il réitéré ses protestations, *à chaque occasion nouvelle,* et avec une si solennelle et pressante *insistance*?

Même en faisant abstraction de la personnalité de Guillaume II et de sa conception particulièrement chatouilleuse de l'honneur, est-ce que jamais un souverain oserait faire de si véhémentes et de si nettes déclarations, s'il risquait d'être, un beau jour, *confondu devant le monde entier,* par la découverte ultérieure d'une preuve décisive?

Qui ne voit dans l'attitude du Kaiser un très simple et très douloureux cas de conscience?

L'Empereur sait, — mieux que personne — l'innocence de Dreyfus; et, sans toutefois vouloir faire courir à son pays le djjiger d'une complication diplomatique, il cherche à le crier aussi souvent et aussi haut qu'il le peut.

Il n'y a pire sourd que celui qui ne veut pas entendre.

LE SEMEUR.

« A M. Marc Elie Luce, Auteuil.

« Rennes, le 5 septembre 1899.

« Mon cher ami,

« Notre découragement est sans bornes.Pratiquement, la cause est perdue. Les deux semaines qui viennent de s'écouler ont décidé de l'Affaire. L'opinion des juges est établie: et ils sentent bien que la majorité est avec eux.

« Woldsmuth me reproche d'avoir trop tardé à publier son article. Je me le reproche aussi, quoique je reste sceptique sur l'efficacité qu'il aurait pu avoir. Comment s'attaquer à une fable qui n'a jamais été clairement formulée par personne? Et, le serait-elle, qu'elle resterait pareillement insaisissable, puisqu'il est admis qu'aucune trace matérielle ne peut subsister des fameux autographes impériaux. C'est le domaine des affirmations gratuites. Devant ces fumées, nous sommes sans armes; pas de lutte possible.

« Si l'opinion avait pû être retournée, elle l'eût été l'autre jour, le lendemain de votre départ, par l'attitude de Casimir-Périer, l'homme de France qui sait le mieux si oui ou non le Kaiser s'est trouvé mêlé à l'Affaire, et qu, fort de son passé intègre, est venu répéter de sa voix loyale, les yeux dans les yeux du colonel-président:

« Vous me demandez de dire la vérité, toute la vérité; je l'ai juré, je « la dirai, sans réticences et sans réserves. Quoi que j'aie déjà dit dans le « passé, on persiste à croire ou à dire, — ce qui, malheureusement, n'est « pas toujours la même chose — que je connais seul des incidents ou des « faits qui pouiraient faire la lumière, et que je n'ai pas jusqu'ici dit tout « ce que la justice a intérêt à connaître. C'est faux... *Je ne veux sortir de « cette enceinte, qu'en y laissant l'inébranlable conviction que je ne sais rien « qui doive être tu, et que j ai dit tout ce que je sais !*»

« Je ne mets pas en doute la bonne foi des juges du Conseil de Guerre. Je les crois aussi impartiaux qu'ils peuvent être. « Mais ce sont des soldats, j--- « Comme toute l'armée, ils sont tenus par leurs journaux dans une ignoj rance absolue de ce qu'est réellement l'Affaire. On a posé devant eux la I question, avec un raccourci criminel: la culpabilité de Dreyfus ou bien L' 1 infamie de l'Etat-Major: voilà dans quel dilemme imbécile on a enfermé ces officiers.

« Si encore ils étaient soustraits à toute influence, seuls avec leur conscience et les faits! Mais non: ils continuent, chaque soir, après les débats, à vivre dans le milieu où la trahison de l'accusé est un axiome invulnérable.

« Je ne dis pas qu'ils soient d'avance inclinés à trouver Dreyfus coupable; mais je puis affirmer dès aujourd'hui, qu'ils voteront la culpabilité. Et il n'en peut être autrement pour ces hommes dont la personnalité humaine ne se dégage plus du revêtement professionnel; dont les vingtcinq ans d'uniforme sont collés à la peau; qui, depuis un quart de siècle, sont façonnés par la discipline, imprégnés du sentiment hiérarchique, fanatiques de cette armée dont l'emblème vivant est là, dans la personne de ses chefs qui comparaissent devant eux. Comment pourraient-ilsse prononcer en faveur du juif, contre l'EtatMajor? Le voudraient-ils par instants, au fond de leurs consciences troublées, que, *physiquement,* ils ne le pourraient pas. Et peut-on leur en faire reproche?

« D'ailleurs je dois convenir que l'attitude de l'accusé n'a rien qui puisse contrebalancer le prestige des uniformes. Il a déçu la plupart même de ses amis. A tort, selon moi. Depuis quatre ans, nous nous battons pour des idées; mais en somme, c'est lui qui les représente: et nous nous étions tous fait, en nous-mêmes, une image arbitraire, mais précise, de cet inconnu. Il débarque: et, ainsi que nous aurions dû nous y attendre, la réalité ne coïncide pas avec notre imagination.

« Beaucoup d'entre nous ne le lui ont pas pardonné.

« C'est un homme simple, dont l'énergie naturelle est tout intérieur. Il arrive, affaibli par la séquestration, par les émotions inouïes qu'il a supportées; il est malade, il grelotte de fièvre, il digère à peine un peu de lait. Comment serait-il au diapason de cet auditoire forcené, dont les trois "T7«ai4e-4MÏsseTïr«mmèTr et dont l'autre quart l'adore comme un symbole? Ce rôle écrasant n'est-il pas au-dessus des forces humaines? Il n'a plus la vigueur de hurler furieusement sonirmpcence, comme il faisait dans la cour de l'Ecole Militaire. Le peu d energie qui lui reste, il l'emploie, non pas contre les autres, mais contre lui-même: à ne pas se laisser abattre, à paraître un homme; il ne veut pas qu'on l'ait vu pleurer,-...

« C'est une conception dont la grandeur héroïque, ingrate, échappe à l'esthétique populaire. Il aurait peut-être conquis la foule par une attitljdejplus théîtrale: mais cet empire qu'il garde au prix d'un dur effort) est taxé d'indifférence, et ceux qui se démènent pour lui depuis quatre ans, lui en font un grief.

« Moi-même, qui ne le connaissais pas, je dois avouer que lorsque je l'ai aperçu à la première audience, malgré l'enthousiasme de nos amis, malgré l'espoir insensé que j'avais triomphalement clamé, le matin même, dans le *Semeur,* j'ai reçu à ce moment-là, l'avertissement intime de la défaite, un je ne sais quoi, le petit ressort qui casse net... Je l'ai caché, même à vous. Mais je puis dire que ce jour-là, j'ai senti tout à coup, avec une «ertitude indiscutable, que l'Affaire était perdue, mal perdue, et qu'elle ne laisserait, au fond de toutes ces âmes enflammées par elle, qu'un peu de cendre nauséabonde.

« Cette amère inquiétude ne me quitte plus.

«Vous avez bien fait de partir. Votre place n'était pas ici, dans le tumulte.

« Nous sommes à la limite de notre résistance. Songez que pour beaucoup d'entre nous c'est le second été torride, sans trêve, dans la sombre hantise de ce drame! Songez à ces journées d'attention exaspérée, dans l'atmosphère irrespirable de la salle du Conseil, où tant de témoignages suent le parti-pris et la haine! Et les soirées, pires que les jours, dans les rues, dans les cafés, pour éviter l'étouffement de la chambre d'hôtel où l'on ne peut plus dormir, des soirées — presque des nuits — à discutailler sans fin, à pointer pour la centième fois les chances de victoire ou de défaite! Si nous avons pu résister jusqu'à présent, c'est que la certitude de notre bon droit nous servait d'armature. .. Mais voici encore une étape douloureuse, et le repos n'est pas au bout! Combien nous en reste_t-il à franchir?
———

« C'est bien dur de voir notre pays, si

beau, dans une pareille déchéance intellectuelle et morale! Penser qu'il y a, en ce moment, une révolte de la conscience universelle, et que la conscience française, pour la première fois depuis des siècles, n'en est pas!

« Au revoir, mon grand ami.

« Voulez-vous dire à Breil-Zoeger, que s'il a envie de revenir ici, Harbaroux propose de le remplacer à la direction du *Semeur*?

Barois. »

« J'apprends ce soir que Labori compte faire une démarche personnelle auprès du.Kaiser, pour obtenir avant la fin de? débats une dernière déclaration impériale de l'innocence de Dreyfus.

« A quoi bon? Il est déjà trop tard... »

« Bar ois. — 103 Lycée. Rennes.

« Paris, 8 septembre. — 11 h. 30.

« Suis averti télégraphiquement nouvelle protestation Gouvernement allemand, parue ce matin en note officielle dans *Moniteur Empire,* pour répondre appel Labori.

« Voici texte:

« Sommes autorisés renouveler déclarations que Gouvernement Impé" rial, afin sauvegarder dignité propre, a faites pour remplir son devoir « d'humanité.

« L'ambassadeur a remis, sur ordre Empereur, en janvier 1894 et « janvier 1895, à Hanotaux, Ministre Affaires Etrangères, à Dupuy, Prési« dent Conseil, et au Président République Casimir-Périer, déclarations « réitérées que l'ambassade allemande en France n'avait jamais entretenu « relations, ni directes ni indirectes, avec capitaine Dreyfus.

Le secrétaire d'Etat de Bulow s'est exprimé en ces termes le 24 jan« vier 1898 devant commission Reicbstag. » Je déclare de la façon la plus « formelle qu'entre ex-capitaine Dreyfus et n'importe quel organe allemand, « jamais existé relations ni liaisons quelque nature qu'elles soient. »

« Ministre Affaires Étrangères, prévenu, s'est engagé à communiquer officiellement cette protestation aux juges avant vote. Espérons encore. Faites répandre nouvelle par tous journaux locaux.

Luce. »

« Luce. Auteuil.

« Rennes, 9 septembre, 6 heures soir.

« Condamnation avec circonstances atténuantes. Dix ans détention. Contradictoire et incompréhensible. « Vive justice quand même! « L'affaire continue! »

Le 9 septembre 1899: le soir du verdict.

En gare de Rennes, trois trains, successivement, ont été pris d'assaut. Un quatrième, formé de tous les wagons de rebut qui restaient dans les garages, a démarré, péniblement, à son tour, dans la cohue d'émeute qui grouille sur les quais.

Barois, Cresteil et Woldsmuth, les épaves du *Semeur,* sont parqués dans un wagon de troisième, ancien modèle: des cloisons, à mi-hauteur, divisent la voiture en compartiments étroits; deux quinquets pour tout le wagon.

Les vitres sont ouvertes sur la campagne endormie. Aucun souffle. Le train roule lentement, charriant à travers l'épaisse nuit d'été un brouhaha de séance électorale.

Des vociférations se croisent dans 1 air empesté des compartiments:

— Tout ça, c'est les Jésuites!

— Taisez-vous donc! Et l'honneur de l'armée?

— Oui: c'est la faillite du Syndicat...

— Ils ont bien fait! La réhabilitation d'un officier qui a été condamné par sept camarades, et déclaré coupable par le Haut-Commandement de l'Armée, compromet le salu. d'un pays bien plus qu'une erreur judiciaire...

— Parbleu! Et je vais plus loin! Moi qui vous parle, admettons que j'aie été du Conseil, et que j'aie su que Dreyfus était innocent... Eh bien, Monsieur, sans hésiter, pour le bien de la patrie, pour l'ordre public, je l'aurais fait fusiller comme un chien!

CRESTEIL D'allize (se dressant, malgré lui, dans la pénombre, et dominant le tumulte de sa voix éraillée). — Il y a un savant français, nommé Duclaux, qui a déjà répondu à cet argument de la sécurité nationale: il a dit, — ou à peu près — qu'il n'y avait pas de raison d'Etat qui puisse empêcher une Cour de

Justice d'être juste!

— Vendu! Lâche! Fripouille! Sale juif! 3

CRESTEIL (insolent). — Messieurs, je suis à vos ordres.

Les injures redoublent. Cresteil reste debout. BAROIS. — Laissez-les donc, Cresteil...

Peu à peu, une torpeur lourde, — causée par la chaleur suffocante, l'oppression de l'obscurité, la dureté des banquettes, le cahotement du vieux matériel, — envahit le wagon.

Le tapage se localise, diminue.

Serrés dans leur coin, Barois, Cresteil et Woldsmuth causent à voix basse.

WOLDSMUTH. — Le plus triste, c'est que cette pensée estimable de rendre service au pays, a été, j'en suis sûr, le principal mobile de beaucoup de nos adversaires...

CRESTEIL. — Mais non! Vous avez toujours tendance, Woldsmuth, à croire que les autres sont mûs par des sentiments élevés, des idées... Ils sont mûs, le plus souvent, par leur intérêt, conscient ou inconscient, et à défaut de calcul, par de simples habitudes sociales...

BAROIS. — Tenez, à propos d'habitudes, je me souviens d'une scène qui m'a beaucoup frappé à la troisième ou quatrième audience.

J'étais en retard. J'arrivais par le couloir de la presse, juste au moment où les juges s'engageaient dans l'entrée. Presque en même temps qu'eux, un peu en arrière, débouchent quatre témoins, quatre généraux en grande tenue. Eh bien, les sept officiers-juges, sans avoir eu le temps de se concerter, d'un même mouvement devenu chez eux machinal et qui révèle un asservissement de trente ans, se sont arrêtés net, le dos au mur, au garde-àvous... Et les généraux, simples témoins, ont passé devant eux, comme à la revue, pendant que les officiers-juges faisaient automatiquement leur salut militaire...

CRESTEIL (spontanément). — Ça a sa beauté!

BAROIS. — Non, mon petit, non.. . C'est l'ancien Saint-Cyrien qui vient dejparler, ce n'est pas le Cresteil d'aujourd'hui.

CRESTEIL,(tristement). — Vous avez raison... Mais ça s'explique, voyezvous... Pour des êtres fiers et énergiques, la discipline demande un tel sacrjfice de toutes les heures, qu'on ne peut pas perdre l'habitude de l'estime au prix qu'elle coûte...

BAROIS (suivant son idée). — D'ailleurs, le verdict de tout à l'heure, c'est la répétition de cette scène du couloir... Cette condamnation d'un traître avec circonstances atténuantes, cela paraît boiteux, inepte... Mais, réfléchissez: la condamnation, c'est le salut militaire qu'ils ont fait sans s'en rendre compte, par discipline professionnelle; et les circonstances atténuantes, ça, c'est, malgré tout, l'hésitation de leurs consciences d'hommes...

L'arrivée à Paris, au petit jour.

Un silence morne emplit les wagons, qui vident sur le quai leur bétail frissonnant et blême.

Luce est là, pâle, son regard doux cherchant les amis. Etreinte silencieuse: une immense affection, une immense tristesse. Les yeux sont pleins de larmes.

Woldsmuth embrasse la main de Luce, en pleurant.

BAROIS (après une hésitation). — Julia n'est pas avec vous?

Breil-Zoeger redresse la tête. ZOEGER. — Non.

Quelques pas silencieux, en groupe serré.

BAROIS (timidement, à Luce). — Quoi de nouveau? (Inquiet de son mutisme.) La cassation?

LUCE. — Non, il paraît que c'est impossible, juridiquement...

BAROIS. — Alors?

Luce ne répond pas tout de suite.

LUCE. — La grâce...

CRESTEIL ET BAROIS (ensemble). — Il la refusera

Luce (fermement). — Non.

C'est un dernier coup, au visage.

Ils restent immobiles, debout sur le trottoir, les lèvres entr'ouvertes, la gorge serrée, sans rien voir. Leurs épaules plient...

WOLDSMUTH. — Ayez pitié de lui... Retourner là-bas? Recommencer le supplice? Et pourquoi faire?

CRESTEIL (pathétique). — Pour rester le symbole!

WOLDSMUTH (patient). — Il en mourrait. Et alors?

LUCE (avec une indulgence infinie). — Woldsmuth a raison... Au moins nous réhabiliterons un vivant...

Le même soir.

Barois a quitté de bonne heure son journal, et il s'est mis à marcher, devant lui, froissant au fond de sa poche le billet de Julia, qu'il a trouvé, le matin, sur son bureau:

« Tu vas revenir de Rennes, tu vas être étonné de ne pas me trouver au *Semeur.*

« Je ne veux pas te tromper.

« Je me suis donnée librement, je me reprends de même. « Tant que je t'ai aimé, je t'ai appartenu, sans restriction. Mais depuis que j'en aime un autre, je te le dis avec franchise, tu ne peux plus exister pour moi. Je te préviens loyalement; c'est ma façon de te prouver jusqu'au bout mon estime.

« Quand tu liras ce mot, j'aurai repris la libre disposition de moi-même. Tu es assez énergique et trop intelligent pour ne pas comprendre, et pour te diminuer par une souffrance inutile. Moi je resterai toujours ton amie,

JULIA. »

Il rentre rue Jacob et se laisse choir tout habillé sur son lit.

Une douleur aiguë, personnelle, malsaine, s'est greffée sur l'autre, sur ce vaste découragement qui la épuisé. Ses tempes sont lourdes et brûlantes.

Soudain, dans cette chambre, mille souvenirs sensuels... Un désir éperdu de revivre, à quelque prix que ce soit, certains instants précis... Il se soulève, hagard, mordant ses lèvres, tordant ses bras; puis il retombe en sanglotant sur son lit.

Il se débat, quelques secondes encore, comme un suicidé qu'un remous emporte...

Puis tout sombre en un noir sommeil.

Un coup de sonnette le réveille, le rejette, d'un saut égaré, en plein désespoir.

Il fait grand jour: dix heures...

Il va ouvrir la porte: sur le palier, Woldsmuth.

WOLDSMUTH (troublé par le visage bouffi et ravagé de Barois). — Je vous dérange...

BAROIS (agacé). — Entrez donc!

Il referme la porte.

WOLDSMUTH (évitant de le regarder). — Je vous avais cherché au *Semeur...* pour ces renseignements que vous m'avez demandés... (Il relève les yeux.) J'ai pu voir Reinach... (Balbutiant.) Je suis... j'ai...

Ils se regardent. Woldsmuth n'a pas le courage de poursuivre Et Barois comprend que Woldsmuth sait tout; il en éprouve un soulagement immense; il lui tend les deux mains.

Woldsmuth (avec simplicité). — Ah... Et Zoeger, un ami!

Barois pâlit, jusqu'à en perdre le souffle.

BAROIS(des lèvres). — Zoeger?

WOLDSMUTH (effaré). — Je ne sais pas... je dis ça...

Barois reste assis, les bras raidis, les poings crispés, la tête en avant, le cerveau vide.

WOLDSMUTH (que ce silence épouvante). — Mon pauvre ami... Je me mêle de ce qui ne me regarde pas... J'ai tort... Mais j'arrive justement... Je voudrais vous aider à moins souffrir...

Sans répondre, sans le regarder, Barois enfonce sa main dans sa poche et lui tend la lettre de Julia.

Woldsmuth la lit avidement, et sa respiration devient sifflante; à travers la barbe, ses lèvres ont un tremblement flasque.

Puis il replie le feuillet, et vient s'asseoir à côté de Barois; maladroitement il lui entoure la taille de son bras trop petit.

WOLDSMUTH. — Ah, cette Julia... Je sais... On souffre, on souffre... On voudrait tuer I (Avec un sourire poignant.) Et puis ça passe...

Tout à coup, sans faire un mouvement, il commence à pleurer, doucement, intarissablement, — comme on ne peut pleurer que sur soi-même.

Barois l'examine. Ces paroles, cet accent, ces larmes... Il soupçonne, et presqu'en même temps, il découvre la vérité.

Et aussitôt, avant toute pitié, c'est une

sorte de satisfaction sombre, une diversion à sa douleur, à lui. Il est moins seul. Une crise de bonté sentimentale lui mouille les yeux.

Ah, la vie est trop cruelle...

BAROIS (humblement, comme si les mots pouvaient effacer). — Mon bon Woldsmuth, comme j'ai dû vous faire du mal...

VI

A l'Exposition.

Le 30 mai 1900.

Sur le bord de la Seine, dans un de ces restaurants de carton, pavoisés et fleuris, en terrasse sur l'eau.

Une trentaine de jeunes hommes, autour d'une table servie.

Les garçons viennent d'allumer les candélabres, et, dans la nuit hésitante, la lueur mate des petits abat-jour jaunes, enveloppant les cristaux et les fleurs qui penchent, crée autour du banquet qui s'achève une atmosphère languissante et recueillie.

Un léger silence.

Marc-Elie' Luce, qui préside, se lève.

Ses yeux clairs, enfoncés sous le front qui fait ombre, promènent sur les convives un regard pénétrant et grave.

Puis il sourit, comme s'il voulait se faire pardonner les feuillets qu'il tient dans sa main.

Son accent franc-comtois souligne le relief des phrase» et donne à son discours une bonhomie provinciale, simple et imposante.

LUCE. — Mes chers amis, 11 y a aujourd'hui un an, c'était pour nous une grande allégresse. M. Ballot-Beaupré venait de lire publiquement son rapport. Nous venions de voir toute l'Affaire revivre sous nos yeux, résumée avec une vigueur de raccourci et une exactitude de détails, qui font de ce travail un impérissable modèle. Un silence sympathique nous garantissait la conversion de ce public, qui, l'année précédente, avait hué Zola. Nous éprouvions une immense confiance à voir enfin soulevé par des mains officielles, ce poids qui nous écrasait depuis trois ans Et nous avions tous sur les lèvres cette parole d'espoir, que M. Mornard, se tournant vers la Cour, prononçait d'une voix anxieuse: « J'attends votre arrêt comme l'aurore du jour qui fera luire sur la patrie la grande lumière de la concorde et de la vérité. »

C'est pour commémorer ces heures sacrées, — qui sont, n est-il pas vrai, parmi les dernières heures pures de l'Affaire? — que nous sommes réunis ce soir.

Je ne reviendrai pas sur le drame douloureux de cet été. Déjà les détails s'estompent. Le souci généreux qu'a eu le Gouvernement de rendre inefficace en fait l'hésitante condamnation du Conseil de Guerre, nous permet d'attendre, avec une patience qui est nouvelle pour nous, l'instant où, par la nécessité même des choses, la vérité anéantira jusqu'aux moindres traces de l'injustice; car la force de la vérité est opiniâtre, et finit par plier les événements sous sa loi." . —

En réalité, la crise est traversée. L'un de nous n'écrivit-il pas, dernièrement: « La violence des hommes est comme les grands vents dans la nature: elle s'enfle et grossit comme eux, puis s'apaise et disparaît, laissant les germes à leur activité... » (i).

C'est un pénible moment de désarroi pour tous ceux qui, depuis plusieurs années, vivent en pleine intensité d'action. Ils s'arrêtent, essoufflés, comme des chiens de meute au soir de la chasse; la journée a été rude; leur rôle est terminé. Et voici qu'une angoisse nouvelle les étreint, une angoisse devant ces ruines et ces morts qui encombrent le champ de bataille... Je crois exprimer ce que nous ressentons tous, n'est-ce pas? Une angoiss"e3evant cette France endolorie où règnent les rancunes et tes dissensions.

Au fort de la lutte nous ne pensions guère aux conséquences. C'était l'argument de nos ennemis. Nous leur répondions, — et à bon escient — que l'honneur national devait passer avant l'ordre public, et qu'une illégalité, manifestement commise, fût-ce au nom de la sécurité de l'Etat, si elle est officiellement acceptée par tous, engendre des maux mille fois plus graves que le trouble passager d'un peuple: elle compromet la seule acquisition dont les hommes puissent avoir quelque fierté, ces libertés sacrées dont le sang français a jadis enrichi les nations; exactement, elle compromet le Droit et la Justice de tout le monde civilisé. (Applaudissements.)

Mais enfin, maintenant que nous avons eu satisfaction, il faut bien reconnaître en quelle posture l'entêtement de l'opinion publique a mis le pays: nous sommes au lendemain d une révolution.

Dans la période confuse qui a précédé l'issue, au cours des derniers assauts, une foule de partisans, que nous ne soupçonnions pas, est venue se mêler au groupe de penseurs actifs que nous formions jusque-là (2).

(1) E. Carrière. (a) D. Halévy. *Apologie pour notre passé*. (Cah. de la quinzaine. XI. 10).

Notre humble et tenace drapeau, ils nous l'ont arraché des mains, pour le brandir ostensiblement à notre place.Jls _ont envahMes espaces libres gue notre travail d'assainjssejnent..£QiiaJLava aujourd'hui aulendemain delà Victoire, ce sont eux qui occupent, en maîtres, le terrain. Voulez-vous me permettre une distinction qui m'est chère: nous étions une poignée de *dreyfusistes* ; et maintenant, *ils* sont une armée de *dreyfusards*...

Que valent-ils? Je n'en sais rien. Ils font des confusions que nous nous étions sévèrement interdites, entre le militarisme et l'armée, entre le nationalisme et la France. Que feront-ils? Que sont-ils capables d'édifier sur les ruines que nous avons voulu faire? Je n'en sais rien. L'ère resplendissante dont nous avions rêvé l'avènement, se lève-t-elle avec eux?

Hélas! Ils ressemblent, par bien des côtés, à ceux que nous avons renversés: mais je ne pense pas qu'ils puissent être pires.

Pour nous, notre tâche est accomplie; la réalisation de ce que nous avons passionnément espéré, n'est pas pour nous. Ce branle-bas dont nous avons sciemment donné le signal, nous le payons presque tous de notre repos, de notre bonheur individuel.

Mes chers amis, c'est dur, c'est très dur. Je le sais comme vous: j'ai perdu mes auditeurs au Collège de France; et si j'ai été réélu au Sénat, je ne dois pas m'illusionner: aucune commission n'a fait appel à mon travail, toute la besogne se fait loin de moi. Ceux qui, actuellement, tirent de notre effort le plus manifeste profit, sont généralement aussi ceux qui se détournent de nous avec la plus inquiète méfiance... Ils ont tort: ils nous feraient supposer, qu'après avoir constaté de près le danger que nous sommes pour qui n'a pas les mains pures, notre voisinage leur fait peur..

(Sourires.)

Les moins à plaindre, ce sont les plus jeunes, ceux qui ont le temps de refaire leur vie. Oh, pour ceux-là, le beau baptême du feu, au seuil d'une existence consciencieuse! La flamme a dévoré tout le factice, tout le décor, tout le carton-peint de leurs caractères: il ne reste plus que la masse essentielle: le roc! Et quelle bienfaisante nécessité ce fut pour eux, d'avoir à choisir, une fois pour toutes, leur direction et leurs amitiés!

J'en connais beaucoup, en somme, qui s'en tireront...

(Il sourit, quitte un instant ses feuillets des yeux, et se penche vers Barois que l'on a placé auprès de lui.) ...Notre ami Barois, tenez, dont la confiance aventureuse et la générosité ne se sont jamais démenties; qui a été, depuis le début, pour chacun de nous, un perpétuel réconfort aux jours de défaillance! (Reprenant la lecture.) Barois demeure au centre de nous tous. C'est lui qui a la garde de notre feu sacrôrJg_Semeur qui est son œuvre, dont il constitue Je foyer central, çt autour duquel nous devons rester groupes. Voyez-le à l'œuvre, et que son exemple soit notre sauvegarde. Depuis des années, il s est consacré à son journal, ne spéculant pas, semant sans arrièrepensée toutes ses idées, tous ses projets, sans avoir la crainte mesquine qu'on s'en empare et qu'on les réalise avant lui; ne ménageant rien, — que sa conscience! Près de lui, il y aura toujours du _±iavail pour les hommes de bonne volonté. Le Semeur, après les tirages inouïs qu'il a eus et qui seront historiques, est revenu à une expansion mieux proportionnée à son objet: il s'adresse à une minorité, et cette minorité intellectuelle lui reste scrupuleuse-

ment attachée. Apportons-lui tous notre concours, Messieurs; apportons-lui cette part d'expérience, dont, parmi nous, les plus jeunes mêmes sont aujourd'hui pourvus, — r rs annTM" troublées valent une-vie entière. Que Barois continue à centraliser nos efforts, et à leur donner cette diffusion qui les aiguillonne et les justifie!

Et surtout, mes amis, ne nous laissons pas atteindre par le stérile découragement, qui déjà rôde et nous guette. Je sais autant que vous, combien la tentation peut être forte. (D'une voix angoissée.) Devant les difficultés que notre pays s'est préparées, lequel de nous n'a pas éprouvé un sentiment d'effroi, et senti planer sur lui l'ombre lourde d'une responsabilité? Comment en serait-il autrement? Comment ne garderions-nous pas de cette épreuve, un indélébile pessimisme? Il nous a fallu joncher le chemin de tant d'illusions!

(Redressant la tête.) Mais un pareil malaise, si légitime soit-il, ne doit as obscurcir notre discernement. Nous nous sommes sacrifiés pour une elle cause, et cela seul importe! Ce que nous avons fait, mes amis, nous devions le faire, et s'il fallait recommencer, nous n'hésiterions pas! Répétons-nous-le, aux heures de doute et de scrupule!

La France est divisée: c'est grave, mais ce n'est pas irréparable; le pire qui puisse en résulter c'est, pour notre pays, un dommage matériel et momentané; tandis que nous lui avons sauvé l'intégrité de ses principes, sans lesquels il n'y a pas de vie pour une nation.

Songeons que, dans quelques cinquante ans, l'affaire Dreyfus ne sera qu'un petit épisode des luttes de la raison humaine contre les passions qui l'aveuglent; un moment, et pas davantage, de ce lent et merveilleux cheminement de l'humanité vers plus de bien.

Notre façon de concevoir la justice et la vérité est infailliblement con damnée à être dépassée dans les âges à venir; nous le savons; et loin d abattre notre courage, cet espoir est le plus efficace stimulant de notre élan actuel. Le devoir strict de chaque génération est donc d'aller dans le sens de la vérité, aussi loin qu'elle peut, à la limite extrême de

ce qu'il lui est permis d'entrevoir,—et de s'y tenir désespérément, comme si elle prétendait atteindre la Vérité absolue. La progression de l'homme est à ce prix.

La vie d'une génération, ce n'est qu'un effort qui en suit et en précède d'autres. Eh bien, mes amis, notre génération a fait le sien. La paix soit sur nous

Il s'assied.

Une grande émotion silencieuse.

LE CALME

Rue de l'Université, plusieurs années après.

L'immeuble entier est occupé par le *Semeur*. L'entrée est encombrée de rames et de ballots. Le rez-de-chaussée et l'entresol servent de locaux aux machines. Les autres étages sont réservés aux bureaux de la revue et de la maison d'édition.

Au 3 étage: RÉDACTION. UN EMPLOYÉ (entrant). — Monsieur Henry vous demande à l'appareil. LE SECRÉTAIRE. — Connais pas. L'employÉ. — C'est pour le *New-York Herald*. LE SECRÉTAIRE. — Ah, Harris? Donnez...

Il prend le récepteur.

LE SECRÉTAIRE. — Allô! Parfaitement... J'en ai parlé à M. Barois, il veut bien: mais pas de phrases, pas d'éloges, les faits, sa vie... A votre disposition; questionnez...

Depuis l'affaire Dreyfus? (Riant.) Pourquoi pas depuis 70?

Oui, la besogne actuelle, ça vaudra mieux...

Si vous voulez... D'abord ses cours du soir, aux mairies de Belleville, de Vaugirard, du Panthéon. Beaucoup d'ouvriers; au Panthéon, une majorité d'étudiants... Oui, insistez: c'est l'idée directrice: tout ce qui peut servir à faire évoluer le cerveau des masses vers la liberté de la pensée..

Maintenant, il y a son cours aux *Etudes sociales,* deux fois par semaine...

Cette année? Sur *la crise universelle des religions*. Ça fait un livre par an.

Enfin il y a le *Semeur*... C'est le gros morceau... deux cents pages tous les quinze jours...

—Je ne sais pas, mais certainement une quinzaine d'articles personnels dans l'année. Et puis, dans chaque numéro, une chronique régulière, toutes ses idées du moment...

Non! Les *Conversations du Semeur,* c'est autre chose. Voilà: chaque semaine il y a une réception ici; on apporte les articles, on combine les numéros suivants. Il a eu l'idée de faire sténographier la conversation, et de publier, sous forme de *Fiches,* les digressions d'ordre général. Les abonnés s'en sont mêlés. Ils ont écrit pour qu'on abordât tel ou tel sujet. C'est très bon, ça met en contact avec le public: on voit les points qui préoccupent... Bref, les *Fiches* sont devenues les *Conversations du Semeur,* presqu'un volume tous les trois mois...

Allo? Soit, mais vous auriez trouvé la liste partout... D'abord les livres sur l'Affaire: *Pour la vérité* (l, 2 et 3 séries), sans compter les brochures; je passe. Ensuite, les conférences, qui paraissent à la fin de chaque année: *Paroles de combat,* six volumes; le septième est sous presse. Et puis, quatre bouquins: son enseignement aux Etudes sociales: *Les progrès de l'instruction populaire. — La libre-pensée hors de France. — Essai sur le déterminisme. — La divisibilité de la matière.*

Allo! Il serait bon de dire que la conférence de dimanche au Trocadéro est tout à fait exceptionnelle, hors des habitudes de M. Barois. Insistez... Que jamais il n'a voulu prendre la parole devant tant de monde...

Hein? je ne sais pas, trois mille places, je crois; et il paraît que la moitié de la salle est déjà louée...

Oui, le nom attire, et puis le su;et: *L'avenir de l'incroyance.*

Merci... A votre disposition... Au revoir!

II

Au Trocadéro.

Le dimanche suivant; l'après-midi.

Grande animation. Des files de fiacres viennent se décharger au bas des escaliers. Un cordon d'agents assuré l'ordre.

Tout à coup, un mouvement se produit parmi les jeunes gens qui stationnent sur le trottoir: une voiture s'est arrêtée devant l'entrée particulière de la salle.

Barois descend, accompagné de Luce.

Les têtes se découvrent.

Les deux hommes s'engagent vivement dans l'intérieur du palais, suivis de quelques intimes.

A trois heures la salle est comble; des gens debout obstruent les dégagements.

Les rideaux s'écartent lentement, découvrant la scène vide, où Barois paraît presque aussitôt. Une immense ovation roule en tonnerre, s'élève, retombe, se relève lourdement, ondule comme un essaim qui hésite avant de prendre son vol, et subitement s'évanouit en un silence total.

Barois gravit lentement les marches de l'estrade.

Il est un nain au centre du vaste hémicycle. On distingue mal ses traits; mais son entrée rapide, la fermeté de son salut, le long et calme regard qu'il promène sur ces milliers de têtes nues concentnquement alignées autour et au dessus de lui, révèlent l'assurance d'un homme qui a le vent en poupe.

Il s'assied sans quitter la salle des yeux.

Barois. — Mesdames, Messieurs...

Une brève angoisse; son cœur se crispe."

Mais le silence de ces visages immobiles, la confiance de ces innombrables regards qui convergent sur lui, desserrent l'étau. Il cède à une inspiration subite: il renonce au préambule préparé, laisse retomber ses notes, et se livre, en souriant, sur un ton de causerie affectueuse.

...Mes chers amis,

Vous êtes ici deux ou trois mille... vous n'avez pas hésité à abandonner vos occupations du dimanche pour entendre parler de *l'Avenir de F incroyance.* A ce seul titre, vous êtes accourus.

Symptôme caractéristique,' et combien émouvant!

Tous les peuples civilisés subissent actuellement la même crise religieuse: dans tous les coins du monde où la culture, où la pensée ont quelque autorité, un même mouvement soulève la conscience humaine, un même courant de réflexion et d'incrédulité rejette les fables des éaises, un même geste

d'affranchissement repousse la tutelle dogmatique d dp tous les dieux. La France qui, par son équilibre intellectuel, son appent de liberté, son besoin de vérification positive, est, depuis deux cents ans, le véritable foyer de la libre-pensée dans le monde, semble avoir donné le signal de cet ébranlement. L'Italie, l'Espagne, l'Amérique du Sud, tous les pays latins où dominait le catholicisme, ont suivi son exemple. Une transformation parallèle travaille les pays protestants, l'Angleterre, l'Amérique du Nord, le sud de l'Afrique. Et ce mouvement est si général qu'il atteint, dès aujourd'hui, les centres instruits de l'Islam et du Bouddhisme, les parties civilisées de l'Afrique, de l'Inde, le Japon tout entier. Partout les églises ont dû renoncer à ce pouvoir civil qu'elles avaient exercé pendant de longs siècles et qui renforçait habilement leur puissance. Elles se sont vu retirer un à un leurs privilèges, et exclure impitoyablement du domaine temporel. En fait, il n'y a pour ainsi dire plus de religions nationales; partout, l'Etat est laïc, et il affirme sa neutralité entre les croyances dont il tolère les cultes.

Cet immense assaut de la pensée contre le bloc des religions est trop complexe pour être étudié en détail: mais j'ai voulu vous rappeler qu'il est *universel,* afin que vous ne fussiez pas tentés de considérer l'évolution irreligieuse de notre pays comme un événement local et sans retentissement; il est étroitement lié au frémissement parallèle de tous les peuples.

Il s'arrête.

Il avait devant lui une agglomération d'hommes, de jeunes gens, de femmes,- c'est maintenant un auditoire. La synthèse est faite. Ses yeux, sa voix, sa pensée, sont maintenant en contact direct avec une masse uniforme, une seule et riche sensibilité, dont la sienne n'est plus distincte, mais forme l'élément central et moteur.

L'Eglise catholique, qui se prétend au-dessus de toute loi humaine, ne s'est pas laissé assujettir au droit commun sans une vive résistance. Elle a dû capituler cependant, et reporter tout ce qu'elle garde encore d'influence, dans le domaine spirituel: dernier retranchement, dont le flot qui monte, malgré certaines apparences momentanées, ronge activement les fondations... Car l'insuffisance de la théodicée à satisfaire les esprits actuels s'accroît, dans des proportions colossales, à mesure que se succèdent les générations: chaque découverte nouvelle ajoute invariablement une objection de plus aux affirmations dogmatiques de la religion, qui, par contre, ne reçoit plus, depuis longtemps, le moindre renfort des études contemporaines.

En lutte contre cet irrésistible courant, il n'y aurait pour l'Eglise qu'un» seule chance de salut:£Uû/uer, _nde rendre ses formules acceptables aux consciences modernes. C est pour elle" question de vie ou de mort. Si ettëTne se transforme pas, elle provoquera infailliblement, en quelques générations, une désertion générale et définitive.

Or je voudrais vous montrer qu'il est littéralement impossible que ses dogmes se modifient, si peu que ce soit. Je voudrais vous montrer que l'Eglise catholique est condamnée. Quoi qu'elle fasse, elle est fatalement vouée à une dissolution totale, que l'on doit, dès maintenant, tenir pour inévitable, et dont on pourrait presque fixer l'échéance!

Une doctrine philosophique peut évoluer; elle est composée de pensées *humaines* qui sont groupées dans un ordre arbitraire, et, par nature, provisoire. Mais une religion *révélée,* — dont le point de départ n'est pas sujet à correction, mais parfait dès l'origine, immuable par définition, comme l'absolu, — une telle religion ne peut varier sans se détruire ellemême. Car, pour elle, s'amender, c'est reconnaître que sa forme précédente n'était pas parfaite, c'est avouer que sa source n'est pas en Dieu, qu'il n'y a pas de révélation à son origine. Ceci est de telle évidence, que l'Eglise n'a cessé d'affirmer son immutabilité comme une preuve de sa provenance divine, et que, récemment encore, le concile de 1870 n'a pas hésité à déclarer: « La doctrine de la foi que *Dieu a révélée* n'a pas été livrée *comme une invention philosophique aux perfectionnements humains,* mais elle a été transmise comme un dépôt divin. » (i).

Le cathoKscime est donc prisonnier de son principe essentiel.

Maîs luTons plus loin. Même s'il lui était loisible d'opérer sans se con ( i) Concile du Vatican Ch. IV tredire quelque réforme dans sa doctrine, il ne pourrait s'assurer par là qu'un sursis passager. Voici pourquoi:

Le plus élémentaire aperçu historique sur le développement des relii. gions nous montre qu'elles sont toutes nées de la curiosité de l'homme en présence de l'univers; leur noyau initial est toujours le même: il est"c5n$= titué par les premières et naïves explications que l'homme a pu trouver aux phénomènes naturels. A ce point que l'on pourrait simplifier, jusqu'à dire: il n'y a pas eu, à proprement parler, de religion primitive; depuis l'humanité balbutiante jusqu'à nous, il n'y a qu'une seulé trame de pensée: la trame scientifique; rudimentaire à son origine, elle s'enrichit peu à peu. Et ce que nous désignons sous le terme de religion, c'est une des étapes de la recherche humaine, l'étape de l'affirmation déiste; c'est une simple minute de l'effort scientifique, stupidement arrêtée et prolongée jusqu'à nous par la crainte du surnaturel; en un mot, l'homme est resté dupe des hypothèses mystiques qu'il avait ébauchées pour s'expliquer le tnonde. Cette cristallisation accidentelle a ralenti pendant plusieurs siècles le cheminement de la science; et, dès lors, le mouvement scientifique s'est trouvé nettement distinct du mouvement religieux.

J'en reviens donc à ce que je voulais vous dire. La religion, c'est la science d'autrefois, desséchée, devenue dogme; ce n'est que l'enveloppe d'une explication scientifique dépassée depuis longtemps. Elle a perdu, en se figeant, son principe de vie; elle est morte. Si, par impossible, elle tentait aujourd'hui de se transformer, de rejoindre le progrès scientifique, — qui représente ce qu'elle devrait être normalement, —.. .eh bien, elle ne le pourrait pas! Elle n'a pu durer tant de siècles qu'en berçant, avec ses mensonges, l'âme apeurée des hommes, en atténuant par des promesses leur effroi de mourir, et en engourdissant leur instinct d'investigation par des affirmations gratuites et invérifiables. Le jour où elle renoncerait à cet appareil qui la rend semblable à une imagerie populaire, il ne resterait plus rien de l'armature qui lui donne encore, pour certains, une apparence de vie. Car le sentiment religieux, sur l'existence duquel elle a spéculé depuis son origine, n'a pas d'équivalent dans les cerveaux vraiment modernes: et ce serait une lourde erreur de prendre pour un résidu des croyances mystiques de nos ancêtres, ce besoin inné de comprendre et d'expliquer, qui est bien antérieur à toute sentimentalité religieuse, et qui trouve aujourd'hui sa large et complète satisfaction dans le développement scientifique de notre temps.

Il ne me semble donc pas douteux qu'une religion dogmatique comme le catholicisme soit condamnée sans recours. La rigidité fondamentale de ses formules la rend de plus en plus suspecte à ces esprits, qui ont trop souvent expérimenté la relativité de leur connaissance, pour admetiie-une doctrine qui se proclame infaillible et immuable.

D'ailleurs le mal qui la mine ne vient pas seulement du dehors: une paralysie progressive l'envahit et la rend inapte à vivre parmi nous.

Non, le courant actuel est indiscutablement orienté vers une société sans Dieu, vers une conception purement scientifique de l'univers!

Il s'aperçoit aussitôt que cette dernière phrase a déclenché quelque chose. La tension des yeux qui le guettent, s'accentue soudain. Il se sent dominé par une pression de la volonté collective.

Il comprend: après avoir suivi jusqu'au bout sa pensée destructive, ils ont soif de quelque mirage, ils attendent, comme des enfants, leur conte de fée.

Il n'a rien préparé, mais il obéit. Son regard devient lumineux; un sourire de visionnaire joue sur ses lèvres.

LQue sera-t-elle, cette irreligion de l'avenir? Ah, qui de nous peut l'entrevoir et la décrire? _Ce que l'on peut affirmer c'est quelle ne sera, à aucun degré, *une religion scientifique.* On répète trop souvent que les savants sont des prêtres aun nouveau culte, qu'ils remplacent une foi par une autre... Il se peut que, dans le désarroi actuel, certains d'entre nous apportent à la science qu'ils servent, un reste de religiosité héritée et sans emploi. N'y attachons pas d'importance. En fait, il n'y a plus de place pour de nouvelles idoles, et la science ne peut en être une; car *l'intelligence est négative,* et c'est une constatation à laquelle il faudra bien que se résignent les imaginations les plus exaltées.

Je crois que le ralliement des esprits et des cœurs, égarés encore, ne saurait tarder; et qu'il se fera, d'une part, sur le terrain de la solidarité sociale, et de l'autre, sur le terrain de la connaissance scientifique. J'entrevois la possibilité de lois morales, basées sur l'analyse de l'individu et de ses rapports avec ce qui l'entoure. Le cœur y trouvera son compte, parce qu'une telle orientation laisse à l'instinct altruiste son plein développement: en face d'une nature indifférente et qui le dépasse, l'homme semble avoir besoin de s'associer; et de ce besoin naissent des obligations morales. J'imagine aisément que ces devoirs, réglés par leur attraction les uns sur les autres, puissent établir, pour un temps, un bon équilibre social.

Pronostics vagues, simples jeux de l'esprit... Je le sais bien! (Souriant.) Mais les temps nouveaux n'ont plus de prophètes...

Ce qui est indubitable c'est que le terrain de ralliement ne sera plus métaphysique. Il nous faut en toutes choses, maintenant, une base expérimentale. Aux religions qui affirmaient connaître le sens de l'univers, succédera sans doute une philosophie positive et neutre, sans cesse alimentée par les découvertes scientifiques, essentiellement mobile, transiloire, modelée sur les mouvements de la réflexion humaine. On peut prévoir, en conséquence, qu'elle ne cessera d'élargir son horizon, et bien au delà des conceptions restreintes auxquelles nous devons actuellement borner notre vue. Remarquez dé-

jà combien nous semble mesquin et incomplet le matérialisme sentimental d'il y a cinquante ans! Le nôtre, plus scientifique, tend déjà à s'élever au-dessus des visions qui satisfaisaient nos pères; le suivant s'en écartera davantage encore. La pensée pousse en plein inconnu son investigation; je crois que nous possédons déjà quelques bonnes méthodes de recherche... Mais que nous sommes loin de pouvoir deviner vers quels nouveaux aspects de la réalité notre élan nous mène!

Courte pause.

Son expression change. L'œil reprend sa dureté naturelle. La voix redevient incisive.

Il baisse la tête, et palpe les feuillets épars devant lui.

Je me laisse entraîner par ces visions hypothétiques... L'heure avance, et je ne veux pas vous quitter sans avoir abordé le second point de cette usene:

Quelle action chacun de nous peut-il avoir sur la réalisation plus ou moins rapide de ces espérances?

Cette action est immense! Pour ingrat que puisse paraître le rôle des hommes d'aujourd'hui, après ce coup d'œil complaisant vers l'avenir, il est capital, et nous ne saurions l'envisager avec trop de fermeté.

Nous sommes l'une de ces quelques générations, auxquelles incombe le soin d'opérer l'évolution scientifique: nous sommes l'une des minutes tragiques de la douloureuse agonie du passé.

Ah, mes amis, si 1 on comprend quels abîmes d'angoisses morales représente chaque génération de consciences, écartelées comme sont tant des nôtres, entre ce qui a été et ce qui sera; si l'on songe que notre option plus ou moins vigoureuse, peut abréger ou prolonger la souffrance de ces milliers de sensibilités, — quelle lourde responsabilité pèse sur nous!

Eh bien, nous avons deux moyens d'agir: par notre attitude personnelle et par l'éducation de nos enfants...

Faisons ensemble notre examen de conscience, voulez-vous?

Combien d'entre nous, dont les convictions sont nettement opposées aux croyances religieuses, supportent

néanmoins que la religion domine tous les actes graves de leur vie, depuis leur mariage, jusqu'à leur mort!

(Sombre.) Oui, je sais, je sais aussi bien que vous... — mieux que vous, peut-être! —. tout ce que l'on peut dire pour excuser cette faiblesse, et quel morne supplice endure souvent l'homme libre qui croit devoir se soumettre à ces gestes rituels... Quels déchirements, quelles rancunes, quelles sourdes luttes entre une conscience qui voudrait être rigide, et tant de forces dissolvantes, les engagements de la tendresse, le respect d'autrui!... Mais il n'est pas moins vrai qu'il y a dans une semblable résignation une immoralité que rien, rien ne saurait légitimer! Aux heures troubles que traverse notre humanité, il n'est rien de plus grave qu'un acte de foi public, non seulement pour la dignité individuelle de celui qui l'accomplit, mais pour la répercussion illimitée qu'il peut avoir sur les irrésolutions voisines. *La probité envers soi-même comme envers ceux qui nous regardent vivre, voilà, pour le moment, la plus certaine, la plus inflexible des règles morales.* Et ceux qui transigent avec elle, qui, par l'incohérence de leur attitude, retardent, dans leur sphère, le cours de l'évolution commettent un crime social mille fois plus redoutable que tous les chagrins sentimentaux qu'ils auraient pu causer! Plus impardonnable encore est leur faute, en ce qui concerne l'éducation de leurs fils.

L'esprit de l'enfant n'est pas capable de prévention: la notion du doute est le résultat d'une longue pratique des phénomènes; elle suppose l'expérience de l'erreur, une défiance de soi et de ses sensations, une défiance d'autrui. L'enfant est crédule, comme tout primitif; le sens du vraisemblable n'existe pas en lui: le miracle ne le surprend pas.

Le prêtre, à qui vous abandonnez cet esprit vierge, y marquera sans peine une empreinte ineffaçable. Il lui inspirera d'abord une crainte arbitraire de son dieu; puis il lui présentera les mystères de son culte, comme autant de vérités révélées, qui échappent et *doivent* échapper à l'entendement humain. Le prêtre affirme plus facilement qu'il ne prouve; l'enfant croit plus facilement qu'il ne raisonne: la concordance est parfaite... Le raisonnement est l'opposé de la foi; un cerveau que la foi a façonné, reste longtemps, sinon toujours inapte aux jugements critiques.

Et c'est l'esprit sans défense de cet enfant que vous allez confier, dès le plus jeune âge, à l'influence religieuse?

Il s'est levé, emporté par la fougue de cette indignation, où vibre un remords personnel.

C'est l'homme d'action: la polémique quotidienne lui a révélé sa puissance: il aime la lutte; si violent est son élan qu'il renverse parfois l'obstacle avant de l'avoir aperçu: une force qui se rue...

Quoi! L'Eglise nous maudit, elle lance l'anathème sur ce qui constitue les réalités les plus vivantes de notre existence; et c'est à elle que nous allons livrer nos enfants? Comment expliquer pareille aberration? Est-ce parce que nous gardons l'espoir secret qu'ils sauront bientôt se dégager de ces superstitions? Alors, comment qualifier cette hypocrisie?

Et puis, la grossière erreur de croire qu'en mûrissant, l'esprit secouera sans peine ces fumées! Ne vous rappelez-vous pas combien peut être tenace une foi d'enfant Hélas, l'homme que la religion a marqué dès l'enfance ne s'en débarrasse pas d'un simple mouvement d'épaule, comme d'un vêtement usé, devenu trop étroit! Les éléments religieux trouvent chez l'enfant un sol préparé par dix-huit siècles d'asservissement consenti; ils se mêlent inextricablement à tous les autres éléments de safoTmation intellectuelle et morale. La dissociation, lorsqu'elle est possible", est longue, irrégulière, souvent incomplète, toujours douloureuse. Et combien sont-ils, ceux qui, dans les conditions actuelles de la vie, ont le loisir ou le courage de procéder à cette refonte totale de leur personnalité?

Encore ai-je jusqu'ici restreint la question: je n'ai envisagé ces dangers de l'enseignement religieux qu'à l'égard de l'individu. Mais ils menacent directement la Société. A notre époque, où les croyances religieuses sont partout ébranlées, il y a un véritable péril à laisser, dans l'âme des enfants, se souder les lois de la morale aux dogmes de la religion. Car, s'ils s'habituent à considérer ces règles de vie sociale comme autant d'ordres divins, le jour probable où la certitude de Dieu vacillera dans leur esprit, tout en eux s'effondrera à la fois, et ils perdront du même coup leur direction morale.

Voilà donc, brièvement résumés, les risques que nous courons, lorsque nous agissons en pères insouciants ou trop faibles. Et sous quels principes retentissants masquerons-nous notre apathie?

Je vous entends... Nous proclamerons généreusement la *neutralité*!

Ah, notre devoir est difficile, je le sais. Mais ne soyons pas dupes des mots... Cette neutralité, nos adversaires ont beau nous reprocher de la violer souvent, — (est-il possible à un enseignement d'être strictement neutre?) — c'est nous seuls qu'elle entrave! Neutralité, cela veut dire aujourd'hui: effacement devant la propagande acharnée de l'Eglise.

Eh bien, cette situation fausse n'a que trop duré. Prenons franchement notre parti d'une lutte qui est inévitable, qui est la grande lutte de notre temps; et au lieu de la mener sourdement, acceptons-la au grand jour, avec des armes égales. Laissons les prêtres libres d'ouvrir des écoles et d'y enseigner que le monde a été créé de rien en six jours; que Jésus-CHrisT" était le fils de Dieu-le-Père et d'une Vierge; et que son cadavre _s est échappé tout seul de son tombeau, trois jours après son ensevelissement, pour monter dans le Ciel, où il est assis, depuis lors, a la droite de DîeiTÎ Mais soyons libres, nous aussi, d'ouvrir des écoles où nous aurons Tè droit de prouver, avec tout l'appui de la raison et de la science, sur quelles inqualifiables crédulités se fonde encore la foi catholique! Quand la vérité est libre et l'erreur aussi, ce n'est pas l'erreur qui triomphe! La liberté, oui, mais pas seulement pour l'abbé du catéchisme: la liberté pour la raison, la liberté pour l'enfant!

Il s'avance sur le bord de l'estrade, le visage dressé, les prunelles ardentes, les mains tendues.

Ah, mes amis, je voudrais terminer sur ce cri: *la liberté pour l'enfant*!

Je voudrais secouer toutes vos consciences, je voudrais surprendre dans vos regards le feu des résolutions nouvelles!

Souvenons-nous de ce que nous avons souffert pour extirper de nous le vieil homme... Souvenons-nous de cet incendie qui nous a dévasté... Souvenons-no de nos terreurs nocturnes, de nos révoltes, de nos confessions désespérées... Souvenons-nous de nos d'angoisses et de nos agenouillements...

Pitié pour nos fils!

,,,''1' La même année, quelques mois plus tard.

Barois hèle un fiatre, place de la Madeleine.

Barois. — Au *Semeur*, rue de l'Université.

Il claque la portière.

La voiture ne démarre pas. Coup de fouet; une ruade.

BAROIS. — Allons! je suis pressé...

Nouveau coup de fouet. Le cheval, une bête jeune et rétive, hésite, se cabre, lève les naseaux et part comme une flèche.

Il enfile la rue Royale, traverse d'un trait la place de la Concorde, et s'élance dans le boulevard Saint-Germain.

Quatre heures de l'après-midi. Circulation intense.

Le cocher, arcbouté sur son siège, incapable de maîtriser l'animal, parvient à le diriger, à grand'peine.

Un tramway poussif barre la route.

Pour le dépasser, l'homme lance sa voiture à gauche, sur les rails libres. Il n'a pas vu le tramway qui vient en sens inverse...

Impossible de ralentir... Impossible de passer entre les deux véhicules...

Barois, blême, se jette en arrière, contre les coussins. La vision de son impuissance au fond de cette boîte, la certitude de l'inévitable, pénètrent en lui, comme la foudre.

Il balbutie: « Je vous salue, Marie, pleine de grâces.., i'

Un fracas infernal de vitres pulvérisées..,

Un choc mortel...

Du noir..

Plusieurs jours après.

Chez Barois, à la tombée du jour.

Woldsmuth, sur une chaise, près de la fenêtre, lit sans faire un mouvement.

Barois est étendu sur son matelas, les jambes noyées jusqu'aux hanches dans du plâtre.

Il n'a recouvré sa pleine conscience que depuis quelques heures; et, pour la dixième fois, il reconstruit mentalement l'aventure:

— « Il y avait la place, si celui de droite n'avait pas accéléré... « Ai-je eu le temps de sentir le frôlement de la mort? Je ne sais plus... J'ai eu peur, une peur atroce.. Et puis le hurlement des freins bloqués... »

Il sourit involontairement: entre la mort et lui, tout le bouillonnement de sa vie présente, reconquise!

— « Curieux, cette peur qu'on a de mourir... Comment peut-on craindre la suppression de toute pensée, de toute sensation, de toute souffrance? Craindre de ne *plus être*?

« Peut-être est-ce uniquement l'inconnu qui terrifie? C'est évidemment la seule sensation qui nous soit *totalement* nouvelle: personne n'a, dans son hérédité, la moindre expérience de ça...

« Et pourtant, un homme de science, qui a le temps de réfléchir quelques secondes, doit se résigner, sans beaucoup de peine. Quand on a bien compris que la vie n'est qu'une suite de transformations, pourquoi s'effrayer de celle-là? Ce n'est pas la première... Ce n'est vraisemblablement pas la dernière...

« Et puis, quand on a su employer son existence, quand on a lutté, quand on *laisse* derrière soi, qu'est-ce qu'on peut regretter?

« Je suis bien sûr, moi, de m'en aller, très calme... »

Soudain, son visage se contracte. Il reste épouvanté, anéanti. Il vient de revivre la minute tragique, et, brutalement, il s'est rappelé le seul cri venu à ses lèvres:

« Je vous salue, Marie... »

Une heure s'écoule.

Woldsmuth tourne ses pages, sans bouger.

Pascal apporte une lampe; il ferme les volets et s approche de son maître; sa figure plate de Suisse, aux cheveux ras, aux yeux larges et clairs, est bonne à regarder. Mais Barois ne l'aperçoit pas; son regard est fixe; son cerveau fonctionne avec une activité déréglée; sa pensée est extraordinairement lucide, clarifiée comme l'atmosphère des montagnes après l'orage.

Enfin son visage, crispé par l'effort cérébral, se détend progressivement.

Barois. — Woldsmuth...

WOLDSMUTH (se levant avec précipitation). — Vous souffrez?

BAROIS (d'une voix brève). — Non. Ecoutez-moi. Asseyez-vous là.

WOLDSMUTH (qui lui a pris le poignet). — Vous avez un peu de fièvre... Restez tranquille, ne parlez pas.

BAROIS (dégageant son bras). — Asseyez-vous là, et écoutez-moi. (Avec colère.) Non, non, je veux parler! Je ne me rappelais pas tout... J'oubliais le plus beau...

Woldsmuth! Au moment où j'ai vu que j'étais perdu, savez-vous ce que j'ai fait?

Eh bien, j'ai prié la Sainte Vierge!

WOLDSMUTH (conciliant). — Ne pensez plus à tout ça... Il faut vous reposer...

BAROIS. — Non, je n'ai pas le délire. Je parle sérieusement, je veux que vous m écoutiez. Je ne serai tranquille que lorsque j'aurai fait ce que je dois faire...

Woldsmuth s'assied. Barois (les yeux briilants, les pommettes rouges). — A ce moment-là, moi, Jean Barois, je n'ai pensé à rien d'autre, j'ai été soulevé par un espoir fou, *j'ai supplié de tout mon être la Sainte Vierge de faire un miracle* !... (Il rit violemment.) Ah, mon cher, après ça, on peut être fier de son armature! TROISIEME PARTIE (Il redresse le buste, resté libre.) Alors, vous comprenez, je suis hanté par l'idée que ça pourrait recommencer... Ce soir, cette nuit, est-ce que je sais, maintenant? Je veux rédiger quelque chose, protester d'avance. Je ne serai pas tranquille avant.

WOLDSMUTH. — Oui, demain, je vous promets. Vous me dicterez...

BAROIS (avec une violence irrésistible). — Tout de suite, Woldsmuth, tout de suite, vous entendez! Je veux tout écrire moi-même, ce soir! Je ne pourrais pas dormir... (Se passant la main sur le front.) D'ailleurs, c'est là, tout prêt, je ne me fatiguerai pas... Le plus dur est fait...

Woldsmuth cède. Il soulève Barois sur deux oreillers, et lui donne son stylographe, du papier. Puis il reste debout, contre le lit.

Barois écrit, sans une hésitation, sans lever les yeux, d'une écriture droite et ferme:

« Ceci est mon testament.

« Ce que j'écris aujourd'hui, ayant dépassé la quarantaine, en pleine force et en plein équilibre intellectuel, doit, de toute évidence, prévaloir contre ce que je pourrai penser ou écrire à la fin de mon existence, lorsque je serai physiquement et moralement diminué par l'âge ou par la maladie. Je ne connais rien de plus poignant que l'attitude d'un vieillard, dont la vie toute entière a été employée au service d'une idée, et qui, dans l'affaiblissement final, blasphème ce qui a été sa raison de vivre, et renie lamentablement son passé.

« En songeant que l'effort de ma vie pourrait aboutir à une semblable trahison; en songeant au parti que ceux dont j'ai si ardemment combattu les mensonges et les empiètements, ne manqueraient pas de tirer d'une si lugubre victoire, tout mon être se révolte, et je proteste d'avance, avec l'énergie farouche de l'homme que je suis, deThomme *vivant* que j'aurai "été, contre les' dénégations sans fondement, peut-être même contre la prière'âgônisahte du déchet humain que je puis devenir. J'ai mérité de mourir debout, comme j'ai vécu, sans capituler, sans quêter de vaines espéTfances, sans craindre le retour aux lentes évolutions de la germination universelle.

f« Je ne crois pas à l'âme humaine, substantielle et immortelle. « Je ne crois pas que la matière s'opposeàl'espnt. L'âme est la sommedes phénomènes psychiques, comme le corps est la somme des phénomènes organiques. L'âme est une résultante occasionnelle de la vie, une propriété 'de la matière vivante. Je ne vois aucune raison pour que l'énergie universelle qui produit le mouvement, la chaleur et la lumière, ne produise pas la pensée. Les fonctions physiologiques et les fonctions psychiques sont solidaires; et la pensée est une manifestation de la vie organique, au même titre que les autres fonctions du système nerveux. Je n'ai jamais constaté de la pensée hors de la matière, hors d'un corps en vie; je n'ai jamais rencontré qu'une substance unique, la substance vivante.

« Que nous l'appellions matière ou vie, je la crois éternelle: la vie a toujours été et produira la vie éternellement. Mais je sais que ma personnalité n'est qu'une agglomération de particules matérielles, dont la désagrégation entraînera la mort totale.

f Je crois au déterminisme universel, et que notre dépendance est absolue. « Tout évolue; tout réagit; la pierre et l'homme;il n'y a pas de matière inerte. Je n'ai donc aucun motif pour attribuer plus de liberté individuelle à mon activité que je n'en attribue aux transformations plus lentes d'un cristal.

« Ma vie résulte d'une lutte incessante entre mon organisme et le milieu où je baigne: j'agis donc, à chaque instant, selon mes réactions particulières, c'est-à-dire pour des raisons qui n'appartiennent qu'à moi seul: ce qui donne aux autres l'illusion que je suis libre de mes actes. Mais en aucun cas je n'agis librement: aucune de mes déterminations ne pourrait être différente de ce qu'elle est. Le libre arbitre équivaudrait au pouvoir d'accomplir un miracle, de dévier les rapports des causes aux effets. C'est une conception métaphysique, qui prouve simplement l'ignorance où nous avons été si longtemps, et où nous sommes encore, des lois auxquelles nous obéissons.

« Je nie donc que l'homme puisse en rien influer sur sa destinée.

« Le bien et le mal sont des distinctions arbitraires. Je concède qu'elles ont une utilité pratique, tant que la notion de responsabilité, qui ne se fonde sur rien de réel, sera nécessaire à l'échafaudage de notre organisation sociale.

« Je crois que, si tous les phénomènes de la vie ne sont pas encore analysés, ils le seront un jour.

« Quant aux causes premières de ces phénomènes, je crois qu'elles sont hors de notre plan de vision, et inaccessibles à nos recherches. L'homme, par suite de sa place limitée dans l'univers, être relatif et fini par essence, "ne peut pas avoir la notion de l'absolu et de l'infini; il s'e '' ' pour exprimer ce qui n'est pas comme lui, mais il n'en est pas plus avancé: il est victime de son langage; ces mots ne correspondent, pour l'entendement humain, à aucune réalité précise. Élément d'un tout, il est nature! que l'ensemble lui échappe.

« Se révolter contre cette nécessité, c'est s'insurger contre les conditions planétaires de ce monde.

« J'estime donc qu'il est vain jjéchafauder, pour expliquer l'inconnaissable, des hypothèses qui n'ont aucune Base expérimentale. Il est temps que nous nous guérissions de notre délire métaphysique, et que nous renoncions enfin aux « pourquoi » sans réponse, que notre hérédité mystique nous incite encore à poser.

« L'homme a, devant lui, un champ d'observation *pratiquement illimité.* Peu à peu, la science reculera si loin les bornes de ce qui n'est pas constatable, que si l'homme s'employait à comprendre tout le réel qui est à sa portée, il n'aurait plus le temps de gémir sur ce qui échappe irrémédiablement à ses facultés.

« Je suis certain que la science, en apprenant aux hommes à *savoir ignorer,* procurera à leurs consciences un équilibre qu'aucune foi n'a jamais su leur offrir.

Jean Barois. »

D'une main lourde, il achève lentement sa signature.

Puis sa volonté tendue se rompt. Sa face congestionnée devient brusquement livide. Il se renverse dans les bras de Woldsmuth.

Les feuillets s'éparpillent sur les draps.

Woldsmuth, d'une voix anxieuse, appelle Pascal. Mais déjà Barois soulève les paupières, et sourit aux deux hommes.

Quelques instants plus tard, sa respiration régulière révèle un profond et calme sommeil.

LA FÊLURE

Un matin.

Barois achève de déjeuner.

Pascal. — Il y a là un abbé, qui voudrait voir Monsieur

BAROIS. — Un abbé?

PASCAL. — Il n'a pas voulu dire son nom.

Barois entre dans son cabinet.

Un prêtre âgé, debout à contre-jour: l'abbé Joziers.

L ABBÉ. — Je ne me suis pas fait nommer, je n'étais pas sûr d'être reçu... (Il rencontre le regard joyeux de Barois, et baisse la tête.) Bonjour, Jean.

Depuis plus de dix ans, aucune voix amie ne l'a appelé « Jean »... Ses yeux s'emplissent de larmes; il tend les mains. L'abbé les saisit.

Ils sont un instant l'un contre l'autre sans parler.

L'abbé Joziers: la soixantaine.

Le corps, maigre et long, est demeuré alerte Mais le visage est d'un vieillard: les cheveux sont tout gris; la peau est jaune, fripée; aux coins des lèvres, deux entailles, par où les joues semblent s'être vidées de leur chair.

Barois, familièrement, avance un siège L'abbé s'y assied avec réserve.

Barois aussi a changé: il a maigri; il porte ses cheveux emmêlés sur le front; le regard est plus pensif; la moustache noire, striée de blanc, masque maintenant la révolte de la bouche.

L'abbÉ. — Je ne viens pas en ami, voas vous en doutez bien... Je viens, parce qu'on me l'a demandé, et qu'il n'y avait personne d'autre pour faire cette démarche...

Vous devinez sans doute pourquoi?

Barois secoue négativement la tête; sa bonne foi est évidente.

L'abbé était venu, indigné; et, devant ce regard loyal, il se sent incliné à plus d'indulgence: « C'est un irresponsable. .. » Mais il reprend son rôle; et l'affection ancienne redescend au fond de son cœur.

L'abbÉ (agressif). — Vous avez récemment fait une leçon publique, je ne sais à quelle occasion, sous ce titre: *Documents psychologiques pour l'évolution contemporaine de la foi.*

BAROIS (intrigué). — Oui.

L'ABBÉ. — Vous y êtes délibérément sorti du domaine des idées générales, pour donner des détails... dont le caractère autobiographique est manifeste. Les fragments que j'ai *dû* lire, font allusion à des circonstances de votre jeunesse, de votre *mariage...* qui y sont étalées... avec une absence de... respect...

BAROIS (sèchement). — Vous allez un peu loin. Les détails dont vous parlez sont anonymes et présentés sous une forme scientifique, qui écarte toute autre interprétation. J'ai étudié un grand nombre de cas psychologiques, dont une partie m'était fournie par des correspondants, médecins en province, et dont quelques autres, je le reconnais, m'étaient personnels...

L'abbÉ (haussant le ton). — C'est *là* où vous vous trompez, Jean. Ces détails n'appartiennent pas à *vous seul.* (Amèrement.) J'ai eu la douleur de perdre, à votre sujet, bien des illusions déjà. Mais je ne croyais pas qu'il me faudrait un jour vous rappeler à votre plus *élémentaire* dignité d'homme. Il y a des analyses intimes dont le secret est inviolable. On n'expose pas à la curiosité d'un public, quel qu'il soit, pour quelque motif que ce soit, les sentiments d'une femme, qui est et qui reste la *vôtre,* qui est la mère de votre enfant!

Barois reçoit le coup au visage, sans un geste de protestation. tT3evient pourpre.

Des souvenirs s'abattent sur lui, en rafale: au fond de sa conscience, un passé, qui n'était qu'enseveli, ressuscite..

L ABBÉ. — Un journal franc-maçon de l'Oise a relevé dans vos paroles ce qui pouvait blesser Mme Barois, et...

Barois n'écoute pas. Il regarde l'abbé avec une expression concentrée, lointaine. Blesser sa femme?... Pas une seule fois, depuis leur séparation, l'idée ne lui est venue qu'elle pût encore être blessée par lui!

Il a besoin de se ressaisir. Il gagne sa table de travail, comme un refuge, et s'assied lourdement, les mains crispées sur les bras de son fauteuil, son fauteuil quotidien.

BROlS. — Oui, je comprends maintenant... Mais c'est si involontaire! Le regard de l'abbé est incrédule.

BAROIS (vivement,. — Vous ne le croyez pas?Ah, rendez-vous compte: je vis ici, seul, depuis plus de dix ans; je ne vois personne; quelques amis, des collaborateurs... Je suis terriblement occupé. .. Je n'ai pas le temps de regarder en arrière; et puis, ce n'est pas dans ma nature... Je n'ai jamais aucune nouvelle de Buis: une fois par an, un clerc de notaire m'avertit que la pension a été versée: et c'est tout.

L'abbé le considère avec stupéfaction.

BAROIS. — Je vous étonne? c'est la pure vérité. Le passé est le passé, j'en suis sorti; il est loin, il est mort pour moi; je n'y pense jamais, jamais.

Quand j'ai préparé le cours en question, j'ai cherché avant tout des documents authentiques, exacts. J'en ai pris dans ma propre expérience, sans hésiter. Evidemment, ces souvenirs ne m'appartenaient pas entièrement... C'est vrai... *Caj.* (S'interrogeant.) Je me suis peut-être conduit comme un goujat. ..

Il fixe le sol.

Ses mains ont un imperceptible tremblement.

Ah, je suis très contrarié, d'avoir été, sans le youloir, la cause.. (Spontanément.) Expliquez-lui, dites-lui bien tout ce que je...

L'abbé (désarmé par tant d'inconscience). — Non, Jean, il vaut mieux que je ne répète pas tout ce que vous venez de me dire là...

Un silence.

L'abbé prend son chapeau.

BAROIS. — Vous n'êtes pas pressé. .. (Il hésite.) Donnez-moi quelques nouvelles. Est-ce que... Cécile vit toujours chez sa mère?

Le visage du prêtre reste fermé; il fait un signe afHrmatif.

BAROIS. — Et elles mènent toujours la même vie? Les patronages, les ouvroirs?

L'abbÉ (désapprobateur). — Mme Barois donne aux œuvres le temps qu'elle ne consacre pas à sa fille.

BAROIS. — Ah, oui, l'enfant... qui a maintenant... voyons... treize ans...? Hein? (Naïvement.) Comment est-elle, cette petite? A-t-elle une bonne santé?

Il croise le regard de l'abbé; sa phrase s'achève dans un sourire gêné.

BAROIS.— Je vous parais être un monstre? Que voulez-vous... (Geste brutal.) J'ai rayé tout ça! C'est passé, c'est fini 1 Ma vie, elle est toute ailleurs, et elle me passionne exclusivement! Pourquoi feindrais-je? Souvenezvous: cette petite, j'étais déjà parti en Angleterre, quand elle est née... Elle ne m'intéresse vraiment à aucun titre, elle n'a rien de moi...

L'abbÉ (qui le considère soigneusement). — Si. J'en suis même frappé depuis ce matin: elle *vous* ressemble.

BAROIS (la voix changée). — Elle me ressemble?

L'abbé. — L'expression générale... Le regard... Le menton...

Nouveau silence.

L'abbé se lève.

Il s'en va, mécontent de Barois, mécontent de lui-même, gar dant pour lui ce qu'il eût aimé dire, emportant de cette visite une rancœur nouvelle.

BAROIS (qui l'accompagne vers la porte). — Et... vous habitez toujours à Buis?

L'abbÉ. — Monseigneur m'a confié la cure de Buis, il y aura quatre ans à la Fête-Dieu...

Barois. — Je ne savais pas.

Ils ont atteint le vestibule.

L'abbÉ (avec une soudaine rancune). — Ah, nous sommes cruellement éprouvés, là-bas, par *votre* nouvelle loi des Congrégations!

BAROIS (souriant). — Ce n'est pas parce que je m'obstine à réclamer la liberté de la pensée, ou parce que j'ai combattu l'injustice, que je suis solidaire de tout ce qui se fait en France...

L'abbé qui avait déjà entr'ouvert la porte du palier, la referme doucement, et se retourne.

BAROIS. — Si vous suiviez, même de loin, le périodique que je dirige.. (L/ abbéJaisse échapper un geste de répugnance qui provoque un nouveau sourire _deBarois.... vous sauriez que je n'ai cessé d'appliquer à l'Eglise les principes qui nous animaient pendant l'Affaire: exactement les mêmes. (Mélancolique.) Nous y avons perdu, d'ailleurs, bien des abonnés... Peu importe. J'ai protesté de toutes mes forces, en voyant le gouvernement s'appuyer sur les dreyfusards de la nouvelle couche, pour trahir le vote de la Chambre et faire exécuter la loi dans un tout autre esprit que celui où elle avait été conçue.

L'ABBÉ (froidement). — J'enregistre avec satisfaction ce que vous me dites là... Mais si vous apercevez combien ce qui se fait aujourd'hui en France est vilje déplore que vous n'en voyiez pas la cause et combien lourde est la responsabilité qui vous en incombe, à vous, et à vos amis... XAvec gravité.J Au revoir.

BAROIS (serrant sa main). — Cette rencontre m'a fait un grand plaisir, je 1 avoue... Quoique je regrette profondément ce qui vous a amené: dites-le à... à Buis...

(Avec un sourire forcé.) D'ailleurs, soyez rassuré pour l'avenir... Oui, il paraît que je me detraque... (la maip sur le cœur)... par là,., Défense de parler en public, ménagements... Un tas de misères.,,

L'abbÉ (affectueux). — Vraiment? Mais rien de grave?

BAROIS. — Non, si je suis raisonnable.

L'abbÉ (ardemment). — Il faut l'être! Votre vie n'est pas terminée,?e ne peut pas finir comme ça...

BAROIS (coupant court). — J'ai plus que jamais la certitude d'être dans ma voie, et de la suivre, comme je dois!

LABBÉ (hochant la tête). — Au revoir, Jean.

A Auteuil.

Une après-midi de printemps.

Luce est assis dans son jardin à l'ombre des marronniers. Des taches de soleil tremblent sur son front et sur sa barbe blanchie. Reposé et triste, il regarde devant lui. Sur ses genoux, un journal déplié.

En caractères gras:

LES CENDRES DE ZOLA AU PANTHÉON CORTÈGE OFFICIEL.

LE PRESIDENT DE LA REPUBLIQUE ET LES MINISTRES.
LES MESURES DE POLICE.
LA BAGARRE.

Tout à coup son visage s'éclaire: à travers les arbustes, Barois. vient vers lui.

Leurs mains s'étreignent.

Pas d'explications superflues...

Ils s'asseyent, en silence; ils sont résolus à ne pas épancher leurs cœurs. Mais la même pensée se croise dans leurs regards: ce défilé théâtral, dont ils ont été exclus, cette parade ds foire pour glorifier leur grand Zolacet_accaparement d'un nom qui.signifie leyauté et justice, pour couvrir une politique d'intérêt!

LUCE (mélancolie profonde). — Le beau soleil, n'est-ce pas?

Barois approuve de la tête, longuement

Peu importent les mots...

Quelques secondes passent.

Puis Luce fait un nouvel effort.

LUCE. — Et vous, cher ami, comment va?

BAROIS. —Pas mal. Depuis que j'ai interrompu mes cours, le vais même bien.

LUCE. — Et le *Semeur*?

Barois regarde Luce; rire silencieux.

BAROIS. — Vous rappelez-vous votre surprise quand vous avez appris les désabonnements, après ma campagne contre les exagérations de Tantimilitarisme?

LUCE. — Eh bien?

BAROIS. — Eh bien, tenez, j'ai voulu tenter une épreuve... (Il rit à nouveau, et tout à coup s'arrête, comme s'il craignait de laisser monter un sanglot.) J'ai choisi vingt des nôtres, vingt combattants de la première heure; depuis trois mois j'ai cessé de leur envoyer le *Semeur.* (Articulant.) Pas un seul ne s'en est aperçu: je n'ai pas reçu *une* lettre de réclamation!

(Une pause.) Tenez, voilà ma liste.

Mais Luce repousse le papier de la main.

BAROIS (quelques allées et venues sous l'ombrage des arbres). — Bah... Ce ne serait rien, si l'on se sentait toujours aussi combattif, aussi jeune...

LUCE (spontanément). — Vous, Barois?

BAROIS (fierté involontaire; souriant). — Je vous remercie...

Mais c'est exact pourtant: je remarque depuis plusieurs mois des symptômes qui me préoccupent... Des heures de fatigue, des tendances à devenir sceptique, trop indulgent... (Avec lassitude.) Il y a des soirs où je me sens terriblement seul...

LUCE (adroitement). — Vous n'êtes pas seul quand vous êtes à votre table de travail!

BAROIS (se redressant). — Ça, c'est vrai!J'ai tant à faire encore!

Il passe ses doigts à travers ses cheveux, et fait quelques pas. Son regard se fixe, s'éteint.

BAROIS. — Oui, mais tenez, quelque chose qui est mauvais signe: maintenant, quand j'ai un prétexte à quitter mon bureau, une démarche, une course, eh bien, au lieu d'enrager, comme autrefois, je... je suis plutôt... Hein? Vous n'éprouvez pas encore ça, vous?...

LUCE (amusé). — Non.

BAROIS. — Et puis, par moments, j'ai l'impression que la part des souvenirs devient plus importante que celle des acquisitions nouvelles... Je résiste, je m'astreins à lire tout ce qui paraît. Mais, malgré tout, je me sens moins souple, comme engourdi par un poids mort...

LUCE. — L'expérience!

BAROIS (sérieux). — Peut-être... Le sentiment qu'on serait encore apte à tout comprendre, et que pourtant, on est un peu entravé, physiquement... Une sorte d'insoumission de l'organisme... Très pénible.

Sourire incrédule de Luce.

BAROIS (sans répondre à ce sourire). — Pendant longtemps on croit que la vie est une ligne droite, dont les deux bouts s'enfoncent à perte de vue aux deux extrémités de l'horizon: et puis, peu à peu, on découvre que la ligne est coupée, et qu'elle se courbe, et que les bouts se rapprochent, se rejoignent... L'anneau va se boucler... (Souriant à son tour.) On va devenir un vieux qui ne sait plus que tourner dans son cercle!

LUCE. — Oh, oh, oh...
(Brusquement il se dresse.) Ah, les braves cœurs, les voilà tous!

Au fond de la cour, trois hommes surgissent de l'ombre de la voûte: Breil-Zoeger, Cresteil d'Allize et Woldsmuth.

LUCE (bas, vivement). — Dites-moi... Est-ce que Cresteil a perdu quelqu'un de proche?

BAROIS (de même). — Personne ne sait. Il est en grand deuil depuis quinze jours.

Effusions silencieuses.

LUCE (simplement, après quelques secondes de gêne). — L'un de vous y a-t-il été?

ZOEGER. — Non.

CRESTEIL (de sa voix rauque). — Ils ont bien senti qu'il fallait choisir: eux, ou nous!

Il est plus décharné que jamais. Le front s'est dégarni, exagérant le port hautain de sa tête. Sa peau, collée sur les méplats du crâne et sur la courbe du nez, a l'aspect du buis.

WOLDSMUTH (exprimant la pensée de tous). — Quand on se rappelle les obsèques de Zola, les vraies!...

LUCE. — Nous n'étions, autour de ce mort, que des cœurs purs...

ZOEGER (ricanant). — Nous n'avions pas besoin de police pour protéger des ministres!

Le noir de ses yeux est dur comme une pierre taillée. Sa maladie de foie le ronge, sans le vaincre: iï la porte au flanc comme un cilice.

BAROIS. — Et, lorsqu'Anatole France s'est levé, vous souvenez-vous de ce frisson, de cette vaillance qui nous a saisis? Quand il a dit: « Je ne dirai que ce qu'il faut dire, mais je dirai tout ce qu'il faut dire... » Et que la France était la patrie de la Justice...

WOLDSMUTH (rassemblant ses souvenirs). — Attendez...

« Il n'y a qu'un pays au monde dans lequel ces grandes choses pouvaient s'accomplir... Qu'elle est belle, cette âme de la France, qui, dans les siècles passés, enseigna le Droit à l'Europe et au monde!... i'

Ils écoutent, les yeux sur sa broussaille qui grisonne, et où luisent deux disques de verre fumé.

Cresteil rompt le charme.

CRESTEIL (rire amer). — Ah, oui, tout était beau, c'était du cristal l Et quen est-il résulté? Hein? Nous avons crevé l'abcès: nous corriptions sur là guérison: et maintenant, c'est la gangrène î

Luce fait un geste de la main.
Breil-Zoeger hausse les épaules.

CRESTEIL. — En avons-nous assez vu I... La gabegie politique, les abus d'autorité, le mercantilisme partout! Les spoliations anticléricales, le contre-sens antimilitariste... Enfin, — faillite générale l

ZOEGER (sèchement). — La politique d'aujourd'hui, je ne là défends pas. Mais elle n'est pas pire, en tout cas, que celle qu'on faisait avant l'Affaire!

BAROIS (après un instant de perplexité). — Ma foi, je ne sais pas...

LUCE (vivement). — Ah, ne regrettons rien, Barois, ne regrettons rien!

ZOEGER. — Si le gouvernement d'alors avait été digne de son poste, ce n'est pas nous qui eussions fait là lumière, c'est lui!

Luce. — Vous ne regardez que les choses mauvaises, mon pauvre Cresteil. Vous ne voyez pas les bonnes qui se préparent. La République porte en elle-même une vertu précieuse: elle est le seul régime perfectible par nature. Laissez la démocratie s'organiser à nouveau...

CRESTEIL. — Il est tout de même inadmissible que ceux dont tous les actes politiques trahissent nos intentions, revendiquent effrontément notre héritage! Rappelez-vous l'histoire des fiches! Ceux qui s'étaient permis d'organiser officiellement la délation dans l'armée, n'ont pas hésité, devant la Chambre, à s'abriter derrière nos principes!

ZOEGER. — Verbiage de tribune!

Barois (tristement). — Et puis, c'est une loi historique: les vainqueurs prennent immédiatement les vices des vaincus. On dirait qu'une immoralité) spéciale et contagieuse suinte directement du pouvoir

CRESTEIL (sombre). — Non. La vérité, c'est que tout ce qui a été touché par cette affaire, tout ce qui est né

d'elle, est resté empoisonné.

LUCE (sur un ton de reproche). — Cresteil...
y

CRESTEIL — Pourquoi nier l'évidence? Depuis le dossier secret de 94, lusqu'au dessaisissement de la Chambre Criminelle, en passant par le procès Esterhazy et par le procès Zola, la route est jalonnée d'irrégularités! (Avec exaspération.) Et ça n'est pas le plus fort! Quand nous avons abouti à la condamnation de Rennes, — et puis, à la grâce... (Il paraît prendre plaisir à rouvrir toutes les blessures)... ceux dont l'activité n'était pas détruite jusque dans ses racines, gardaient, malgré tout, l'espérance d'un triomphe final. Mais c'était encore trop pour notre destinée de laisséspour-compte! Il fallait que nous fussions irrémédiablement trahis! Alors, tout le sens de l'Affaire, tout ce pour quoi nous avions sacrifié notre vigueur, notre repos, tout a sombré dans l'acceptation d'une illégalité définitive: la cassation sans renvoi d'un tribunal qui n'avait pas le droit de la prononcer, et qui n'a pas reculé, pour faire la justice, devant le viol flagrant de la Loi!Ah, ah...

LUCE. — Cresteil...

ZOEGER (de sa voix atone et sarcastique). — Estimez-vous qu'un nouveau conseil de sept officiers quelconques, improvisés juges, eût été plus qualifié que la Cour de Cassation, la plus haute juridiction civile?

Barois croise le regard de Luce et détourne le sien sans prendre la parole.

CRESTEIL. — Ce n'est pas ainsi que la question doit être poseie, Zoeger. On a raconté que la Cour de Cassation était cuisinée depuis deiïx ans, — et il est positif qu'en ces deux ans, bien des sièges ont reçu de rouveaux titulaires... Mais ce n'est pas à ces points de vue-là que je désire m\$ placer.

(Avec une élégance dédaigneuse.) Je dis seulement qu'il y aviait une façon plus propre de conclure, sans obtenir, en dernier ressort, l'assentiment de juges civils, après d'interminables ergotages de juristeset de scribes autour de l'article 445. Je dis que pour annuler l'injustice de Rennes, il fallait le verdict éclatant d'une autre juridiction militaire. Et je dis que l'Affaire en est restée, pour toujours, comme une plaie qui suppure, et qui ne pourra pas se fermer!

BAROIS (sans conviction). — C'était tout recommencer.

CRESTEIL. — Tant pis!

Barois. — Les forces humaines ont des limites.

CRESTEIL. — Barois, vous pensez exactement comme moi, à ce sujet vous l'avez assez souvent répété dans votre *Semeur*!

Barois baisse la tête en souriant.

CRESTEIL. — D'autant plus que l'occasion d'un nouveau conseil de guerre était magnifique!... Les généraux, ceux-là mêmes dont les réticences avaient emporté la condamnation de 99, venaient de démentir formellement, à l'enquête de la Chambre Criminelle, l'histoire du bordereau annoté par le Kaiser! Il eût donc suffi de leur faire répéter leurs dépositions devant les juges-officiers, et l'acquittement était assuré!

LUCE. — A quoi sert de récriminer? Votre pessimisme est excessif, Cresteil, — même aujourd'hui!

BAROIS (se levant). — Nous avons l'air d'être venus là tout exprès, pour étaler les déceptions de nos cinquantaines...

ZOEGER (montrant le journal déplié à terre; rire bref). — C'est notre jour des cendres...

Sourires.

Barois s'approche de Luce pour prendre congé.

CRESTEIL (brusque, à Barois). — Vous rentrez par le Bois? Je vous accompagne...

LUCE. — Voyez-vous, le grand mal, c'est que le peuple français n'est pas un peuple moral: et pourquoi? parce que, depuis des siècles, la politique et l'intérêt priment le droit. C'est une nouvelle éducation à faire... Notre but n'est pas atteint, c'est vrai, mais il n'est pas manqué pour ça, il est en voie de réalisation. (Serrant la main de Cresteil.) Vous aurez beau dire, Cresteil, c'est un fameux siècle, celui qui a commencé par la Révolution et qui finit par l'Affaire!

CRESTEIL (avec une sombre désin-

voiture). — C'est aussi celui de la fièvre, des utopies et des incertitudes, des échafaudages hâtifs et des malfaçons. Nous ne savons pas. On l'appellera peut-être le siècle de la câmé-' lote!, v

Une allée du Bois.

Fin de journée, très douce.

Cresteil, énervé, presse le pas.

CRESTEIL (sur Un ton différent, confidentiel). — Quand je me retrouve avec les autres, vous avez vu, je m'emballe, j'ai des airs convaincus... Mais quand je suis rendu à moi-même, ah la la! Non, mon cher, c'est fini, je ne peux plus me payer de mots... J'en ai trop vu, je sais trop bien ce qu'est la vie. la foire que c'est, la vie!... Le bien, le devoir, la vertu, allons donc! Des déguisements de nos instincts égoïstes, notre seule réalité. Ah, fantoches!

BAROIS (ému). — Voyons, voyons, mais c'est pitoyable, ce que vous me racontez-là!

CRESTEIL (durement). — On est comme on est. Encore une chose que je n'ai bien comprise que depuis peu. Je n'ai pas demandé à vivre, ni surtout à vivre la vie que j'ai vécue...

BAROIS (en dernier recours). — Vous ne travaillez donc pas en ce moment?

CRESTEIL (éclatant de rire). — Oui, mes livres! Je suis un beau type de raté, hein?... L'artJ C'est comme la Justice et comme la Vérité, c'est _un_de. ces mots qui ne représentent rien, qui sont plus creux qu'une noix véreuse, et pour lesquels je me suis enivré d'abnégation!L'Art!L'homme, cet infirme, veut ajouter à la nature, il tient à *créer* ! Créer! Lui! C'est du dernier grotesque!...

Barois écoute, le cœur serré, comme on écoute la rafale, les arbres tordus, tous les gémissements de la tempête... rCRESTEIL. Vg Savez-vous, mon cher? Si j'avais mon existence à recommencer, j'anéantirais en moi toute ambition, je me « payerais ma tête », jusqu'à ce que j'aie bien renoncé à croire en quoi que ce soit! Je m'appliquerais à n'aimer la vie que sous ses formes minimes, — les seules qui ne; j contiennent pasftrop d'am;rtume à ava-

ler en unejfois... Ramasser le bonheur par miettes... C'est la seule chance que l'homme ait d'en récolter un peu... avant de mourir... puisqu'il faut toujours en arriver la... au trou...

Il a prononcé les derniers mots avec une angoisse poignante. Barois l'examine, surpris.

Cresteil s'est tu. Il fait quelques pas, et tout à coup, comme s'il était à bout de souffle et de volonté, il étend le bras vers une allée transversale.

CRESTEIL. — Je vous quitte, je vais par là...

Barois le regarde fuir, dans son deuil, dégingandé, le dos rond, les basques au vent.

## L'ENFANT

### I

« A Monsieur l'Abbé Jozjers
« Curé de Buis-la-Dame (Oise).

« 26 décembre.

« Mon cher ami,

« Maître Mougin, sur la demande de Madame Barois, vient de me rappeler, qu'au terme de nos conventions, je suis en droit d'exiger que ma fille passe un an auprès de moi, puisqu'elle atteint dans quelques semaines sa dix-huitième année. Je veux éviter que ma réponse ne soit transmise par voie de notaire: ai-je eu tort de penser que vous ne refuseriez pas ce rôle d'intermédiaire?

« Je vous serais donc reconnaissant de remereier Madame Barois de l'initiative qu'elle a prise, et de lui exprimer, sous la forme que vous jugerez la meilleure, les raisons qui me font décliner cette offre.

« Ces raisons, je vous les donnerai avec ma sincérité coutumière.

« Au moment de notre rupture, j'ai voulu me réserver la possibilité d'intervenir, à un moment donné, dans l'éducation de ma fille. Mais les circonstances ont bien changé. Depuis dix-huit ans, vous le savez, je n'ai revu ni ma femme, ni l'enfant. J'abuserais vraiment de mon droit, en réclamant aujourd'hui la moindre parcelle d'une existence dans laquelle je n'ai tenu jusqu'ici et ne tiendrai jamais aucune place. D'ailleurs, pour vous dire toute ma pensée, les sentiments que ma fille doit nécessairement éprouver pour ce

Père inconnùTtûî rendraient, comme à moi-même, un parell rapprochement intolérable, II n'y a donc pas lieu de changer quoi que ce soit à nos situations respectives, et j'ai compté sur vous pour délier ma femme de tout engagement à ce sujet.

« Je vous prie de croire à ma gratitude, et d'accepter l'assurance de ma sympathie dévouée.

Barois, »

Quelques jours après. Neuf heures du matin.

Barois, levé tard, achève en flânant sa toilette.

Il n'a rien à faire: c'est le 1 janvier.

Pascal apporte un paquet de cartes et de lettres.

PASCAL. — Monsieur dînera-t-il ici?

Barois s'est approché du plateau et trie le courrier,

BAROIS. — Non, non... disposez de votre soirée. (Coup d'œil hésitant.) Vous devez avoir de la famille, des amis?

PASCAL (placide). — Ma foi, non: si Monsieur n'est pas là, je dînerai de bonne heure et j'irai au cinéma.

BAROIS (le rappelant). — Eh bien, alors, Pascal, préparez-moi donc à dîner ici... Hein? N'importe quoi, à l'heure que vous voudrez: je ne bouge pas de la journée. Les restaurants sont si bêtes, les jours comme aujourd'hui...

Il ouvre quelques lettres. Puis il aperçoit le timbre de Buis, et, sans hâte, déchire l'enveloppe.

« Presbytère de Buis-la-Dame.

« 31 décembre.

« Mon cher Jean,

« Je serai toujours prêt, en souvenir du passé, à être votre porte-paroles.

« Je me suis acquitté de la présente tâche avec d'autant plus de zèle, que toute autre solution m'eût semblé singulièrement inconsidérée. Votre décision épargne à Madame Barois de nouvelles épreuves, et c'est justice: la pauvre femme mérite d'être un peu récompensée du digne renoncement de sa vie.

« Je croirais cependant manquer envers vous d'une certaine loyauté, en vous cachant que c'est Marie qui a obligé sa mère à vous faire écrire par Maître

Mougin. Vous, voyez à queLpp.int les sentiments filiaux que vous prêtez t la chère enfant, sont.différents de ceux qu'une éducation profondément chrétienne a su développer en elle. "TM"

« Je vous serre la main,

M. L. Joziers, pr. »

Barois est debout contre la fenêtre; il lui faut un instant pour se ressaisir. Il regarde l'enveloppe, puis la chambre, puis la rue.

Il reprend la lettre, posément, cherchant de bonne foi à concentrer sa pensée:

— « Pourquoi Joziers dit-il: *Je manquerais d'une certaine loyauté* ?C'est qu'il a bien le sentiment que ce dernier paragraphe change du tout au tout mon point de vue

« Si c'était une exigence de ma part, un caprice, je dirais non... Ou bien, si j'avais eu le dessein d'avoir sur elle une influence secrète, je dirais non... Mais ce n'est pas ça: c'est elle qui...

« Alors? Pourquoi pas? »

Il sourit.

— « C'est tout de même curieux que ce soit elle qui ait tenu à me rappeler l'échéance. Et malgré sa mère, en somme, puisque mon refus épargne à Cécile *de nouvelles épreuves* ? Cécile a donc très peur que je ne renonce pas à nos conventions; et la petite a dû avoir à lutter ferme... Il faut qu'elle y tienne bien!

« Du diable, par exemple, si je devine pourquoi! Curiosité? Invraisemblable... Elle doit avoir très peur de quitter Buis, sa mère, sa grand' mère, ses habitudes; et surtout pour venir ici! _Qu'est-ce qui s'est passé dans cette tête de dix-huit ans? « En tous cas, il à fallufurie" volonté extraordinaire pour obtenir le consentement de Cécile. Ça prouve qu'elle a de l'énergie, des idées à elle.. . C'est bien étrange... Joziers m'a laissé entendre, autrefois, qu'elle me ressemblait un peu... Nous avons peut-être, aussi des traits de caractère communs, la même ténacité? Qui / sait?Peut-être certaines tournures d'esprit qui sont les mêmes?../ Elle cherche peut-être à comprendre, à reviser ce qu'on lui a appris Elle se débat peut-être là-bas. comme moi jadis

Elle vient peut-être vers moi, pour respirer Rihs librement» p©"' s'affranchir? »

II s'attarde complaisamment; il aperçoit en lui un foyer de tendresse inemployée qu'il ignorait... Puis, il hausse les épaules.

— « Mais non... *Les sentiments que l'éducation chrétienne a su développer en elle...,.* Ah, je divague, ils la tiennent bien! »

Un geste d'impatience.

— « Bon... Je souffre maintenant à l'idée que cette gamine inconnue est de l'autre côté de la barricade! Et il y a dix minutes, rien ne m'était plus indifférent que sa piété! Je deviens stupide (Souriant-) C'est qu'il n'y a pas plus de dix minutes qu'elle existe pour moi, qu'elle a manifesté son_sxistence, qu'elle est autre chose qu'un nom... Mariev:.',,»

Il déplie la lettre pour la troisième fois.

Et à mesure qu'il la relit, il sent sa réflexion impuissante contre la décision irrévocable que chaque mot de cette lettre incruste davantage en lui.

II

Un après-midi de février.

Pascal, entendan); la clé dans la serrure, s'avance vers la porte. Barois. — Me voilà, Pascal! tout est prêt? Pascal sourit familièrement.

Parois fait le tour de son cabinet, comme s'il passait l'inspection. Rien ne traîne; le bureau seul est en désordre. Sur la cheminée, *L'Esclave enchaîné* de Michel-Ange s'épuise toujours en son effort stérile,

Il gagne hâtivement l'autre partie de l'appartement: deux chambres, communiquant par un cabinet de toilette; la plus grande est tendue de toile claire, et meublée à peuf.

Regard d'ensemble angoissé et satisfait,

Il redresse un abat-jour, tâte le radiateur, consulte sa montre, et retourne dans son cabinet,

BABQIS. — Pascal, nous avons oublié quejque chose!... Vous allez descendre quatre à quatre... Une belle botte de fleurs blanches,,. (Montrant la grosseur.) Et blanches, vous entendez?

Cinq minutes plus tard.

On a sonné.

Barois, qui errait de long en large, pâlit.

— « Et cet imbécile n'est pas revenu I v

Il se dirige yart le vestibule, hésite, et ouvre la porte.

L'abbé Jozieri entre le premier, précédant une jeune fille et une femme de cinquante ans. simplement mise.

BAROIS. — Mon domestique est justement (Poussant la porte de son cabinet.) Entrez donc...

L'abbé passe, puis la jeune fille.

Barois s'apprête à les suivre; mais la femme de chambre marche résolûment dans les pas de sa maîtresse, et frôle Barois, sans s'effacer.

L'abbÉ (gravement). — Bonjour Jean. Je vous amène votre fille... Et Julie, la fidèle Julie... (Geste ecclésiastique.) Deux de mes meilleures paroissiennes...

Barois ébauche un mouvement vers Marie, qui se tient droite, le visage empourpré. Elle est petite, brune, fraîche de teint.. Une image s'impose à lui, aiguë: Cécile à vingt ans 1

Elle avance une main qu'il serre.

Puis, un court silence.

La porte s'ouvre. Pascal paraît, un bouquet à la main. Il s'arrête, et, tranquillement, sourit.

BAROIS. — Je l'avais envoyé chercher quelques fleurs... (Vers Marie.) C'est si sévère, un appartement d'homme...

Ils sont debout, les uns devant les autres, inertes. Marie baisse à demi les paupières. Julie ne quitte pas Barois des yeux. L'abbé promène un regard désapprobateur.

Barois sent qu'il faut à tout prix rompre ce mutisme

BAROIS (à Marie). — Voulez-vous.. . que je vous montre votre chambre? (Il fait un pas vers la porte, et se retourne vers l'abbé.) Venez-vous avec nous?

Son coup d'œil signifie: « Venez voir où elle habitera, pour pouvoir en parler là-bas... » L'abbé les suit.

Dans cette chambre pleine de jour, ils sont encore plus mal à l'aise que dans le cabinet aux teintes neutres; et ils restent pareillement plantés au milieu de la pièce.

Barois prodigue des renseignements.

BAROIS. — Ici, votre cabinet de toilette. Et ici, la chambre de... Julie Vous voyez, vous ne serez pas trop isolée... (A Pascal qui apporte les bagages.) Devant la fenêtre...

Sa joie est tombée, il n'en peut plus: une amertume envahissante... Il faut en finir.

BAROIS (à Marie, dont le regard fuit). — Eh bien, nous allons vous laisser... n'est-ce pas?... Vous devez avoir envie de déballer vos affaires...

L'abbÉ. — D'ailleurs, il va falloir que je reprenne mon train. Ma chère petite, je vais vous dire au revoir.

Marie le regarde, et ses yeux grands ouverts se mouillent lentement. Immobile, elle paraît prête à s'élancer dans les bras du vieil abbé, qui s'approche, et, paternellement, l'embrasse au front.

L'abbÉ. — Au revoir, Marie.

Le ton est affectueux et ferme. On y sent cette indifférence pour la vie quotidienne de ceux qui ont toujours vécu pour J'autre. Il semble dire: « Je vous plains, mais vous avez appelé cette épreuve; et Dieu n'est-il pas avec vous?»

Barois conduit l'abbé dans son cabinet.

Ses lèvres tremblent, sa volonté est tendue, à se briser. Il sourit péniblement.

BAROIS. — A quelle heure est votre

Il ne peut achever; il s'assied lourdement à son bureau, la tête dans ses mains, le corps brusquement secoué de sanglots.

Ce souvenir obsédant de Cécile jeune Ces yeux d'enfant, pleins d'anxiété Et lui, qu'une tendresse sans issue étouffe soudain Ah, la responsabilité de créer jine autre chair, capable de souffrir T

L'abbé assiste, impassible, les bras joints, les doigts enfouis sous les manches. Il pense au roc frappé par Moïse; mais sa pitié est volontairement contenue.

Barois se relève, s'essuie les yeux

BAROîS. — Excusez-moi... Tout ça m'a secoué; je suis si nerveux maintenant... (L'abbé a repris son bréviaire et son chapeau.) A quelle heure est donc votre train?

Deux heures plus tard.

Barois n'a cessé d'aller et de venir de la fenêtre à la porte, prêtant l'oreille à tous les bruits de la maison.

Il n'y tient plus. A pas rapides, il se dirige vers la chambre de Marie.

Silence.

Il frappe.

Quelques mouvements effarés. Marie. — Entrez.

Debout, dans le soir, deux ombres se détachent sur la pâleur de la croisée. Elles viennent de se lever précipitamment; leurs deux chaises sont là, deux épaves au milieu de la pièce.

Le cœur de Barois se serre.

BAROIS. — Vous êtes donc sans lumière?

, v»'... T j j 11 tourne le commutateur, et reçoit au visage le regard de Julie; un chapelet pend au bout de son bras. Marie, les paupières rougies et baissées, esquisse un geste gauche.

BAROIS. — Vous avez déjà défait vos malles? Vous manque-t-il quelque chose? (A Julie.) Demandez bien tout ce dont vous aurez besoin... Pascal est un brave garçon, il vous rendra tous les services possibles...

(A Marie.) Eh bien, voulez-vous que nous allions dans mon cabinet, en attendant le dîner?... Je vous montre le chemin.

Elle le suit, résignée.

Il se retourne.

Barois. — J'ai l'air de vous mener à la guillotine..

Elle essaye de sourire, mais cette Voix affectueuse lui dorme envie de pleurer.

Dans le cabinet, Barois allume toutes les lumières et avance gaiement un fauteuil, sur le bord duquel Marie s'assied.

Il se sent aussi gêné qu'elle, — et ridicule, à cause de son âge.

Marie:

Le front est étroit, un peu bombé. Une peau de brune, avec des roseurs transparentes et des pourpres soudaines, d'Un éclat de fleur. Des yeux clairs et-sagS-Jeceur, d'Urt gris bleu inattendu sous les sourcils noirs, qui ontJemême dessin toufmenté que ceux de son père. Le menton accuse une volonté "cPhomme. Mais la finesse du nez, la gaieté qui erre autour de la bouche, corrigent ces duretés.

Le charme d'une jeunesse saine et fière.

BAROIS.- Oui, je comprends très bien que ce soit dur, très dur, cette séparation, Paris, cet appartement inconnu... et puis nïoi.v... (Elle esquisse un mouvement de politesse intimidée.) Si, si, je me rends bien compte

Moi-même, tenez, je suis là, devant vous, je ne sais plus comment aire ce que je pense... (Elle sourit gentiment. Il s'enhardit.) Et pourtant, c'est vous qui avez eu l'idée de passer deux mois ici... Je n'aurais jamais ôSé' le demander... Eh bien, vous y voilà, il n'y a aucune raison pouf cfuêî nous ne fassions pas bon ménage... Aucune, n'est-ce pas?

Elle tente un visible effort.

MARIE. — Non, mon père.

Il pense avec humeur: « Comme au confessionnal. »

Sa physionomie devient sérieuse.

BAROIS. — Je ne sais pas du tout ce que...on vous a râcOrtté sur moi...

Elle rougit brusquement, et l'interrompt pâf un geste de protestation. Il heurte un regard qui résiste. Il continue, sur un ton camarade.

BAROIS. — En tous cas, puisque Voué avez désiré me connaître (Irtterrogatwft sous-entendue.), je suis décidé à (n'expliquer franchement. Je puis paraître avoir eu des torts irréparables vis-à-vis de votre mère et de vous. Je ne nie pas que j'aie certains reproches à me faire mais il y a du pour et du contre... Vous êtes bien jeune, Marie, pour être mêlée à ces questions: je le ferai le plus discrètement, le plus loyalement possible.

Au mot « loyalement » elle a relevé le front.

PASCAL (solennel). — Mademoiselle est servie.

Elle se tourne à demi, surprise.

BAROIS (souriant). — Vous voyez, je ne compte déjà plus... Vous êtes chez vous. (Se levant.) Allons à table. Ce soir si vous n'êtes pas fatiguée, nous causerons de tout ça.

Après le dîner.

La glace est rompue.

Marie entre la première dans le cabinet et aperçoit les fleurs enveloppées.

MARIE. — Oh, il fallait les mettre dans l'eau...

BAROIS (à Pascal qui porte le café). — Tenez, Pascal, donnez-donc vos fleurs à Julie, elle saura les...

MARIE (vivement). — Mais non, donnez... Avez-vous un vase assez grand?

Pascal lui apporte ce qu'elle demande; il la regarde faire le bouquet, et sort sans cesser de sourire.

BAROIS. — Marie, vous avez fait la conquête de Pascal.

Elle rit.

BAROIS. — Du café?

MARIE. — Non, jamais.

BAROIS. — Eh bien, voulez-vous me servir le mien, puisque vous êtes maîtresse de maison? Une demi-tasse... C'est tout ce qu'on me permet maintenant... Merci.

Ils sourient, comme deux enfants qui jouent aux grandes personnes.

BAROIS (brusquerie affectueuse). — Voyez-vous, Marie, depuis que vous êtes là, je me pose la même question: pourquoi a-t-elle désiré venir?

Un silence.

BAROIS (de sa voix chaude). — Oui, pourquoi?

Marie ne sourit plus. Elle subit, sans un clignement de cil, le regard de Barois; puis elle secoue la tête. Elle semble dire: « Non. Plus tard peut-être... Aujourd'hui, non. »

III

Six semaines après.

Aux bureaux du *Semeur,* dans le cabinet du Directeur.

SECRÉTAIRE DE LA RÉDACTION. — L'article de M. Breil-Zoeger sur les instituteurs?

BAROIS (regardant l'heure). — Faites passer autre chose.

Il se lève.

LE SECRÉTAIRE. — C'est qu'il va y avoir quatre mois bientôt...

BAROIS (debout). — Je ne dis pas le contraire. Mais je ne veux pas publier ça, sous cette forme... Il faudra que je voie Breil-Zoeger.

LE SECRÉTAIRE. — Eh bien, l'article de Bernardin?

BAROIS. — Si vous voulez.

LE SECRÉTAIRE. — Je voulais vous demander aussi ce qu'il faut répondre à Merlet.

BAROIS. — Ça ne presse pas, mon ami. Je n'ai pas le temps ce soir. Nous verrons demain.

Il prend son chapeau et son pardessus.

/ En passant devant la gare d'Orsay, il lève la tête:

/ — « Quatre heures moins le quart... Je rentre tous les jours un peu plus tôt... Je finirai par ne plus sortir de chez moi...

« Je *finirai...* Non I puisqu'elle va. partir dans trois semaines...»

Une angoisse déchirante. Il hâte le pas. Il entrevoit un coin de son cabinet, et, sous la lampe, un front dans l'ombre, une nuque caressée de lumière.

Il sourit en marchant.

— « Elle s'est installée là comme chez elle!Ce petit air décidé, cette assurance, ces timidités! Et sachant toujours ce qu'elle veut... Elle m'en impose. Elle a quelque chose de sain, de parfaitement équilibré: c est un tout, un anneau fermé.

« Non, je n'ai aucunement les sentiments d'un père... J'ai un sentiment paternel, ce qui n'est pas la même chose. Un père se sent une autorité, des droits. Rien de semblable. J'ai cinquante ans passés, elle en a dix-huit: voilà ce qu'il y a de paternel entre nous. Ce que j'éprouve pour elle, au fond, c'est tout bêtement une inclination sentimentale, une sympathie... amoureuse... Mais oui, pourquoi avoir peur des mots?... »

Il gravit l'escalier, allègrement. Il répète avec complaisance:

— « Une inclination amoureuse... »

Le visage rond de Pascal. BAROIS. — Mademoiselle est là?

PASCAL. — Non, Monsieur. Mademoiselle n'est pas rentrée.

Une déception; puis une poignante tristesse: dans trois semaines, ce sera tous les jours ainsi.

MARIE. — Bonjour, Père.

Elle entre, en toilette sombre, les joues fraîches, les yeux vifs.

BAROIS (souriant de plaisir). — Comme vous rentrez tard aujourd'hui...

Il regrette déjà sa phrase: il vient d'apercevoir la tranche dorée du paroissien qu'elle dépose sur la cheminée, pour enlever son chapeau

Marie (simplement). — C'est le premier jour de la retraite..

Quelques minutes plus tard, elle revient portant deux années reliées du *Semeur*. Elle fait glisser sa charge sur le bureau.

MARIE. — Voilà: j'ai fini. Qu'est-ce que vous me donnerez, maintenant, père?

BAROIS. — Je ne sais pas. Qu'est-ce que vous désirez?

Le ton signifie: « Vous savez bien que je ne comprends rien à vos lectures. »

MARIE (gaiement). — La suite.

BAROIS. — Ce volume-là va jusqu'en décembre dernier. Il n'y a eu que huit numéros depuis. (Se tournant vers un casier.) Ils sont là. Mais si vous ne voulez lire que mes articles, ce n'est pas le peine, je n ai rien publié depuis janvier. (Il rit.) Vous devinez pourquoi?

MARIE. — Est-ce que vraiment je vous empêche de travailler?

BAROIS (souriant). — Non, vous ne m'empêchez pas de travailler, ce n'est pas ça... Mais depuis que vous êtes là, je travaille moins, voilà tout... Je n'en ai plusTe même désir...

Il la regarde. Elle semble éprouver un réel remords. Cependant, quelle importance pour elle, qu'il écrive ou non? Au contraire, elle devrait' se réjouir d'interrompre la production maudite...

Barois (repris par la pensée du départ). — Je peux bien le dire. Vous avez mis dans ma vie quelque chose qui n'y était pas, dont je ne soupçonnais même pas le prix... Une présence, une affection... Je parle de l'affection que je ressens, moi... (Elle esquisse une rectification, et rougit.) Enfin, il n'y a pas à dire: l'idée que vous allez bientôt me quitter, m'est très dure, très dure...

Marie (gentiment). — Je reviendrai...

Il la remercie d'un sourire âgé.

Un temps.

BAROIS. — Je me suis attaché à vous, Marie, et pourtant vous m'êtes une énigme, vous êtes indéchiffrable!

Elle fronce les sourcils: sur la défensive.

BAROIS (montrant du doigt le paroissien). — Je sens qu'il *y a là* un

abîme entre nous: je le sens tous les matins, quand je vous vois revenir de la messe... Et, à d'autres moments, quand vous êtes ici, le soir, près de moi, recherchant dans le *Semeur* tout ce que j'ai écrit, lisant mes livres, demandant des explications, et les écoutant sans broncher comme si vous étiez curieuse de libre-pensée, — il me semble alors que vous n'êtes pas si loin!... Ah, c'est vrai, je ne vous comprends pas...

Marie est debout, le genou sur un fauteuil, les mains nouées sur sa jupe, le corps abandonné. Son regard seul est actif. Elle jette un coup d'œil aux *Semeur* qu'elle a rapportés, semble brusquement prendre un parti, et se laisse glisser dans le fauteuil.

MARIE. — J'ai voulu tout lire, d'abord..

Elle s'arrête. Sa voix alourdie marque la contraction de cette petite âme, au seuil de l'entretien toujours reculé.

Barois rencontre son regard bleu: et il a l'intuition qu'elle s'est interrompue pour lancer vers Dieu un appel de courage.

Il cherche à l'aider.

BAROIS. — Si je comprenais seulement pourquoi vous avez désiré venir?

Elle le fixe, l'œil chargé de pensées.

MARIE. — Par épreuve.

Il ne réprime pas son amertume. Elle s'empourpre et baisss les yeux: son front est rond comme un bouclier.

MARIE (vite). — Je veux être religieuse, père...

Barois sursaute. Elle relève la tête.

MARIE. — Je savais que vous aviez perdu la foi. Alors j'ai voulu vous connaître, vivre de votre vie, étudier vos œuvres, subir votre influence: c'était l'épreuve décisive de ma vocation... (Fièrement.) Et je suis contente d'être venue!

Long silence.

BAROIS (morne). — Vous voulez être religieuse, Marie?

Il surprend alors une certaine façon qu'elle a de spurir: une crispation des lèvresépouillçe de joie; et, en même temps, un regard qui se fige, assuré, légèrement ironique, mais terne et sans vie.

BARQJS (soulevant les bras, d'un

geste las, sans la regarder), «t Js ne m'y attendais guère... Je me disais: « Pourquoi est-elle là? ¥ JV fait vingt hypothèses. Finalement je m'étais dit: « Elle va essayer de me convertir,., »

Son rire éclate, puéril, nerveux, trop vif.

BAROIS (agacé). — Eh bien, ce n'aurait pas été si mal, pour une future religieuse!

Marie a repris son sérieux. Elle va chercher son paroissien, le feuillete, et le tend à 6pn père.

BAROIS (lisant). — « Je voudrais que vous fussiez tous comme moi; mais chacun a son don particulier, selon qu'il le reçoit de Dieu. »

MARIE (souriant).—Vous me croyez bien orgueilleuse! Si Dieu vous désirait pour lui, est-ce qu'il aurait besoin de moi? C'est donc qu'il a d'autres vues sur vous... (Secouant la tête.) Non, non, chacun cherche son devoir où il peut. Moi j'ai le bonheur de l'avoir trouvé devant moi, simple et facile. Vous pas. Je vous plains... (Hésitation.) Je ne peux que vous plaindre, père... Mais essayer, *moi,* de vous convertir, *vous*!

BAROIS. — Et vous n'avez pas craint, en soumettant votre foi à mon influenceMarie secoue la tête.

MARIE. — D'abord, je savais bien que si vous aviez ces idées-là, c'était, comment dire... — d'une façon élevée... On ne peut pas vous en vouloir..

BAROIS. — Comment le saviez-vous?

MARIE, — Je le savais.

Marie rougit brusquement et fait un imperceptible signe d'assentiment. Il n'insiste pas.

11 va vers sa bibliothèque, l'ouvre, et, pensif, manie quelques volumes.

BAROIS, — Voyons, Marie... Vous avez lu: *Les raisons de ne pas croire,* huit articles qui se suivent?

MARIE. — Oui.

BAROIS. — Et ça: *Le dogme devant la science* ?... Et ça: Les *origines comparées des religions* ?...

MARIE, — Oui.

BAROIS (repoussant le battant vitré). — Vous avez lu tout ça, en y appliquant votre esprit, — et ce que vous aviez cru vrai jusque-là ne vous a pas semblé...

Il voudrait dire: « Vous ne me ferez pas croire que tout le aDeur d une vie comme là mienne,"èmplflyée à combattre la "religion par des arguments précis, puisse se briser contre votre foi d'enfant! »

Mais il s'arrête: il vient de reconnaître le sourire et le regard butés de Marie.

MARIE (cherchant à formuler sa pensée). —-Mais, père, si ma certitude était à la merci des objections, ce ne serait plus une certitude,..

Elle sourit, naïvement cette fois. Et Barois entrevoit une vérité pscHychologique, Il pense: .—- Une certitude qui n'offre pas de prise aux objections... Qu'est-ce qu'elle veut dire? Que les difficultés de, la rpfjgion _ne peuvent pas, «ristgrjjour ejle, parce qu'elle ppssède, *a priori*, une certitude? Ce qui veut dire qu'elle a mis d avance sa foi au-dessus de tout raisonnement; et que, même si sa raison se laissait convaincre par les objections, sa foi n'en serait pas même. effleurée, parce qu'elle est *au-desKu-Hots d'atteinte*. 1. «,'C'e»t enfantin,., et inattaquable I »...

BAROIS (doucement). — Mais cette certitude, Marie, sur quoi donc l'asseyez-vous si solidement?

Elle se contracte; mais elle ne veut pas se dérober.

MARIE. — Quand on a éprouvé ce que j'ai éprouvé, père... Je ne sais pas comment vous dire... La présence même de Dieu... Dieu qui pénètre l'âme, qui l'inonde d'amour, de bonheur... Ah, quand on a éprouvé ça, ne fût-ce qu'une fois dans sa vie, tous ces raisonnements que vous échafaudez pour vous prouver à vous même que votre âme n'est pas immortelle, u'elle n'est pas une parcelle de Dieu, tous vos raisonnements, père... ! ''n sourire souverain...)

Barois ne répond pas.
Il pense:
— « *Ce que j'ai éprouvé...* Là-contre, il n'y a rien à faire, il. n'y aura jamais rien à faire!

« Si seulement je _p.Quv.ais empêcher qu'elle ne prenne . résol

BAROIS. — Est-ce que votre mère vous encourage dans cette voie?

Marie baisse la tête avec une expression douloureuse et têtue. BAROIS (stupéfait). — Comment? Vous ne lui avez rien dit encore?

Marie ne répond pas. BAROIS — Mais pourquoi? Vous pensez donc qu'elle s'y opposerait?

Un temps.

BAROIS. — Voilà le meilleur des avertissements: il est en vous-même.. Quel que soit votre désir d'être religieuse, vous sentez, devant une pareille décision, tant de chagrins à franchir, que vous n'avez même pas osé...

MARIE (prête à pleurer). — Pourquoi lui aurais-je fait cette peine dès maintenant? J'ai pitié. Maman n'a jamais été heureuse...

Elle a parlé vite, sans réfléchir. Elle rougit.

Barois ne semble pas avoir compris. Il se penche vers elle.

BAROIS. — Marie, écoutez-moi... Je ne veux pas discuter avec vous: Y il ne s'agit pas de votre foi. Vous avez lu dans mes articles tous les arguments que je pourrais développer; ils ne vous ont pas convaincue, — n'en parlons plus... (Longue aspiration.) Vous voyez, ce n'e pas le libre-penseur qui parle... C'est simplement l'homme de cinquante ans, l'homme de bon sens, qui a vu des idées se modifier au cours d'une même vie!S'engager, à vingt ans, se lier pour toujours... Quelle folie! Des serments *éternels* ! Songez à tout ce qui peut encore se passer en vous et que vous ne soupçonnez pas, à tout ce que l'âge, et la réflexion, et les circonstances, pour-y ront modifier... /
Geste de Marie: « Oh, je suis bien sûre de moi!"

BAROIS. — Mais rien que votre atavisme devrait vous faire frémir d'inquiétude! Tous les instincts qui m'ont affranchi, moi, quand j'avais votre âge, ils sont en vous, quoi que vous fassiez, plus ou moins obscurs, plus ou moins mâtés, mais ils sont, et ils peuvent remonter brusquement à la surface et bouleverser votre vie!

Voyons, Marie, comment pouvez-vous affirmer que vous ne douterez pas? Pouvez-vous soutenir que vous n'ayez jamais eu un seul doute? Rentrez en

vous, voyons... Il n'est pas possible que jusqu'ici... (Il montre les tomes du *Semeur*.) Aucun, aucun doute ne vous a frôlée?

MARIE. — Aucun, je vous assure... Jamais.

Ses yeux brillent de candeur. Il la considère en silence.
Un temps.

MARIE. — Non, le monde est trop vide... Rien n'est grand, rien ne dure...

BAROIS. — Croyez-vous qu'il n'y ait pas de place sur terre pour un cœur qui veut s'agrandir?

Elle l'examine longuement, avec respect, avec compassion.

MARIE. — Oui, père, j'ai souvent pensé à vous, depuis que je suis ici... . Vous n'avez pas eu la chance de connaître la grâce, vous n'avez pas senti ce que c'est qu'un regard de Dieu: et pourtant vous êtes bon, et juste. Mais comme vous avez dû vous donner du mal! C'est tellement plus simple d'être bon pour l'amour de Dieu!

BAROIS. — Croyez-vous qu'il soit plus beau d'abdiquer toutes les responsabilités, tout le labeur de la vie, de s'en remettre une fois pour toujours à une règle monastique, — plutôt que de prendre courageusement la tâche qui se présente, et de l'accomplir, par les chemins de tout le monde? Ce que vous désirez, c'est un suicide de la pensée et de l'action!

MARIE (souriant à son rêve). — Le don de soi...

BAROIS. — Ah, qu'est-ce qu'il est, ce don de soi, au seuil d'une vie qui sera dure, comme toute vie humaine, si ce n'est le sacrifice des devoirs les plus élémentaires? Et ne vantez pas les mérites de la soumission! c est un anesthésiant qui endort la douleur à mesure qu'elle la cause. Vous êtes jeune, ardente, intelligente, et vous aspirez au néant de la vie contemplative? Est-ce digne de vous?

MARIE. — Vous parlez comme tous les autres; vous ne pouvez pas deviner. .. (S'exaltant avec des réminiscences.) Je suis une privilégiée, cela crée des devoirs.. Toutes ne sont pas appelées; mais celles que Dieu choisit, doivent se donner sans restriction. Elles sont le rachat de tous ceux qui vivent en faisant à Dieu la plus petite part possible... et de ceux qui ne lui en font pas du tout...

BAROIS (brusque). — C'est ma rançon que vous voulez payer?

MARIE. — Je ne vous demande pas de me comprendre, père...

Oui, ces vœux, ils acquittent un peu la dette de la famille, ils réparent un peu... ce que vous avez pu faire par vos livres... (Tendrement.) Et qui sait si cette vocation n'a pas été voulue par Dieu, en échange d'une âme qui est belle, très belle, et qui, sans ça, serait damnée?

Son regard est devenu une surface plate et dure où le regard /d'autrui, où l'interrogation et le doute d'autrui, ne pénètrent 'plus.

— As- f -/ i-'y

Barois pense. —. / — « Quelle religion, celle qui peut amener des cerveaux humains à un tel écart de la réalité, et les y faire tenir! '——r Ça ne repose sur rien... Le plus humble bon sens en aurait raison, si les esprits ne se trouvaient pas d'avance préparés par des siècles de servitude sereine...

« Ça mijote dans les âmes d'enfants, tenu à feu doux par les surexcitation du catéchisme, les communions brûlantes.. . Ça monte à un tel degré de chaleur artificielle qu'une vie toute entière peut en être réchauffée!...

«_Ejç'est là que Marie trouve cet équilibre qui fait mon admiration dej- Duisjjue je la vois _Yiyre_?

« Dans combien (Tannées, après combien de générations hésitantes, la vérité scientifique donnera-t-elle cet apaisement total?

« Jamais peut-être...

« Mon cher ami,

« Je pensais vous rencontrer cet après-midi à notre réunion, et vous annoncer que je profite des vacances de Pâques pour faire une absence de quinze jours. J'ai tant de questions à régler avant de quitter Paris que je ne suis pas sûr de pouvoir aller vous serrer la main.

« J'aurais eu pourtant bien des choses à vous dire. J'ai passé, ces dernières semaines, par des émotions bien inattendues, bien cruelles.

« Ma fille désire entrer au couvent...

« Vous imaginez ce que j'ai pu éprouver. Rien ne melelaissaitsoupçonner. Au contraire, l'intérêt qu'elle avait pris, depuis son arrivée, à lire tout ce qui porte atteinte au cathohscisme, me faisait illusion. Je vous en ai parlé déjà. Je me trompais étrangement. Le sentiment religieux a pris chez elle une forme qui le rend invulnérable à nos raisonnements. Je crois que sa nature résolue et intuitive a souffert de la vie de province, et qu'elle s'est défendue en se donnant une activité intérieure démesurée. La religion dogmatique de l'Eglise n'est plus pour elle qu'un cadre, précis mais large, dans lequel son sentiment personnel s'est exagérément développé; et ce qui domine aujourd'hui sa sensibilité, ce n'est pas le dogme, c est l'élan spontané de sa petite âme vers l'infini, — et l'illusion qu'elle l'embrasse!

« Il n'est pas douteux, qu'avec le fond de santé et l'intelligence claire qu'elle possède, sa croyance d'enfant eût pu évoluer si elle avait attaché au dogme l'importance qu'elle accorde aux aspects sentimentaux de la foi. Mais il n'en est rien. Et l'état mystique où elle atteint aujourd'hui est *autoritatif*, au point de lui donner une certitude absolument irréfutable du monde spirituel.

« Nous qui sommes habitués à plier notre sensibilité au travail de notre raison, nous n'avons aucune idée de ces certitudes-là. Marie a *éprouvé* le contact de Dieu, et nous sommes aussi désarmés devant une auto-suggestion de cette espèce, que nous sommes impuissants à convaincre un malade de l'irréalité de ses hallucinations. Rien ne fera comprendre à Marie, que ce milieu surnaturel où elle a projeté le meilleur d'elle-même (et que ses dispositions extatiques lui permettent de percevoir nettement) n'est qu'un mirage, un égarement de sa sensibilité, un conte de magicien qu'elle se répète à elle-même depuis des annees.

« Mon cher ami, je sais que vous ne m'approuverez pas. Mais en présence de cette situation *sans issue,* les dispositions où vous m'aviez laissé, les conseils que vous m'aviez donnés pour amener cette enfant à substituer progressivement une vérité féconde à son

erreur, m'ont paru sans objet. J'ai vu mon impuissance à la convaincre, et en même temps, quelle force elle puise à se tromper. Elle m'est apparue façonnée par la religion et pour la religion... Devant un ensemble si fort, j'ai reculé... Une telle foi, c'est évidemment un mensonge, mais c'est aussi du bonheur humain: *son* bonheur! Vous êtes père— et plus que moi; vous me comprendrez peutêtre. Autrefois j'aurais dit: la vérité d'abord, fût-ce au prix de la souffrance. Aujourd'hui je ne sais pas, je ne peux plus dire de même. Je me tais, et je crois l'aimer plus en me taisant, malgré mon chagrin, qu'en m'acharnant à détruire ce qui est le secret de son activité.

« J'ai obtenu de passer encore les vacances de Pâques avec elle. Ce séjour, qui aura été dans ma vie quelque chose d'inattendu et de délicieux, je veux le finir comme un beau rêve, par un voyage dans un pays de lumière et de fleurs.

« Nous partons après-demain pour les lacs italiens.

« A mon retour, je sais d'avance l'amertume que je trouverai à ma solitude. Je ne veux pas y penser. J'aurai bien besoin de vous, et je sais que vous ne vous refuserez pas: c'est la pensée consolante qui me permettra de revenir seul.

Au revoir, mon grand et cher ami. Je vous serre la main très affectueusement.

Barois. »

A Pallanza.

Avril. Six heures du soir.

Une barque plate sur l'eau.

Marie et Barois sont assis à l'arrière, côte à côte, tournant le dos à la ville, dont l'animation ne les atteint plus.

Autour d'eux, le lac palpite à peine. Un glissement mou et lent, dans une lumière grise, à la rois intense et voilée. La lune est si haut dans le ciel qu'il faudrait renverser la tête pour la voir; son éclat, diffus dans la buée, isole la barque au centre d'une immensité silencieuse et blême.

A l'avant, le torse du rameur s'incline et se relève; la chemise, le pantalon de toile, forment deux clartés nébuleuses; son visage, ses mains, ses pieds nus, sont noirs comme ceux d'une icône.

Barois ne peut détacher sa pensée de

la séparation prochaine.

Marie, le front renversé, hors du temps et de l'espace, diluant son âme dans la fluidité du ciel et de l'eau, s'enivre, comme s'il n'y avait plus rien entre elle et Dieu.

Soudain, une bouffée odorante, chaude comme l'haleine d'une bouche: les roses, les giroflées, les iris, les citronniers, les eucalyptus de l'île San Giovanni. La main de Barois cherche celle de Marie, qui, penchée en arrière, laisse traîner dans le sillage son bras nu; la fraîcheur résistante de l'eau encercle leurs deux poignets.

Sept coups sonnent à un campanile; sur l'autre rive, un écho répète les sept coups, durement, comme un gong.

Ils reviennent vers Pallanza.

*i* Julie les attend sous le péristyle, deux dépêches à la main: Mme Pasquelin vient de mourir.

Neuf heures, le même soir.

Barois, ayant bouclé sa malle, s'accoude au balcon de sa chambre.

Devant lui, le lac couleur de perle. Au-dessous de lui, la place: une vie désordonnée: des chants, un orchestre, des trompes de tramways, un bruit de foire.

Un gros vapeur illuminé verse sa fourmillière sur le ponton.

— « Pauvre petite... Ces quinze jours qu'elle m'a donnés... Ah!... Ce que je vais me sentir seul... »

Le vapeur, d'un coup, s'éteint. Il était sombre et semé de lumières; il devient blanchâtre et percé de trous noirs, comme une carcasse abandonnée. Il tremblote lourdement au clapotis de l'eau, et le peu de vie qui lui reste s'exhale dans le panache hésitant de sa fumée.

A Buis.

Veillée mortuaire: deux cierges; le lit; les cornettes des religieuses.

Cécile, épuisée par un long agenouillement, est prostrée dans un fauteuil. Ses paupières irritées se ferment à demi: sa pensée s'évade, s'élance au-devant de Marie:

« A l'aube, elle sera là, je ne serai plus seule... »

Mais, au fond d'elle-même, sa pensée est: « A l'aube, *ils* seront là... »

Elle se remémore ce qu'elle a appris sur Jean, par sa fille, par Julie. Elle se passe la main sur le visage. — « Il va me trouver changée... »

Elle ne l'a pas revu depuis dix-huit ans, et soudain son image surgit, dans l'épanouissement de la trentaine...

Elle se lève précipitamment; et, pour ne plus penser qu'à la morte, elle retourne s'agenouiller au bord du lit.

Depuis son arrivée à Buis, Barois n'a pas quitté sa chambre d'hôtel.

Une moisissure, qui tombe sur les épaules, suinte des murs comme un brouillard.

Il est resté assis tout le jour devant son feu, les joues brûlantes, le dos transi, tournant entre ses doigts la lettre de Marie:

« Mon cher Père,

« Le service a lieu demain matin, mais maman vous demande de ne pas y assister. Elle a été sensible à votre sympathie et elle me charge de vous dire que si vous êtes encore à Buis demain, elle sera heureuse de vous remercier elle-même de ce que vous avez fait pour moi. Venez à six heures, il n'y aura plus personne.

« Je vous embrasse tristement.

Marie. »

La nuit tombée, Barois n'y tient plus, et se glisse dehors.

D'abord la ville basse, comme s'il fuyait le coin qui l'attire. La vie paisible des rues, le soir; les étalages qu'on rentre, automatiquement, depuis un demi-siècle; le même vacarme sur le passage de l'omnibus branlant; les mêmes enseignes, grinçant aux mêmes angles... Tant de fixité 1...

Il remonte maintenant vers l'église. Il ne se souvenait pas que la pente fût si raide. Essoufflé, le cœur battant, il passe devant le presbytère, il arrive à *sa* rue...

Elle est déserte. Un courant d'air glacé la balaye toujours. La maison de la grand'mère Barois... Une à une, les fenêtres des chambres, celle où il couchait, celle où son père est mort... Le grand portail: A LOUER. Et, debout, le beffroi noir.

Puis, quelques pas: la maison des Pasquelin.

Cécile est là, avec Marie... Marie, qui

va demeurer ici maintenant!

Cette lueur derrière les volets, le corps sans doute...

Il s'immobilise, envahi par son enfance... L'horloge du clocher... Il sourit; les larmes lui viennent aux yeux.

Autour de lui, la bise impitoyable; il relève en frissonnant le col de son pardessus d'Italie.

Puis, grelottant, il regagne son hôtel.

Le feu s'est éteint. On le rallume. Il allonge les probes vers la maigre flambée. Le passé danse dans les flammes: l'abbé Joziers, Cécile, les fiançailles...

— « Je me suis marié comme un imbécile!... »

Il tremble de froid, d'angoisse. Des souvenirs l'accablent.

— « C'est difficile, de vivre... »

Le lendemain; six heures du soir.

Barois, rongé de fièvre, toussotant, arrive devant la porte close des Pasquelin.

Le même timbre, les mêmes socques de la servante sur le carrelage. Un mot de province lui vient aux lèvres: la *coutume* d'une maison...

Dans le petit salon, Cécile, en noir, est assise sous la lampe, devant une pile de faire-part.

Il la reconnaît si mal qu'il n'a pas de peine à être comme un étranger.

BAROIS. — J'ai bien compati à votre chagrin...

Elle s'est levée. Elle le regarde: elle ne s'attendait pas à cette maigreur; et, dans la physionomie quelque chose d'inconnu la déroute.

CÉCILE. — Merci Jean.

Elle tend la main. Il la serre avec une ejfusion polie, comme à des obsèques.

Il est surpris qu'elle ait tant changé; il n'avait pas réfléchi qu'elle continuait, depuis dix-huit ans, à vivre, un à un, les mêmes jours que lui. C'est bien elle, cependant: le front bombé, le regard inégal, ce zézayement intimidé... Tout à l'heure, il ne l'imaginait même pas: et maintenant, il ne conçoit pas qu'elle aurait pu se faner autrement. Marie rompt le silence:

MARIE. — Prenez ce fauteuil, père.

CÉCILE (s'asseyant).—Je vous remercie de la façon dont vous avez reçu Marie... Vous avez été très bon pour elle, je vous remercie.

BAROIS (machinalement). — C'était tout naturel.

Il rougit aussitôt.

BAROIS. — Est-ce que votre mère s'est vu mourir?

CÉCILE. — Non. Elle avait tant de fois reçu les sacrements depuis sa première attaque... D'ailleurs, le dernier jour, elle n'avait plus sa tête, la paralysie gagnait. (Pleurant.) Elle n'a reconnu personne.

Cette voix larmoyante réveille en lui une résonnance inattendue.

MARIE. — Maman, il faudrait donner à père une des dernières photographies de grand'mère?

Cécile jette un regard biais vers Jean, qui a baissé le front.

CÉCILE (hésitation). — Si tu veux, mon enfant.

Ils restent seuls.

Ce tête-à-tête, dans ce cadre...

I Leurs regards se croisent, se fuient. Ensemble, obscurément,

(ls espèrent le mot d'oubli, d'amitié...

Mais la porte s'ouvre. De nouveau Marie est entre eux.

La minute est passée.

Ils peuvent se séparer, maintenant, ils n'ont plus rien à sedire.

VI

« Paris, le 25 avril.

« Je m'adresse à Mademoiselle pour lui annoncer que depuis son retour. Monsieur est bien malade d'une pleurésie. Il est si faible qu'il ne parle presque plus. Le médecin est revenu ce matin avec deux autres; ils sont restés longtemps auprès de Monsieur, ils ont dit qu'ils enverraient une garde, et ils m'ont demandé si Monsieur avait de la famille.

« Je crois bien faire en prévenant Mademoiselle,

« Votre serviteur dévoué,

Pascal. »

Deux jours après. Le soir.

Marie est dans la chambre de Barois, avec le médecin.

Cécile est assise sur la banquette du vestibule. Rien ne la retenant plus à Buis, elle a voulu accompagner sa fille à Paris. Mais devant la gravité du mal, Marie s'est réinstallée chez son père.

Et Cécile, déracinée, s'est cloîtrée dans la chambre d'une pension voisine, d'où elle ne sort que pour venir aux nouvelles.

Le médecin paraît, suivi de Marie.

MARIE. — Revenez vite, docteur, ne nous laissez pas seuls...

Ses traits sont décomposés. Elle s'effondre sur l'épaule de sa mère.

Cécile n'ose plus interroger.

MARIE. — Il a changé, depuis midi, d'une façon effrayante. Le docteur ne répond plus de rien. Il a demandé une autre consultation, pour ce soir Il ne veut pas essayer une nouvelle ponction, sans l'avis des autres...

CÉCILE (voix brisée). — Il souffre?

MARIE. — Un peu moins. (Sanglotant.) La garde dit que c'est mauvais signe... Ah, laissez, ça me fait du bien de pleurer! C'est affreux... Il m'a appelée tout à l'heure... Il a prononcé votre nom, deux fois...

MARIE (brusquement). — Maman, entrez le voir...

Cécile ne résiste pas; c'est la dernière fois, la mort est dans la maison. Elle est épouvantée de cet irréparable qui va sceller leur j. rupture pour l'éternité. _Jr (Jamais elle n'a si douloureusement senti ses torts...

Elle traverse, en évitant de regarder, le cabinet de travail; elle entre dans la chambre; elle aperçoit le lit, le visage livide.

Il ouvre les yeux et la reconnaît sans la moindre surprise. Elle saisit sa main, elle veut y mettre ses lèvres. Mais il l'attire, il se soulève vers elle, et la regarde jusqu'au fond des yeux, avec désespoir.

BAROIS. — Cécile, tu sais, je vais mourir...

Elle secoue la tête, crispant sa volonté pour ne pas fondre en

Mais l'infirmière s'approche avec des ventouses.

Pascal soutient le corps. Marie écarte les plaques d'ouate. Ils sont tous trois penchés sur le malade. Cécile aperçoit un peu de chair pâle.

Elle s'est reculée. Elle est là, en visiteuse, avec son voile de crêpe, ses gants noirs. Un accablement sans borne...

Elle gagne la porte, jette un dernier regard vers le lit, et s'enfuit en sanglotant.

Un silence.

larmes.

Trois semaines plus tard.

Barois est dans son bureau, étendu sous une couverture. Il fixe avec anxiété Breil-Zoeger, debout devant lui.

ZOEGER. — Nous y étions tous.

BAROIS. — Qui conduisait le deuil?

ZOEGER. — Le père Cresteil, en colonel.

BAROIS. — Ah, il avait encore son père? Il n'en parlait jamais...

ZOEGER. — Tout était mystérieux dans sa vie.

BAROIS. — Et tu ne sais toujours pas ce qu'il allait faire à Genève?

ZOEGER. — Non. Mais je suppose qu'il allait se tuer, simplement. Il devait logiquement "en arriver là... (Un temps.) Des détails poignants: il avait brûlé tout ce qui pouvait le faire reconnaître: il s'était même rasé la moustache, en wagon I La police a mis quatre jours à retrouver son identité... Hein? cette hantise, non seulement de mourir, mais de disparaître...

BAROIS (les yeux pleins de larmes) — Ah, mon pauvre ami, que la vie est...

Il n'achève pas. Breil-Zoeger ne répond rien; de son œil jaune, il mesure les ravages de la pleurésie.

Barois avait des cheveux noirs, emmêlés; beaucoup sont tombés, en quelques jours. Les yeux sont creusés, le regard est las, les paupières alourdies; le corps se tasse au fond de la chaiselongue. Les mains reposent, molles.

BAROIS (triste sourire).

— Tu me trouves changé?

ZOEGER (de sa voix douce et coupante). — Oui.

Un silence.

BAROIS. — J'ai été très touché, vois-tu, très touché..

Breil-Zoeger l'examine froidement, sans répondre. Puis il se lève pour partir.

ZOEGER. — Woldsmuth s'est chargé de l'article nécrologique. Je lui dirai de te l'apporter.

BAROIS. — Non, je t'assure, je ne peux encore m'occuper de rien. Prends toutes les décisions... Avant de t'en aller, voudrais-tu me donner un tome du *Semeur...* 1900, le deuxième semestre... Merci.

Resté seul, il feuillète le volume avec une préoccupation maladive. Enfin il retrouve cet article dont le souvenir l'obsède; il le parcourt; puis, lentement, il relit la dernière page:

« Pourquoi craindre la mort? Est-elle si différente de la vie?__No.tie existence n'est qu'un passage incessant d'un état à un autre: la mort n'est qu'une transformation de plus. Pourquoi la craindre? Qu'y a-t-îî de redoutable à cesser d'être ce *tout,* momentanément cordonné, que nous sommes? Comment peut-on s'effrayer d'une restitution de nos éléments au milieu inorganique, puisque c'est en même temps un retour assuré à l'inconscience?

« Pour moi, depuis que j'ai compris le néant qui m'attend, le problème de la mort n'existe plus. J'ai même... plaisir... à penser que ma personnalité n'est pas durable... Et la certitude que ma vie est limitée... augmente singu

Pascal ouvre la porte.

Cécile paraît, suivie de Marie.

MARIE. — Comment vous trouvez-vous, père, aujourd'hui?

BAROIS. — Mieux, mieux... Bonjour Cécile. Vous êtes bonne de venir me voir.

Marie se penche.

Il l'embrasse, et s'adresse à elle, en souriant.

BAROIS. — La maladie nous apprend combien nous avons besoin des autres...

Cécile s'est assise sur le bord d'un fauteuil. Le jour l'éclairé durement. Barois remarque son visage bouleversé.

Marie reste debout, contre la fenêtre; elle aussi, a pleuré.

MARIE (répondant au regard de Barois). — Père, j'ai parlé à maman de ma vocation religieuse... Je lui ai dit que vous consentiez...

BAROIS (vivement). — Moi, Marie?... Mais je n'ai pas à consentir!

Cécile fait un mouvement.

CÉCILE. — Vous avez connu le projet de Marie avant moi, Jean. Est-il possible que vous ne l'en ayiez pas détournée?

MARIE (fixant Barois). — Dites tout ce que vous pensez, père!

Il fait un effort pour rassembler ses idées.

BAROIS (à Cécile). — Je lui ai fait des objections. Une telle vocation est trop loin de moi pour que je puisse comprendre... Mais j'ai trouvé Marie si résolue... et, d'avance, si heureuse...

Il ne peut s'expliquer davantage sans rouvrir des blessures dont il respecte maintenant les cicatrices; et il regarde tristement sa femme et sa fille, qui souffrent l'une par l'autre.

Marie est toujours debout; le regard est terne; elle tend son front, où la pensée semble volontairement figée.

Une image s'impose à Barois: Cécile, l'année de la rupture...

Et c'est alors qu'il découvre combien Cécile a changé: plus rien d'obstiné, rien d'inerte: une douleur qui palpite... Les larmes coulent sur ses joues.JJn atroce débat la divise: l'instinct _ se révolte contre la foi: ellène peut se résoudre à livrer son enfant, même à Dieu.

CÉCILE (dont le cœur éclate). — Ah, vous avez cédé, vous, mais ça ne vous est pas difficile! Qu'elle soit avec moi à Buis, ou bien qu'elle soit dans un couvent... (Zézayant.) Mais moi, si seule aujourd'hui, qu'est-ce que vous voulez que je devienne, si elle s'en va?...

Marie esquisse un geste involontaire; ses yeux vont de l'un à l'autre...

Ils ont compris, tous les deux, et se détournent.

Un silence.

## L'AGE CRITIQUE

*"Nostra vita a che val?* Leopardi.

I

Dix-huit mois plus tard.

Aux bureaux du *Semeur,* un jeudi, jour de réception du Directeur.

Barois, dans son cabinet, avec Portal.

PORTAL. — Vous y écrivez moins souvent.

BAROIS. — C'est vrai, mais je n'ai pas la fatuité de croire que ce soit la vraie cause... D'autant que le *Semeur* s'est renouvelé, et que nous avons maintenant quelques jeunes, de premier ordre.

PORTAL. — Parbleu, vous avez

contre vous, la réaction nouvelle. Dans tous les domaines, c'est le même recul.

Barois s'approche frileusement du brasier de coke, et s'assied dans la cheminée, les épaules basses, les coudes sur les genoux.

BAROIS. — La mode n'y est plus; ça tourne, c'est la loi de la vie. On n'a qu'un temps... (Il tend ses mains au foyer.) Moi-même, quand j'écris maintenant, je n'ai plus la spontanéité d'autrefois! J'y mets la même conviction, mais, comment dire, malgré moi, par le seul effet du temps qui s'est écoulé, cette sincérité est devenue quelque chose de tout fait, un outil, un procédé...

Pause.

PORTAL (enjoué). — Et votre enquête sur la jeunesse? Vous ne l'abandonnez pas, je pense?

BAROIS. — Non, j'attends même aujourd'hui une visite à ce sujet. (Las.) Mais, au fond, j'ai eu tort d'entreprendre ça; les jeunes sont des énigmes pour moi. Voilà plus d'un mois que je n'ai touché à cet article...

Il est vrai que mon déménagement m'a mis en retard pour tout.

PORTAL. — Vous êtes tout à fait installé?

BAROIS (assombri). — A peu près... (Il se dirige vers la croisée.) Tenez, vous voyez, là-haut, ces trois fenêtres?... Ça n'est pas grand, mais je m'y ferai. Mon appartement était vraiment devenu trop lourd. (Souriant.) Les affaires ne sont pas brillantes...

(Il continue, avec la visible satisfaction de confier les détails de son existence.) En somme, mon cher, j'ai eu de la chance de trouver ça dans la maison! Les jours de brouillard, ou même d'humidité, j'étais obligé de rester confiné chez moi. Tandis que, de là-haut, vous comprenez... en me couvrant bien... je peux toujours descendre jusqu'ici...

Portal (gagnant la porte). — Allons, je viendrai vous surprendre un de ces soirs; nous bavarderons...

BAROIS. — Oui, comme autrefois...

Resté seul, il regarde le feu. Puis il se lève, cherche des papiers dans un carton, et s'installe à son bureau.

Quelques minutes.

Il griffonne dans les marges.

Brusquement il repousse les feuillets, et sonne.

BAROIS (au garçon).— Voulez-vous voir si M. Dalier est à la rédaction?

Peu après, entre un jeune homme de vingt-cinq ans.

Dalier: petit, les jambes courtes, mais le buste dilaté; la tête forte.

Visage blanc et maigre, entièrement rasé. Lèvres fines, un peu dédaigneuses. Lorgnon.

Barois l'enveloppe d'un coup d'œil, et se renverse légèrement en arrière.

Barois. — Je viens de parcourir votre article, mon ami. Ça ne va pas, mais pas du tout... (Mouvement de Dalier.) Je ne dis pas qu'il soit mal construit: mais il ne peut pas être publié tel quel, dans notre revue.

Dalier debout: surpris, réservé.

Barois choisit quelques feuilles et les lui tend.

BAROIS. — Tenez... Si c'est là votre conception personnelle du sentiment religieux, tant pis pour vous. *Le Semeur* ne peut pas s'en faire l'écho.

DALIER. — Mais, monsieur, je ne comprends pas; c'est bien dans ce sens-là que M. Breil-Zoeger m'avait dit...

BAROIS (brusquerie inattendue).— M. Breil-Zoeger a le droit d'envisager la question comme bon lui semble! Mais le Directeur de la revue, c'est moi. Et jusqu'à nouvel ordre, je ne laisserai pas paraître, dans un périodique que je dirige, un article aussi étroitement sectaire!

Son visage s'empourpre, puis pâlit.

Un silence.

Dalier fait un pas en arrière pour se retirer. Barois passe sa main sur son front; d'un geste, il invite Dalier à s'asseoir.

BAROIS (ton voulu de causerie). — Voyez-vous Dalier, vous escamotez une partie de la réalité... C'est trop commode.

Moi aussi j'ai proclamé toute ma vie la faillite des religions, — et je crois même y avoir contribué, dans ma sphère... Mais la faillite des religions dogmatiques: et non la faillite du sentiment religieux. (Hésitant.) Ou, si j'ai

fait la confusion, ce qui est possible, c'est que je n'avais pas compris ce qu'est le Sentiment religieux, et qu'il échappe, par définition, à l'action de l'esprit critique. (Il regarde Dalier bien en face.) La forme *dogmatique* des religions, voilà ce qui ne compte pas; mais le sentiment religieux, lui, subsiste, et c'est une ânerie de le nier, mon ami, croyez-moi: je puis le dire» puisque je l'ai fait-.. Quand une forme artistique est périmée, l'art ne disparaît pas avec elle, n'est-ce pas? Eh bien, c'est exactement la même chose.

Dalier se tait, mais sa physionomie exprime un avis nettement opposé.

BAROIS. — D'abord vous êtes trop jeune pour pouvoir parler de ces questions-là. Vous venez de traverser la première crise, vous en êtes à l'affranchissement absolu, sans restriction...

DALIER (positif). — Il n'y a pas eu la moindre crise religieuse dans ma vie jusqu'à présent, et je crois pouvoir prétendre qu'il n'y en aura pas.

Barois: sourire incrédule.

DALIER (mécontent). — Je vous affirme, monsieur, que je ne sais pas ce que vous voulez dire. Chez moi, l'athéisme est inné. Mon père, mon grand-père étaient athées. Ma raison n'a jamais eu à lutter contre ma sensibilité, pour me faire accepter que le ciel soit vide; et, dès que j'ai eu l'âge de réfléchir, j'ai compris que les causes s'engendrent, les unes les autres, aveuglément, sans but, et que rien dans l'univers ne nous permet de supposer une direction, ni un progrès... Ce sont des mouvements, voilà tout.

BAROIS (après l'avoir considéré). — Il y a peut-être des gens absolument dénués de sens religieux, comme il y a des daltoniens par exemple... Mais il est évident que ce sont des exceptions: ils ne doivent pas généraliser d'après eux. Et puisque vous ignorez tout du sentiment religieux, pourquoi en parlez-vous?Qu'est-ce que vous pourriez en dire?Votre logique vous amène à des solutions qui vous paraissent simples, rationnelles, définitives: et pourtant, toute conscience religieuse les rejettera, je vous l'affirme, comme absolument

insuffisantes à expliquer l'intensité de la vie intérieure!

DALIER. — Mais monsieur, vous-même, vous avez soutenu, vingt fois, devant moi...

BAROIS (soucieux). — Eh bien, c'est possible. Mais aujourd'hui je vous dis que si l'on déracine les dogmes, le sentiment religieux persistera. Il prendra une forme différente. Regardez autour de vous: tout l'effort de la raison n'a pu l'ébranler, au contraire!Le sentiment religieux, il se laïcise déjà, il est partout!Dans tout ce qu'on tente, d'un bout à l'autre du monde, pour défendre le droit, pour préparer un avenir social meilleur, une répartition plus équitable des biens et des devoirs! La charité, l'espérance et la foi... Mais c'est exactement ce que, sans employer les mêmes termes, je m'efforce de pratiquer depuis que je suis affranchi. Alors? N'est-ce qu'une question de mots? Qu'est-ce qui me guide obscurément vers le bien, sinon la permanence en moi d'un sentiment religieux qui a survécu à ma foi? Et d'où vient qu'il y ait, en chacun de nous, ce même principe de perfectionnement?

Non, non, la conscience humaine est religieuse, en son essence. Il faut l'admettre comme un fait... Le besoin de croire à quelque chose!... Ce besoin-là est en nous comme le besoin de respirer.

(A Dalier, qui semble prêt à l'interrompre.) Dites!

DALIER. — C'est au nom de ce besoin-là qu'on a toujours légitimé les préjugés, — les erreurs!

Barois le regarde longuement. Il semble hésiter.

BAROIS. — Et s'il y avait des erreurs... qui fussent utiles, — du moins pour l'état actuel de l'humanité... — est-ce que ces erreurs-là... à notre point de vue humain... ne ressembleraient pas singulièrement à des vérités?...

DALIER (sourire imperceptible). — J'avoue que je suis surpris, monsieur, de vous entendre plaider le droit à l'erreur...

Barois ne répond pas tout de suite.

BAROIS (penché en avant, sans regarder Dalier). — C'est parce que je me suis rendu compte, mon ami, qu'il existe des êtres, des êtres qui vivent, qui aiment, — des êtres qui sont aimés! — auxquels l'erreur est mille fois plus nécessaire que la vérité, pour cette raison qu'ils l'assimilent entièrement, qu'elle les fait vivre! Tandis que la vérité les laisserait mourir d inanition, comme des poissons tirés sur la terre ferme... Et à ces êtres-là, nous n'avons pas le droit.. non, nous n'avons pas le droit..

Il lève la tête et heurte le regard de Dalier.

Vous me regardez? Vous vous dites: « Décidément le patron est fini... » (Sourire indifférent.) Je n'en sais rien, vous avez peut-être raison.

La vérité, oui... La vérité quand même! C'est le grand mobile des consciences, tant qu'elles sont jeunes. Plus tard, on perd cette assurance: on admet la possibilité d'erreurs provisoires, individuelles; on préfère l'indulgence à la stricte justice...

Un temps.

Que voulez-vous, on est à peu près forcé de se contredire en vieillissant... On s'est donné, trente ans de suite, la tâche de rendre la vie plus complète, plus harmonieuse: et on s'aperçoit qu'en somme, on n'a pas perfectionné grand'chose... On se demande même quelquefois si, à la pratique, le neuf vaut toujours l'ancien?... Alors, on ne sait plus... Comment ne pas se contredire? Quand on est sincère, quand, année par année, on a acquis le sens total de la réalité, il est impossible de n'être que logique...

DALIER (dur). — Vous sembleriez dire que l'homme n'est pas capable de profiter jusqu'au bout des enseignements de la raison seule!

Barois le regarde longuement. Pause.

BAROIS (inattentif). — On est jeune — je l'ai été! — on va, on va... Jusqu'au moment où l'on comprend qu'il y aura une fin à tout ça...A partir de ce moment-là!... Oh, on est prévenu longtemps d'avance, on a tout le temps de s'y habituer... Même, au début, on ne sait pas ce que c'est; la confiance, 1 entrain fléchissent; on se dit: « Qu'est-ce que j'ai donc, maintenant? » Et puis, doucement, peu à peu, on se sent tiré

en arrière... Et il n'y a pas de résistance possible!

A partir de ce moment-là, vous verrez, mon petit, comme on considère différemment les choses...

Il sourit péniblement...

Dalier sent vibrer sa jeunesse: un plaisir sportif, à arracher le flambeau aux mains qui tremblent!

DALIER (vivement). — En tous cas, je ne vois vraiment aucun moyen de modifier mon article selon vos vues actuelles.

Un garçon remet à Barois une carte de visite.

BAROIS. — Faites attendre, je sonnerai.

Un temps.

DALIER. — Il faudrait refaire tout le travail. (Ferme.) Je ne le pourrais plus.

Barois, distrait, roule la carte entre ses doigts. Pui« il se tourne vers Dalier avec lassitude.

Barois. — Eh bien, faites comme vous voudrez

Dalier sorti, il s'approche de la cheminée, active les charbons, et sonne.

Tout à coup, il hausse les épaules.

— « C'est stupide... J'aurais dû m'y opposer carrément. »

Le garçon introduit deux jeunes gens d'une vingtaine d'années BAROIS. — Monsieur de Grenneville?

GRENNEVILLE. — C'est moi, monsieur. Permettez-moi de vous présenter mon camarade Maurice Tillet, un normalien.

De Grenneville: mince, taille moyenne: sobre élégance. Un visage fin, sans dominante. Très français. Petite moustache blonde.

Regard sincère, décidé. Sur les lèvres, une nuance de fatuité ironique.

Dans l'ensemble, ce mélange d'assurance et de retenue, que le bon élève d'une institution religieuse conserve jusqu'à sa première aventure.

Tillet: grand, robuste, un peu gauche.

La figure largement taillée; des yeux bruns, vivants et précis; un grand nez; la bouche fendue; une barbe noire, peu fournie.

De fortes mains qui disparaissent dans les poches dès qu'il veut parler, et qui, par réflexion, en ressortent aussitôt.

GRENNEVILLE. — La lettre que vous avez reçue en réponse à votre enquête, est de nous deux.

Barois. — Veuillez vous asseoir, messieurs. Je vous remercie de vous être dérangés. (A Grenneville.) Comme je vous l'ai écrit, j'ai l'intention de publier votre étude in-extenso. Elle est de beaucoup la plus intéressante que nous ayons reçue jusqu'ici. Mais, puisque je dois l'accompagner d'un commentaire.. . (Souriant)... critique, j'ai été très heureux d'avoir cette occasion de causer avec vous.

(A Tillet.) Vous êtes encore à l'Ecole Normale?

TILLET. — Oui, monsieur. Je commence ma seconde année.

Barois. — Normale-lettres, naturellement?

Tillet. — Normale-sciences.

BAROIS (à Grenneville). — Et vous, monsieur, je crois que vous prépa. rez l'agrégation de philosophie?

GRENNEVILLE. — Non, monsieur. Je ne suis que licencié. Je fais mon Droit, et ma dernière année de Sciences politiques.

Barois prend sur son bureau un dossier qu'il feuillette. Il fait un effort pour concentrer son attention.

BAROIS.' — Il y a d'abord dans votre réponse quelque chose qui, je l'avoue, m'a choqué infiniment: c'est le mépris manifeste en lequel vous tenez vos aînés, quoi qu'ils aient fait. Croyez qu'il n'y a dans cette observation rien de personnel: c'est le principe qui me surprend. Car ce n'est pas seulement insouciance de jeunesse: votre arrogance a quelque chose d assuré, de réfléchi, d'intentionnel. (Souriant.) Nous aussi, nous étions convaincus d avoir raison; mais il me semble que nous respections davantage ceux qui nous avaient précédés. Nous avions, — comment dire?... — une certaine modestie; ou, plus exactement, le sentiment que nous pouvions nous tromper... Vous, au contraire, vous paraissez certains de représenter seuls la partie saine de la jeunesse...

Et pourtant, il y a bien à dire! Car enfin le nationalisme que vous prêchez, est, par définition, une anomalie; ce n'est pas une attitude naturelle pour un peuple; c'est une posture de combat, une parade défensive!

GRENNEVILLE (voix jeune, un peu caustique). — Tout à fait exact. Il est en effet regrettable que la France soit, en ce moment, obligée de se contracter pour expulser d'elle un germe qui serait mortel, — exactement comme un organisme vigoureux dans lequel se serait introduit un corps étranger.

BAROIS. — Ce germe, c'est?

GRENNEVILLE (offensif). — L'anarchie.

Il s'arrête, prêt à la riposte.

Barois le regarde placidement.

GRENNEVILLE (demi-sourire). — Vous ne nierez pas, monsieur, que notre pays soit en proie à une véritable anarchie? Anarchie raisonnée, sans éclats, mais généralisée, et progressivement destructive... La cause n'en est pas secrète: la majorité, lorsqu'elle a perdu ses croyances traditionnelles, a perdu en même temps sa mesure d'appréciation, les éléments les plus nécessaires à son équilibre.

BAROIS. — Mais ce que vous appelez anarchie, c'est tout simplement la vitalité intellectuelle d'une nation! Il n'y a pas plus de dogmes en morale qu'en religion. La loi morale, ce n'est qu'un ensemble de convenances sociales, et cet ensemble est, par nature, provisoire, puisqu'il doit, pour garder sa valeur pratique, évoluer en même temps que la société: or cette évolution n'est possible que s'il y a, dans la société, ce ferment que vous appelez anarchique, ce levain sans lequel aucun progrès ne peut lever.

TILLET. — Si vous appelez progrès cette succession de soubresauts incohérents!

BAROIS, — Les transitions sont brusques parce que les états se succèdent à intervalles de plus en plus rapprochés: jadis la morale variait d'un siècle à l'autre; actuellement, elle varie d'une généralion à la suivante: c'est un fait, il faut l'accepter.

Léger silence.

Les jeunes gens échangent un coup d'œil.

TILLET. — Nous ne sommes pas autrement surpris, de vous voir défendre cette anarchie. Vous avez été, comme vos contemporains, élevé par des écrivains révolutionnaires, insurgés contre tout ce qui avait une stabilité...

BAROIS (plaisantant). — Taine?

TILLET. — Parfaitement! Depuis Gœthe jusqu'à Renan, Flaubert, Tolstoï, Ibsen, tous!...

Barois hausse les épaules sans cesser de sourire.

GRENNEVILLE (pitié tranquille). — Le xiX siècle tout entier, de» *Déclarations de* 89 à Jaurès, en passant par Lamartine et par Gambetta, est empoisonné par ce romantisme: d'un bout du siècle à l'autre, c'est le même verbiage, pittoresque peut-être, mais dénué de direction et de pensée...

TILLET. —...ou plutôt gonflé de pensées généreuses, mais sans la moindre compréhension du réel. Rien de logique: des nuées. Aucun rapport entre les mots et la vérité sociale.

BAROIS (conciliant). — Ne pensez-vous pas que les mots, quels qu'ils soient, s'appauvrissent mécaniquement de leur sens, quand on les agite à tous les carrefours, pendant un siècle?Ces mots que vous rejetez aujourd'hui comme des coques vides, vous en avez assimilé, malgré vous, le suc...

Ils font, ensemble, le même geste de protestation.

BAROIS. — Et vous-mêmes? Croyez-vous que vous ne vous grisez pas à votre tour de mots creux?

(Il saisit sur son bureau le dossier de l'enquête, et le soulève.) « Discipline », « Héroïsme », « Renaissance », « Génie national »!... Croyez-vous qu'avant quinze ans d'ici ce tintamarre verbal ne paraîtra pas dépourvu de toute pensée précise?

Grenneville. — Les termes passeront peut-être de mode, mais les fortes réalités qu'ils expriment, dureront. « Nationalisme », t Classicisme », ce ne sont pas des formules vagues: ce sont des pensées claires j ce sont même les pensées les plus claires et les plus riches de. notre civilisation!

TILLET (précis). — Le malentendu vient peut-être de ce que nous employons le mot *pensée* dans une acception différente de la vôtre. Pour nous, toute pensée qui ne se concilie pas avec la vie active jusqu'à se confondre avec elle, n'est pas une pensée: elle n'est rien, elle n'existe pas. On peut, j'en conviens, dire que la pensée doit diriger la vie; mais il faut que ce soit la vie qui fasse naître cette pensée directrice, et qui l'alimente, et qui la règle.

GRENNEVILLE. — Votre génération, contrairement à la nôtre, se contentait de théories abstraites, qui, non seulement ne développaient pas en elle le désir d'agir, mais contribuaient à le stériliser. (Fat.) Ce jeu de mandarin, qui aboutit a une complète inactivité) répugne aujourd'hui à la France nouvelle, à la France de la menace allemande, a la Franc d'Afadiri.i

BAROIS (se révoltant enfin). — Mais vous considérez toujours vos aînés comme des rêveurs, incapables de vouloir et d'agir!C'est une monstrueuse injustice, — j'allais dire une monstrueuse ingratitude!

Est-ce que la génération qui a fait affaire Dreyfus mérite d'être qualifiée *i'inacHvei* Aucune génération, depuis la Révolution, n'a eu davantage que la nôtre à lutter, à payer de sa personne!Beaucoup d'entre nous ont été des héros! Si vous l'ignorez, allez apprendre votre histoire contemporaine! Notre goût de l'analyse était autre chose qu'un stérile dilettantisme, et notre passion pour certains mots qui vous semblent aujourd'hui sonores et vides, comme « Vérité » et « Justice », a pu âtre, à son heure, inspiratrice d'action!

Courte pause.

GRENNEVILLE (respectueux et froid). — Vous revendiquez bien haut ce court moment, où certains d'entre vous ont consenti — et pour quelle cause! — à descendre dans l'arène. Remarquez justement combien cette crise a été brève, et vite suivie de découragements célèbres..

Barois ne répond pas.

GRENNEVILLE (avec douceur). — Non, Monsieur, cette génération-là n'était pas taillée pour la lutte: elle n'était pas susceptible de durée.

TILLET. — La preuve, c'est que son activité, pendant ces heures troubles de l'Affaire, s'épanchait au hasard. A tel point au'auiourd'hui l'Affaire Dreyfus paraît, à ceux qui n'y étaient pas, une mêlée d'énergumènes sans doctrines et sans chefs, se lançant au visage des mots à majuscules!

GRENNEVILLE (sans lâcher prise). — Et voyez les résultats! Qu'est devenu notre régime parlementaire? Vous avez reconnu vous-même, dans *Le Semeur,* la faillite de vos espérances, et que les réalisations de vos amis avaient trahi vos intentions 1

Barois ébauche un geste vague.

Que leur dirait-il? Ils se servent d'armes qu'il a lui-même forgées. D'ailleurs, empêcherait-il ces esprits simplistes de juger l'arbre à ses seuls fruits?

TILLET (concluant). — Les mœurs de la politique actuelle, voilà où nous ont conduits ceux qui, depuis tant d'années, méconnaissent notre génie national. U est grand temps de nous soumettre à une discipline. Il nous faut une république, où les droits et les devoirs soient différemment répartis.

Barois (surpris). — Seriez-vous républicains?

TILLET. — Certes!

BAROIS. — Je ne le croyais pas.

TILLET (vivement). — Malgré de sérieuses divergences d'opinion, malgré le développement incontestable du parti monarchique, la majorité de la jeunesse reste ardemment démocrate.

BAROIS. — Tant mieux...

GRENNEVILLE. — C'est d'ailleurs le sentiment intime de la nation.

BAROIS. — Je m'étonne que vous n'estimiez pas le gouvernement républicain incompatible avec vos principes de hiérarchie et d'autorité.

GRENNEVILLE. — Pourquoi donc? Il s'agirait seulement de l'améliorer.

TILLET. — Il s'agirait de réformer le régime parlementaire pour épurer les habitudes politiques; et de dévier le principe de la souveraineté nationale, qui ne correspond en fait à rien de précis, vers la souveraineté des syndicats professionnels ou autres groupements corfstitués. Cela reviendrait au même, du reste, avec l'ordre et la mesure en plus.

BAROIS (souriant). — C'est encore

sur ces points-là, voyez-vous, que nous pourrions nous entendre le mieux. Je souhaite que la jeune couvée parvienne à réglementer notre régime, et à faire passer les préoccupations sociales avant les agitations des partis politiques...

GRENNEVILLE (avec assurance). — Ce but, nous l'atteindrons tout naturellement, lorsque nous aurons davantage accrédité dans le pays notre morale traditionnelle.

BAROIS (souriant toujours). — Et qu'est-ce que vous appelez « notre morale traditionnelle? »

GRENNEVILLE. — La morale catholique.

Barois ne sourit plus; il les regarde posément.

BAROIS. — Car vous êtes tous deux catholiques? Catholiques pratiquants?

GRENNEVILLE. — Oui.

BAROIS. — Ah...

Une pause.

BAROIS (avec une angoisse soudaine). — Répondez-moi loyalement, messieurs: est-ce que vraiment, aujourd'hui, la grande majorité des jeunes gens est catholique?

GRENNEVILLE (brève hésitation). — Je ne sais pas; je sais seulement que nous sommes très nombreux. Parmi les plus jeunes, parmi ceux qui sortent du collège, je crois qu'il y a une majorité incontestable de pratiquants. Parmi nous, leurs aînés de quatre ou cinq ans, je crois pouvoir affirmer qu'il y a approximativement autant de croyants que d'incrédules; mais ceux qui n'ont pas la foi le regrettent pour la plupart, et agissent en toutes circonstances comme s'ils l'avaient.

BAROIS. — Je vous avoue que cette restriction enlève, selon moi, à cette moitié d'entre vous, toute autorité pour une propagande catholique!

TILLET. — C'est parce que vous ne comprenez pas leur sentiment. S'ils défendent une foi qu'ils ne partagent pas, — mais qu'ils voudraient pouvoir partager, — c'est qu'ils ont reconnu ses vertus actives. Ils ont eux-mêmes expérimenté ces vertus; ils éprouvent une recrudescence d'activité à être enrôlés parmi les défenseurs de la religion. Et, tout naturellement, ils contribuent, par

leur effort raisonné, à l'épanouissement d'un ensemble moral qu'ils savent le meilleur possible.

BAROIS (après réflexion). — Non, je ne puis admettre que la protestation religieuse d'un individu qui n'a pas la foi, ait quelque sens. Votre explication est spécieuse, mais elle n'atténue pas ma sévérité pour certains de vos chefs spirituels... Ils n'ont vraiment pas assez voilé le mépris aristocratique que leur inspirent les masses. Toutes les fois qu'ils sont acculés au mur, leur échappatoire équivaut à cet aveu: « La religion est faite pour le peuple, comme le bât pour l'âne; mais nous ne sommes pas bêtes de somme. » Ce qui revient à dire, sans plus, qu'ils considèrent le catholicisme comme une excellente garantie sociale. Mais eux, ils préfèrent se réserver le privilège de la vérité , (5'anirnaBt.) J'ai toujours obéi à un prjncipe 4iarnétralement opposé: j'estime que toute vérité doit d abord être répandue; qu'il faut attranphjr les hommes aussi largement qu'on le peut, sans se préoccuper s'ils sont prêts à faire tout de suite un bon emploi de leur affranchissement; enfin, que la liberté est un bien dont on n'apprend à se servir que petit à petit, et seulement par un usage démesuré!

Silence courtois et désapprobateur.

Barois (haussant les épaules). — Mais je vous demande pardon de cette profession inutile... Il s'agit seulement de vous. (Un temps-)

Votre lettre montre assez bien ce qui peut vous attacher au catholicisme; mais elle n'explique pas le chemin qui vous y a mené. Sans doute une foi d'enfant, qui n'a jamais été ébranlée?

Grenneville. — En effet, — pour moi du moins. J'ai reçu une éducation catholique; j'ai même eu une enfance assez feryente. Pourtant, vers les quinze ans, j'ai subi une éclipse... Mais la foi était en moi, et elle a reparu d'elle-même, pendant que je suivais à la SorbonnP le? çours pour la licence de philosophie.

BAROIS. — Pendant que vous suiviez les cours de philosophie à la Sprbonne?

GRENNEVILLE (très naturel). — Oui, monsieur.

Barois n'insiste pas,
Il se tourne vers Tillet.

Barois. — Vous aussi, monsieur, vous avez toujours été pratiquant?

TILLET. — Non. Mon père était professeur de sciences naturelles, en province, et il nous a élevés dans une libre-pensée absolue. Aussi ne suis-je venu au catholicisme que très tard, pendant ma préparation à Normale...

BAROIS. — Une véritable conversion, alors?

TILLET. — Oh non, rien de brusque, aucune exaltation. Je suis arrivé au port, ntellernent, après avoir cherché à atterrir un peu partout... Et j'ai compris ensuite que j'aurais pu, par la seule logique, m'éviter tous ces tâtonnements; il est tellement évident que seul le catholicisme apporte à notre génération ce dont elle a besoin!

BAROIS. — C'est là ce que je comprends mal...

TILLET. — Rien n'est plus simple, cependant. Pour stimuler notre volonté d'action, il nous faut, de toute nécessité, une discipline morale. Il nous faut un cadre immuable et tout fait, pour endiguer définitivement ces restes de fièvre intellectuelle qui nous viennent de vous, et dont nous avons, malgré tout, quelques traces dans le sang.

Eh bien, la religion catholique nous offre tout ça. Elle étaye notre personnalité de son pouvoir et de son expérience, fondés sur une épreuve de vingt siècles. Elle exalte notre sens de l'action, parce qu'elle s'adapte à toutes les nuances de la sensibilité humaine, et qu'elle confère un merveilleux supplément de vie à ceux qui l'embrassent sans marchander. Or, tout est là: il nous faut aujourd'hui une foi capable de décupler notre activité.

BAROIS (qui a suivi attentivement). — Soit. Mais enfin, cette défaveur que vous affichez complaisamment pour l'intelligence spéculative, ne va pas jusqu'à vous laisser dans l'ignorance de certaines vérités, acquises aujourd'hui par la science, et qui ont ruiné les bases de cette religion dogmatique?

Comment l'acceptez-vous alors, dans son intégrité? Comment conciliez-vous, par exemple...

TILLET (vivement). — Mais noua ne cherchons pas à concilier, monsieur... La religion est sur un plan; la science est sur un autre. Les savants ne pourront jamais atteindre la religion, dont les racines sont hors de leur portée.

BAROIS, — Mais l'exégèse attaque directement... dans ses origines mêmes...

GRENNEVILLE (sourire tranquille). — Non, nous ne nous comprenons pas...

Ces difficultés auxquelles vous faites allusion, elles n'existent pas pour nous. Quelle valeur peut avoir la contestation d'un professeur d'hébreu, qui tire ses arguments d'une comparaison de vieux textes, à côté de la certitude intime de notre foi? (Riant.) Je vous assure, je suis stupéfait de penser que des affirmations de cette qualité ont pu avoir une influence décisive sur la croyance de nos aînés!

TILLET, — Au fond, la logique d'un raisonnement historique ou philologique n'est qu'apparente: elle ne peut rien contre le cri du cœur. Lorsqu'on a éprouvé *personnellement* l'efficacité pratique de la foi...

BAROIS. — Permettez. Cette efficacité, à laquelle vous revenez toujours, il y a bien des convictions philosophiques qui...

TILLET. — Mais nous les avons passés en revue, tous vos systèmes! Depuis votre fétichisme de l'évolution, jusqu'au mysticisme romantique de vos philosophes athées! Non! Notre vitalité renaissante exige d'autres appuis que ceux-là! Nous aspirons à nous passionner, mais nous voulons que ça en vaille la peine! Votre génération ne nous a rien légué qui puisse servir de règle à une existence pratique.

BAROIS. — Toujours ce même refrain: la vie pratique! Vous ne paraissez pas vous douter que cette recherche exclusive de résultats palpables et immédiats, est au détriment de votre noblesse intellectuelle!

Nous étions moins intéressés!

GRENNEVILLE. — Pardon, monsieur, pardon... C'est qu'il ne faudrait pas confondre vie active et vie simplement pratique... (Souriant.) Je vous affirme que nous continuons à penser, et même que nos pensées s'élèvent assez haut. Mais elles ne se perdent plus dans les nuages, et c'est un incontestable progrès. Nous les asservissons à des besoins précis. Tout ce qui est abstraction stérile nous fait horreur, comme une lâcheté devant la vie et devant les responsabilités qu'elle impose.

BAROIS. — C'est la faillite de l'intelligence.

TILLET. — De l'intellectualisme, tout au plus...

BAROIS. — Tant pis pour vous, si vous ne connaissez plus l'ivresse de la raison et de la pensée pure...

TILLET. — C'est consciemment que nous avons substitué le goût du devoir présent à ces méditations fumeuses qui n'aboutissaient qu'à faire des sceptiques et des pessimistes.

Nous avons une superbe confiance en nous.

BAROIS. — Je le vois bien. Nous aussi, nous avions confiance!

TILLET. — Ce n'était pas une confiance de même nature, puisque la vôtre ne vous a pas empêchés de sombrer dans le doute...

BAROIS. — Mais le doute n'est pas uniquement cette position négative que vous croyez! Allez-vous nous faire un grief de ne pas avoir trouvé la clef de l'énigme universelle? Les recherches de ces cinquante dernières années ont établi que la plupart des affirmations dogmatiques qui passaient pour exprimer la vérité, ne la renfermaient pas. Et c'est déjà quelque chose, à défaut de posséder la vérité, que d'avoir bien repéré les endroits où elle n'est pas!

GRENNEVILLE. — Vous vous êtes heurté à l'inconnaissable, et vous n'avez pas su lui faire dans votre vie sa véritable place, en y découvrant un principe de force. Vous étiez parti de cette conviction *a priori,* que l'incrédulité était supérieure à la foi, et vous...

BAROIS. — Ainsi vous êtes assez peu conscients pour parler de convictions *a priori* ! Vous qui êtes les dupes de la première théorie toute faite que l'on vous a proposée! Vous me faites penser au bernard-l'ermite, qui s'installe dans la première coquille inhabitée qu'il rencontre... C'est comme lui, que vous êtes entrés dans le catholicisme! Et vous vous y êtes moulés, au point de vous imaginer maintenant, — et de faire croire — que cette enveloppe vous est naturelle!

GRENNEVILLE (souriant). — C'est un procédé qui peut avoir de grands avantages... Il suffit pour le justifier qu'il nous vaille un accroissement de courage.

TILLET. — Pour vivre, il faut une direction. Le principal est d'en choisir une qui ait fait ses preuves, et de s'y tenir!

BAROIS (pensif). — Je n'ai pas encore compris ce que vous y gagnez...

GRENNEVILLE. — Nous y gagnons une sécurité qui vous a toujours manqué!

BAROIS, — Je ne vois pas davantage ce que vous apportez de nouveau ou d'utile. Tandis que je vois fort bien ce que vous apportez de nuisible: une agitation volontairement perturbatrice, qui interrompt, qui compromet l'effort de vos devanciers, et qui risque de retarder, sans profit,

GRENNEVILLE. — Nous apportons notre goût de l'action, capable, à lui seul, de régénérer l'esprit français!

BAROIS (perdant patience). — Mais vous parlez toujours de l'action, de la vie, comme si vous en aviez acquis le monopole!Nul n'a plus passionnément aimé la vie que moi I Et pourtant cet élan m'a jeté exactement à l'opposé de vous: il vous a donné la nostalgie de la foi; et moi, il m'en a irrémédiablement détaché 1

Long silence.

BAROIS (avec lassitude). — L'homme n'est peut-être pas capable de profiter, plusieurs générations de suite, des enseignements de sa raison...

Il s'arrête. Il a prononcé cette phrase machinalement, et voici qu'il la reconnaît: c'est celle que Dalier lui opposait, il y a une heure...

Dalier 1

Suffit-il maintenant qu'on le contredise," dans un sens ou dans un autre, pour provoquer de sa part une égale révolte? Toujours fuyante, la vérité?

Il passe la main sur son front. II aperçoit ces deux enfants, raidis dans leur certitude...

Ah, non, certes, ce n'est pas là qu'elle est, la vérité!

BAROIS. — Ça tourne... Je pourrais être votre père, et nous ne nous comprenons plus: c'est la loi...

Ils échangent un bref sourire, qui le blesse à vif.

Il les toise: il les découvre enfin tels qu'ils sont.

Barois. — Mais ne vous faites pas d'illusion, messieurs, sur votre rôle... Vous n'êtes pas autre chose qu'une *réaction*. Et cette réaction était tellement inévitable, que vous n'avez même pas la gloriole de l'avoir provoquée: c'est l'oscillation du pendule, le reflux mécanique, après le flux... Un moment à attendre: la mer monte quand même!

GRENNEVILLE (agressif). — A moins que nous ne soyons le début d'une évolution dont vous ne soupçonnez même pas les conséquences!

BAROIS (sèchement). — Non. Une évolution n'aurait pas cet aspect brusque, arbitraire, défensif...

Il est debout et il se met à rire en sentant renaître la combativité de jadis. Il arpente la pièce, les poings aux poches, l'œil vif et direct, la lèvre moqueuse.

Barois. — Vous représentez un mouvement social, c'est indéniable; mais un mouvement isolé, sans tenants et sans aboutissements possibles: vous n'avez qu'un intérêt documentaire. Vous parlez haut; vous voulez re-créer l'Univers; vdûs datez le monde d'urie ère nouvelle, qui correspond ingénûment avec votre vingtième année... Vous affirmez.
— avant rl'avoir prjs le temps maild'apprendre etde juger.

Voulez-yeus Hlè pertnèttre d'aller plus loin encore?. "il y â, à l'origine de votre attitude, un sentiment que vous h'avouez paS, — peut-être parcé qu'il n'est pas très glorieux, — irials surtout, je crois, parce' qu'il ést obscur et què vbùs h'èrt avèz *pài* pris conscience: t'est un vague sentiment de peur...—'

Mouvement des jeunes gens.

BAROIS. — Oui... Sous ces grands mots d'ordre, de courage national, il y a un peu ce que vous croyez y mettre; mais il y a encore autre chose: un assez vulgaire instinct de conservation!

Depuis votre naissance, vous avez senti que les hardiesses du XIX siècle finiraient par ébranler une à une les bases, sur lesquelles l'équilibre social est encore assis; vous avez senti qu'en sapant l'arbre malade sur lequel vous avez votre nid, les aînés, — ces mandarins, ces dilettantes, ces impuissants! — allaient vous faire faire un plongeon un peu trop brusque dans l'avenir... Et vous vous êtes raccrochés, d'instinct, à tout ce qui peut étayer votre instabilité, pour quelque temps encore: vive la force, messieurs, vive l'autorité, la police, la religion! Ce sont les seules digues aux libertés des autres; et vous avez clairement compris que ces libertés-là ne pouvaient s'exercer qu'au détriment de votre situation personnelle 1 Le progrès marchait un peu trop vite: vous bloquez les freins... Vous n'avez pas le cœur assez solide, vous avez le vertige...

Vos protestations d'activité masquent un affaiblissement de la pensée français, qui a besoin de repos, peut-être, pour avoir trop longtemps de suite poussé sa pointe dans l'inconnu. Soit; c'est d'ailleurs une vieille histoire: il a existé une autre société de privilégiés, qui n'a pas osé faire la Révolution, et qui l'a payé de quelques têtes...

Les jeunes gens se sont levés; leur attitude déférente et hostile exaspère Barois. Sa fougue vient se briser contre le sourire impertinent de deux gamins.

Un silence.

GRENNEVIIXE. — Vous nous excuserez de ne pas vous suivre sur ce terrain-là... Je crois que nous avons dit tout ce que nous avions à dire. Barois leur tend la main.

Barois. — Je vous remercie de votre visite. Votre lettre paraîtra tout entière. Le public jugera.

GRENNEVILLE (à la porte). — Vous avez la certitude, monsieur, que votre génération « a poussé une pointe dans l'inconnu? » (Il sourit.) C'est fort heureux, sans quoi la vieillesse de vos amis s'annoncerait bien amère... Je remarque seulement combien ces vérités soi-disant libératrices, ont mal affranchi la plupart de vos contemporains!

BAROIS (tranquille). — Peut-être. Mais elles libèreront complètement nos descendants... (Souriant.) — et les vôtres, messieurs!...

II Dans l'escalier du *Sapeur*.

Marie, en montant, croise un petit vieillard.

Marie. — Bonjour, docteur.

LE MÉDECIN (se découvrant avec politesse). — Mademoiselle...

Marie. — Je suis la fille de M. Barois

LE MEDECIN (souriant, la main tendue). — Excusez-moi, Mademoiselle,

MARIE. — Je suis bien heureuse de vous rencontrer, docteur. Je voudrais tant être renseignée sur la santé de mon père! (Poussant la porte d'un bureau vide.) Puis-je vous retenir un instant?

LE MÉDECIN (la suivant). — Mais, Mademoiselle, il me semble que vous vous inquiétez à tort. Notre malade va ce soir aussi bien que possible. Dans quelques jours...

Marie l'arrête et le regarde franchement, de ses yeux masculins.

MARIE. — Vous pouvez me dire la vérité, docteur. Je me trouve dans des circonstances spéciales: je suis à la veille d'entrer au couvent, en Belgique. Dans quelques mois, j'aurai vu mon père pour la dernière fois... (Se dominant.) Je vous donne ces détails pour que vous compreniez... Ce n'est pas la crise actuelle qui me préoccupe. Je sens que mon père a quelque chose de grave, de très grave: il a tant changé depuis deux ans!

LE MÉDECIN. — Mon Dieu, Mademoiselle, c'est certain... M. Barois est atteint dans son état général... (Il se reprend aussitôt.) Mais c'est un mal qui ne l'empêchera pas de vivre longtemps encore, avec des précautions, une bonne hygiène... A l'âge de M. Barois, il faut bien s'attendre a quelques misères...

MARIE (pressante, le masque dur). — Il ne peut pas guérir, n'est-ce pas?

Le médecin hésite, mais un coup d'œil le décide à la franchise; il secoue négativement la tête. Court silence

LE MÉDECIN. — Je vous le répète. Mademoiselle, c'est un mal à très. longue échéance... L'excès de travail, la parole en public surtout, ont attaqué peu à peu le cœur. D'autre part, votre père a présenté, étant enfant, des signes de... d'anémie. Il a été traité énergiquement,

et on était parvenu à enrayer le mal, puisqu'il ne s'en est pas ressenti pendant plus de quarante ans! Malheureusement il a eu cette pleurésie, que nous avons soignée ensemble, voici...

MARIE. — Deux ans.

LE MEDECIN. —...Alors, il s'est produit une chose qui arrive quelquefois: l'infl'mmation des bronches facilite la pénétration des germes, et , fait évoluer totlt à coup la tuberculose assoupie... (Mouvement de Marie.) Oui, même après quarante années d'arrêt, c'est fréquent; des lésions anciennes se réveillent... Mais, je voes le répète, Mademoiselle, chez les vieillards ces maladies-là sont très lentes, avec des symptômes atténués, de longs arrêts, puis des reprises.;;

Marie (les yeux fixés sur le médecin). — Et, ce qu'il vient d'avoir, c'est une de ces reprises?

LE MÉdecin. — Oh, très bénigne... Votre père a pris froid, l'autre jour; il n'en faut pas davantage pour que l'état général s'en ressente.

Marie. — Je vous remercie, docteur C'est tout ce que je voulais savoir.

Le logement de Barois: detax pièces basses, une cuisine.

Bârois est allongé près «te là fenêtre. Â'&i il s'ifrféfesse àë allées et venues de la cour.

Marie, les Manches relevées» un ta-Wier sur sa robe, remet de l'ordre dans la chambre.

BAROIS. — Je vous en conjure, Marie; La femme de mériage rangera ça demain matin.

MARIE. — Elle rie revient donc pas le soir?

BAROIS (souriant). — Non.

MARIE. — Et qu'est-ce qui fait votre dîner?

BAROIS.— La concierge. (Gaiement.) Vous savez, quand on est seul, ce n'est pas long, un dîner...

MARIE (après une pause). — Avouez, Père, que Pascal vous manque? Je vous l'avais bien dit...

BAROIS (gêné). — Mais non. Je suis parfaitement soigné, je ne manque de rien... D'ailleurs je n'avais pas la place de loger un domestique ici.

Un silence.

Marie reprend ses rangements. Barois la suit des yeux.

Elle passe à sa portée: il saisit sa main et l'appuie à ses lèvres.

Elle sourit; mais leurs regards sont lourds d'arrière-pensées.

BAROIS (jouant avec la main de Marie). — Moi qui me faisais une fête de ces huit jours à Paris, avant votre noviciat!Et toutes vos visites auront été des séances de garde-malade!

MARIE. — Vous viendrez me voir à Wassignies...

A l'évocation du couvent, ses pommettes rosissent.

BAROIS. — Les novices ne sont donc pas cloîtrées?

MARIE. — Si. Mais on vient leur dire adieu, la veille de la prise du voile..

Une larme glisse sur son sourire.

Barois lâche sa main.

Barois. — Votre mère ne se soucierait guère de me rencontrer là-bas...

Sa voix est indifférente, à peine interrogative. Mais il la dévisage de biais, anxieusement.

Elle fait un signe de protestation.

BAROIS (ton léger, où perce du plaisir). — Et puis, ma pauvre Marie, je ne suis plus en état de voyager...

III

Un appartement modeste, rue de Passy.

Luce, à sa table de travail.

Il retire hâtivement ses lunettes en voyant entrer Barois, et va vers lui.

LUCE. — Je suis bouleversé, mon cher ami... Que s'est-il passé?

Barois, essoufflé par les trois étages, s'assied lourdement, le poing sur le cœur; son sourire demande quelque répit.

Luce (après un instant). — Je n'ai trouvé dans votre mot aucun motif plausible...

BAROIS. — Je vous en prie, mon vieil ami, ne cherchez pas à me convaincre. Ma décision est prise.

Luce fait un geste d'incompréhension, et va s'asseoir à son bureau.

BAROIS. — J'y pensais depuis longtemps, ce n'est pas un coup de tête.

LUCE (attentif). —Remettez-vous à

un nouveau travail, Barois, et vous verrez, vous retrouverez vite l'équilibre!

BAROIS. — Je suis incapable de faire un projet. (Soucieux.) D'ailleurs je vais avoir à m'absenter bientôt... Vous savez, cette cérémonie en Belgique... Ma fille...

LUCE (vivement). — Ah... Eh bien, attendez, croyez-moi; ne prenez aucun parti avant votre retour.

Barois devine sa pensée; il sourit péniblement.

BAROIS. — Non, ce n'est pas ça. .. Je ne suis plus, ni physiquement ni moralement, le chef qu'il faut au *Semeur.* L'entrain n'y est plus. Le public s'en aperçoit bien. Et les collaborateurs! En fait, la direction m'échappe de jour en jour: ce sont les jeunes venus qui donnent le ton, maintenant. Moi je suis le vieux, débordé et suspect... (Sourire amer.) Et puis, voilà assez longtemps que Breil-Zoeger attend la place...

Il tire de sa poche un manuscrit plié qu'il pose sur le bureau.

BAROIS. — Tenez. J'ai voulu vous soumettre ça: une sorte de confession, de testament... J'ai l'intention d'y consacrer un numéro du *Semeur.* Pour ne pas m'en aller comme un vaincu, vous comprenez? Un dernier numéro, tout entier pour moi seul. Après, je me tairai.

Luce. — Vous ne pourrez pas!

BAROIS. — Pourquoi donc? Justement, les médecins me prescrivent le repos; ils veulent que je quitte Paris, que je m'installe en banlieue, au grand air...

LUCE. — Un homme comme vous ne se condamne pas volontairement au silence!

BAROIS. — Oh si!... Il y a des stations, dans la vie, où il faut savoir s'arrêter, se tourner sur soi-même et prendre une détermination.

LUCE (penché). — Supposez un instant que les rôles soient renversés; que je sois venu vous dire: « Je quitte tout, je renonce à vivrf... »

BAROIS. — Ah, vous, vous n'en auriez pas le droit! Mais ce n'est pas la même chose

LUCE. — Je n'ai rien que vous n'ayez vous-même...

BAROIS. — Vous avez une sagesse qui accepte tout ce qui arrive... C'est la différence qu'il y a entre le bonheur et le malheur.

LUCE (souriant). — Il est si facile de ne chercher son bonheur que dans les satisfactions de la raison!

BAROIS (farouche). — Elles ne me suffisent plus!
Une pause.

BAROIS. — J'en ai assez 4e me débattre dari6 une vie dont le seris *m'é-J* chappe... /

Luçe est assis, les bra§ croisés, les yeux à terre. Aux derniers mots de Barois, il lève son regard pensif et reste un instant avant de répondre.

LUCE. —T Voilà le point malade... Mais pourquoi vouloir à tout prix porter us jugement définitif sur la vie?Pourquoi toujours poser ces problèmes insolubles.?

BAROIS (violence soudaine), — Pourquoi? Mais parce que, si je disparais, moi, avant d'en avojr la clef, mon effort n'aura abouti à rien! Qu'est-ce que vous voulez que ça me fasse, à moi, Barois, de penser que dans deux mille ans, on en saura peut-être un peu plus que nous? Cette énigme, c'est moi seul qu'elle oppresse!

Luce. — Il faut se rappeler que Moïse n'est pas entré en Terre promise...

Barois (avec une animosité involontaire). — Ah, je ne sais vraiment pas comment vous êtes fait! On dirait que vous ne vous êtes jamais trouvé en tête à tête avec la mort!Vous avez eu des chagrins, pourtant, des deuils. Après (a mort 4e votre femme,,.

LUCE (d'une voix subitement voilée). — Oui, à ce moment-là, j'ai désespéré de tout... Pendant plusieurs semaines. (Relevant le front.) Et puis un matin, dans le jardin,:— nous habitions encore Auteuil, — e me souviens, j'ai vu à nouveau les arbres, le soleil, les petits... Peu a peu, j'ai remonté la pente.

BAROIS. — Moi, voyez-vous, je n'ai plus une heure de paix;, depuis que je sens mon tour approcher I Autrefois je me disais: « Oui, e//e viendra, e//e me prendra, comme les autres... » (La main au cœur.) Mais maintenant je sais *par où,* et tout est changé! Je sens son crampon qui a mordu là, qui m'attire par ce lambeau de chair malade, qui m'attire, moi, mon œuvre, la joie que j'aurais à vivre...

Ah, je ne peux pas rne résigner à ce néant!

Un silence.

LUCE. — Nous ne vqyons pas les choses de même. Pour moi, la vie et a mort se sont toujours confondues. C'est la suite du même mystère... Et j'envisage ainsi le problème depuis tant d'années, que je n'ai plus la moindre vel'éité de révolte.

BAROIS. — Votre consentement est au-dessus de mes forces I

LUCE. — Je ne consens pas! Mais je ne m'insurge pas non plus. Je me sens si peu de chose dans 1 agencement des lois universelles... Je me suis habitué à n'être qu'une parcelle d'univers qui accomplit sa destinée; je me relie au passé et à l'avenir; je me devine, par avance, prolongé par ceux qui feront, après moi, la même œuvre que moi. (Souriant.) Je vous répète que les satisfactions de la raison ont pour moi une extrême importance: ce que la mort a de rationnel, quand on l'envisage ainsi, me la fait accepter aussi naturellement que la naissance

Barois. — Je vous envie.

LUCE. — Mais ce calme est à la portée de chacun!
Barois secoue la tête.

LUCE (ton de reproche). — Je vous assure que si j'étais, comme vous, paralysé par la mort, je me contraindrais à réagir. Nous sommes un fragment de vie universelle, — peut-être le seul qui ait conscience de luimême: cette conscience nous fait un devoir de *vivre* le plus possible.

Vous, Barois, vous qui aimiez tant la vie!

BAROIS (avec désespoir). — Mais je l'aime plus que jamais, mon ami, et c'est bien ce qui m'empêche d'accepter qu'elle puisse finir!Plus j'aime la vie, et moins je me résigne aux conditions dans lesquelles il faut vivre. Pourquoi la conscience, si c'est pour contempler le néant?

Luce le regarde sans répondre.

BAROIS.—Le néant... J'ai beau me raisonner, je ne peux plus sortir de là!

LUCE. — Vous vous laissez dominer par votre moi. C'est fréquent, lorsqu'on vieillit: la personnalité devient plus précise, plus pesante; on est moins sollicité par l'extérieur, on concentre ses facultés sur soi... Il faut lutter contre cette ankylose!

BAROIS (s'abandonnant). — Ah, mon pauvre Luce, comment ne pas désespérer de tout? Voyons! A quoi ont abouti nos efforts? Récapitulez nos déceptions, depuis l'Affaire! Partout le mensonge, l'intérêt, l'injustice sociale, comme avant! Où est-il le progrès? Y a-t-il une seule de nos certitudes qui se soit imposée, grâce à nous? Au contraire, je constate I plutôt un recul, puisque les jeunes nous renient, et qu'ils ont pris le con. trepied de tout ce qui nous avait paru définitif! Quelle pitié! Voilà que I beaucoup d'entre eux se soumettent intégralement au catholicisme! Est-ce qu'ils ignorent nos attaques? Non, mais ils y ont trouvé des réponses en accord avec les besoins de leurs tempéraments, et ils sont assurés, autant que nous l'étions nous-mêmes! Ils ont même découvert de subtils détours pour réhabiliter le libre arbitre, et pour s'en faire une raison d'agir! Ce sont des faits, mon cher...

Nous aurons beau travailler à améliorer le sort des autres, à les affranchir, toute la nature travaille contre nous: toutes les injustices, toutes les erreurs renaissent avec chaque couvée neuve, et c'est toujours la même lutte, et toujours la même victoire du fort sur le faible, du jeune sur le vieux, éternellement!

LUCE (très ferme). — Non, je ne peux pas vous suivre, je ne peux pas voir le monde si mauvais que vous le faites... Non... Au contraire, je vois qu'en somme, malgré des écarts, qui me désespèrent autant que vous, c'est tout de même l'ordre et le progrès qui finissent par gagner, peu à peu... Vue d'ensemble, l'humanité avance. C'est incontestable. Aucun esprit de bonne foi ne pourra le nier.

Barois se met à rire.

BAROIS. — Avouez donc que la croyance au progrès est un postulat optimiste qui est nécessaire à votre équilibre personnel!

Le progrès? L'outillage, les méthodes, oui, tout ce qui dépend de l'observation et de l'exercice, a progressé... Mais dans le fond qu'y a-t-il de nouveau depuis les philosophes grecs?Sur la vie, sur la mort, nous n'en savons pas plus qu'eux... Conjectures! Impossible d'affirmer ni de nier avec certitude l'existence de l'âme, la liberté...

LUCE. — C'est déjà beaucoup d'avoir bien prouvé que tout se passe somme si l'âme et la liberté n'existaient pas.

»

Bii-KOIS. — Ces acquisitions négatives et provisoires ne me contentent plus/!

U.UCE (tristement). — Vous aussi, Barois, vous voilà atteint par la contagion? Ah, je reconnais que nous vivons à une époque bouleversée... Mais comment ne sentez-vous pas que c'est l'avenir qui germe sous cette souffrance! Tu enfanteras dans la douleur...

Vous n'avez pas prononcé le cri du ralliement actuel, mais il était déjà sur vos lèvres: *la faillite de la science...* Formule commode! Une classe ignorante la répèteapuis dix ans, et la jeune génération s'en est emparée, sans revision; car c'est plus facile à affirmer qu'à vérifier... (Avec orgueil.) Pendant ce temps-là, elle travaille, la science en faillite, et son apport s'accroît peu à peu: les théories qu'elle avait provisoirement ébauchées, elle les retouche quotidiennement, elle les consolide par de nouvelles découvertes... Elle avance sans répondre, — et c'est elle qui aura le dernier mot!

11 se lève et fait quelques pas, les mains derrière le dos.

LUCE. — C'est une réaction inévitable... Stupidement, on a voulu exiger de la science beaucoup plus qu'elle ne pouvait donner à ses débuts, — peut-être même plus qu'elle n'est susceptible de donner jamais. On a cru tout possible d'elle. Et maintenant il y a des esprits scientifiques, comme vous, qui se laissent aveugler par leur point de vue individuel: ils se disent naïvement, quand sonne leur soixantaine: « Voilà trente ans que je travaille. En ces trente

années, mon existence à moi s'est chargée d'événements... Eh bien, pendant ce temps, la science, qu'a-t-elle fait? Je ne vois guère qu'elle ait progressé. »

La faillite de la science, mon ami, résulte tout simplement de la disproportion qui existe entre la brièveté de notre vie d'hommes, et la lente évolution des connaissances. Vous et les autres, vous êtes le jouet d'une apparence: vous êtes comme nos ancêtres qui ont affirmé pendant des siècles l'inertie du monde minéral, parce qu'au cours de leur rapide existence ils n'arrivaient pas à observer de modification sensible dans la composition d'un caillou 1

Barois l'écoute avec une incurable indifférence.

BAROIS. — Oui... autrefois ce genre de raisonnement me satisfaisait. Maintenant non. J'y vois un agencement logique: mais rien de tout ça ne m'atteint à l'endroit où je souffre...

Un silence. jrs

"est

BAROIS. — (Les larmes aux yeux.) Ah, c'est affreux de vieillir... t LUCE (vivement). — Mais vous êtes plus jeune que moi I .1

BAROIS (grave). — Je me sens très vieux, mon cher. Je suis une machirre usée: les leviers n'obéissent plus. Le cœur bat la breloque. J'ai lài.. (il touche sa poitrine) comme un soufflet percé... Le moindre refroidissement me met au lit, avec la fièvre... Je suis fini, je me sens incapable de fournir une étape nouvelle...

Luce (sans conviction). — Vous traversez une période de dépression qui passera...

BAROIS (avec rancune). — Mais vous ne sentez donc pas les années, vous! Le cerveau qui fléchit, les habitudes qui se figent... L'isolement, le vide sentimental, l'impossibilité de prendre quelque chose à cœur... Ah, sapristi, je les sens bien, moi! Ma vie est bloquée; c'est une impression atroce. Je suis incapable d'activité: je n'ai plus qu'une mortelle envie... d'avoir envie d'agir!

Et quand je me retourne vers le passé, qu'est-ce que j'y trouve?Qu'estce que j'ai fait?

Mouvement de Luce.

BAROIS (l'interrompant). — Evidemment, j'ai écrit, j'ai aligné des mots, j'ai échafaudé des argumentations... Je laisse des livres, des articles qui ont eu leur actualité... Mais croyez-vous que je sois dupe? que je m'illusionne sur la pauvreté de tout ça?

LUCE. — Vous méconnaissez votre vie, Barois, ce n'est pas digne. Vous avez cherché; vous avez trouvé des parcelles de vérité; vous les avez divulguées généreusement; vous avez contribué à extirper quelques erreurs, et à préserver quelques certitudes qui vacillaient; vous avez défendu la justice, avec une ferveur communicative, qui a fait de vous, pendant quinze ans, l'âme vivante d'un parti...

(Simplement.) Je trouve votre vie très belle.

Une fierté dans les yeux de Barois.
Il sourit et tend la main.

BAROIS. — Merci, mon ami... Autrefois, ces paroles-là m'auraient remis dapfes»b... Je ne rêvais pas d'autre oraison funèbre... H Mais maintenant. IT-I

Un silence.

ta BAH OIS. — A quoi pensez-vous?

LUCE. — Je viens d'avoir, en vous regardant, cette idée: que beaucoup de ceux qui nous ont précédés ont dû éprouver cette angoisse.. Ces hommes, — à qui nous sommes redevables de tout ce que nous avons pu faire — ont dû avoir ce même désespoir, ont dû s'imaginer que leur effort était inutile...

(Un temps.) Allez, allez, Barois, la vérité, c'est qu'i' l n'y a pas une bonne graine qui se perde, pas une idée qui ne germe un, jour, pas une parcelle de conscience *acquise,* qui disparaisse. Savons-nous si l'une des pensées que nous avons émises, vous ou moi, ne sera pas le point de départ d'une découverte, qui libèrera davantage l'avenir? Il suffit, pour avoir fait du bon ouvrage, de s'être donné, humainement, toute sa vie. Quand on a semé le mieux et le plus possible, on peut s'en aller en paix, et céder la place à d'autres...

BAROIS (sombre). — Mais je ne suis pas aussi sûr que vous d'avoir semé le bon grain...

Luce le considère avec un découragement infini.

TBAROIS. — J'ai totalement changé d'attitude devant l'univers. Je ne sais plus où j'en suis, voilà la vérité...

Certains jours, comme aujourd'hui, je ne peux plus accepter comme vrai ce que j'ai défendu jusqu'ici. Je sens bien que je n'arriverais pas à me prouver logiquement l'inanité de mes convictions passées: mais, — je ne sais comment dire, — c'est presque *physiquement* que je les repousse: je les repousse parce qu'elles ne m'ont apporté que des déceptions!

( y LUCE. — Vous ne raisonnez plus...

BAROIS. — Ah, on peut raisonner quand on a trente ans, quand on a la vie devant soi pour changer d'opinion, une sève qui bouillonne, du bonheur plein les veines! Mais quand on se sent près du terme, on est tout petit devant l'infini...

(Très lentement, les yeux perdus.) On a, par dessus tout, un désir vague... le désir d'on ne sait quoi... qui serait le remède à toutes les transes...

Un peu de paix, un peu de confiance... quelque chose sur quoi s'appuyer... pour n'être pas trop malheureux, pendant le temps qui-'-e encore... V v,

Il redresse la tête.

Luce, qui souriait mélancoliquement, rencontre son re son sourire s'évanouit. V

Long silence.

Après un instant, Barois semble se ressaisir. Il tend son ma nuscrit à Luce.

BAROIS. — Tenez, lisez ça, voulez-vous?
/ /

Vingt minutes passent.
Le jour décroît.

Luce s'est levé, pour s'approcher de la fenêtre. Une symphonie de blancheurs: la vitre blême, le rideau de mousseline, son front pâle, sa barbe, les feuillets...

Les coins de la chambre s'emplissent de grisaille.

Barois, les yeux fixes, attend.

Luce tourne la dernière page. Il la lit jusqu'au bout, attentivement; la main qui tient le manuscrit s'abaisse; il retire ses lunettes; ses paupières se plissent à

chercher Barois dans la pénombre.

LUCE. — Mon pauvre ami, que voulez-vous que je vous dise? Je ne peux plus rien pour vous, maintenant...

(Après une pause.) Non... je ne peux plus rien pour vous, moi...

Bit

A Wassignies-sur-Lys, près de Gand.

La voiture de Barois longe un mur de couvent et s'arrête devant un portail, qui s'entr'ouvre aussitôt. Il traverse une cour déserte, hésite, et se dirige vers le perron central; lorsqu'il atteint la dernière marche, la porte close s'ouvre devant lui.

Vestibule dallé. Le battant se referme. Une ombre s'approche, le visage caché sous un voile noir.

Il la suit.

Elle marche vite, agitant sans interruption une claquette de bois. Des couloirs. La religieuse pousse une dernière porte, s'efface pour qu'il passe, et donne un tour de clef derrière lu.

Le parloir: vaste salle au carrelage luisant, divisée en deux, sur toute la hauteur, par un lattis de bois à claire-voie.

Une femme est là, en noir, immobile, écroulée sur une chaise. Il reconnaît Cécile; il s'avance. Elle tressaille et tend la main, sans pouvoir articuler un mot.

Il s'assied près d'elle.

Quelques minutes.

Dans la cour, un carillon léger, se met à sonner ses quatre heures.

Aussitôt, de l'autre côté du grillage, paraissent troiis religieuses, de même taille, la figure voilée de noir. Deux dVentre elles vont s'agenouiller devant une statue de la Vierge. La. treisième s'approche, et, à l'aide d'une clef, fait jouer un panuieau de la clôture; puis elle va rejoindre les autres, qui récitentune dizaine de chapelet.

Cécile et Barois sont debout, les nerfs à vif.

Cécile écarte les lèvres comme si elle allait mourir.

La dizaine s'achève...

L'une des religieuses se signe, et s'avance. Elle écarte son voile...

Cécile pousse un cri étouffé et l'étreint convulsivement; puis elle se détache brusquement pour la dévisager, comme si elle craignait d'être trompée; et, gémissant de tendresse, elle la serre de nouveau contre son cœur.

Marie se redresse, et sans se dégager, tend la main à son père; il l'embrasse en pleurant. Leurs yeux se rencontrent: Barois retrouve ce regard anxieux, durci, ce sourire crispé, qui est chez elle le signe extérieur de la foi; mais, dans son expression passée, il n'y avait pas tant de lumière.

MARIE. — Par pitié, maman, ne pleurez pas... Dieu vous donnera la force, la consolation... (La voix a perdu son timbre. Elle ajoute, malgré elle:) Si vous saviez comme je suis heureuse!

Cécile halète sur son épaule, zézayant des plaintes vagues.

CÉCILE. — Qu'est-ce que je vais devenir, Marie... Qu'est-ce que je vais devenir...

Marie tient sa mère doucement appuyée contre elle, et lui caresse le front.

MARIE (se tournant vers Barois). — Père, j'ai lu votre manifeste... Oui, c'est la dernière faveur que j'aie demandée. . (Elle le considère, les yeux dans les siens. Et, brusquement, avec un éclat d'espoir:) Père, ces pages-là appellent Dieu!...

Barois secoue négativement la tête.

Cécile sanglote toujours, n'écoutant rien, balbutiant:— «Qu'estce que je vais devenir... Qu'est-ce que je vais devenir. .. »

Les regards de Marie vont de l'un à l'autre. Son cœur s'amollit une dernière fois de pitié humaine. Elle se penche pour atteindre la main de son père, et l'attire doucement près de sa mère.

M ARIE (bas). — Ah, j'ai tant prié... (A peine perceptible:) Ne vous sep? /rez plus, maintenant...

*I* Les religieuses, au fond de la pièce, se sont relevées, i Elles approchent.

Marie les entend venir derrière elle; son corps frémit; son i. masque s'épouvante. Elle s'arrache des bras de Cécile, et glisse dans ceux de son père: à peine a-t-il le temps de sentir sous ses lèvres la soie du petit front bombé.. . Elle se détache: d'un geste Jf.' éperdu, elle étreint encore une fois sa mère, qui la regarde avec f des yeux fous...

Puis elle se recule vivement.

Le voile retombe.

Une religieuse referme soigneusement le grillage.

Personne ne verra plus ce visage vivant. Cécile reste foudroyée, les mains tendues, les lèvres ouvertes.

Tout à coup elle chancelle, et se serait abattue si Barois ne l'avait saisie.

Elle s'accroche à lui.

CÉCILE (dans un souffle). — Ne me quittez pas, Jean... ne me quittez pas..

La porte s'ouvre.

La tourière fait entendre sa claquette.

Barois soutenant Cécile, l'entraîne vers la sortie.

Une heure plus tard.

Dans une arrière-salle de l'auberge. On a traîné deux fauteuils devant le poêle. Une lampe suspendue éclaire un souper auquel ils n'ont pas touché..
4 reli

Barois, assis en retrait, aperçoit Cécile de dos, courbéel'entre chapeau cabossé glissant sur les bandeaux défaits; par instaitroi- elle tourne la tête, et, pour étouffer une reprise de sangloWau ; presse son mouchoir sur ses lèvres enflées. «une

Il est abattu par la fièvre; chaque pulsation du cœur lui f; i, mal; sa sensibilité est à nu. Le bruit de ces larmes ressusciti des émotions lointaines.
11 songe au passé, sans amertume: la solitude d'hier, celle qui l'attend demain, sont pires que la mésentente de jadis.

— « Elle a dit: Ne *me quittez pas*... Un cri de désespoir peutêtre?

« Ah, si elle veut...

« Mais pratiquement, c'est bien difficile...

« Qu'elle vienne habiter avec moi dans la banlieue? Elle ne pourrait pas s'y faire; sa vie active, ses patronages...

« Alors? Je ne peux pourtant pas aller habiter dans la maison de la mère Pasquelin... »

Involontairement il termine sa pensée à voix haute:

Barois. —...ça ne serait possible, que si vous consentiez à quitter votre maison... à venir habiter celle de ma grand'mère...

Cécile se retourne.

Barois rougit.

Elle hésite, le temps de bien comprendre. L'émotion la fait loucher.

Puis, de son fauteuil, avec un abandon reconnaissant, elle allonge la main jusqu'à la sienne, s

CRÉPUSCULE

«...pareil à qui suivrait pour se guider une lumière que lui-même tiendrait en sa main... »
A. Gide.

«...N'éteins pas le lumignon qui fume... Son odeur même nous sert de guide.. »
Ibsen.

I

A Buis, dans la vieille maison Barois. Premiers jours de l'été.
Dix heures du matin.
La chambre de Cécile.

Elle a rassemblé là tous les meubles du petit salon de Mme Pasquelin.

Elle est assise à son bureau. Robe noire. Bandeaux lisses. Un livre de comptes ouvert devant elle. D'autres registres, étiquetés: *Quêtes, Vestiaire.*

CÉCILE. — Entrez...

C'est Jean.

Elle achève son addition, appuie le buvard, et tourne la tête. Sourire affectueux.

CÉCILE. — Comment vous sentez-vous, ce matin?

JEAN. — Pas mal.

CÉCILE. — Un temps merveilleux...

Jean s'avance vers la fenêtre.

L'appui est chaud. La cour est pleine de lumière. JEAN. — Il doit faire bon au soleil...

Cécile range ses cahiers, avec des gestes étroits. Puis elle pique un chapeau sur sa tête, et glisse un cahier sous son bras.

CÉCILE. — Je vais porter ça à l'abbé Lévys.

Jean descend l'escalier derrière elle. La porte du vestibule est ouverte; l'éclat du perron est éblouissant.

Quelques pas, aveuglé. Le soleil cuit la chair des épaules.

Les premières pivoines, les premières fraises; les feuilles vertes de la treille.

Une demie sonne au clocher.

Il lève les yeux; son regard longe le pan de pierre ocre et se perd dans la profondeur bleue: un ciel qui vient de loin et qui passe, un ciel qui fait le tour du monde.

Il gagne, à petits pas, le banc de la tonnelle. Il écarte les bras sur le dossier tiède, pour que toute cette clarté, toute cette chaleur le baignent. Ses mains sont roses de soleil.

Apaisement.

Il pense:

— « Je suis là, dans ce printemps... Je ne le comprends pas. Mais il s'empare de moi, il me soumet à lui.

« Il doit y avoir d'immenses cycles d'idées dans lesquels notre pensée ne s'est pas aventurée encore... Des idées qui dépassent nos hypothèses de l'âme, de Dieu; des idées qui accorderaient nos contradictions... Ah!... »

Quelques minutes plus tard.

Jean regagne lentement la maison.

Le timbre du portail.

Un abbé pénètre dans la cour, aperçoit Jean et s'approche. JEAN. — Mme Barois vient de sortir, Monsieur.

Le prêtre hésite.

L'abbÉ. — Permettez-moi de me nommer: l'abbé Lévys.

JEAN (du haut du perron). — Mme Barois sera désolée. Je crois qu'elle allait justement vous voir.

L'abbÉ (geste évasif, qui relègue Mme Barois et ses œuvres à l'arrière-plan de ses préoccupations). — Je m'en voudrais, Monsieur, de ne pas saisir cette occasion... Mon arrivée à Buis est encore très récente. Mais depuis que j'habite la même ville que vous, j'ai le désir de vous rencontrer.

Jean s'incline légèrement.

L'ABBÉ. — Oh, je sais que vous vivez très seul. Mais je me serais fait un titre, pour enfreindre la consigne, d'avoir été pendant douze ans, — je ne dis pas un de vos abonnés (il montre sa soutane) — mais l'un de vos lecteurs...

JEAN (stupéfait). — Vous suiviez le *Semeur*?

L'ABBÉ. — Régulièrement. (Baissant les yeux.) J'y ai même collaboré, si l'on peut dire, par des lettres non signées, que vous avez publiées à plusieurs reprises...

JEAN (redescendant deux marches). — Vraiment? Ah, je ne me doutais guère...

Mais je vous tiens debout sous ce soleil... Voulez-vous entrer un instant? Mme Barois ne tardera pas.

Il guide l'abbé jusqu'à l'ancien salon, son cabinet, qu'il a meublé avec les épaves de sa vie active: ses bibliothèques, son bureau, et, sur la cheminée, seul et nu, le douloureux *Esclave enchaîné* de Michel-Ange, immuablement arrêté dans son effort.

L'abbé Lévys: long, maigre.

Masque régulier, zébré de tics nerveux. Une peau jaune, bossuée. Un regard tantôt distrait, tantôt fixe. Des lèvres mobiles, dont le sourire est une grimace triste.

JEAN (intrigué). — Je suis si surpris que nous avions eu un prêtre parmi nos correspondants!... Dans quel esprit lisiez-vous donc notre *Semeur*?

L'ABBÉ. — En y faisant, le plus souvent, de graves restrictions; mais toujours avec intérêt, et souvent avec sympathie...

Jean fait un geste d'étonnement.

L'ABBÉ. — Ne croyez-vous pas qu'à un certain niveau de pensée, lorsqu'on est décidé à prendre au sérieux la vérité et à suivre sa conscience, il est bien difficile d'être de son parti, sans être aussi un peu de l'autre?

Jean l'examine, sans répondre.

L'abbÉ (après un temps). — C'est M. Breil-Zoeger qui a pris votre succession?

JEAN. — Non. C'est un jeune, un nommé Dalier, un sectaire. Mais il n'est que le prête-nom de Zoeger, qui a toujours aimé se tenir dans la coulisse.

L'abbÉ. — Vous ne vous en occupez plus du tout?

JEAN (brusque). — Oh, non, plus du tout! Et je vous prie de croire que je désapprouve entièrement la tournure anarchiste, de plus en plus accusée, qu'ils donnent à leur revue!

L'abbé garde le silence.

JEAN. — D'ailleurs, je n'ai plus aucune relation avec eux. J'ai rompu définitivement. (Prenant des brochures sur une étagère.) On m'envoie les fascicules, par habitude; mais, voyez, je n'ai même pas coupé les derniers... A quoi bon? Je n'y trouve que des sujets d'irritation!

(Il fronce les sourcils, et éparpille les revues devant lui; puis il cherche à dévier la conversation.) Je ne suis plus en correspondance qu'avec MarcElie Luce, et un vieil ami des mauvais jours, Ulric Woldsmuth.

L'abbÉ. — Le chimiste?

JEAN. — Vous le connaissez?

L'abbÉ. — J'ai lu son livre.

Jean sourit, enchanté

JEAN. — Ah, voilà un beau caractère! Trente ans, qu'il cherche l'origine de la vie... Trente ans, sans une défaillance...

L'abbÉ (coup d'œil circulaire) — Mais... vous travaillez toujours?

JEAN (haussant les épaules). — Non. Je m'occupe. En ce moment, je traduis, — pour moi — le journal d'un mystique anglais...

(Sourire pénible.) J'ai mis quelque temps à m'habituer à cette existence de mollusque... Mais ma santé ne me permet plus autre chose. Je vivote, en prenant des précautions, l'hiver au coin du feu, l'été au soleil... (L'éclat des yeux contraste avec la résignation des paroles.) Que voulez-vous, Monsieur l'abbé, c'est la vie...

Il soulève quelques numéros du *Semeur* et les laisse tomber un à un sur la table.

JEAN. — Ah, les jeunes ont vite fait de vous désarçonner!

Une pause.

JEAN (Le front baissé).—Voyez-vous, on est trop sévère pour les ratés... Leur effort n'aboutit pas directement, c'est vrai; mais il n'est pas perdu pour ça... Hein?... Aucun effort n'est perdu...

L'abbÉ (étonné). — Je ne pense pas que vous fassiez allusion à une expérience personnelle?

Jean le remercie d'un sourire.

L'abbé regarde curieusement ce Barois qu'il ne soupçonnait pas.

JEAN (après quelques minutes de réflexion, repris par une hantise familière). — J'ai trop longtemps cru que la science, à elle seule, pourrait établir, entre les hommes, la paix, l'unité... Eh bien, non.

L'abbÉ (prudemment). — Pourtant... si vous ne vous placez qu'à ce point de vue du rapprochement des peuples, la science, en moins de cent ans, a fait à peu près autant que le bouddhisme — et même que le christianisme — en vingt siècles!

JEAN. — Peuh... Voyez les résultats pratiques: qu'est-ce que le peuple y a gagné? Un matérialisme au ras du sol, qui est vraiment sans beauté.. Qui, surtout, est stérile...

L'abbé hésite. Ce n'est pas lui pourtant qui doit plaider pour la science...

JEAN (distrait). —...Ce qui semblerait prouver, au fond, que l'homme ne vit pas seulement de travail, de vérité. Il lui faut son *dimanche* : peu importe la formule...

L'abbÉ. (Passion soudaine). — Oui, peu importent les formules, puisqu'aucune n'est encore assez vaste pour contenir tout le Parfait, l'Infini, Dieu.. . Ce ne sont en somme que des façons différentes de nommer une attraction, qui est la même pour tous!

Jean le regarde avec attention.

JEAN. — Alors, si je vous comprends bien, vous, prêtre catholique, vous ne condamneriez pas irrémédiablement un être, qui, toute sa vie, aurait préféré sa formule à la vôtre?...

L ABBE (instinctivement). —. Non.

Sous l'insouciance de la voix, il a perçu l'anxiété de l'interrogation.

Un silence.

L ABBE. — Je me souviens d'un personnage d'une pièce Scandinave, qui disait...

Il se lève: Cécile vient d'entrer.

Elle ne laisse pas paraître sa surprise.

L ABBE. — J'espérais vous éviter cette course, Madame, mais je suis arrivé trop tard.

CECILE (lui remettant le registre). — Voici nos comptes à jour.

Elle éprouve une gêne à parler devant Jean, et dans cette pièce inhospitalière, dont elle ne franchit jamais le seuil.

CECILE. — j'aurais aussi diverses décisions à prendre pour la souscription des écoles... Voulez-vous m'accompagner là-haut un instant?

LABBÉ. — Je vous suis. (A Jean.) Je m'excuse, Monsieur, d'avoir ainsi abusé...

JEAN (spontanément). — Votre visite m'a fait beaucoup de plaisir.

Cécile est sortie, laissant la porte ouverte.

JEAN (d'un autre ton). — Vous n'avez pas achevé ce que disait votre Scandinave...

L'ABBÉ. — « Quand il s'agit de la foi, c'est l'affaire du bon Dieu. Notre devoir, à nous, est d'être sincères. » (i).

JEAN. — C'est une belle parole...

Bjornstjerne Bjoknson. *Au delà des forces.*

II

« 12 octobre, (après un long entretien avec M. Barois.)

« J'allais à lui, dans un mouvement de sympathie coupable: j'allais au polémiste dont le nom était pour moi le symbole de la pensée libre. J'allais à lui comme au seul être d'ici à qui parler de mes préoccupations.

« Et j'ai trouvé un pauvre homme, plus malheureux que moi, plus déchiré, plus pitoyable!

« Je ne l'ai pas vu tout de suite tel qu'il est.

« J'espaçais mes visites, par discrétion: c'est lui qui m'envoyait chercher, sans but, pour me voir. Je remarquais son souci d'aiguiller la conversation vers les questions religieuses. Je ne m'y dérobais pas; je cherchais même à lui faire deviner le pénible état de ma conscience. Mais il ne me semblait ças pouvoir distinguer l'homme sous le prêtre: mon caractère sacerdotal 1 attirait seul. Pourtant il ne se départait pas d'une attitude agressive à l'égard du catholicisme. Il ne cessait de m'opposer des arguments d'ordre scientifique, dont, pour mon supplice, je connaissais bien la valeur: mais il le faisait avec je ne sais quelle restriction, et comme s'il s'attendait bien à les voir réfuter. Ce que je faisais, d'instinct.

«Peu à peu, j'ai compris. Physiquement, il est rongé par la tuberculose pulmonaire des vieillards: c'est un fantôme, aux yeux brillants, miné presque chaque jour par la fièvre, et périodiquement repris par des poussées congestives qui aggravent ses lésions. Moralement, son état est pire encore: il est rongé par le doute de ce qu'il a cru vrai, et par la peur de mourir. Il se cramponne à ses convictions passées: mais

elles ne sont plus pour lui qu'un sujet d'angoisse.

« Je pensais trouver en lui un conseil: et c'est moi qui peux lui porter secours!

« Je ne songe pas à me soustraire à ce devoir inattendu: mais les circonstances ont quelque chose de tragique... Pourquoi faut-il que le prêtre, appelé à guider cet athée vers Dieu, soit un pauvre tourmenté, que les doutes ravagent lui-même depuis dix ans î

« Peut-être est-ce bien ainsi, peut-être suis-je mieux préparé qu'un autre à soigner cette plaie?

« Je m'y appliquerai de tout mon cœur, et je ferai en sorte qu'il ne soupçonne jamais de quelles mains incertaines, de quelles mains tremblantes, je lui apporte ce Dieu qu'il cherche!

« 2 novembre.

« Il a des moments de lucidité terribles, dès qu'il passe quelques jours sans fièvre.

« Aujourd'hui il m'a interrompu avec un regard singulier:— « A certaines heures, — tenez, en ce moment, — je parviens à me dédoubler, et une partie de moi-même juge, comme j'aurais jugé il y a quinze ans, ce que je suis devenu. .. Je me demande alors si je n'étais pas, de toute éternité, voué à la servitude? »

« En parlant, il tendait la main vers un plâtre de Michel-Ange qui est sur sa cheminée: — « *Regardez-le! Il ne peut pas lever un bras libre!... Peut-être n'ai-je fait, comme lui, pendant des années, que le simulacre de l'affranchissement...* »

« 10 novembre.

« Ce matin:

— « J'en ai assez des négations scientifiques! elles n'ont pas plus d'autorité pour nier que d'autres pour affirmer. Mais votre dogmatisme religieux me rebute, au même titre. Je sais ce qu'il vaut: j'y ai été pris, assez longtemps! » 16 janvier.

« Je l'ai trouvé couché, sans courage.

« Sur son lit, il y avait un numéro du *Semeur* qu'il venait de recevoir, m a ouvert. A la dernière page, un écho intitulé: *Une nouvelle conversion,* et quelques lignes mordantes qui le visaient; Il a haussé les épaules; mais je 1 ai senti profondément blessé.

« Il a changé la conversation. Nous n'avons abordé aucun sujet précis.

« Comme j'allais me retirer, après un silence, il m'a regardé:— Jè Suis un mystique, au fond... Et pourtant je ne crois à rien... »'

« Je lui ai répondu: — « Vous ne croyez à rien? On croit toujours à quelque chose. Chacun, au fond de soi, a son Dieu caché auquel il retourne pieusement, auquel il se sacrifie tous les jours. »

« Mais il a secoué la tête, d'un air sombre: « — Non, je vous dis que je ne crois à rien... J'erre dans le noir, je voudrais... » Il a baissé la voix, mais je crois avoir entendu: «... la paix... pour mourir. »

« 25 janvier.

« J'ài pu revenir sur le même sujet. Nous discutions encore une fois les preuves de l'existence de Dieu.

« Il m'a dit:— « Vos preuves ne prouvent rien, sinon que vous, Lévys, vous croyez en Dieu. Et elles ne prouvent absolument rien d'autre. Si ces preuves avaient quelque valeur, croyez-vous qu'il y aurait des athées?»

« J'ai répliqué:— « Màis il n'y a pas de véritables athées! Vous-même, vous ri'àvez jamais cessé d'être un croyant I Votre confiance dans le progrès, dans l'avenir de la science, votre croyance même au triomphe de l'athéisme, qu'était-ce, sinon un principe de foi?

« Vous croyez qu'il y a un but dans la nature.vous croyez à l'ordre éternel des lois; cet ordre-là, il a produit la conscience humaine, la vôtre; et par là, il a introduit dans l'univers l'idée de justice: cet ordre-là, c'est Dieu!»

« Il a réfléchi quelques secondes:—« Oui. Mais un Dieu indéterminé Le vôtre est déterminé. Et c'est là que la superstition commence. »

« Que répondre?

« 7 mars.

« Chaque fois que je le quitte, je me reproche de n'avoir pas su trouver,dans ma foi qui hésite, le mot, l'accent qu'il eût fallu. Et, chaque fois que je le revois, je suis stupéfait du résultat inespéré de mes froides paroles.

« Non que mes raisonnements l'aient convaincu. Mais, ils sont une *réponse* aux difficultés qu'il avait soulevées. Je m'aperçois que le pire serait de rester coi, et qu'à toutes ses attaques il fautopposer Une contradiction, même chancelante. Avant tout il a besoin d'une solution simple) une, et surtout categorique.

« Rien ne m'a si bien fait comprendre que la foi n'est pas seulement un acte de l'intelligence, une conviction, mais un acte de la sensibilité et de la volonté, un sentiment de confiance, un désir de soumission.

« 19 mars.

« L'Evangile prend une grande importance dans sa vie intérieure. Il en tire de fréquentes citations. Il a contracté l'habitude d'y recourir quotidiennement, comme à l'unique source de poésie qui le satisfasse.

« D'ailleurs il lit peu, et de moins en moins. Je le trouve généralement seul, dans un fauteuil de son cabinet, les pieds au feu, et sur les genoux, un journal qu'il n'a pas déplié.

« 3 juin.

« Jusqu'ici je lui développais surtout les raisons sentimentales de croire: le besoin de consolation; la nécessité d'une justice finale, d'un dédommagement; le désir d'une direction dans la vie.

« Il est particulièrement sensible à la beauté de la vie chrétienne;je lui en multiplie les exemples. Il me considère alors, de ses yeux vitreux, avec une expression d'envie. L'autre jour il m'a dit: — « Cette beauté, à elle seule, suffirait à justifier la foi, — si le fruit suffisait à justifier l'arbre... Et peut-être est-ce défendable, après tout?... »

« Aujourd'hui, l'entretien a été particulièrement animé. Il se sèntait réconforté par ces premiers beaux jours, qui lui permettent de sortir. Nous avons fait une promenade, au soleil, en causant. Il m'a demandé de préciser certains dogmes. Il a paru très frappé d'apprendre que là théologie comprend des éléments divers, dont la valèuf est fort inégale; qu'il ne faut pas confondre les dogmes essentiels de la foi, relativement peu nombreux, avec les doctrines communément reçues; et, qu'à tout prendre, il y a beaucoup de questions, comme l'efficacité des indulgences par exemple, sur lesquelles les catholiques sont libres d'avoir des opinions très différentes. Je lui ai même dit combien les dogmes du purgatoire et de l'enfer sont moins explicites qu'on ne te croit généralement, et combien il reste de marge aux croyants les plus orthodoxes, pour l'interprétation de ces dogmes.

« J'ai peut-être insensiblement forcé la note, tant j'ai senti que mes paroles le rasérénaient. D'ailleurs je ne pensé pas être sorti des limites que 1 apologétique moderne s'est fixée...

« 28 juin.

« Je rentre, le cœur serré. Il m'a inspiré aujourd'hui une pitié indicible.

« Il était couché, très affaibli par les accès de fièvre de la nuit. Cette semaine pluvieuse et malsaine a provoqué une petite toux qui l'épouvante.

« Mme Barois m'a dit que le médecin ne s en inquiétait pas outre mesure, et qu'il comptait sur l'été pour en venir à bout. Mais lui, avait un visage ravagé. Il m'a dit, avec un frisson: « — Ah, j'ai cru mourir cette nuit »; puis, d'une voix angoissée, comme une confidence: « — J'ai peur de la mort... »

« Jamais encore il n'avait directement abordé ce sujet.

« Je le regardais, subissant la contagion de cette terreur, et ne voulant pas le laisser paraître. J'étais resté debout contre le lit. Il avait gardé mes doigts dans sa main.

« — La première fois que j'en ai eu peur, tenez, c'était ici, dans la cour... devant le cercueil de ma grand'mère. J'avais onze ou douze ans, je venais d'être très malade. J'étais devant le catafalque, je regardais les fleurs, les bougies, et brusquement je me suis dit: *Et si elle n'est plus du tout, du tout, du tout ?...* »

« Il a ajouté d'une voix bizarre:« Qu'est-ce que c'est, la mort? La désorganisation de l'être que je suis, dont ma conscience fait toute l'unité... Alors? Disparition de la conscience, de l'âme?... »

« Il me dévisageait en parlant. Je le sentais parvenu à ce point de faiblesse morale où 1 on ne peut plus supporter que les hypothèses consolantes.

« Jamais je n'ai si fortement éprouvé

la puissance sacerdotale dont je suis revêtu, moi, si indigne... Je lui ai crié, presque violemment: « — Ah, moi aussi, j'aurais beau m'étourdir, si je n'avais pas une foi absolue en la vie future, l'idée de la mort paralyserait toutes mes forces!Mais la croyance à l'immortalité fait partie de ma conscience, et les pires obstacles qu'on puisse lui opposer sont des objections faciles à anéantir! »

« Il n'abandonnait pas ma main. Il m'écoutait avec une anxiété qui faisait mal. J'ai continué:

« — D'où vient ma conscience? D'une simple organisation nerveuse de mon cerveau? Le cerveau, les nerfs, — la vie, la mort? Mais vous ne voyez pas que ce sont des *mots* qui tous renferment un égal mystère! Ce sont des étiquettes, ce ne sont pas des explications!

« Je sens en moi une notion du divin, un sentiment de la perfection, qui ne *peuvent* pas être de pures sécrétions de mon cerveau imparfait et périssable. Je sens en moi l'existence d'une vie idéale, dont je ne trouve le point d'origine dans aucune partie de mon corps. Je sens eh moi deux sortes de rapports, absolument distincts: ceux que j'ai avec le monde matériel, par l'intermédiaire de mes organes, et ceux que j'ai avec le monde spirituel. La mort, par la désagrégation des éléments matériels, supprime toute la première série de ces rapports; mais elle ne supprime pas la seconde. Et c'est là que je mets toute ma foi en la survivance de ma personnalité morale! »

« C'est alors qu'il m'a dit, lentement, avec un regard suppliant qui quêtait une réponse décisive: — « Mais... une conscience n'existe qu'avec cette double forme de relations... Qu'est-ce que c'est qu'une conscience qui n'a plus de relation avec le monde matériel?»

« J'ai balbutié: — « Peu importe de se faire de la vie future une idée nette; l'important est que cette vie future soit certaine!»

« Il a lâché ma main.

« J'ai deviné que je l'avais atrocement déçu. La pitié m'a permis un suprême effort.

« Je me suis penché vers lui, répondant à sa pensée plus qu'à ses paroles:

— « Vous avez soif de certitude. Puisque la faiblesse de notre intelligence vous a refusé la vérité stable, pourquoi ne la demandez-vous pas à Dieu? »

« Il a fait un geste de désespoir..

« J'ai continué: — « Moi, prêtre, je ne puis vous apporter que des raisonnements. Mais Dieu peut vous toucher de sa grâce!... » Et avec toute l'autorité convaincante dont j'étais capable: — « Espérez, espérez... Ne vous défendez pas contre la foi... Ouvrez votre cœur, ne vous contractez pas, laissez pénétrer l'amour infini du Consolateur... »

« Puis j'ai pris les Evangiles qui étaient sur la table, et j'ai cherché le passage de St Marc: « *Il en est du royaume de Dieu comme d'un homme qui a jeté de la semence en terre. Qu'il dorme, qu'il se lève de nuit et de jour, la semence germe et croît sans qu'il sache comment.* »

« A mesure que je parlais, je voyais ses traits se détendre et son angoisse fondre. Il a renversé la tête, il pleurait.

« Moi, je ne pouvais détacher mes yeux de ce visage. Ainsi, c'est là que vient aboutir l'élan d'une pareille existence! Trahi par ce corps ravagé qui l'abandonne à moitié de sa course... Trahi par sa pensée, qui le portait vers un but inaccessible... Ah, trahison, trahison universelle! *s*

« Le même soir.

« Comme elle est belle la religion qui apporte un remède à de pareilles souffrances! Elle seule peut donner le courage de vivre et de mourir, elle qui transforme 1 effroi du mystère en une attraction sublime... Là p'upart d'entre nous ont bien davantage besoin de paix intérieure que de vérité; la religion leur est une autre nourriture que la science. Et c'est une belle mission que d'être ce messager d'espoir.

« Non, je ne quitterai pas l'Eglise. Je ne la perdrai pas... Je ne pourrais pas la perdre... Comment renier la tradition qui a fait l'humanité ce qu'elle est?

« J'étais insensé! Me séparer d'elle parce qu'elle est en retard sur la science humaine? Je comptais pour rien cet attachement de cœur, qu'aucune volonté pourtant ne parviendrait à rompre!

« Evidemment le sens littéral des dogmes me paraît aussi difficile à accepter aujourd'hui qu'il y a un an. Mais je me sens incapable de me créer hors de leur ombre, une unité, un équilibre.

« Je me contenterai, pour pouvoir vivre, de m'attacher à l'esprit plus qu'à la lettre. L'efficacité morale de la foi reste pour moi intacte.

« Ah, j'ai trop donné à l'Eglise de moi-même, j'ai trop connu la sueur d'agonie du jardin des oliviers! L'Eglise m'a trop supplicié, elle m'a fait verser trop de larmes, et elle m'a fait trop de bien...

« Nous sommes rivés l'un à l'autre,-indissolublement... »

II

Fin de juillet.

Un matin.

L'abbé Lévys traverse hâtivement la cour. Visage bouleversé'

Cécile l'attend. Elle lui saisit les deux mains; elle ne peut articuler un mot; ses yeux s'emplissent de larmes.

L'abbé monte rapidement l'escalier. Jean habite la chambre dans laquelle son père est mort.

Il est couché, les bras étendus, les traits apaisés. En apercevant l'abbé, il sourit.

JEAN. — Je vous remercie d'être venu tout de suite. Je ne pouvais plus attendre...

Un sourire joyeux, confiant, extraordinaire. C'est la grâce aujourd'hui, qui rayonne sur ces lèvres, dans ce regard...

L'abbé comprend; son cœur bat, ses mains tremblent; tout l'équivoque de sa foi s'évanouit; il redevient, en un instant, pour un instant, le prêtre fervent qu'il a été.

Alors il s'approche de Jean et prend sa main.

L'abbÉ. — Dites-moi tout... tout...

Le regard de Jean s'attarde dans la fenêtre ouverte: puis, de très loin, vient se poser sur l'abbé.

JEAN. — Ce qui s'est passé? (Un effort pour démêler les souvenirs d'un rêve.) Laissez-moi reprendre... Hier soir, nous nous sommes rencontrés au presbytère, n'est-ce pas? Mais vous n'avez rien remarqué, et je ne pouvais rien vous dire...

Devant le corps de ce pauvre abbé Joziers.je venais d'avoir...(son œil s'illumine)... la perception nette de l'âme!

Mouvement dë l'abbé.,

JEAN. — J'étais assis, je ne pouvais pas détacher mes yeux de ces traits pétrifiés; je cherchais l'ancienne ressemblance: mais il y avait *une différence essentielle* que je ne découvrais pas. Je cherchais une comparaison. Je me disais: « Ce corps est là comme une boîte vide... » Vide! ç'a été une révélation: le corps était là, et ce n'était plus rien. Pourquoi? parce qu'il avait perdu *ce qui l'animait...* L'heure saisissante de la dissociation était arrivée; la personnalité, ce qui faisait l'homme, s'était évanouie, *était ailleurs* ! Autant l'idée de survivance spirituelle me paraissait inexplicable, autrefois; autant l'idée contraire me paraît maintenant absurde.

Oui, l'âme existe! Il m'a suffi d'un regard sur ce lit pour constater sa disparition, et pour être frappé par la plus élémentaire, la plus indubitable évidence!

L'abbé serre fébrilement sa main.

JEAN. — Je commençais à souffrir; mais je dominais mon mal pour ne pas interrompre ce tête-à-tête, qui m'ouvrait la possibilité d'une vie éternelle...

Enfin le domestique m'a ramené ici. Il m'a couché tout de suite; une crise effroyable... Oppressions, arrêts du cœur, étouffements... J'ai cru que j'allais mourir.

Alors je me suis adressé à Dieu, de toutes mes forces: mais je sentais qu'il ne m'écoutait pas... J'ai voulu être seul. Ma femme ne voulait pas me quitter; je l'ai suppliée de s'éloigner. J'ai encore essayé de prier, sans pouvoir... Enfin les douleurs se sont calmées, j'ai éprouvé un soulagement sensible. Mais j'étais faible, faible... Je me sentais inerte, et si peu de chose, un souffle... J'étais certain que j'allais mourir...

Ah, l'atroce nuit! J'avais la tête en feu et le cœur tout refroidi, tout resserré, comme si l'ombre l'écrasait... Mon cerveau travaillait, à vide... J'étais pris entre deux courants contradictoires: je cherchais à prier, je faisais des efforts désespérés pour appeler l'attention de Dieu; et, à chaque élan, une voix, en

moi, me disait: « Non, non, non... Personne ne te répondra!... Personne... Tu vois bien qu'il n'y a personne... »

Il parle lentement, sans amertume, sa main dans celle du prêtre, son regard ne quittant pas le ciel matinal.

j'étais si faible, j'ai perdu conscience, j'ai dormi sans doute. Mais, tout en dormant, je rie cessais de sentir une lutte au-dessus de moi, et j'avais la certitude obscure que la Volonté de Dieu finirait par triompher.

Et puis, il m'a semblé qu'on parlait, «t j'ai ouvert les yeux J'aijnême Cru entendre si distinctement mon nom, que j'ai dit: « Quoi? » pensant que c'était ma femme... Mais j'étais seul.

J'avais dormi longtemps. Il faisait petit jour. J'entendais la respiration du domestique, dans le cabinet... Moi qui ai maintenant le sommeil si lourd et le réveil si lent, je me suis trouvé tout de suite lucide, extraordinairement lucide, et comme allégé d'une façon miraculeuse.

Alors j'ai fait un nouvel effort pour prier.

La voix qui disait: « Non, non... » s'était tue. A la place de mon impuissance, de cet affreux sentiment du néant, j'avais une espèce de certitude imprécise, une confiance... Je percevais sur moi comme un secours, comme une affection...

(Sourire radieux.) Je ne sais pas comment expliquer... L'impression de sortir de léthargie après plusieurs années de sommeil... L'impression de sortir d'un tunnel, de trouver la lumière, de commencer vraiment une nouvelle vie!...Un immense bonheur intérieur... La paix surtout, la paix... le calme...

Je sens que je n'ai plus à chercher, que ma volonté est comme fondue, que je vais obéir avec délices, que tout est clair, que tout est pur... *Tout a un sens...*

Il tourne la tête. Son regard rencontre celui de l'abbé, dont le visage anxieux reste incliné vers lui.

JEAN (ouvrant les bras). — Alors je vous ai fait venir, mon ami, pour me confesser...

Marc-Elie Luce est introduit dans le salon de Buis, où se trouve l'abbé Lévys.

L'abbÉ (s'avançant). — Je suis chargé, monsieur, par Mme Barois, de vous prévenir que notre malade est à peine remis de sa dernière rechute... Il a besoin de ménagements...

LUCE (inquiet). — Mais je ne demande qu'à lui serrer la main. Si vous supposez qu'une conversation...

L'abbÉ (embarrassé). — Non, monsieur, je ne pense pas qu'une conversation... sur des "sujets... Enfin, sans rien qui puisse provoquer un effort cérébral...

Luce sourit: une indulgence nuancée d'amertume.

LUCE. — Vous pouvez rassurer Mme Barois, monsieur l'abbé... Barois m'a prévenu de sa conversion, et je ne viens pas ici pour le contredire..

L'abbé rougit. Tics nerveux.

LUCE (froid). — D'ailleurs, je n'ai que peu de temps: je compte reprendre le train de trois heures.

L'abbÉ (vivement). — La gare est très proche, par le raccourci... Et si vous voulez bien, je vous montrerai moimême le chemin...

Jean a voulu se lever.

Il s'est fait habiller, et asseoir devant son bureau, qui est maintenant dans sa chambre, — car il ne descend plus.

Ses vêtements de drap noir, boutonnés, flottent autour de lui. Une parade mortuaire: le col baille; la peau colle au crâne; une barbe peu fournie comble la cavité des joues; les lèvres brident sur les dents; les ongles sont en corne jaune.

A l'entrée de Luce, il cherche à deviner le progrès de son mal. Mais Luce vient vers lui, souriant, impassible.

JEAN (tout de suite). — Vous vous demandez, n'est-ce pas, comment c'est arrivé?

Luce ne comprend pas.
Cette voix éteinte et rauque...

Jean soulève un petit crucifix, qui est près de son mouchoir, sur le bureau désert.

Une gêne.

JEAN (buté). — Comment c'est arrivé? Je n'en sais rien... Mais ce n'est pas le premier *comment* ni le premier *pourquoi* qui nous échappent! (Il sourit bizarrement.) « *Invocavi et venit in me spiritus sapientiæ.* » Depuis longtemps je ne croyais plus aux idées...

LUCE (évasivement). — Oui, c'est le cœur qui mène à la foi...

JEAN. — Ah, mon ami, c'est bon. .. On sent qu'on pénètre enfin la vie, qu!on voit l'univers par le dedans... (Vivement, comme s'il craignait une objection.) Et puis c'est une solution pratique qu'il nous faut...

Luce acquiesce par un sourire affectueux.

Jean a glissé au fond de son fauteuil. Son regard a la fixité d'yeux de verre, enchâssés dans un masque de cire.

Luce évoque le Barois, qui, pour discuter, se campait, les jambes écartées, tête de biais, sourcils dressés...

Jean le regarde; et tout à coup, un petit rire silencieux.

JEAN. — Je vous plains, mon pauvre ami... Vous résistez encore, vous... Vous vous débattez...

Luce, surpris, proteste doucement. Mais le sourire de Jean est obstiné.

JEAN. — Vous vous débattez, comme je faisais... Je connais ça... (Haussant les épaules.) A quoi bon?Vous savez bien que vous y viendrez aussi...

Il saisit la petite croix et la soulève à nouveau.

JEAN. — Voyez comme je me suis résigné à mourir, pour revivre auprès de Lui!

L'intonation est angoissée.

Luce l'examine d'un regard compatissant: il a mesuré d'assez près l'abîme, pour ne plus mépriser ceux qui ont le vertige. Mais il ne trouve rien à répondre.

Quelques minutes s'écoulent.

Luce se lève.

Jean le voit partir, presque sans regret. Une couche d'impressions neuves s'interpose maintenant entre son équilibre actuel, sa foi, — et son passé. Il prend la main tendue. Luce est très pâle.

JEAN. — Nous avons été deux semeurs de doutes, mon vieil ami. Que Dieu nous pardonne...

Luce descend l'escalier, le cœur serré.

Il entre dans le salon; la fuite d'une jupe.

LUCE (à l'abbé). — Pourrai-je saluer Mme Barois?

L'abbÉ. — Je ne pense pas que Mme Barois soit rentrée... D'ailleurs si nous voulons gagner la gare à pied, il va être l'heure...

Luce n'insiste pas.

Dehors, froid vif et sec.

Aussitôt franchi le portail, l'abbé se tourne. L'abbÉ. — Eh bien, comment l'avez-vous trouvé?

Luce fait un arrêt, à peine sensible, regarde l'abbé, et reprend sa marche. Il n'a plus, avec ce prêtre, les mêmes motifs qu'avec Jean pour dissimuler.

LUCE. — Il est méconnaissable... Il ne reste plus rien de son intelligence: il vit aujourd'hui, d'une faible lueur de sensibilité...

L'abbe (défensif). — Vous faites erreur: croyez bien qu'il a longuement discuté, avant de trouver sa voie!

Luce (avec amertume). — Discuter? Mais il ne le pouvait déjà plus lorsqu'il a quitté Paris!

(Posément.) Non. Ce pauvre Barois est, comme tant d'autres, une victime de notre époque. Sa vie, a été celle de beaucoup de mes contemporains: elle est tragique...

Il se tourne vers l'abbé, oubliant le prêtre; dans son regard, cette curiosité amoureuse et perspicace, qui a été la poésie de son existence.

LUCE. — Son éducation catholique s'est brisée, un jour, contre la science: toute la jeunesse cultivée passe par là. Malheureusement, notre conscience morale, dont nous sommes si vaniteux, nous la tenons, par hérédité, de plusieurs centaines de générations mystiques. Comment rejeter un pareil patrimoine? C'est lourd... Tous n'arrivent pas à fortifier suffisamment leur raison pour qu'elle reste jusqu'au bout victorieuse. Aux jours de tempête, tant d'instincts, tant de souvenirs, l'assaillent! Toutes les faiblesses sentimentales d'un cœur humain...

La plupart, en pleine force d'âge, donnent bien, comme Barois, le coup d'épaule qu'il faut pour s'affranchir. Mais viennent les déceptions, viennent les maladies, la menace finale, c'est la déroute: vous les voyez recourir bien vite aux contes de fées qui consolent...

L'abbé, le menton dans sa cape, hâte le pas.

LUCE (triste). — Vous lui avez offert la survie, et il s'y est accroché désespérément, comme tous ceux qui ne peuvent plus croire en eux, qui ne peuvent plus se contenter de la vie réelle...

Mouvement de l'abbé.

C'est votre mission, je sais bien... Et je dois reconnaître que l'Eglise a ecquis en ces matières une incomparable expérience! Votre au-delà est 27 une invention merveilleuse: c'est une promesse placée si loin, que la raison ne peut pas interdire au cœur d'y croire, s'il en a envie, puisqu'elle échappe, par définition, à tout contrôle...

An, c'est la trouvaille de votre religion, monsieur l'Abbé, d'avoir su convaincre l'homme qu'il ne doit plus chercher à comprendre!

L'abbÉ (relevant la tête). — C'est la loi de Jésus lui-même, monsieur. Il ne démontre pas, il ne raisonne pas; il dit: « Croyez en moi. » Il dit, plus simplement encore: « Si quelqu'un a soif, qu'il vienne à moi, et qu'il boive.., »

Un temps.

LUCE (malgré lui). — Une belle conversion! Vous pouvez être fier. L'abbÉ (s'arrêtant). — Oui, j'en suis fier!

Une bise soudaine, au tournant de la rue, fait claquer son manteau. Il brave Luce d'un regard sombre, ambigu.

L'abbÉ. — Etiez-vous capable de le consoler? Moi, je lui ai apporté le calme; je lui ai montré des horizons de clarté. Vous n'avez su lui proposer que des visions sans espérance!

LUCE (avec mesure). — Pourquoi « sans espérance »?

Mon espérance, c'est de croire que mes efforts vers le bien sont indestructibles! Et elle est si forte, ne vous en déplaise, que les triomphes partiels du mal ne la découragent pas...

Mon espérance, à moi, n'exige pas, comme la vôtre, l'abdication de ma raison: au contraire, ma raison l'étaye. Elle me prouve que notre vie n'est ni un mouvement à vide, ni une simple occasion de souffrir, ni une course au bonheur individuel; elle me prouve que mes actes collaborent au grand effort universel; et partout elle me fait découvrir des motifs d'espérer! Partout je vois la vie naître de la mort, l'énergie naître de la douleur, la science naître de l'erreur, l'harmonie naître du désordre... Et, en moi-même, ces évolutions-là se produisent tous les jours.

Oui, je lui ai offert une foi, moi aussi, et qui valait bien la vôtre, monsieur l'Abbé.

L'abbÉ. — Elle n'a pu lui suffire: c'est un fait!

(Violence inattendue.) Et même si vous pensez que je lui ai offert un mensonge, vous devriez être heureux que j'aie pu, par n'importe quel moyen, lui rendre la paix!

LUCE. — Je ne connais pas deux morales. On doit arriver au bonheur, sans être dupe d'aucun mirage, par la seule vérité.

Un temps.

LUCE. — Ah, nous aurons été un moment pathétique de l'histoire de la science, le moment le plus aigu sans doute de son conflit avec la foi!

L'abbÉ (brusque impatience). — Vous êtes d'un autre temps, monsieur Luce... du temps où l'on coupait inconsidérément les ponts qui nous relient au passé. Vous croyez à la régénération sociale, et vous avez pu renoncer à la prière, à la survivance spirituelle... Mais vous ne savez pas voir autour de vous: ce temps-là est déjà loin! Vous n'avez pas aperçu le réveil général d'un besoin religieux, que vos sèches théories ne pourront jamais satisfaire!

(Rire révolté.) Un athée ne comprendra jamais ce qui se passe dans l'âme d'un homme qui prie...

LUCE (souriant). — Ce sont des défaillances inévitables. Mais cette incroyance raisonnée que nous avons conquise, au prix souvent de pénibles souffrances, ne peut pas être perdue: elle s'imprime, peu à peu, jusqu'au fond des moelles de notre race, et libère d'autant l'humanité à venir!

L'abbÉ (farouche). — Non, l'homme ne pourra jamais se passer de Dieu... La vie est dominée par la mort; et seule la religion apprend à l'attendre, à la subir, — quelquefois même à la désirer.

LUCE (le masque contracté). — La mort est dans la logique de la vie. J'accepte l'idée de mort comme j'accepte l'idée de naissance.

L ABBÉ (sourire cruel). — Oui, pour le moment! Oui, vous vous portez assez bien pour « accepter » la mort!

Mais je vous le dis, monsieur Luce, le jour où vous sentirez *qu elle* approche, qu'*elle* est là, ah! vous verrez quel piètre appui vous trouverez dans vos négations stériles!

La place de la gare, que sillonne un va-et-vient de piétons et de véhicules.

Luce s'arrête. Une ombre s'est creusée sous ses yeux gris. LUCE (voix lourde). — A mon âge, — autant dire au seuil de la mort — on est sincère, n'est-ce pas? Ce n'est pas l'heure où l'on a envie de faire des phrases...

Eh bien, je vous affirme que j'envisage la mort avec toute la sérénité dont l'homme est capable, — avec la même sérénité que vous!

L'abbé détourne la tête.

LUCE. — Qu'est-ce qui vous adoucira le moment fatal? c'est la paix d'une conscience tranquille... Cette sérénité-là, je puis l'avoir au même titre que vous...

L'abbÉ (ton âpre, sans regarder Luce). — Mais ce que vous n'aurez pas, vous, c'est un prêtre, un envoyé de Dieu, pour venir se pencher sur votre agonie, et, d'un seul geste d'absolution, effacer jusqu'au souvenir de ce que vous aurez fait de pire!...

LUCE (doucement). — Je n'en ai pas besoin.

Il est devenu blême, tout à coup.

Un sourire d'orgueil. Il tend sa main à l'abbé.

LUCE. — Au revoir, monsieur l'Abbé... Sans rancune... Et pourtant vous venez de me faire mal... J'avais presqu'oublié que je suis condamné, et vous venez de m'en faire souvenir, — durement...

Geste de l'abbé.

LUCE (souriant toujours). — Je sais que dans deux, trois, quatre mois,, tout au plus, il faudra que je subisse une opération, qui est sans espoir... Et si je suis venu voir Barois, c'est parce que je me sais encore plus sûrement perdu que lui-

même...

L'abbé (bouleversé). — Vous vous exagérez, peut-être...

LUCE (cessant de sourire). — Oh, ce n'est pas que je regarde la mort sans épouvante... Non... Mais je la regarde! (Il frissonne.) J'en ai peur, autant qu'un autre, parce que ma chair est lâche: mais c'est une peurphysique.

Moralement, allez, je reste bien d'aplomb!

Il traverse le trottoir, d'un pas ferme.

L'abbé le suit des yeux jusqu'à ce qu'il ait disparu.

« Mon cher Barois,

« Depuis que Luce est mort, je veux vous écrire. Mais j'ai eu le côté droit ankylosé à la suite d'une petite congestion, et j'ai été retardé.

« Les médecins avaient résolu de tenter l'opération. Il s'y était soumis sans illusion. Il avait demandé quinze jours pour ranger ses papiers. Il m'a prié de l'aider, et je ne l'ai plus quitté.

« Un jour, en classant les notes du livre qui reste inachevé, il a vu que je pleurais. Il est venu à moi, et il m'a dit un mot qui le résume: — « Vous, Woldsmuth? Mais quoi? c'est la vie.. . *Ne nous laissons pas aveugler par l'individuel...* »

« L'opération a eu lieu.

« Elle a réussi au delà de toutes les espérances. Le chirurgien lui-même semblait oublier que ce n'était qu'une rémission; nous tous avec lui. Le dix-huitième jour, Luce était debout, on le laissait rentrer chez lui. Il disait: « Je vais me remettre au travail, j'ai tant à faire encore!»

« C'est à partir de ce moment-là que le mieux a cessé, brusquement. Il l'a senti tout de suite: les symptômes reparaissaient, un à un. Il reculait toujours le moment d'avertir ses enfants; et eux, qui s'apercevaient du.changement, feignaient de croire à sa guérison.

« J'y allais tous les jours. Avec moi, il parlait de sa mort, sans répit. « Il me disait:

— a J'ai de la chance d'être ainsi prévenu d'avance, de pouvoir me préparer à l'acceptation. C'est le dernier acte qui me reste à accomplir pour avoir fait ce que je devais. Je me suis toujours efforcé de rendre ma vie conforme à mes idées, pour donner à celles-ci leur maximum de force; il me reste à mourir, sans dévier; il me reste à montrer que je n'ai pas peur de la mort, que je la vois venir, que je l'accueille, que je meurs *en confiance...*

« Le retentissement d'une fin sereine est immense, sur notre pauvre troupeau affolé de condamnés à mort! Socrate l'avait bien compris. Plus on relit le récit de ses derniers jours, plus il est clair que Socrate n'a pas.consenti à se faire acquitter. Il avait soixante-dix ans; il avait fini d'enseigner; il a eu la suprême sagesse de vouloir agir, une fois encore, par une mort qui ne fût pas passive, qui fût la preuve dernière de l'assurance de son cœur. Je me souhaite une pareille fin. » «Puis un trouble passait sur son visage:

— « Et pourtant, on dit que souvent ceux qui l'ont attendu avec le plus de calme, sont justement ceux qui, au moment de mourir, se laissent aller à la plus grande révolte... »

« Mais il ajoutait, précipitamment:

— « Une révolte *nerveuse,* bien entendu... »

« Pas un seul jour je n'ai vu fléchir cette adhésion à la vie et à la mort. Et pourtant il a bien souffert!

« Il faisait le bilan de son existence. Un matin, après une nuit d'insomnie, il m'a dit:

— « C'est une consolation pour moi de m'apercevoir combien ma vie aura été harmonieuse. Pendant que l'on vit, on se désespère de ne pas pouvoir mettre plus d'unité dans ses actions. Mais maintenant, je vois que je n'ai pas à me plaindre. J'ai rencontré tant d'êtres tourmentés, insatisfaits, sans cesse emportés en deçà ou au delà de leur centre de gravité!

« Mon existence, à moi, n'a pas connu ces secousses; elle pourrait s'exprimer par deux ou trois mots simples et clairs. Cela me donne, en m'en allant, un sentiment de paix. Je suis né avec de la confiance en moi, en l'effort quotidien, en l'avenir des hommes. J'ai eu l'équilibre facile. Mon sort a été celui d'un pommier de bonne terre, qui porte régulièrement ses fruits.

»

« La dernière semaine a été particulièrement cruelle.

« Puis, la veille du jour où il est mort, les souffrances ont diminué.

« Ses petits enfants, les aînés, sont entrés un instant dans sa chambreIl ne parlait déjà presque plus. Il les a vus venir, il leur a dit: — Allezvous-en, mes petits, adieu, il ne faut pas que vous voyiez ça... »

Vers six heures, on allumait les lampes, il a regardé autour de lui comme pour s'assurer que tous ses enfants étaient réunis. Il avait un regard extraordinaire. Il semblait pouvoir dire la vérité sur tout. Il semblait que s'il avait pu s'expliquer encore, il eut dit, sur lui, sur sa vie, sur la vié de tous les hommes, la parole décisive, libératrice. .. Mais il s'est soulevé sur un coude, et il a seulement dit, d'une voix étouffée, comme s'il s'éveillait:

— « Ah, c'est la mort, cette fois... »

« Ses filles n'ont pu retenir leur douleur. Elles étaient à genoux autour de son lit. Alors il a posé ses mains sur toutes ces têtes, et il a murmuré,, pour lui seul:

— « Qu'ils sont beaux, mes enfants! »

"Puis il s'est renversé sur l'oreiller.

« C'était le soir. Il est mort, au matin, sans avoir rouvert les yeux.

« Voilà ce que je voulais vous écrire, mon cher Barois, parce que je sais ue cette mort peut vous faire du bien, comme à moi. Elle nous console e toutes les choses mauvaises que nous avons rencontrées sur notre chemin.

« J'ai la certitude après avoir vu mourir Luce, que je n'ai pas eu tort, d'avoir foi en la raison humaine.

«Pour moi, j'ai de si faibles yeux maintenant, que je ne travaille plus guère au laboratoire. J'écris: je récapitule mes recherches sur l'origine de la vie. Elles n'ont pas atteint leur but, mais je lègue à ceux qui me suivent, les résultats que j'ai acquis. Le temps est un facteur essentiel du progrès; il est vraisemblable qu'un jour un autre trouvera ce que j'ai cherché; et c'est une pensée très apaisante.

« Votre dévoué,

Ulric Woldsmuth. »

Depuis le matin, Jean délire.

Huit heures du soir.

Il s'éveille. Lassitude extrême.

La pièce est sombre.

Autour du lit, le va-et-vient des vivants prolonge son cauchemar.

Tout à coup, près de Cécile qui tient la lampe, l'abbé Lévys.

étole au cou: entre ses doigts, les burettes.

Une frayeur folle: la réalité...

Son regard court d'un visage à l'autre.

JEAN. — Je vais mourir? Dites? Je vais mourir?

Il n'entend pas la réponse. Une quinte le prend à la gorge, lacère ses poumons, l'étouffe.

Cécile se penche. Il l'enserre de ses deux bras, passionnément.

Elle le force à s'allonger. Il se laisse faire, épuisé, les yeux clos, le souffle sifflant.

A travers sa fièvre, des phrases latines... La fraîcheur de l'huile sur ses oreilles, sur ses paupières, sur ses paumes...

Sa transpiration baigne les draps.

JEAN. — Ah, délivrez-moi!... Ne me laissez pas souffrir!...

Ses mains battent l'air.

Elles rencontrent les manches de l'abbé et s'y cramponnent, comme à Dieu.

JEAN. — Vous êtes sûr qu'Il m'a pardonné? (Un effort surhumain. Il se dresse.) L'enfer!...

Sa bouche s'ouvre pour un cri d'épouvante.

Un râle mouillé...

L'abbé tend le crucifix. Il le repousse, hagard. Puis il aperçoit le Christ: il s'en empare, il se renverse en arrière, et, frénétiquement l'écrase sur ses lèvres.

La croix trop lourde, glisse de ses doigts.

Ses membres n'obéissent plus, s'éloignent. Le cœur bat à peine. Le cerveau fonctionne à une vitesse déréglée.

Une brusque tension de tout l'être: en chaque point du corps, en chaque parcelle vivante, le summum de la souffrance humaine!

Quelques soubresauts..

L'immobilité.

A l'aube.

Cécile et l'abbé, seuls dans la chambre.

Cécile prie, le front dans les mains.

Elle revoit sa vie, année par année. Dans cette même chambre, un matin de sa jeunesse, elle a communié avec Jean, au chevet du docteur...

Le jour naissant pénètre par les volets entr'ouverts. Un feu vif dans la cheminée; sur le mur, derrière le cadavre plus rigide, des reflets de flamme dansent.

L'abbé est assis. Il regarde le mort: les muscles du visage sont raidis; la peau est gélatineuse; les cheveux gris sont durs, piqués dans le crâne; le cou ne semble pas avoir pu porter la tête.

Une incomparable sérénité.

Cécile ouvre successivement les tiroirs du bureau. Elle cherche quelque volonté posthume. Elle ne trouve rien.

Mais, dans le cartonnier, sous les dossiers, une enveloppe:

« A OUVRIR APRÈS MOI. »

Elle rompt le cachet, parcourt les premières lignes, pâlit.

Elle marche vers l'abbé, et lui tend les papiers.

Il s'approche de la fenêtre.

Une grande écriture, ronde et ferme:

« Ceci est mon testament.

« Ce que j'écris aujourd'hui, ayant dépassé la quarantaine, en pleine force et en plein équilibre intellectuel, doit, de toute évidence, prévaloir contre ce que je pourrai penser ou écrire à la fin de mon existence, lorsque je serai physiquement et moralement diminué par l'âge ou par la maladie. Je ne connais rien de plus poignant que l'attitude d'un vieillard, dont la vie tout entière a été employée au service d'une idée, et qui, dans l'affaiblissement final, blasphème ce qui a été sa raison de vivre, et renie lamentablement son passé.

« En songeant que l'effort de ma vie pourrait aboutir à une semblable trahison, en songeant au parti que ceux dont j'ai si ardemment combattu les mensonges et les empiétements, ne manqueraient pas de tirer d'une si lugubre victoire, tout mon être se révolte, et je proteste d'avance, avec l'énergie farouche de l'homme que je suis, de l'homme vivant que j'aurai été, contre les dénéga-

tions sans fondement, peut-être même contre la prière agonisante du déchet humain que je puis devenir.

« J'ai mérité de mourir debout, comme j'ai vécu, sans capituler, sans quêter de vaines espérances, sans craindre le retour aux lentes évolutions de la germination éternelle... »

L'abbé frissonne. Ce rappel si net, si volontaire...

Il tourne la page:

« Je ne crois pas à l'âme humaine, substantielle et immortelle... » « Je sais que ma personnalité n'est qu'une agglomération de particules matérielles, dont la désagrégation entraînera la mort totale... »

« Je crois au déterminisme universel. .. »

« Le bien et le mal sont des distinctions arbitraires... »

Il n'achève pas.

Il replie les feuillets, et les rend à Cécile.

Il fuit l'interrogation de son regard.

Elle recule délibérément vers la cheminée. Il devine son geste. Il pourrait l'empêcher.

Mais ses yeux restent fixés sur la mort, et il ne fait pas un mouvement.

Il pense que depuis longtemps déjà, Barois ne peut plus se défendre... Il pense à l'Eglise, qui a su alléger ce départ, et à qui le sacrifice est dû, — peut-être...

Une flamme claire illumine la chambre.

*Le Verger d'Augy,*
Avril igio. — Mai 1913.

SOMMAIRE

CH.-L. PHILIPPE LETTRES DE JEUNESSE in-16 3.50

J. KEATS LETTRES A FANNY BRAWNE (Trad. des Garets) in-16 2.50 *ROMANS ET CONTES*:

HENRI BACHELIN JULIETTE LA JOLIE in-iô 3.50

J. RICHARD BLOCH LÉVY in-16 3.50

G.-K. CHESTERTON LE NOMMÉ JEUDI (Trad. J. FloRence) in-i5 3.50

G.-K. CHESTERTON LE NAPO-LÉON DE NOTTING

HILL. (Trad. J. Florence) in-16 3.50

BERNARD COMBETTE DES HOMMES in-16 3.50

ANDRÉ GIDE ISABELLE, récit in-16 3.50

ANDRÉ GIDE ISABELLE (1" édition sur vergé d'Arches, tirée à 500 exemplaires).

Epuisé in-8 7.50 *LITTÉRATURE:*

HENRI GHÉON NOS DIREC-TIONS (Réalisme et

Poésie. — Notes sur le Drame poé-tique. —. Du Classicisme. — Sur le vers libre)

ANDRÉ GIDE SOUVENIRS DE LA COUR D'AS-SISES

JACQUES RIVIÈRE ÉTUDES (Baudelaire, Claudel, Gide,

Ingres, Cézanne, Gauguin, etc.)..

ANDRÉ SUARÈS TROIS HOMMES (pascal, Ibsen,

Dostoievsky)

ANDRÉ SUARÈS ESSAIS

ANDRÉ SUARÈS PORTRAITS

ALBERT THIBAUDET LA POÉSIE DE STÉPHANE MAL-LARMÉ

. LBERT THIBAUDET.... LES HEURES DE L'ACROPOLE..

in-16 3.50 in-16 3. 50 in-16 3.50 in-16 3.50 in-16 3.50 in-16 3.50 in-8 10. in-16 2.50 in-16 2.50 in-16 3.50 in-16 3. 50 in-16 2.50 in-16 3.50 in-16 3.50 in-16 3.50 in-8 10. « in-16 3.50 ACHE-VÉ D'IMPRIMER LE DIX MAI MIL NEUF CENT DIX-HUIT PAR L'IMPRIMERIE LA SEMEUSE, ÉTAMPES.

Lightning Source UK Ltd.
Milton Keynes UK
UKOW07f0843301115

263800UK00011BA/453/P